New Frontiers in Dermatology

New Frontiers in Dermatology

Edited by Nicolas Webb

hayle
medical

New York

Hayle Medical,
750 Third Avenue, 9th Floor,
New York, NY 10017, USA

Visit us on the World Wide Web at:
www.haylemedical.com

ISBN: 978-1-63241-577-6

Cataloging-in-Publication Data

New frontiers in dermatology / edited by Nicolas Webb.
p. cm.
Includes bibliographical references and index.
ISBN 978-1-63241-577-6
1. Dermatology. 2. Skin--Diseases. I. Webb, Nicolas.
RL72 .N49 2019
616.5--dc23

Contents

Preface

The field of medicine, which deals with the health of nails, skin, hair and scalp, and their associated disorders, is known as dermatology. It is a clinical specialization, which integrates both surgery and medicine. Skin diseases are generally skin neoplasms and skin infections. Acneiform eruptions, autoinflammatory syndromes, dermatitis, erythemas, congenital anomalies, chronic blistering, lichenoid eruptions, genodermatoses, etc. are some of the skin conditions treated in dermatology. The therapies typically used in clinical dermatology include laser hair removal, cryosurgery, cosmetic filler injections, intralesional treatment, liposuction, vitiligo surgery and allergy testing, besides many others. This book is compiled in such a manner, that it will provide in-depth knowledge about the current techniques and procedures of dermatology. It aims to present the new researches that have transformed this discipline and aided its advancement. It is a vital tool for all researching or studying dermatology as it gives incredible insights into emerging trends and concepts.

This book is a comprehensive compilation of works of different researchers from varied parts of the world. It includes valuable experiences of the researchers with the sole objective of providing the readers (learners) with a proper knowledge of the concerned field. This book will be beneficial in evoking inspiration and enhancing the knowledge of the interested readers.

In the end, I would like to extend my heartiest thanks to the authors who worked with great determination on their chapters. I also appreciate the publisher's support in the course of the book. I would also like to deeply acknowledge my family who stood by me as a source of inspiration during the project.

Editor

Preface

Eczema in early childhood is strongly associated with the development of asthma and rhinitis in a prospective cohort

Laura B von Kobyletzki[1,2*], Carl-Gustaf Bornehag[2], Mikael Hasselgren[3,4], Malin Larsson[2], Cecilia Boman Lindström[2] and Åke Svensson[1]

Abstract

Background: This study aimed to estimate the association between eczema in early childhood and the onset of asthma and rhinitis later in life in children.

Methods: A total of 3,124 children aged 1–2 years were included in the Dampness in Building and Health (DBH) study in the year 2000, and followed up 5 years later by a parental questionnaire based on an International Study of Asthma and Allergies in Childhood protocol. The association between eczema in early childhood and the incidence of asthma and rhinitis later in life was estimated by univariable and multivariable logistic regression modelling.

Results: The prevalence of eczema in children aged 1–2 years was 17.6% at baseline. Children with eczema had a 3-fold increased odds of developing asthma (adjusted odds ratio [aOR], 3.07; 95% confidence interval (CI) 1.79–5.27), and a nearly 3-fold increased odds of developing rhinitis (aOR, 2.63; 1.85–3.73) at follow-up compared with children without eczema, adjusted for age, sex, parental allergic disease, parental smoking, length of breastfeeding, site of living, polyvinylchloride flooring material, and concomitant allergic disease. When eczema was divided into subgroups, moderate to severe eczema (aOR, 3.56; 1.62–7.83 and aOR, 3.87; 2.37–6.33, respectively), early onset of eczema (aOR, 3.44; 1.94–6.09 and aOR, 4.05; 2.82–5.81; respectively), and persistence of eczema (aOR, 5.16; 2.62–10.18 and aOR, 4.00; 2.53–6.22, respectively) further increased the odds of developing asthma and rhinitis. Further independent risk factors increasing the odds of developing asthma were a parental history of allergic disease (aOR, 1.83; 1.29–2.60) and a period of breast feeding shorter than 6 months (aOR, 1.57; 1.03–2.39). The incidence of rhinitis was increased for parental history of allergic disease (aOR, 2.00; 1.59–2.51) and polyvinylchloride flooring (aOR, 1.60; 1.02–2.51).

Conclusion: Eczema in infancy is associated with development of asthma and rhinitis during the following 5-year period, and eczema is one of the strongest risk factors. Early identification is valuable for prediction of the atopic march.

Background

The prevalence of eczema has increased to levels of public health relevance in the Western world, especially in children [1]. As the most frequent inflammatory condition in childhood, eczema affects physiological and psychological wellbeing of affected children and results in substantial costs [2,3]. It has been suggested that early life eczema is a risk factor for the development of asthma later in life [4]. However, evidence for the progression to asthma comes mainly from cross-sectional studies [5]. There are only a few prospective cohort studies that have investigated the association between early life eczema and later onset of asthma and rhinitis [6-11]. Some of the existing longitudinal studies found no association between eczema and later onset of asthma [6-8], and other prospective studies found an eczema/asthma relationship much weaker than expected

* Correspondence: laura.vonkobyletzki@liv.se
[1]Lund University, Institute of Clinical Research in Malmö, Skåne University Hospital, Department of Dermatology, Malmö, Sweden
[2]Karlstad University, Department of Public Health Sciences, Karlstad, Sweden
Full list of author information is available at the end of the article

[9]. This overall weak association might be partly explained by a different effect across eczema subgroups on allergic airway diseases [12]. The severity of eczema has been found to be more closely associated with the risk of developing asthma than the timing of onset, or duration of eczema symptoms [12-14]. We examined whether eczema in early childhood predicts the later onset of asthma and rhinitis in children and determined the importance of severity, time of onset and persistency of the childhood eczema by analysing data from a large prospective population-based cohort with a follow-up period of 5 years.

Methods

Data collection

The methods of the population-based Swedish Dampness in Buildings and Health (DBH) study have been published by Bornehag et al.. and Larsson et al. [15,16].

The DBH study started in 2000, and a questionnaire based on an International Study of Asthma and Allergies in Childhood (ISAAC) protocol [17] was given to parents of all children aged 1 to 5 years living in the county of Värmland (DBH-I). Follow-up was performed in 2005 in children who were aged 1 to 3 years in 2000 (DBH-III). In this study we investigated the children initially aged 1–2 years.

Four thousand and twenty children initially aged 1–2 years had answered a baseline questionnaire in 2000 based on an ISAAC protocol. The cohort of the current study consisted of 3,124 children who responded both to the baseline and a follow-up questionnaire in 2005 (response rate: 77.7%).

Inclusion criteria of the baseline survey were all children living in Värmland aged 1–5 years whose parents gave consent to participate and who answered a postal questionnaire. The study was approved by the regional ethical committee in Örebro.

Definition of variables

The original ISAAC questions were used. In addition, questions on doctor-diagnosed asthma and doctor-diagnosed rhinitis were included. The additional questions were: "Has your child been diagnosed with asthma by a physician?" and "Has your child been diagnosed with rhinitis by a physician?" The main outcomes were "5-year cumulative incidence of asthma" and "5-year cumulative incidence of rhinitis". The "5-year cumulative incidence of asthma" was defined as no report of physician-diagnosed asthma and no wheezing at baseline in 2000, but physician-diagnosed asthma was reported in 2005. The "5-year cumulative incidence of rhinitis" was defined as no report of physician-diagnosed rhinitis in 2000, but physician-diagnosed rhinitis was reported in 2005.

The main explanatory variable was eczema. Eczema in early childhood was defined by affirmative responses to the question "Has your child had an itchy rash at any time in the last 12 months?" in the baseline questionnaire in 2000.

Secondary analysis was performed for subgroups of eczema, persistent eczema, severe eczema and early onset of eczema, and their association with later development of allergic airway diseases. Persistent eczema was assumed when children reported signs of eczema both at baseline and at follow-up; the questions asked were: "Has your child ever had an itchy rash (eczema) which was coming and going for at least 6 months" and "Has your child had this itchy rash at any time in the last 12 months?" in 2000, and "Has your child had this itchy rash at any time in the last 12 months?" in 2005. The onset of eczema was determined form the question "At what age did this itchy rash first occur?" in 2000, and it was categorised into "early onset" if symptoms occurred before the age of 1 year. The question "In the last 12 months, how often, on average, has your child been kept awake at night by eczema?" was included in the ISAAC eczema questionnaire as a measure of the severity of eczema, where sleep loss several times per week was considered to be severe eczema [17,18]. To simplify analysis, the severity of eczema was re-categorized, by using "any awakening at night" as an identifier for moderate to severe eczema, and "no awakening" was considered to be mild eczema. Information on single parenthood was obtained via the question "How many adults are currently living with the child"; two adults caring for the child could be any two adults.

Statistical analysis

The association between eczema in early childhood and the development of asthma and rhinitis was estimated by using univariable logistic regression and expressed as odds ratios (ORs) with confidence intervals (CIs). Statistical significance was assessed using the likelihood ratio test (LRT; $p < 0.05$). Characteristics of participants and non-participants were compared in drop-out analysis using the chi-square test ($p < 0.05$). Crude analysis of the association between all other risk factors, and asthma and rhinitis were performed. Linear trends of variables with several categories were evaluated. In multivariable logistic regression analysis, the ORs were adjusted for sex, age of the child, socioeconomic variables (parental smoking, number of adults living with the child, and type of house), and potential confounding variables, which included all other factors (see Table 1). The potential confounding variables were added in descending order of strength of crude association (smallest p-value first). Factors still associated with asthma and rhinitis were kept in the model. The interaction between

Table 1 Crude associations between risk factors at baseline and the incidence of asthma and rhinitis*

Risk factor at baseline	Total number in category n (%)	Number with asthma n	Asthma OR (95% CI)	P-value	Number with rhinitis n	Rhinitis OR (95% CI)	P-value
Eczema				<0.001			<0.001
No	2,573 (82.4)	101	1.0		107	1.0	
Yes	551 (17.6)	49	2.85 (1.72-4.71)		65	3.14 (2.27-4.36)	
Persistence of eczema							<0.001
No	2,886 (92.4)	58	1.0	<0.001	135	1.0	
Yes	238 (7.6)	15	4.20 (2.31-7.64)		37	3.92 (2.64-5.82)	
Onset of eczema							<0.001
No	2,483 (80.6)	46	1.0	<0.001	98	1.0	
Age ≥ one year	216 (6.9)	6	1.87 (0.7-4.45)		8	0.96 (0.46-2.00)	
Age < one year	386 (12.6)	21	3.63 (2.12-6.22)		66	5.02 (3.58-7.05)	
Eczema severity							<0.001
No	2,478 (79.47)	45	1.0	<0.001	98	1.0	
Mild	468 (15.0)	17	2.42 (1.36-4.29)		47	2.74 (1.90-3.95)	
Moderate to severe	173 (5.5)	11	4.55 (2.27-9.12)		27	4.74 (2.98-7.55)	
Gender							0.001
Female	1,546 (49.5)	25	1.0	0.002	65	1.0	
Male	1,579 (50.5)	48	2.16 (1.32-3.54)		107	1.67 (1.21-2.29)	
Age of the child							0.727
12-23 month	1,557 (49.8)	41	1.0	0.325	88	1.0	
24-35 month	1,568 (50.2)	32	0.79 (0.49-1.27)		84	0.95 (0.70-1.29)	
Parental history of allergic disease							<0.001
No parent	1,594 (51.0)	26	1.0	<0.001	47	1.0	
One parent	1,199 (38.4)	32	1.92 (1.14-3.25)		83	2.45 (1.69-3.53)	
Two parents	332 (10.6)	15 (7.2)	3.67 (1.90-7.08)		42	4.85 (3.12-7.55)	
Asthma in the child							<0.001
No	2,843 (91.4)	–	–		147	1.0	
Yes	269 (8.6)	–	–	–	25	4.10 (2.57-6.54)	
Length of breastfeeding							0.791
Longer than 6 month	2,043 (65.9)	44	1.0	0.021	112	1.0	
Up to 6 months	974 (31.4)	23	1.14 (0.68-1.90)		54	1.02 (0.73-1.43)	
No breastfeeding	82 (2.7)	6	3.32 (1.36-8.11)		6	1.35 (0.57-3.16)	
Number of bedrooms with PVC							0.116
No PVC in bedroom	1,300 (42.8)	23	1.0	0.184	60	1.0	
PVC in one bedroom	558 (18.4)	14	1.42 (0.72-2.79)		38	1.51 (0.99-2.30)	
PVC in two bedrooms	1,183 (38.9)	34	1.65 (0.96-2.82)		70	1.31 (0.92-1.87)	
Type of building							0.453
Single-family house	2,522 (82.4)	58	1.0	0.902	137	1.0	
Multi-family house	538 (17.6)	12	1.04 (0.55-1.96)		33	1.13 (0.75-1.70)	
Parental smoking							0.357
No	2,431 (77.8)	56	1.0	0.691	139	1.0	
Yes	694 (22.2)	17	1.12 (0.64-1.94)		33	0.83 (0.56-1.23)	

Table 1 Crude associations between risk factors at baseline and the incidence of asthma and rhinitis* *(Continued)*

Number of adults living with the child							0.830
Two or more adults	2,853 (93.8)	66	1.0	0.320	157	1.0	
One adult	190 (6.2)	6	1.54 (0.65-3.62)		11	1.07 (0.57-2.01)	

3,124 children aged 1–2 in 2000 in Värmland, Sweden, were included in the analysis.
*during the 5-year follow-up period.

eczema and sex was explored. The effect of different subgroups of eczema on asthma and rhinitis was examined. Because of the strong association between persistence, early onset and severe eczema, three adjusted models for these groups are reported.

Clustering by families was considered. No clustering effects were found after statistical assessment. The results obtained using robust standard errors, generalised estimating equations, and random effect modelling were similar to those obtained from the analysis of single subjects in terms of the exposure outcome relationship, and no evidence for significant intra-cluster correlation was found. Therefore, ordinary logistic regression models are shown that ignore clustering. The Hosmer and Lemeshow goodness-of-fit test statistic provided evidence that the models were a good fit to the data [19]. We undertook a sensitivity analysis and used questions that asked about symptoms of asthma/rhinitis (wheezing and runny nose) and questions that asked about doctors' diagnoses (asthma and rhinitis). This was performed in case people's perceptions of symptoms are stronger indications of health than reports of doctors' diagnoses.

Power

Assuming that 7.3% of children with eczema and 2.5% of children without eczema develop asthma later in life, this study had the power to detect an odds ratio of 2.8 with 96% power.

All analyses were carried out using STATA, version 11 (STATA Corp., College Station, TX).

Results

The study population consisted of 3,124 children, aged 1–2 years from 2,526 families due to siblinghood. The study population showed equal distribution regarding age and sex. Most children were breastfed (97.4%), and living with two adults (93.8%) in a single-family house (82.4%), with non-smoking parents (77.8%). A high proportion of children had at least one parent with a history of allergic disease (49.0%, Table 1). In the 1–2-year-old children, the prevalence of baseline eczema was 17.6% (n = 551; 95% CI, 16.3–19.0%). The cumulative 5-year incidence of asthma was 3.1 % (2.5–3.9) and rhinitis was 5.6% (4.8–6.5).

Drop out in the study

Of 4,020 children aged 1–2 years, who participated in the baseline survey in 2000, 3,124 children participated in the follow-up in 2005. A total of 896 children did not continue participating in the study. There were no differences in background (age and sex) and health factors (prevalence of eczema, asthma, wheezing and rhinitis, and parents with history of allergic disease) measured at baseline between the children participating in both surveys compared with the "drop-outs" ($p > 0.05$). However, there was a higher prevalence of socioeconomic risk factors, parental smoking (30.5% vs. 22.2%; $p < 0.001$), one adult living with a child (11.1% vs. 6.2%; $p < 0.001$), and living in a multifamily house (27.0% vs. 17.6%; $p < 0.001$) in drop-outs compared with that in participants.

Odds of developing asthma and rhinitis

Unadjusted analyses showed that children with eczema at baseline had more than a 2-fold increase in the odds of developing asthma (OR, 2.85; 95% CI, 1.72–4.71) and a 3-fold increase in the odds of developing rhinitis (OR, 3.14; 2.27–4.36) compared with children without eczema at baseline. The odds for developing asthma and rhinitis remained increased after adjustment (aOR, 3.07; 1.79–5.27 and aOR, 2.63; 1.85–3.73, respectively) for eczema, sex, age, family history of allergic disease, asthma, length of breastfeeding, PVC-flooring material in the home, type of building, environmental tobacco smoke, and number of adults living with the child (Table 2).

Different subgroups of children with eczema

In adjusted analysis, children with persistence of eczema, early onset of eczema, or moderate to severe eczema had even higher odds of developing asthma and rhinitis than children with eczema in general. The odds of developing asthma and rhinitis was 5-fold in children with persistence of eczema compared with the absence of eczema (aOR, 5.16; 2.62–10.18 and aOR, 4.00; 2.53–6.22, respectively). Early onset of eczema was a strong risk factor for the incidence of asthma (aOR, 3.44; 95% CI, 1.94–6.09) and the incidence of rhinitis (aOR, 4.05; 95% CI, 2.82–5.81) compared with children without eczema, whereas there was no significant

Table 2 Factors associated with the 5-year cumulative incidence of asthma and incidence of rhinitis in eczema patients aged 1–2 years in Sweden

Risk factor at baseline	Incidence of asthma (N = 2063)		Incidence of rhinitis (N = 2751)	
	Adjusted odds ratio* (95% confidence interval)	P-value	Adjusted odds ratio* (95% confidence interval)	P-value
Eczema at baseline				<0.001
No	1.0	<0.001	1.0	
Yes	3.07 (1.79-5.27)		2.63 (1.85-3.73)	
Gender				0.006
Female	1.0	0.003	1.0	
Male	2.20 (1.30-3.72)		1.59 (1.14- 2.23)	
Age of the child				0.290
12-23 month	1.0	0.340	1.0	
24-35 month	0.78 (0.47-1.30)		0.84 (0.60-1.16)	
Parental history of allergic disease[&]				<0.001
No parent with allergic disease	1.0	<0.001	1.0	
Parent(s) with history of allergic disease	1.83 (1.29-2.60)		2.00 (1.59-2.51)	
Asthma in the child				<0.001
No	–	–	1.0	
Yes			2.80 (1.66-4.70)	
Breastfeeding[&&]				0.446
Breastfeeding longer than 6 month	1.0	0.044	1.0	
Breastfeeding up to 6 month	1.57 (1.03-2.39)		1.13 (0.83-1.54)	
Number of bedrooms with PVC				0.106
No PVC in bedroom	1.0	0.288	1.0	
PVC in one bedroom	1.36 (0.65-2.83)		1.60 (1.02- 2.51)	
PVC in two bedrooms	1.57 (0.89-2.78)		1.30 (0.90-1.90)	
Type of dwelling				0.546
Single family house	1.0	0.605	1.0	
Multi family house	1.21 (0.60-2.44)		1.15 (0.73-1.81)	
Smoking by parents				0.707
No	1.0	0.810	1.0	
Yes	0.92 (0.47-1.79)		0.92 (0.60-1.42)	
Number of adults living with the child				0.942
Two or more	1.0	0.208	1.0	
One	0.43 (0.10-1.81)		1.03 (0.50-2.11)	

*Adjusted by logistic regression for all other variables listed in the table.
[&]linear effect aOR, with reference category no parent; other categories one parent, and two parents.
[&&] linear effect aOR, with reference category longer than 6 months; other categories up to 6 months, and no breastfeeding.

association between the late onset of eczema and the incidence of asthma (aOR, 2.07; 0.78–5.49) and rhinitis (aOR, 0.96; 0.45–2.03). Both mild and moderate to severe eczema were associated with the incidence of asthma and rhinitis compared with children without eczema, with a higher odds of developing asthma and rhinitis in moderate to severe eczema (aOR, 3.56; 1.62–7.83 and aOR, 3.87; 2.37–6.33, respectively) than mild eczema compared with children without eczema (aOR, 2.85; 1.57–5.19 and aOR, 2.37; 1.60–3.51, respectively) (Table 3).

Other risk factors for development of asthma and rhinitis during a 5-year period

In adjusted analysis, a parental history of allergic disease increased the odds of developing asthma and rhinitis by 2-fold. The odds of developing asthma was 2-fold and that of developing rhinitis was 59% higher in boys

Table 3 Subgroups of eczema in children and the 5-year cumulative incidence of asthma and rhinitis$

Eczema group	Crude OR (95% CI)	P-value	Adjusted OR# (95% CI)	P-value
		Incidence of asthma (N = 2063)		
Duration of eczema				
Never eczema	1.0	<0.001	1.0	<0.001
Eczema only in 2000	1.94 (0.93-4.06)		2.17 (1.01-4.65)	
Eczema only in 2005	1.97 (0.94- 4.13)		1.77 (0.77-4.11)	
Persistence of eczema##	4.95 (2.65-9.25)		5.16 (2.62-10.18)	
Onset of eczema				
Late onset of eczema###	1.87 (0.78-4.45)	<0.001	2.07 (0.78-5.49)	<0.001
Early onset of eczema ###	3.63 (2.12-6.22)		3.44 (1.94-6.09)	
Severity of eczema				
Mild eczema###	2.42 (1.36-4.29)	<0.001	2.85 (1.57-5.19)	<0.001
Moderate to severe eczema ###	4.55 (2.27-9.11)		3.56 (1.62-7.83)	
		Incidence of rhinitis (N = 2751)		
Duration of eczema				
No eczema	1.0	<0.001	1.0	<0.001
Eczema only in 2000	2.52 (1.61-3.94)		2.25 (1.40-3.61)	
Eczema only in 2005	1.96 (1.20-3.21)		2.00 (1.19-3.37)	
Persistence of eczema##	4.91 (3.23-7.46)		4.00 (2.53-6.22)	
Onset of eczema				
Late onset of eczema###	0.96 (0.46-2.00)	<0.001	0.96 (0.45-2.03)	<0.001
Early onset of eczema ###	5.02 (3.58-7.05)		4.05 (2.82-5.81)	
Severity of eczema				
Mild eczema###	2.74 (1.90-3.95)	<0.001	2.37 (1.60-3.51)	<0.001
Moderate to severe eczema###	4.74 (2.98-7.55)		3.87 (2.37-6.33)	

$ If not otherwise stated, the comparisons are dichotomous with the referent category being the low-odds group (aOR = 1), and the high-odds group data shown in the table.
#Adjustments were made for gender, age, family history of allergic disease, asthma, length of breastfeeding, PVC-flooring material in the home, type of building, environmental tobacco smoke, and number of adults living with the child.
Defined as eczema ever for at least 6 months, and current eczema in both 2000 and 2005.
no eczema in 2000 as reference.

compared with girls. Further, asthma increased the odds of developing rhinitis by nearly 3-fold, and a period of breastfeeding shorter than 6 months increased the risk of developing asthma by 57% (Table 2). PVC-flooring material in the bedroom increased the incidence of asthma and rhinitis, but statistical significance was only reached for the relationship between PVC flooring-material and rhinitis. Interestingly, PVC-flooring material had a higher effect on girls for the incidence of asthma and rhinitis in all models (data not shown). Interactions between eczema and sex were explored and there was no effect of eczema on the incidence of asthma and rhinitis across sex strata (interaction p-values: 0.747 for asthma and 0.664 for rhinitis).

Sensitivity analysis

For assessing the relationships between asthma and rhinitis and remission, we used different assessments of asthma and rhinitis to ensure that the relationship was stable and not dependent on which questions were used. We used both reports of symptoms and reports of doctors' diagnoses. Both of these reports were similar in both crude and adjusted analysis; eczema increased the odds of developing rhinitis symptoms (OR, 2.81; 2.23–3.55 and aOR, 2.39; 1.86–3.08) and wheezing symptoms (OR, 2.10; 1.37–3.23 and aOR, 1.97; 1.24–3.12).

Discussion

Our study found that eczema in early childhood was strongly associated with the development of asthma and rhinitis during the following 5-year period. Eczema was one of the strongest independent risk factors. Interestingly, when eczema was divided into subgroups, children with early onset of eczema, moderate to severe eczema, and persistence of eczema had the highest odds of developing asthma and rhinitis.

This population-based prospective study confirms that early eczema affects later development of asthma and rhinitis.

Although some previous prospective studies were not able to show an association between early childhood eczema and later development of asthma and rhinitis [6,8], our findings are robust and in line with the study by Arshad et al [9]. In addition, similar results regarding severity have been found in both Gustavsson's and Ricci's eczema cohorts [12,13], which reported that eczematous children with high severity scores were at increased risk of developing asthma. To the best of our knowledge, our study is the first prospective cohort to show that early onset of eczema or persistent eczema increases the odds of later onset of asthma in both boys and girls, which is in contrast to a previous study that only showed a relationship in boys [20]. Definitions of asthma and rhinitis are important for the interpretation of results [15]. Our sensitivity analysis confirmed that the association between eczema and asthma/rhinitis remained when symptom-based criteria for asthma and rhinitis were used.

Possible explanations for the relationship between eczema and asthma and rhinitis

Evidence from several experimental studies has suggested that impaired epithelial function results in increased sensitization and IgE production [21]. In humans, the theory of epicutaneous sensitization is supported by the observation that exposing atopic children to topical emollients containing peanut protein leads to an increased risk of airway peanut sensitization [22]. Genetic factors, such as the common loss of function mutations within the filaggrin gene, are a risk factor for incident eczema and account for skin barrier dysfunction [23,24]. Recently, it has been shown that filaggrin mutations affect asthma, which supports the hypothesis that impaired skin function acts as a gateway for allergens, increasing the risk of atopic airways diseases [25].

Advantages and limitations

A major advantage of our study was its prospective design, which made results less subject to recall bias and allowed assessment of temporal relationships. Our study had a large sample size compared with earlier studies [6,8]. Our results should be less prone to selection and ascertainment bias because of its population-based design. We also had a high response rate and limited loss to follow-up. There were no differences between the analysed sample and drop-outs in health-related variables; therefore results might have been biased towards 1. A higher prevalence of socioeconomic risk factors in children leaving the study, while assuming that low socioeconomic status is a risk factor for the incidence of asthma, might have biased the results towards 1 as well. Therefore, our conclusions that eczema is associated with later onset of asthma and rhinitis would not change if all children had participated. The advantages of the study design and performance allow generalization of results.

Reporting of eczema by questionnaire might have advantages compared with assessment by physicians, because eczema can be intermittent [26]. The term *"itchy flexural rash in the last 12 months"* has been shown to correlate well with diagnosis by a physician in a validation study performed in the UK on children aged 3–11 years [18]. Sensitivity in this previous study was 84% and specificity was 93% [18]. In addition, the ISAAC eczema questionnaire has been used for studies on pre-school children [26]. Although questions for diagnosis have been validated for eczema in 4–11-year-olds and for asthma in children aged 1–6 years [27], the ISAAC questionnaire has not been validated for parental information regarding preschool children. However, we consider that it is unlikely that there was differential misclassification; random misclassification would mean that any bias in our estimates was towards null.

Currently, there is no clear definition of persistence of eczema, which is consistent as reported by Williams [28]. Illi [7] and Möhrenschlager [29] considered eczema as persistent when signs of the disease were present at different points of time. In our study, persistence of eczema was defined as having had eczema at least three times. Therefore, the risk of including children with "short-term rashes only" might be low, but we cannot exclude the possibility that some children classified as having persistent eczema had longer symptom-free intervals. It would have been advantageous to assess the prevalence of eczema more often during the study period.

Implications

Based on the results of our study, further evidence is required to unravel the underlying mechanisms of eczema in early childhood leading to asthma. Although we confirmed a relationship between childhood eczema and incident asthma and rhinitis, the association between childhood eczema and later asthma and rhinitis might still be separate and sequential, but are otherwise unrelated in the background of an atopic phenotype. Because the relationship between childhood eczema and incident asthma and rhinitis was temporal, strong, and linear, our findings suggest that the relationship might be causal. In this regard, impaired skin function might hypothetically be one explanatory factor [21], and the effect of early and successful treatment of eczema should be explored regarding the incidence of asthma as one outcome measure [30,31]. Further, it might be beneficial to estimate if objective measured sensitization (IgE) modifies or confounds the eczema/asthma relationship in future studies. Our study results have important implications for patient management since asthma can lead to high impairment and costs.

Conclusions

Eczema in infancy independently increases the odds of developing asthma and rhinitis during the following 5-year period. This association is present for children with eczema at baseline; however when they are divided into subgroups (severe eczema, early onset of eczema and persistence of eczema) the odds of the incidence of asthma and rhinitis further increases. Identifying risk groups is important for healthcare planning.

Abbreviations

DBH: Dampness in Building and Health; ISAAC: International Study of Asthma and Allergies in Childhood; PVC: Polyvinyl chloride.

Competing interests

There is no conflict of interest among the authors Laura B. von Kobyletzki, Carl-Gustaf Bornehag, Mikael Hasselgren, Malin Larsson, Cecilia Boman Lindström, and Åke Svensson, between reporting of the study findings, and financial or non-financial interests that might bias the report.

Authors' contributions

LVK, AS and CGB take responsibility for the integrity of the data. LVK performed data analysis. LVK, AS, and CGB participated in the concept and design of the study. CGB, MH, ML, LVK, and CBL were involved in acquisition of data. LVK, AS, CGB, and ML interpreted the data. LVK drafted the manuscript. AS, CGB, MH, ML, and CBL critically revised the manuscript for important intellectual content. AS and CGB supervised the study. All authors read and approved the final manuscript.

Author details

[1]Lund University, Institute of Clinical Research in Malmö, Skåne University Hospital, Department of Dermatology, Malmö, Sweden. [2]Karlstad University, Department of Public Health Sciences, Karlstad, Sweden. [3]Örebro University, School of Medicine, Örebro, Sweden. [4]County Council of Värmland, Primary Care Research Unit, Karlstad, Sweden.

References

1. Williams H, Stewart A, von Mutius E, Cookson W, Anderson HR: **Is eczema really on the increase worldwide?** *J Allergy Clin Immunol* 2008, **121**:947–954.
2. Lewis-Jones S: **Quality of life and childhood atopic dermatitis: the misery of living with childhood eczema.** *Int J Clin Pract* 2006, **60**:984–992.
3. Carroll CL, Balkrishnan R, Feldman SR, Fleischer AB Jr, Manuel JC: **The burden of atopic dermatitis: impact on the patient, family, and society.** *Pediatr Dermatol* 2005, **22**:192–199.
4. Spergel JM, Paller AS: **Atopic dermatitis and the atopic march.** *J Allergy Clin Immunol* 2003, **112**:S118–S127.
5. Beasley R, Keil U, von Mutius E, *et al*: **Worldwide variation in prevalence of symptoms of asthma, allergic rhinoconjunctivitis, and atopic eczema: ISAAC. The International Study of Asthma and Allergies in Childhood (ISAAC) Steering Committee.** *Lancet* 1998, **351**:1225–1232.
6. the Group Health Medical Associates, Martinez FD, Wright AL, Taussig LM, Holberg CJ, Halonen M, Morgan WJ: **Asthma and wheezing in the first six years of life.** *N Engl J Med* 1995, **332**:133–138.
7. Illi S, von Mutius E, Lau S, Nickel R, Gruber C, Niggemann B, *et al*: **The natural course of atopic dermatitis from birth to age 7 years and the association with asthma.** *J Allergy Clin Immunol* 2004, **113**:925–931.
8. Klinnert MD, Nelson HS, Price MR, Adinoff AD, Leung DY, Mrazek DA: **Onset and persistence of childhood asthma: predictors from infancy.** *Pediatrics* 2001, **108**:E69.
9. Arshad SH, Kurukulaaratchy RJ, Fenn M, Matthews S: **Early life risk factors for current wheeze, asthma, and bronchial hyperresponsiveness at 10 years of age.** *Chest* 2005, **127**:502–508.
10. Burgess JA, Dharmage SC, Byrnes GB, Matheson MC, Gurrin LC, Wharton CL, Johns DP, Abramson MJ, Hopper JL, Walters EH: **Childhood eczema and asthma incidence and persistence: a cohort study from childhood to middle age.** *J Allergy Clin Immunol* 2008, **122**:280–285.
11. Martin PE, Matheson MC, Gurrin L, Burgess JA, Osborne N, Lowe AJ, Morrison S, Meszaros D, Giles GG, Abramson MJ, *et al*: **Childhood eczema and rhinitis predict atopic but not nonatopic adult asthma: a prospective cohort study over 4 decades.** *J Allergy Clin Immunol* 2011, **127**:1473–1479. e1471.
12. Ricci G, Patrizi A, Baldi E, Menna G, Tabanelli M, Masi M: **Long-term follow-up of atopic dermatitis: retrospective analysis of related risk factors and association with concomitant allergic diseases.** *J Am Acad Dermatol* 2006, **55**:765–771.
13. Gustafsson D, Sjoberg O, Foucard T: **Development of allergies and asthma in infants and young children with atopic dermatitis–a prospective follow-up to 7 years of age.** *Allergy* 2000, **55**:240–245.
14. Queille-Roussel C, Raynaud F, Saurat JH: **A prospective computerized study of 500 cases of atopic dermatitis in childhood. I. Initial analysis of 250 parameters.** *Acta Derm Venereol Suppl (Stockh)* 1985, **114**:87–92.
15. Larsson M, Hagerhed-Engman L, Sigsgaard T, Janson S, Sundell J, Bornehag CG: **Incidence rates of asthma, rhinitis and eczema symptoms and influential factors in young children in Sweden.** *Acta Paediatr* 2008, **97**:1210–1215.
16. Bornehag CG, Sundell J, Sigsgaard T: **Dampness in buildings and health (DBH): Report from an ongoing epidemiological investigation on the association between indoor environmental factors and health effects among children in Sweden.** *Indoor Air* 2004, **14**(Suppl 7):59–66.
17. Asher MI, Keil U, Anderson HR, Beasley R, Crane J, Martinez F, *et al*: **International Study of Asthma and Allergies in Childhood (ISAAC): rationale and methods.** *Eur RespirJ.* 1995, **8**:483–491.
18. Williams H, Robertson C, Stewart A, Aït-Khaled N, Anabwani G, Anderson R, *et al*: **Worldwide variations in the prevalence of symptoms of atopic eczema in the International Study of Asthma and Allergies in Childhood.** *J Allergy Clin Immunol* 1999, **103**:125–138.
19. Lemeshow S, Hosmer DW Jr: **A review of goodness of fit statistics for use in the development of logistic regression models.** *Am J Epidemiol* 1982, **115**:92–106.
20. Lowe AJ, Carlin JB, Bennett CM, Hosking CS, Abramson MJ, Hill DJ, *et al*: **Do boys do the atopic march while girls dawdle?** *J Allergy Clin Immunol* 2008, **121**:1190–1195.
21. Kolarik B, Naydenov K, Larsson M, Bornehag CG, Sundell J: **The association between phthalates in dust and allergic diseases among Bulgarian children.** *Environ Health Perspect* 2008, **116**:98–103.
22. Cookson W: **The immunogenetics of asthma and eczema: a new focus on the epithelium.** *Nat Rev Immunol* 2004, **4**:978–988.
23. Weidinger S, Illig T, Baurecht H: **Loss-of-function variations within the filaggrin gene predispose for atopic dermatitis with allergic sensitizations.** *J Allergy Clin Immunol* 2006, **118**:214–219.
24. Weidinger S, O'Sullivan M, Illig T: **Filaggrin mutations, atopic eczema, hay fever, and asthma in children.** *J Allergy Clin Immunol* 2008, **121**:1203–1209.
25. Lack G, Fox D, Northstone K, Golding J: **Factors associated with the development of peanut allergy in childhood.** *N Engl J Med* 2003, **348**:977–985.
26. Peroni DG, Piacentini GL, Alfonsi L, Zerman L, Di Blasi P, Visona G, *et al*: **Rhinitis in pre-school children: prevalence, association with allergic diseases and risk factors.** *Clin Exp Allergy* 2003, **33**:1349–1354.
27. Hederos C-A, Hasselgren M, Hedlin G, Bornehag C-G: **Comparison of clinically diagnosed asthma with parental assessment of children's asthma in a questionnaire.** *Pediatr Allergy Immunol* 2007, **18**:135–141.
28. Williams HC: *Atopic dermatitis: the epidemiology, causes and prevention of atopic eczema.* Cambridge: Cambridge University Press; 2000.
29. Mohrenschlager M, Schafer T, Huss-Marp J, Eberlein-Konig B, Weidinger S, Ring J, *et al*: **The course of eczema in children aged 5–7 years and its relation to atopy: differences between boys and girls.** *Br J Dermatol* 2006, **154**:505–513.

30. Brown SJ, Asai Y, Cordell HJ, Campbell LE, Zhao Y, Liao H, *et al*: **Loss-of-function variants in the filaggrin gene are a significant risk factor for peanut allergy.** *J Allergy Clin Immunol* 2011, **127**:661–667.
31. Simpson EL, Berry TM, Brown PA, Hanifin JM: **A pilot study of emollient therapy for the primary prevention of atopic dermatitis.** *J Am Acad Dermatol* 2010, **63**:587–593.

2

Low rate of dermatology outpatient visits in Asian-Americans: an initial survey study for associated patient-related factors

Bharathi Lingala, Shufeng Li, Ashley Wysong, Allison K Truong, David Kim and Anne Lynn S Chang*

Abstract

Background: Asian-Americans represent the fastest growing minority group in the United States, but are under-represented patients in outpatient dermatology clinics. At the same time, skin cancer rates in individuals of Asian descent are increasing, but skin cancer detection appears to be delayed in Asian-Americans compared to white individuals. Some health-care provider related factors for this phenomenon have been reported in the literature, but the patient-related factors are unclear.

Methods: This exploratory study to identify patient-related factors associated with dermatology visits in Asian-Americans was performed after Institutional Review Board (IRB) approval. An anonymous, online survey utilizing validated items was conducted on adults who self-identified as Asian-American in Northern California. Univariate and multivariate logistic regression for dermatology visits as indicated by responses to the question of "ever having had skin checked by a dermatologist" were performed on survey responses pertaining to demographic information, socioeconomic factors, acculturation, knowledge of melanoma warning signs and SSE belief and practice.

Results: 89.7% of individuals who opened the online survey completed the items, with 469 surveys included in the analysis. Only 60% reported ever performing a SSE, and only 48% reported ever having a skin examination by a dermatologist. Multivariate models showed that "ever performing SSE" ($p < 0.0001$), marital status ($p = 0.02$), family history of skin cancer ($p = 0.03$) and generation in the United States ($p = 0.02$) were significant predictors of the primary outcome of "ever had skin checked by a dermatologist".

Conclusions: Identification of patient-related factors that associate with dermatology clinic visits in Asian-Americans is important so that this potential gap in dermatologic care can be better addressed through future studies.

Keywords: Dermatology, Skin cancer, Early detection, Acculturation, Asian-Americans, Skin self-examination, Dermatology visits, Prevention, Ethnic skin

Background

According to the 2012 United States Census Bureau, Asian-Americans currently represent the fastest growing minority group [1]. However, data from the National Ambulatory Medical Care Survey (NAMCS) in 2010 showed that Asian-American represent only 1.07% of ambulatory care visits to dermatologists even though they comprise 3% of the American population. This is potentially concerning as the overall incidence rate of melanoma appears to be rising at 2.4% per year from 1999–2006 in the U. S. in all races [2,3], a trend also seen in worldwide populations where Asians are the majority [4-6]. In the U. S., data from the National Cancer Institute Surveillance, Epidemiology and End Results Program (SEER) database 2007–2011 showed age-adjusted new melanoma cases per 100,000 persons was 8.1 for Asian/Pacific Islanders (52.3 for whites). However, Asians and Pacific Islanders had a higher rate of thicker and distant melanomas compared to whites and Hispanics [2,7-10]. Asians/Pacific Islanders in the U.S. also had lower 5-year survival rates than whites [2].

Factors related to delayed diagnosis could be either patient-related or provider-related. Provider-related factors

* Correspondence: alschang@stanford.edu
Department of Dermatology, Stanford University, Pavilion C, 2nd Floor, 450 Broadway St, Redwood City 94063, CA, USA

Table 1 Characteristics of study participants, with n = 469 responses included unless otherwise indicated

Demographic and socioeconomic factors	Number (%)
Age in years, mean (SD)	37.2 ± 15.9
Gender	
Male	147 (31%)
Female	322 (69%)
Marital status	
Single	240 (51%)
Married	187 (40%)
Separated, Divorced, Widowed	28 (6%)
Domestic union (living together)	14 (3%)
Education	
High School	34 (7%)
College	249 (53%)
Graduate or Professional	180 (38%)
Grade school or no formal education	6 (1%)
Annual household income (n = 441, missing data n = 18)	
< $25,000	67 (15%)
$25,000 - $50,000	77 (17%)
$50,001 - $75,000	73 (17%)
$75,001 - $100,000	62 (14%)
> $100,000	162 (37%)
Has health insurance	419 (89%)
Acculturation, n = 410	
Generation in the United States	
First generation (born outside US)	160 (39%)
Second Generation	175 (43%)
Third Generation	41 (10%)
Fourth Generation	26 (6%)
Fifth Generation	8 (2%)
Self-rated acculturation, n = 410 (missing response n = 59)	
Very Asian	46 (11%)
Mostly Asian	72 (18%)
Bicultural	159 (39%)
Mostly Westernized	88 (21%)
Very Westernized	45 (11%)
Additional parameters	
Personal history of skin cancer	8 (1.7%)
Family history of skin cancer	19 (4.1%)
Co-worker or friend with history of skin cancer	116 (25%)
Has heard of ABCDEs of melanoma	79 (16.8%)
Belief in skin self-examination (n = 466, missing response n = 3)	
Disagree	82 (18%)
Neutral	97 (21%)
Agree	287 (61%)

Table 1 Characteristics of study participants, with n = 469 responses included unless otherwise indicated *(Continued)*

Ever performed skin self-examination (SSE)	
Never	159 (34%)
1-3 times	144 (31%)
4-6 times	39 (8%)
7-9 times	5 (1%)
10 or more times	94 (20%)
Not sure	28 (6%)
Ever had skin checked by dermatologist	
Never	237 (51%)
1-3 times	155 (34%)
4-6 times	38 (8%)
7-9 times	5 (1%)
10 or more times	23 (5%)
Not sure	11 (2%)
Self-assessed risk for getting skin cancer during lifetime, n = 465	
Mildly agree	185 (40%)
Mildly disagree	41 (9%)
Neither agree nor disagree	72 (15%)
Strongly agree	144 (31%)
Strongly disagree	23 (5%)
Skin burns when exposed to strong sunshine without protection, n = 460	
Not at all	32 (7%)
Somewhat	203 (44%)
Very little	118 (26%)
Yes (red, painful burn)	107 (23%)
Skin tans when exposed to strong sunshine without protection, n = 452	
Not tan at all - I just burn	15 (3%)
Tan Slightly	86 (19%)
Tan deeply	140 (31%)
Tan moderately	211 (47%)
Number of blistering sunburns in lifetime, n = 468	
0	206 (44%)
1 - 2	168 (36%)
3 - 4	65 (14%)
5 or more	29 (6)

reported include a lowered index of suspicion among clinicians and different anatomic sites leading to advanced stages at presentation and a poorer prognosis [2]. Patient-related factors are less clear. One hypothesis is that Asian-Americans visit dermatology clinics at a lower rate than other races, as suggested by the NAMCS data. Although there is data on patient characteristics such as personal skin cancer history, skin type, psychosocial factors that

Table 2 Univariate and multivariate analyses on the primary outcome variable of "ever had skin checked by a dermatologist"

Demographic and socioeconomic factors	Univariate OR (95% CI)	P	Multivariate OR (95% CI)	P
Age (1 year)	1.02 (1.01 - 1.04)	**<0.0001**	1.00 (0.97 - 1.03)	0.89
Gender (Female (ref = Male))	1.63 (1.09 - 2.43)	**0.02**	1.17 (0.62 - 2.21)	0.64
Marital status				
Single	Ref		Ref	
Married	2.02 (1.37 - 2.97)	**<0.001**	2.52 (1.06 - 5.99)	0.09
Separated, Divorced, Widowed	3.90 (1.65 - 9.22)		3.05 (0.65 - 14.3)	
Education				
High School	Ref		Ref	
College	1.12 (0.55 - 2.31)	0.83	1.84 (0.55 - 6.11)	0.60
Graduate/Professional School	1.00 (0.48 - 2.10)		1.62 (0.46 - 5.72)	
Annual household income				
< $25,000	Ref		Ref	
$25,001-50,000	1.61 (0.79 - 3.28)		1.83 (0.65 - 5.14)	
$50,001-75,000	3.24 (1.59 - 6.61)	**0.004**	3.01 (1.03 - 8.79)	0.21
$75,001-100,000	2.98 (1.43 - 6.23)		3.33 (1.10 - 10.07)	
> $100,000	2.68 (1.44 - 4.99)		2.19 (0.86 - 5.62)	
Has health insurance	0.77 (0.38 - 1.57)	0.47	0.62 (0.21 - 1.84)	0.39
Acculturation				
Generation in the United States				
First Generation (born outside US)	Ref		Ref	
Second Generation	1.92 (1.23 - 2.99)	**<0.0001**	1.83 (0.92 - 3.61)	0.40
Third Generation	3.68 (1.77 - 7.65)		1.52 (0.45 - 5.15)	
Fourth or more Generation	2.99 (1.37 - 6.52)		1.63 (0.52 - 5.04)	
Self-rated acculturation				
Very Asian	Ref		Ref	
Mostly Asian	2.52 (1.12 - 5.67)		0.94 (0.34 - 2.56)	
Bicultural	2.15 (1.03 - 4.47)	**0.001**	1.09 (0.37 - 3.22)	0.44
Mostly Westernized	4.82 (2.17 - 10.67)		1.81 (0.59 - 5.58)	
Very Westernized	3.76 (1.52 - 9.34)		1.83 (0.48 - 6.92)	
Additional parameters				
Personal history of skin cancer	7.71 (0.94 - 63.11)	0.06	NR*	
Family history of skin cancer	3.92 (1.27 - 12.05)	**0.02**	5.67 (0.94 - 34.08)	0.06
Co-worker or friend with history of skin cancer	2.37 (1.52 - 3.69)	**0.001**	1.05 (0.54 - 2.05)	0.89
Has heard of ABCDEs of melanoma	1.78 (1.08 - 2.94)	**0.03**	1.20 (0.57 - 2.53)	0.64
Belief in SSE				
Disagree	Ref		Ref	
Agree	2.44 (1.45 - 4.12)	**<0.0001**	1.29 (0.50 - 3.32)	0.23
Neutral	1.05 (0.56 - 1.97)		1.98 (0.84 - 4.67)	
Ever performed SSE	4.28 (2.79 - 6.59)	**<0.0001**	2.99 (1.54 - 5.80)	**0.0012**
Self-assessed risk for getting skin cancer during lifetime, n = 465				
Strongly disagree	Ref		Ref	
Mildly agree	1.34 (0.54 - 3.35)	0.0099	1.18 (0.28 - 5.00)	0.13
Mildly disagree	1.58 (0.54 - 4.61)		1.72 (0.33 - 8.98)	

Table 2 Univariate and multivariate analyses on the primary outcome variable of "ever had skin checked by a dermatologist" *(Continued)*

Neither agree nor disagree	1.17 (0.43 - 3.15)		0.60 (0.13 - 2.76)	
Strongly agree	2.69 (1.06 - 6.82)		1.99 (0.45 - 8.73)	
Skin burns when exposed to strong sunshine without protection				
Not at all	Ref		Ref	
Somewhat	1.46 (0.67 - 3.17)	0.54	1.37 (0.43 - 4.40)	0.05
Very little	1.70 (0.76 - 3.81)		2.53 (0.76 - 8.46)	
Yes (red, painful burn)	1.52 (0.67 - 3.45)		0.77 (0.22 - 2.74)	
Skin tans when exposed to strong sunshine without protection				
Not tan at all - I just burn	Ref		Ref	
Tan Slightly	1.61 (0.51 - 5.12)	0.20	0.37 (0.06 - 2.25)	0.13
Tan deeply	2.45 (0.80 - 7.55)		0.85 (0.15 - 4.84)	
Tan moderately	1.76 (0.58 - 5.34)		0.57 (0.10 - 3.15)	
Number of blistering sunburns in lifetime				
0	Ref		Ref	
1 - 2	1.13 (0.75 - 1.71)	0.78	1.28 (0.67 - 2.43)	0.73
3 - 4	1.30 (0.74 - 2.28)		1.32 (0.58 - 3.01)	
5 or more	1.28 (0.57 - 2.85)		1.92 (0.49 - 7.49)	

*Not included in multivariate analysis due to small number of skin cancers (n = 8).
Multivariate analysis was based on n = 324 unless otherwise indicated.
Bolded numbers indicate significance at a level P<0.05.

associate with clinical skin examinations [11], there is no data in Asian or Asian-American populations. Furthermore, cutaneous examination by a dermatologist is known to impact skin cancer stage at initial presentation [12-17].

This study examines factors that correlate with "ever having skin checked by a dermatologist" in a Northern California Asian-American population. Because of the overwhelmingly outpatient nature of dermatology, having skin checked by a dermatologist almost always occurs in the setting of an outpatient dermatology clinic visit. In addition, we acknowledge that the guidelines for frequency and utility of dermatologists' cutaneous examinations particularly in asymptomatic people of color continues to be debated due to the lack of high quality evidence for this practice [3,15-18].

Methods

The study was approved by the Stanford Human Subjects Panel and the need for a written consent was waived as the study was anonymous and voluntary. An online survey study of adults in Northern California who self-identified as Asian-American was performed and included items on demographic information, socioeconomic factors, acculturation, belief in SSE, having heard of melanoma warning signs, SSE practices and ever having skin checked by dermatologist. Survey items were adapted from previously published skin cancer survey instruments [19] and previously published acculturation tools [20-22]. Additional file 1: Figure S1 shows the actual survey instrument, with items used in the study analysis highlighted. Because of the many languages spoken within the Asian population in northern California, the survey was available in English only. To minimize bias toward Asian-Americans with access to dermatologic care, this study was conducted completely online rather than at dermatology clinics. The survey was placed online via the Stanford University Surveyor Web site. The web site address was distributed to leaders of Northern California community groups that were likely to contain a large portion of Asian-Americans for circulation among community group members to identify participants for this study. These group members were all adults. Because of technical limitations, we could not prevent individuals who were under 18 years of age or not Asian-American from accessing the survey. These individuals were excluded prior to statistical analysis (see Results section).

Because of the online format, a conventional response rate could not be calculated. However, we did track the number of participants who completed the survey divided by the number of clicks (hits) from unique Internet Protocol (IP) addresses for this web site regardless of whether any survey items were completed.

Characteristics of the study subjects were summarized using descriptive statistics. Clinically meaningful variables were chosen for analysis and based on review of the medical literature [23-25]. Univariate and multivariate logistic regressions were performed on the primary outcome variable of "ever had skin checked by a dermatologist".

A final multivariate analyses model on the primary outcome variable of "ever had skin checked by a dermatologist" was generated after checking for multicollinearity or interactions between any two variables, then applying stepwise selection, plus the variables of interest. Of note, while "generation in the United States" and "self-rated acculturation" did not meet the threshold for collinearity, there was a significant association between these two variables. Hence, only "generation in the United States" was included in the final model. All statistical analyses were conducted using SAS statistical software package (Version 9.1, SAS Institute, Inc., Cary, North Carolina).

Results

Of the 564 individuals who visited the survey website, 506 (89.7%) completed the survey. To ensure an Asian-American population, individuals who self-identified as only "white" (n = 27) or "other" (n = 10) were excluded from the study. The final study sample included 469 individuals. Table 1 shows the demographic characteristics of this group. The most common self-identified races in the study sample were Chinese (39%), Japanese (18%), Taiwanese (8%), Filipino (7%), Korean (7%), and Vietnamese (6%). Other groups represented (<6% each) include Pacific Islander, Thai, Laotian, Cambodian, African-American, and Caucasian (individuals were allowed to select more than one race or ethnicity to allow for mixed race). Thirty-four percent of individuals were born outside of the United States (first-generation), while 37%, 9%, 6%, and 2% self-identified as second, third, fourth, and fifth generation Americans, respectively. To further assess the degree of cultural identification, respondents were also asked to self-rate their acculturation, with 15% identifying their acculturation as "mostly Asian", 10% as "very Asian", 34% as "bicultural", 19% as "mostly westernized", and 10% as "very westernized".

Overall, only 48% of respondents reported ever having their skin checked by a dermatologist. Univariate analyses on the primary outcome of "ever had skin checked by a dermatologist" are presented in Table 2. In multivariate analysis, the only variable significantly associated with "ever having skin checked by dermatologist" was "ever performed a skin self-examination", ($p < 0.0012$) (Table 2). Only 60% of respondents had ever performed an SSE. In multivariate analysis, a family history of skin cancer and "ever having skin checked by dermatologist" showed a trend toward significance ($p = 0.06$).

To explore predictors of "having skin checked by a dermatologist", multiple multivariate analyses varying the variables were performed, after accounting for multicollinearity or interaction (results shown in Table 3). Significant predictors of "having skin checked by a dermatologist" included Ever Performed SSE ($p < 0.0001$), marital status ($p = 0.02$), generation in the United States ($p = 0.03$), and family history of skin cancer ($p = 0.03$).

Table 3 Final multivariate analyses model on the primary outcome variable of "ever had skin checked by a dermatologist"

Characteristic	Multivariate OR (95% CI)	P
Education		
High School	Ref	0.24
College	2.19 (0.80 - 6.00)	
Graduate/Professional School	1.64 (0.57 - 4.74)	
Annual household income		
< $25,000	Ref	0.07
$25,001-50,000	1.93 (0.79 - 4.72)	
$50,001-75,000	**3.19 (1.24 - 8.23)**	
$75,001-100,000	**3.70 (1.41 - 9.71)**	
> $100,000	**2.60 (1.13 - 6.02)**	
Has health insurance	0.55 (0.22 - 1.41)	0.22
Ever performed SSE	**3.32 (1.95 - 5.65)**	**<0.0001**
Marital status		
Single	Ref	**0.02**
Married	**2.04 (1.13 - 3.70)**	
Separated, Divorced, Widowed	**3.56 (1.01 - 12.61)**	
Family history of skin cancer	**6.50 (1.15 - 36.69)**	**0.03**
Generation in the United States		
First Generation (born outside US)	Ref	**0.02**
Second Generation	**2.11 (1.20 - 3.72)**	
Third Generation	2.21 (0.85 - 5.80)	
Fourth or more Generation	**3.14 (1.17 - 8.42)**	

This model was selected after checking for multi-collinearity or interactions between any two variables, then applying stepwise selection, plus the variables of interest. Analysis based on n = 349 responses.
Bolded numbers indicate significance at a level P<0.05.

Discussion

The rates of "ever had skin checked by dermatologist" in our Asian-American study population are difficult to directly compare with other minority groups. Perhaps the most similar study in the literature was an online survey of Hispanics living in the United States, which showed only 9.2% had a total cutaneous examination [10]. As the overall purpose of our study was to examine patient-related factors associated with dermatologic clinic visits, our current survey did not ask if a patient had a total cutaneous examination, only whether they ever had skin checked by dermatologist. This would likely include skin checks for benign skin disease as well as skin cancer surveillance, hence, accounting for our higher percentage of individuals "ever having skin checked by dermatologist" compared to total cutaneous examinations reported in other studies. It is also difficult to directly compare our study with existing studies in other minority groups due to differences in geographic locales and survey methods.

The study participants were similar to the local Asian-American community with respect to household income, education and health insurance status. For instance, the median household income for single race Asian households in Santa Clara County, the location of our institution, was $68,780 (by the U.S. Census, 2009); for our study, 50% of participants reported incomes above $75,000. For education level in single race Asians in Santa County Clara County, 50% have a bachelors or some college degree; this is 53% in our study. For health insurance in single race Asians in Santa Clara County, 17.2% did not have health insurance; 11% in our survey did not. Hence, this study is likely generalizable to the local Asian-American community.

This study was conducted only in English (due to the large number of languages spoken by Asian-Americans in Northern California) and is therefore biased in favor of those proficient in English. In addition, this study was performed online, hence accessible only to those with computer literacy and Internet access. Finally, the Asian-American community is very heterogeneous and therefore, this study does not necessarily represent the demographic and clinical factors and practices of each subgroup.

Finally, SSE and cutaneous examinations by dermatologists have been significantly linked in previous studies that did not primarily focus on Asian-Americans [26]. Nevertheless, the ideal frequency of SSE and cutaneous examinations in asymptomatic persons of any race has not been established, in part due to the lack of high quality studies to support these measures [3,15-18]. Nevertheless, a recent expert opinion article by Agbai *et al.* in persons of color did suggest monthly self-skin examinations, though no recommendations were made for cutaneous examinations by dermatologists [3].

Conclusion

Future research is needed to determine the optimal frequency of skin examinations in Asian-Americans and whether increased dermatology clinic visits lead to earlier detection of skin cancers in Asian-Americans.

Competing interests

The authors have no competing interests to declare.

Authors' contributions

BL contributed to conception, design, statistical analysis and data interpretation. AW and AC contributed to the conception, design, data acquisition, statistical analysis, data interpretation, manuscript draft and revision. SL contributed to design, statistical analysis, data interpretation, manuscript draft and revision. AT contributed to data interpretation and manuscript draft and revision. DK contributed to data acquisition and manuscript draft. All authors read and approved the final manuscript.

Authors' information

Anne Lynn Chang is an Assistant Professor of Dermatology at Stanford University School of Medicine. She is Director of the Stanford Dermatology Adult Dermatological Clinical Trials, the Advanced Basal Cell Carcinoma Clinic and a member of the Stanford Cancer Institute.
Bharathi Lingala and Shufeng Li are co-first authors.

References

1. US Census Bureau Population Division: *Projections of the resident population by race, Hispanic origin, and nativity: middle series, 1999–2100.* Washington (DC): US Census Bureau; 2000.
2. Wu XC, Eide MJ, King J, Saraiya M, Huan Y, Wiggins C, Barnholtz-Sloan JS, Martin N, Cokkinides V, Miller J, Patel P, Ekwueme DU, Kim J: **Racial and ethnic variations in incidence and survival of cutaneous melanoma in the United States, 1999–2006.** *J Am Acad Dermatol* 2011, **65**:S26–S37.
3. Agbai ON, Buster K, Sanchez M, Hernandez C, Kundu RV, Chiu M, Roberts WE, Draelos ZD, Bhushan R, Taylor SC, Lim HW: **Skin cancer and photoprotection in people of color: a review and recommendations for physicians and the public.** *J Am Acad Dermatol* 2014, **70**(4):748–762.
4. Ishihara K, Saida T, Yamamoto A: **Updated statistical data for malignant melanoma in Japan.** *Int J Clin Oncol* 2001, **6**(3):109–116.
5. Koh D, Wang H, Lee J, Chia KS, Lee HP, Goh CL: **Basal cell carcinoma, squamous cell carcinoma and melanoma of the skin: analysis of the Singapore Cancer Registry data 1968–97.** *Br J Dermatol* 2003, **148**(6):1161–1166.
6. Sng J, Koh D, Siong WC, Choo TB: **Skin cancer trends among Asians living in Singapore from 1968 to 2006.** *J Am Acad Dermatol* 2009, **61**(3):426–432.
7. Chen YJ, Wu CY, Chen JT, Shen JL, Chen CC, Wang HC: **Clinicopathologic analysis of malignant melanoma in Taiwan.** *J Am Acad Dermatol* 1999, **41**(6):945–949.
8. Cress RD, Holly EA: **Incidence of cutaneous melanoma among non-Hispanic whites, Hispanics, Asians, and blacks: an analysis of california cancer registry data, 1988–93.** *Cancer Causes Control* 1997, **8**(2):246–252.
9. Johnson DS, Yamane S, Morita S, Yonehara C, Wong JH: **Malignant melanoma in non-Caucasians: experience from Hawaii.** *Surg Clin North Am* 2003, **83**(2):275–282.
10. Coups EJ, Stapleton JL, Hudson SV, Medina-Forrester A, Rosenberg SA, Gordon M, Natale-Pereira A, Goydos JS: **Skin cancer surveillance behaviors among US Hispanic adults.** *J Am Acad Dermatol* 2013, **68**(4):576–584.
11. Kasparian NA, Bränström R, Chang YM, Affleck P, Aspinwall LG, Tibben A, Azizi E, Baron-Epel O, Battistuzzi L, Bruno W, Chan M, Cuellar F, Debniak T, Pjanova D, Ertmanski S, Figl A, Gonzalez M, Hayward NK, Hocevar M, Kanetsky PA, Leachman S, Bergman W, Heisele O, Palmer J, Peric B, Puig S, Schadendorf D, Gruis NA, Newton-Bishop J, Brandberg Y, Melanoma Genetics Consortium (GenoMEL): **Skin examination behavior: the role of melanoma history, skin type, psychosocial factors and region of residence in determining clinical and self-conducted skin examination.** *Arch Dermatol* 2012, **148**(10):1142–1151.
12. Emmons KM, Geller AC, Puleo E, Savadatti SS, Hu SW, Gorham S, Werchniak AE: **Skin cancer education and early detection at the beach: a randomized trial of dermatologist examination and biometric feedback.** *J Am Acad Dermatol* 2011, **64**(2):282–289.
13. Aitken JF, Janda M, Elwood M, Youl PH, Ring IT, Lowe JB: **Clinical outcomes from skin screening clinics within a community-based melanoma screening program.** *J Am Acad Dermatol* 2006, **54**(1):105–114.
14. Hamidi R, Peng D, Cockburn M: **Efficacy of skin self-examination for the early detection of melanoma.** *Int J Dermatol* 2010, **49**(2):126–134.
15. Berwick M, Begg CB, Fine JA, Roush GC, Barnhill RL: **Screening for cutaneous melanoma by skin self-examination.** *J Natl Cancer Inst* 1996, **88**(1):17–23.

16. Pollitt RA, Geller AC, Brooks DR, Johnson TM, Park ER, Swetter SM: **Efficacy of skin self-examination practices for early melanoma detection.** *Cancer Epidemiol Biomarkers Prev* 2009, **18**(11):3018–3023.
17. Brady MS, Oliveria SA, Christos PJ, Berwick M, Coit DG, Katz J, Halpern AC: **Patterns of detection in patients with cutaneous melanoma.** *Cancer* 2000, **89**(2):342–347.
18. **United States Preventative Services Task Force 2009 guidelines for skin self-examination and population based screening in asymptomatic persons by primary care physicians at.** http://www.uspreventiveservices taskforce.org/uspstf09/skincancer/skincanrs.htm, accessed May 20, 2014.
19. Gorell E, Lee C, Munoz C, Chang AL: **Adoption of Western culture by Californian Asian Americans: attitudes and practices promoting sun exposure.** *Arch Dermatol* 2009, **145**(5):552–556.
20. Suinn RM, Ahuna C, Khoo G: **The Suinn-Lew Asian Self-Identity Acculturation Scale: Concurrent and Factorial Validation.** *Educ Psychol Meas* 1992, **52**(4):1041–1046.
21. Lee S, Chen L, He X, Miller MJ, Juon HS: **A cluster analytic examination of acculturation and health status among Asian Americans in the Washington DC metropolitan area, United States.** *Soc Sci Med* 2013, **96:**17–23.
22. Lee S, Chen L, Jung MY, Baezconde-Garbanati L, Juon HS: **Acculturation and cancer screening among Asian Americans: role of health insurance and having a regular physician.** *J Community Health* 2014, **39**(2):201–212.
23. Weinstock MA, Martin RA, Risica PM, Berwick M, Lasater T, Rakowski W, Goldstein MG, Dube CE: **Thorough skin examination for the early detection of melanoma.** *Am J Prev Med* 1999, **17**(3):169–175.
24. Hamidi R, Cockburn MG, Peng DH: **Prevalence and predictors of skin self-examination: prospects for melanoma prevention and early detection.** *Int J Dermatol* 2008, **47**(10):993–1003.
25. Coups EJ, Geller AC, Weinstock MA, Heckman CJ, Manne SL: **Prevalence and correlates of skin cancer screening among middle-aged and older white adults in the United States.** *Am J Med* 2010, **123**(5):439–445.
26. Mitchell J, Leslie KS: **Melanoma death prevention: moving away from the sun.** *J Am Acad Dermatol* 2013, **68**(6):169–175.

3

Improved emollient use reduces atopic eczema symptoms and is cost neutral in infants: before-and-after evaluation of a multifaceted educational support programme

James M Mason[1], Julie Carr[2], Carolyn Buckley[3], Steve Hewitt[3], Phillip Berry[3], Josh Taylor[4] and Michael J Cork[5,6,7*]

Abstract

Background: Parents and carers of children with eczema often underuse emollient therapy, essential to repairing and protecting the defective skin barrier in atopic eczema. Educational interventions delivered by specialist dermatology nurses in hospital settings have been shown to improve emollient use and reduce symptoms of atopic eczema, but benefits of community-based interventions are uncertain. Support and information about appropriate care may often be inadequate for patients and carers in the community.

Methods: A multifaceted educational support programme was evaluated as a method of increasing emollient use and reducing atopic eczema in children. Support provided for parents and carers included an educational DVD, online daily diary and telephone helpline. The before and after study included 136 British children and their parents, providing baseline and 12 week follow-up data while receiving the programme. Measures included emollient use, POEM and PEST scores, and cost of care.

Results: Average emollient use increased by 87.6 g (95% CI: 81.9 to 119.5 g, $p = 0.001$) from baseline with the change being immediate and persistent. The POEM score reduced on average by 5.38 (95% CI: 4.36 to 6.41, $p = 0.001$), a 47% reduction from baseline. Similarly the PEST score reduced on average by 0.61 (95% CI: 0.47 to 0.75, $p = 0.001$), a 48% reduction from baseline. Sleep disturbance was reduced by 1.27 nights per week (95% CI: 0.85 to 1.68, $p = 0.001$) and parental feeling of control improved by 1.32 points (95% CI: 1.16 to 1.48, $p = 0.001$). From the NHS perspective, the programme was cost neutral overall within the study period.

Conclusion: A community-based multifaceted educational support programme greatly increased emollient use, reducing symptoms of atopic eczema and general practitioner contacts, without increasing cost. Significant benefits may accrue to the families and carers of children with atopic eczema due to improved sleep patterns and greater feeling of control. PEST, a new simple measure of acute and remitting atopic eczema severity designed to help parents and children to monitor and manage eczema, merits further evaluation.

Keywords: Atopic eczema, Children, Emollient therapy, Compliance, Symptoms, Measurement, Community study, Health economics, Patient support, Educational support

* Correspondence: m.j.cork@sheffield.ac.uk
[5]Academic Unit of Dermatology Research, School of Medicine & Biomedical Sciences, University of Sheffield, Sheffield, UK
[6]Department of Dermatology, Sheffield Teaching Hospitals NHS Foundation Trust, Sheffield, UK
Full list of author information is available at the end of the article

Background

Atopic eczema (synonym atopic dermatitis) in children is unpredictable in its course and may have a profound impact on the quality of life [1-3] of patients and their family, as well as being time-consuming for healthcare professionals to manage. However, the primary care setting is not often well equipped for patient education and support. Twenty years ago, in 1993 a survey of members of the National Eczema Society asked what members wanted healthcare professionals to do to improve the control of childhood atopic eczema [4]. The majority wanted more time to be spent explaining the nature of eczema and advice about how to use the treatments prescribed. In 83% of consultations with general practitioners (GPs) and 74% of first consultations with a dermatologist, the expectations of parents/patients had been only partially met or not met at all.

Education of parents and children with atopic eczema is now recognised as one of the most important interventions in the management of atopic eczema [1,5-10]. The largest RCT of an education programme was conducted in Germany, including 823 children or adolescents with atopic eczema and their families [7]. A six-week education programme for the management of moderate to severe atopic eczema was evaluated, with dermatological, nutritional and psychological facets; it was delivered as a two hour, once-weekly session by a multi-professional team. At one year, improvement in the severity of atopic eczema (SCORAD) in children who received the education programme was significantly greater than in the control group. There were also significant improvements in subjective assessments of severity, itching behaviour and emotional coping in the group receiving education compared to control.

A cost-effectiveness analysis was performed using the data from the German trial as part of the NICE guidelines for treatment of atopic eczema [2]. This demonstrated that if an atopic eczema education programme, similar to that detailed in the German RCT could be provided at less than about £800 per child, then it would be highly likely to be cost effective. NICE also concluded that if a less-resource intensive (and less effective) programme could be implemented in the NHS then this was also likely to be cost-effective.

The impact of specialist dermatology nurse-led education has been evaluated in children with mild/moderate atopic eczema [5,6,11]. These studies showed a significant improvement in the control of atopic eczema in children receiving education. For example Cork and colleagues [6] found that 24% of children with atopic eczema were receiving no emollient treatment, with an average use of emollient of just 54 g per week. Dermatology clinic-based specialist nurse-led educational intervention resulted in an 800% increase in the use of emollients with a corresponding 89% reduction in the severity of the atopic eczema. Although much less resource intensive than the German RCT, these studies were in populations of children with less severe, mild/moderate atopic eczema.

There have been no comparisons of different education programmes for atopic eczema in children apart from a recent comparison of face-to-face care and an e-health intervention [12]. Children (with their parents) and adults with moderate severity atopic eczema attended for a first consultation with a dermatologist and specialist dermatology nurse. Subsequently, they were randomised to face-to-face follow-up treatment in the dermatology department or to internet-guided monitoring and on-line self-management training. There were no significant differences in severity of the atopic eczema, quality of life and intensity of itching between the two groups. Compared to routine care, the e-health intervention led to non-significant changes in health and broader societal costs although estimates were imprecise.

Atopic eczema arises as a result of gene-environment interactions leading to a defective skin barrier [13-15]. Thus, emollient creams, ointments and wash products are the first line treatment to repair the skin. In mild atopic eczema, effective management consists of complete emollient therapy plus occasional treatment of flares with mild potency topical corticosteroids [2,16]. Educational interventions for atopic eczema are provided most commonly in the secondary care hospital setting, while the large majority of children have mild atopic eczema and are treated in primary care [17,18]. Guidelines emphasize the importance of using sufficient emollient: 250 to 500 grams per week [2], the more emollient being used the less the need for mild potency topical corticosteroids [5]. However, the actual use of emollients in the UK is far less than this recommended amount.

Rather than designing an intervention that influenced the selection of prescribed products, we designed a study to assess and improve emollient use and outcomes in children who had currently been prescribed a proprietary emollient, E45 Cream (Reckitt Benckiser Healthcare, UK). Using this design, the amount of emollient could be tracked, along with co-treatment over a 3-month period, allowing the support programme to be assessed. The support programme used a multifaceted approach since evidence from a number of fields supports an integrated, supportive approach for patients as more effective than single or simple measures in achieving behavioural change [19-21].

Methods

Objective

To investigate the effectiveness of a multifaceted educational support programme to increase emollient use and reduce atopic eczema symptoms in children.

Design

Using a before and after study design, a purpose-designed multifaceted educational support programme (ESP) was provided for parents or carers of children with atopic eczema. The programme included an educational DVD, easy-to-use diaries to record eczema condition and daily use of emollients, and telephone support line with dermatology nurses provided regular and on-demand phone support. Data were collected in a 2-week baseline period and 12-week follow-up period (3 months in all). Parents and carers were also asked to recall use of health services in the 12 weeks prior to starting the programme.

Study population

Parents of children were identified by the Bounty® Database system operating in the United Kingdom, and sent an email introducing the study. Those interested in participating contacted a free telephone call centre number for further details and to assess eligibility. Parents providing informed consent verbally were provided with a link to the study website and the child's GP was notified of their participation in writing. The study website provided a second confirmatory electronic consent and access to a baseline diary.

Eligible children were male or female aged 3 months to 6 years; with mild to moderate atopic eczema; and, currently using E45 Cream as their primary emollient.

Children were ineligible where there was a planned absence from home for more than 21 days during the study period; where parents were unable to complete the patient diaries or questionnaires; if receiving systemic medication (e.g. Ciclosporin A, methotrexate) or UV light treatment for their atopic eczema in the 3 months preceding the study; if receiving oral steroids or any new atopic eczema-specific treatment regimen in the 4 weeks preceding the study.

In the original design, referral in the preceding 3 months to a Dermatologist, a Specialist Dermatology Nurse or a GP with a Specialist Interest in Dermatology or receiving specific atopic eczema education or training was an exclusion criterion. However it was not possible pragmatically to exclude patients with a prior visit to an eczema specialist and these were subsequently included. The analysis plan was modified prospectively to include these subjects, with the effect of inclusion explored by sensitivity analysis.

Discussion with the National Research Ethics Service (NRES) established that Independent Ethics Committee approval was not required. The study was considered to be non-interventional service evaluation assessing patient support as an aid to ensure use of emollient according to NICE recommendations and thus not requiring regulatory approval. Products prescribed to patients were not influenced by the study, only the frequency of their use.

Multifaceted educational support programme

Parents or carers ('parents') reported baseline data (weeks −2 to 0) on the study website. On completion of the baseline assessment, parents received by mail an introductory support pack designed to educate, motivate and correct the use of emollient therapy, followed by the first of several telephone interviews and counselling sessions by a dermatologist nurse specialist. Depending on the support needs of the family, further telephone support calls were made on demand, along with optional SMS messaging reminding parent or carers of the patient support eczema management regime.

The support pack included an instructional DVD on the use of emollients in eczema management, featuring the lead dermatology nurse; a booklet on eczema management co-written with the National Eczema Society, London; a hooded towel designed for child use after bathing to improve the experience of emollient application, and a set of daily diaries. Each diary covered a 4-week period and the total follow-up period covered was 12 weeks. On completion, diaries were returned to the agency conducting the study (Partizan International, London, UK). Components of the support programme are available online [22].

During the study, prescribing of E45 Cream by the child's GP continued in accordance with routine clinical practice. Parents were encouraged to use E45 Cream by depressing the pump 3 times (approximately 12 g), three times a day, or the equivalent for non-pump packs which is 3 level teaspoons (approximately 12 g), three times a day. If followed, this advice would provide approximately 250 g per week. Parents were advised repeatedly to avoid soap and all harsh detergent-based products, replacing these with emollient wash products.

Outcomes

Baseline and follow-up measures included the following:

Emollient use (grams per week) was estimated in an initial telephone questionnaire based on the emollient pack weight and how long this would usually last. This provided the only estimate of baseline use, in order to avoid the risk of the parent altering their pre-programme practice. Once the support programme had begun, emollient use was captured (as at baseline) at each 4-weekly telephone assessment. Additionally, the number of pumps of emollient used daily was recorded in diaries and the weekly use estimated directly.

Severity of eczema was captured using the POEM (Patient Oriented Eczema Measure) [23]. This recorded the days in a week affected by seven signs of eczema:

dryness, itching, bleeding, weeping, flaking, cracking of skin, and by sleep loss.

Additionally a new simple measure called the Patient Eczema Severity Time (PEST) score was developed for this study, reflecting observations in the clinic that patients' own summative severity perceptions very closely correlated with conventional severity scores. Thus a simple daily score of 'overall unhappiness' with eczema might provide a form of monitoring and feedback to patients and their carers as well as sensitively integrating the sum of eczema experience over time, in a condition with relapsing and remitting severity patterns. The daily diary provided pictorials for users ranging from 'not at all unhappy' to 'extremely unhappy' scoring 1 to 5 respectively. The PEST score was also designed to be easy for parents to assess in patients too young to vocalise this for themselves (see Figure 1).

Healthcare contacts. The number of GP visits by patients in relation to their eczema was recorded; in the 12 weeks prior to and during the 12 weeks of the programme. Eczema-related visits to a dermatology specialist were recorded during the programme period.

Parent measures. The level of control the parent felt in managing the child's eczema was captured by telephone questionnaire at baseline and during the programme phase. It was scored from 1 to 5, with 1 being 'not in control' to 5 'fully in control'.

Concurrent medication. Telephone surveys recorded any concurrent treatments used during baseline and the 12 week follow-up, with particular attention to topical corticosteroid use.

Statistical analysis

There were no reliable estimates for the underuse of emollient and thus potential for improvement in the study population, consequently no formal power calculation was performed. The per-protocol intention was to recruit 150 eligible children age 3 months to 6 years. Given the matched (before-after) data design this would give adequate study power to find small standardized effects in continuous measures (post-hoc: 90% power to detect at effect size of 0.27).

Summary measures were reported for study measures at baseline and in each of the follow-up weeks. Average values were estimated for the 12 week follow-up period to reflect the average effects of the patient support programme and to assess the before-after effect. Changes in paired continuous measures were estimated using the bootstrapping method (with 1,000 replications) to avoid parametric assumptions and changes in paired proportions were evaluated using Fisher's exact test. Patients with complete data at all points contributed to average period values and differences.

Economic analysis

Incremental within-study cost analysis was performed from the NHS perspective using nationally reported unit costs for resource items for 2011. The emollient (E45 Cream POM 500 g) was costed at the average English Prescription Pricing Authority-reimbursed rate of £4.89 [24]; GP visits were costed at £36 per visit [25] [D]. The cost of providing the ESP programme was estimated to be £32 per child based on a resource analysis of providing the service.

Results

Study population

Programme diaries were completed by 136 British children between August 2011 and March 2012. Subjects were evenly split as Caucasian and non-Caucasian and all parents spoke adequate English. One child was excluded as they did not provide any baseline data, leaving 135 children evaluable. Of these, 18 subjects visited an eczema specialist in the three months prior to joining the programme and thus might have already received additional education on eczema management: these were excluded in a sensitivity analysis.

During the baseline period (−2 to 0 week) the average weekly use of emollient was 79 g (range 4 g to 700 g) (see Table 1). Just 4 children (3%) received at least the NICE minimum dose of 250 g and 12.9% received 125 g/wk. The baseline POEM score was 11.3 (SD: 6.3), and PEST score 2.3 (SD 0.8), 40% and 32% of maximum on each respective scale. Children experienced dryness, redness and itching on average 5.7, 4.1 and 4.7 days a week. Sleep disturbance occurred on average 2.4 nights a week with 21% of parents reporting sleep disturbance at least one night in two. Parental sense of feeling in control of eczema scored an average of 3.3 where 22% of parents reported low levels of control (scoring 1 or 2).

Figure 1 Patient Eczema Severity-Time Score (PEST) graphic.

Table 1 Changes in emollient use and measures of eczema severity

	Baseline[1]			1-4 weeks			5-8 weeks			9-12 weeks			Mean change[2]			
	Mean	(SD)	N	Mean	(SD)	N	Mean	(SD)	N	Mean	(SD)	N	Mean	95% CI[3]	*N*	p[3]
Emollient Use (g/wk)[4]																
Daily diary	-			165.2	(95.4)	135	168.4	(113.2)	135	167.8	(109.5)	135	87.6	(81.9 to 119.5)	132	0.001
Time to use	79.2	(79.2)	132	173.5	(114.3)	122	195.2	(112.1)	128	197.4	(106.5)	129	110.0	(94.6 to 131.3)	115	0.001
Severity Scores																
POEM[5]	11.34	(6.27)	135	7.52	(5.71)	135	5.50	(5.05)	135	4.85	(5.04)	135	−5.38	(−6.41 to −4.36)	135	0.001
PEST[6]	2.26	(0.81)	135	1.82	(0.73)	135	1.59	(0.78)	135	1.53	(0.68)	135	−0.61	(−0.75 to −0.47)	135	0.001
Individual Scores																
Dryness [A] [7]	5.66	(1.97)	135	4.09	(2.38)	135	3.22	(2.45)	135	2.86	(2.39)	135	−2.28	(−2.67 to −1.90)	135	0.001
Redness [B] [7]	4.12	(2.44)	135	2.74	(2.42)	135	1.95	(2.18)	135	1.82	(2.13)	135	−1.95	(−2.37 to −1.53)	135	0.001
Itchiness [C] [7]	4.73	(2.54)	135	3.38	(2.56)	135	2.63	(2.67)	135	2.37	(2.53)	135	−1.94	(−2.36 to −1.52)	135	0.001
[A] + [B] + [C]	14.51	(5.64)	135	10.21	(6.35)	135	7.79	(6.24)	135	7.04	(6.24)	135	−6.17	(−7.17 to −5.20)	135	0.001
Sleep disturbance [7]	2.36	(2.44)	135	1.49	(2.12)	135	0.98	(1.62)	135	0.80	(1.59)	135	−1.27	(−1.68 to −0.85)	135	0.001
Bleeding[7]	1.34	(1.99)	135	0.68	(1.35)	135	0.42	(1.05)	135	0.33	(1.03)	135	−0.86	(−1.18 to −0.56)	135	0.001
Weeping or oozing[7]	0.86	(1.74)	135	0.40	(1.15)	135	0.24	(0.87)	135	0.18	(0.76)	135	−0.59	(−0.87 to −0.35)	135	0.001
Cracking[7]	2.44	(2.50)	135	1.41	(1.90)	135	1.02	(1.79)	135	0.89	(1.81)	135	−1.34	(−1.77 to −0.97)	135	0.001
Flaking[7]	2.26	(2.63)	135	1.37	(1.96)	135	0.80	(1.47)	135	0.76	(1.57)	135	−1.28	(−1.69 to −0.85)	135	0.001
Roughness[7]	5.49	(2.07)	135	4.25	(2.40)	135	3.32	(2.54)	135	3.56	(2.10)	135	−1.93	(−2.33 to −1.55)	135	0.001
Severity[7]	4.65	(5.16)	135	2.49	(3.86)	135	1.68	(3.17)	135	1.39	(3.02)	135	−2.80	(−3.63 to −2.03)	135	0.001
Other																
Parental Control[8]	3.30	(0.99)	135	4.43	(0.66)	134	4.61	(0.57)	135	4.81	(0.41)	135	1.32	(1.16 to 1.48)	134	0.001
GP Visits[1]	1.90	(2.13)	135	0.46	(0.54)	135	0.25	(0.44)	135	0.13	(0.36)	135	−1.06	(−1.49 to −0.70)	135	0.002
Steroid Prescribed (%)[9]	51/135	(37.8%)		73/135	(54.1%)		82/135	(60.7%)		82/135	(60.7)%		20.8%	(8.9% to 32.1%)	135	0.001

[1] Weeks −2 to 0, except GP visits which included the previous 12 weeks to week 0.
[2] The mean change is the average of the programme period scores minus the baseline period score in subjects with complete data.
[3] Estimated by bootstrapping with 1,000 replications.
[4] Emollient use was estimated using two methods: the time to use a reported weight of emollient (500 g); and, a daily diary record of counts of pumps of emollient used by weight; – the latter method was not available for the baseline period.
[5] POEM score from 0 to 28, including seven signs of eczema at four levels of frequency in the past week at the end of each period.
[6] PEST score, the child's unhappiness with eczema: score 1 (not at all) to 5 (very unhappy), daily diary score averaged over each period.
[7] Number of days in the previous week has the child had this sign of eczema: score 0 to 7 days, at the end of each period.
[8] Parental confidence in managing the child's eczema: score 1 (not being in control) to 5 (being totally in control), at the end of each period.
[9] Proportion of children prescribed topical corticosteroids during each period.

Clinical outcomes

Change in emollient use

Diary recorded emollient cream use increased significantly during the 12 weeks of the programme (see Figure 2 and Table 1). On average emollient use increased by 87.6 g (95% CI: 81.9 to 119.5, p = 0.001) with the change being immediate and persistent with 8.9% of children receiving 250 g/wk at 12 weeks and 61.5% receiving 125 g/wk.

Emollient use was also estimated, as at baseline, as the time taken in each period to use a prescribed emollient cream pack of known weight. The estimated increase in emollient was higher at 110 g/wk (95% CI: 94.6 to 131.3, p = 0.001) although only 85% of parents reported this measure.

From a baseline of 37.8% of patients, prescription of topical corticosteroids increased significantly by 20.8% (95% CI: 8.9% to 32.1%, p = 0.001) during the programme. The volume of use of steroid was not recorded but hydrocortisone 1% accounted for 70% of total use and clobetasone butyrate 0.05% (in various preparations) for 25%. Although topical steroids were prescribed, parents reported that they used these in minimal quantities due to concerns about side effects. An increase in topical steroid use was not planned as part of the educational support provided, but often arose in telephone support sessions.

Changes in measures of eczema severity

Eczema severity reduced significantly during the 12 weeks of the programme. The POEM score reduced on average by 5.38 (95% CI: 4.36 to 6.41, p = 0.001), a 47% reduction from the baseline score (see Figure 3 and Table 1). Individual signs of eczema consistently followed the pattern of improvement seen in the aggregated POEM score (see Table 1).

Similarly the PEST score reduced on average by 0.61 (95% CI: 0.47 to 0.75, p = 0.001), a 48% reduction from the baseline score (see Figure 4 and Table 1). During the programme, 45.9% of children were reported as having an average POEM score of 0 to 2 compared to 4.4% at baseline; similarly 56.3% of children were reported with a PEST score of 1 compared to 13.3% at baseline. POEM and PEST scores were strongly correlated with Pearson correlation coefficients at baseline, 4, 8, and 12 weeks of 0.56, 0.51, 0.63 and 0.71 (P < 0.01 in all instances).

Of particular note are two measures which may have broader implications for the families of children suffering with eczema. Loss of sleep if persistent may have significant knock-on consequences for the health and well-being of family members. On average, the number of nights per week experiencing sleep disturbance was reduced during the 12 week programme by 1.27 nights (95% CI: 0.85 to 1.68, p = 0.001), a halving of the

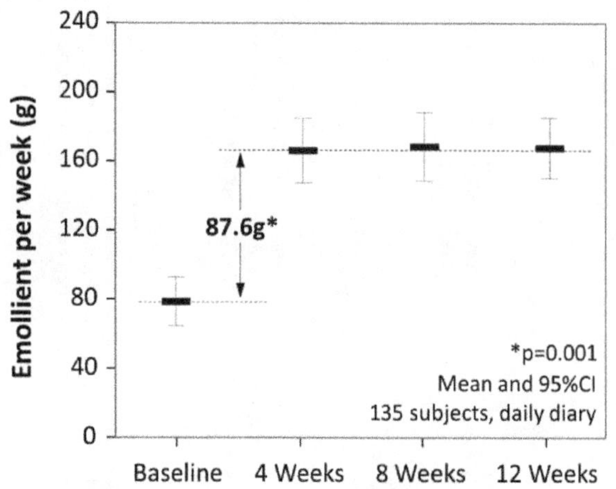

Figure 2 Emollient use before and during the intervention (Means and 95% confidence intervals shown).

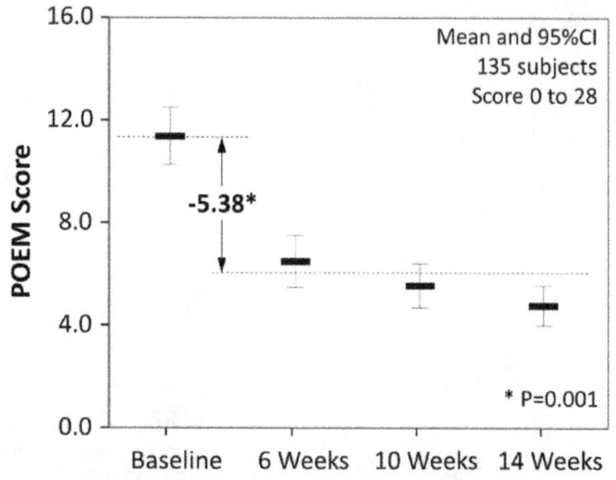

Figure 3 Patient-Orientated Eczema Measure (POEM) before and during the intervention (means and 95% confidence intervals shown).

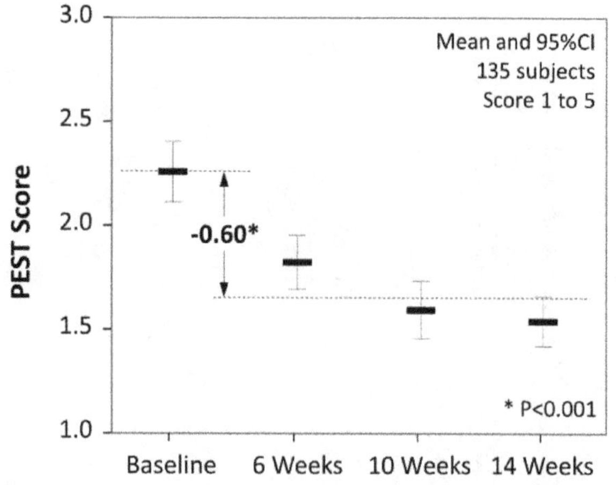

Figure 4 Patient Ezcema Severity-Time Score (PEST) before and during the intervention (means and 95% confidence intervals shown).

baseline level of disturbance. Secondly, parental feeling of control of their child's eczema improved by 1.32 points (95% CI: 1.16 to 1.48, p = 0.001) with 91.5% of parents reporting the highest level of control.

Health economic outcomes

Costs of care in the periods preceding and during the patient support programme are tabulated in Table 2. There was a statistically significant increase in the cost of emollient by about £10 using the diary method, or about £13 using the 'time-in-use' method. GP visits fell on average by about 1 visit per child (Table 1) leading to no overall or significant change in net cost. The finding was similar regardless of the method of estimating emollient use.

Sensitivity analysis

Analyses were repeated in 117 subjects, excluding 18 subjects who had visited an eczema specialist in the three months prior to joining the programme. Qualitatively, findings were unchanged in this subgroup (Table 3).

Discussion

Given the considerable underutilisation of emollients for atopic eczema in children, effective training for parents in the use of topical therapy is a key issue. Our experience within the dermatology clinic has underlined the importance of a comprehensive approach to support and education, including printed, verbal and visual components to achieve the broadest effect [6]. The study findings demonstrate the potential utility of providing a patient-centric support package to enhance concordance with treatment goals and improve patient outcomes.

Primary care practitioners are sometimes concerned about the practicality of delivering multifaceted interventions in routine care. The current study demonstrates that a coherent multifaceted programme, delivered at a distance using a specialist dermatology nurse, may be a cost-neutral use of NHS resources. Primary care commissioners might consider an appropriate local adaptation of the ESP to address patients' needs, while accepting the need not to subtract from the components, which may work synergistically. Details of the ESP are available online to assist those developing services [22]. Education regarding the use of topical products including emollients is an essential part of the management of many other skin diseases such as psoriasis [26]. Similar ESPs to that evaluated in this study for atopic eczema could enhance adherence with topical treatment regimens and improve outcomes in these skin diseases.

Topical steroid prescriptions increased during the study, although it is unlikely that steroid use profoundly affected the study findings. In common with our clinical experience, parents in the study reported using steroids minimally and change in availability only occurred in 20% of patients. However, volume of use of prescriptions was not measured formally.

Two measures within the study captured aspects of the impact of childhood eczema on the broader family. Increased emollient use was significantly related to reduced sleep disturbance and greater sense of parental control through a greater understanding of the disease and their child's symptoms. Parents expressed frustration at the inconsistency of information and advice provided in primary care about eczema and its management. A qualitative analysis of patient narratives will be published separately.

Within the duration of the programme the overall cost was cost-neutral while providing tangible health benefits to children and their families. It is likely that cost savings would continue to accrue beyond the duration of the study hence the within-programme analyses presented should be viewed as conservative. If savings are

Table 2 Costs of care in the baseline and programme periods

	Pre-Programme[1]		Programme[2]		Change[3,4]			
	Mean	(SD)	Mean	(SD)	Mean	95% CI[4]	N	p
Cost (£, 2011)								
Programme			32.00	-	32.00	-	-	-
Emollient [A]	9.29	(9.30)	19.57	(12.03)	10.28	(7.93 to 12.64)	132	0.001
Emollient [B]	9.72	(9.69)	22.64	(12.21)	12.91	(10.72 to 15.10)	115	0.001
GP visits	68.53	(76.70)	30.40	(31.67)	−38.13	(−52.58 to −23.68)	135	0.001
Overall cost [A]	78.29	(79.34)	82.66	(34.16)	4.37	(−10.55 to 19.30)	132	0.62
Overall cost [B]	80.32	(82.48)	84.37	(31.29)	4.06	(−12.00 to 20.11)	115	0.56

[1] Estimated for the 12 weeks preceding intervention, using 2 week baseline data and 12 week recall (GP visits).
[2] Twelve weeks while receiving the patient support programme.
[3] Difference in costs in the two periods (negative denotes a reduction).
[4] Estimated by bootstrapping with 1,000 replications.
A Emollient use costed using the daily diary method.
B Emollient use costed using the estimated time taken to use a 500 g pot of emollient.

Table 3 Sensitivity analysis: excluding children who had recently seen a specialist

	Pre-Programme[1]		Programme[2]		Change[3,4]			
	Mean	(SD)	Mean	(SD)	Mean	95% CI[4]	N	p[4]
Emollient Use (g/wk)								
Daily diary	69.7	(49.5)	170.3	(99.0)	100.6	(81.9 to 119.5)	114	0.001
Time to use	72.2	(49.6)	184.3	(97.6)	112.2	(94.6 to 131.3)	99	0.001
Severity Scores								
POEM	11.03	(6.49)	5.83	(4.67)	−5.20	(−6.39 to −4.34)	117	0.001
PEST	2.26	(0.82)	1.66	(0.62)	−0.60	(−0.74 to −0.47)	117	0.001
Cost (£, 2011)								
Programme			32.00	-	32.00	-	-	-
Emollient [A]	8.18	(5.80)	19.98	(11.61)	11.81	(9.81 to 14.01)	114	0.001
Emollient [B]	8.47	(5.82)	21.63	(11.46)	13.16	(10.94 to 15.39)	99	0.001
GP visits	63.23	(63.80)	30.46	(30.86)	−32.77	(−45.77 to −19.77)	117	0.001
Overall cost [A]	71.81	(66.37)	83.25	(33.75)	11.44	(−1.99 to 24.86)	114	0.123
Overall cost [B]	72.11	(68.24)	83.45	(33.75)	11.35	(−3.14 to 25.83)	99	0.239

[1] Estimated for the 12 weeks preceding intervention, using 2 week baseline data and 12 week recall (GP visits).
[2] Twelve weeks while receiving the patient support programme.
[3] Difference in costs in the two periods (negative denotes a reduction).
[4] Estimated by bootstrapping with 1,000 replications.
A Emollient use costed using the daily diary method.
B Emollient use costed using the estimated time taken to use a 500 g pot of emollient.

extrapolated then, under a range of assumptions, the ESP is likely be both cost saving and symptom-reducing in children with mild to moderate atopic eczema.

Limitations

While introduction of the ESP provided a strong contemporaneous improvement in emollient treatment and subsequent atopic eczema symptoms, the study design lacked the protection against bias afforded by a randomised controlled design. The major threat to attribution is regression to the mean where a concerned subgroup of parents enrol children with naturally recurring and remitting eczema at a point of acute symptoms, which tend naturally to lessen. A control group selected by randomisation would separate out programme and regression effects. However the changes in emollient use and in measures of eczema severity are dramatic, consistent and contemporaneous with the programme and are thus likely to preclude a pure regression effect. A further threat lies in the generalizability of findings if a highly selected population with atypical characteristics (in the parent or child) have volunteered to participate in the study, although this is mitigated by the broad inclusion by ethnicity and socioeconomic group. Finally, parents were asked to recall visits to primary care and specialists in the 12 weeks preceding baseline, a long period of recall potentially introducing recall bias.

Conclusions

The educational support programme (ESP) provided coherent messaging and support to parents and their children with atopic eczema. During the 12 week course of the programme there was a dramatic and significant increase in emollient use and also a small associated increase in mild potency steroid use. The ESP dramatically reduced signs of eczema, sleep disturbance and parental feelings of lack of control. Analysis at 12 weeks provides evidence that the ESP is a cost-neutral strategy although this will be further explored at 12 months. A new, simple measure of eczema severity (PEST score) designed to help parents and children to monitor and manage eczema showed similar sensitivity and high correlation with the POEM [23] measure, and thus merits further evaluation.

Competing interests

The research was funded by an educational grant to participating academic and NHS institutions from Reckitt Benkiser Healthcare. Partizan International is an agency specialising in patient support programmes.

JM Mason received institutional funding from Reckitt Benckiser Healthcare UK to support his participation in the study and attendance at BAD, Birmingham 2012.

MJ Cork has acted as a consultant and has given lectures for Reckitt Benckiser Healthcare UK.

C Buckley, S Hewitt and P Berry are employees of Reckitt Benkiser Healthcare UK, which makes and distributes the emollient product provided to patients in this study.

Authors' contributions

JMM provided methodological, statistical and economic oversight to the study. He led the analyses and writing of the paper. MJC provided study concept, design, clinical and methodological oversight. He participated in the analysis and writing and interpretation of the findings. CB, SH and PB are employees of RB Healthcare UK. All contributed to the study design, writing and interpretation of the findings. JT led the service conducting telephone interviews. He contributed to the study design, writing and interpretation of the findings. All authors read and approved the final manuscript.

Authors' information

Professor Michael Cork is Head of Academic Dermatology Research in the Department of Infection & Immunity at The University of Sheffield Medical School and Honorary Consultant Dermatologist to both Sheffield Children's and Teaching Hospitals. He has published extensively in basic and applied science with particular research interests in atopic dermatitis (atopic eczema), psoriasis, alopecia areata and vitiligo. Internationally, his unit is one of the leading groups translating basic dermatological science into new treatments, including 'Skin Protease Inhibitors' and 'Vitamin A Metabolic Pathway Inhibitors.

Professor James Mason is a health economist for Durham University who has published extensively using health economics, health service research and statistical methodologies. He is health economist for a number of ongoing and published dermatological trials. He is Director of Durham Clinical Trials Unit and co-Director of the Research Design Service for the North East.

Acknowledgements

The study team gratefully acknowledge Nora Tebbutt MBE (telephone and organisational support) and Chris Longton (telephone support) for their contribution to the study. The team also gratefully acknowledge preliminary analyses provided by the Robertson Centre for Biostatistics, University of Glasgow, UK. The emollient used in this study was E45 Cream, manufactured by Reckitt Benckiser Healthcare Ltd.

Author details

[1]School of Medicine, Pharmacy & Health, Durham University, Durham, UK. [2]Sheffield Children's NHS Foundation Trust, Sheffield, UK. [3]Reckitt Benckiser Healthcare UK, Slough, UK. [4]Partizan International, London, UK. [5]Academic Unit of Dermatology Research, School of Medicine & Biomedical Sciences, University of Sheffield, Sheffield, UK. [6]Department of Dermatology, Sheffield Teaching Hospitals NHS Foundation Trust, Sheffield, UK. [7]Department of Infection and Immunity, The University of Sheffield Medical School, Beech Hill Road, Sheffield S10 2RX, UK.

References

1. Carroll CL, Balkrishnan R, Feldman SR, Fleischer AB Jr, Manuel JC: **The burden of atopic dermatitis: impact on the patient, family, and society.** *J Invest Dermatol* 2005, **22**:192–199.
2. National Institute for Health and Clinical Excellence: *Management of atopic eczema in children from birth up to the age of 12 years. December 2007.* http://guidance.nice.org.uk/CG57/Guidance/pdf/English (last accessed 25/04/13).
3. Kawakami T, Soma Y: **Questionnaire survey of the efficacy of emollients for adult patients with atopic dermatitis.** *J Dermatol* 2011, **38**:531–535.
4. Long CC, Funnell CM, Collard R, Finlay AY: **What do members of the national Eczema society really want?** *Clin Exp Dermatol* 1993, **18**:516–522.
5. Broberg A, Kalimo K, Lindblad B, Swanbeck G: **Parental education in the treatment of childhood atopic eczema.** *Acta Derm Venereol* 1990, **70**:495–499.
6. Cork MJ, Britton J, Butler L, Young S, Murphy R, Keohane SG: **Comparison of parent knowledge, therapy utilization and severity of atopic eczema before and after explanation and demonstration of topical therapies by a specialist dermatology nurse.** *Br J Dermatol* 2003, **149**:582–589.
7. Staab D, Diepgen TL, Fartasch M, Kupfer J, Lob-Corzilius T, Ring J, Scheewe S, Scheidt R, Schmid-Ott G, Schnopp C, Szczepanski R, Werfel T, Wittenmeier M, Wahn U, Gieler U: **Age related, structured educational programmes for the management of atopic dermatitis in children and adolescents: multicentre, randomised controlled trial.** *BMJ* 2006, **332**:933–938.
8. Lawton S: **Practical issues for emollient therapy in dry and itchy skin.** *Br J Nurs* 2009, **18**:978–984.
9. Hanifin JM, Tofte SJ: **Patient education in the long-term management of atopic dermatitis.** *Dermatol Nurs* 1999, **11**:284–289.
10. Coenraads PJ, Span L, Jaspers JP, Fidler V: **Intensive patient education and treatment program for young adults with atopic eczema.** *Hautarzt* 2001, **52**:428–433.
11. Grillo M, Gassner L, Marshman G, Dunn S, Hudson P: **Pediatric atopic eczema: the impact of an educational intervention.** *Pediatr Dermatol* 2006, **23**:428–436.
12. van Os-Medendorp H, Koffijberg H, Eland-de Kok PC, van der Zalm A, de Bruin-Weller MS, Pasmans SG, Ros WJ, Thio HB, Knol MJ, Bruijnzeel-Koomen CA: **E-health in caring for patients with atopic dermatitis: a randomized controlled cost-effectiveness study of internet-guided monitoring and online self-management training.** *Br J Dermatol* 2012, **166**:1060–1068.
13. Palmer CN, Irvine AD, Terron-Kwiatkowski A, Zhao Y, Liao H, *et al*: **Common loss-of-function variants of the epidermal barrier protein filaggrin are a major predisposing factor for atopic dermatitis.** *Nat Genet* 2006, **38**:441–446.
14. Cork MJ, Danby SG, Vasilopoulos Y, Hadgraft J, Lane ME, Moustafa M, Guy RH, Macgowan AL, Tazi-Ahnini R, Ward SJ: **Epidermal barrier dysfunction in atopic dermatitis.** *J Invest Dermatol* 2009, **129**:1892–1908.
15. Danby SG, Cork MJ: **The skin barrier in atopic dermatitis.** In *Ch 27 in Harper's Textbook of Pediatric Dermatology.* 3rd edition. Edited by Irvine AD, Hoeger PH, Yan AC. U.K: Blackwell Publishing Ltd; 2011.
16. Cork MJ: **The importance of skin barrier function.** *J Derm Treat* 1997, **8**:S7–S13.
17. Hoare C, Li Wan Po A, Williams H: **Systematic review of treatments for atopic eczema.** *Health Technol Assess* 2000, **4**:1–191.
18. Williams HC: **Epidemiology of atopic dermatitis.** *Clin Exp Dermatol* 2000, **25**:522–529.
19. Gruen RL, Weeramanthri TS, Knight SSE, Bailie RS: **Specialist outreach clinics in primary care and rural hospital settings.** *Cochrane Database System Rev* 2004, **Art. No**(1):CD003798. doi:10.1002/14651858.CD003798.pub2.
20. Kendrick D, Barlow J, Hampshire A, Polnay L, Stewart-Brown S: **Parenting interventions for the prevention of unintentional injuries in childhood.** *Cochrane Database System Rev* 2007, **Art. No**(4):CD006020. doi:10.1002/14651858.CD006020.pub2.
21. Maas T, Kaper J, Sheikh A, Knottnerus JA, Wesseling G, Dompeling E, Muris JWM, van Schayck CP: **Mono and multifaceted inhalant and/or food allergen reduction interventions for preventing asthma in children at high risk of developing asthma.** *Cochrane Database System Rev* 2009, **Art. No**(3):CD006480. doi:10.1002/14651858.CD006480.pub2.
22. Components of the patient support programme used in this study are available at www.eczemaadvice.co.uk (last accessed 25/04/13).
23. Charman CR, Venn AJ, Williams HC: **The patient-oriented eczema measure: development and initial validation of a new tool for measuring atopic eczema severity from the patients' perspective.** *Arch Dermatol* 2004, **140**:1513–1519. Erratum in: Arch Dermatol 2005;141:381.
24. HM Government: Data.gov.uk. Prescription Cost Analysis: England 2011. http://data.gov.uk/dataset/prescription-cost-analysis-england (last-accessed 25-4-13).
25. Curtis L: *The unit costs of health and social care 2011.* France: University of Kent, PSSRU; 2011. http://www.pssru.ac.uk/archive/pdf/uc/uc2011/uc2011.pdf (last-accessed 25-4-13).
26. Pouplard C, Gourraud PA, Meyer N, Livideanu CB, Lahfa M, Mazereeuw-Hautier J, Le Jeunne P, Sabatini AL, Paul C: **Are we giving patients enough information on how to use topical treatments? Analysis of 767 prescriptions in psoriasis.** *Br J Dermatol* 2011, **165**:1332–1336.

4

Exploring patterns of recurrent melanoma in Northeast Scotland to inform the introduction a digital self-examination intervention

Rhona Auckland[1], Patrick Wassell[2], Susan Hall[3*], Marianne C Nicolson[4] and Peter Murchie[3]

Abstract

Background: Melanoma incidence is growing and more people require follow-up to detect recurrent melanoma quickly. Those detecting their own recurrent melanoma appear to have the best prognosis, so total skin self examination (TSSE) is advocated, but practice is suboptimal. A digital intervention to support TSSE has potential but it is not clear which patient groups could benefit most. The aim of this study was to explore cutaneous melanoma recurrence patterns between 1991 and 2012 in Northeast Scotland. The objectives were to: determine how recurrent melanomas were detected during the period; explore factors potentially predictive of mode of recurrence detection; identify groups least likely to detect their own recurrent melanoma and with most potential to benefit from digital TSSE support.

Methods: Pathology records were used to identify those with a potential recurrent melanoma of any type (local, regional and distant). Following screening of potential cases available secondary care-held records were subsequently scrutinised. Data was collected on demographics and clinical characteristics of the initial and recurrent melanoma. Data were handled in Microsoft Excel and transported into SPSS 20.0 for statistical analysis. Factors predicting detection at interval or scheduled follow-up were explored using univariate techniques, with potentially influential factors combined in a multivariate binary logistic model to adjust for confounding.

Results: 149 potential recurrences were identified from the pathology database held at Aberdeen Royal Infirmary. Reliable data could be obtained on 94 cases of recurrent melanoma of all types. 30 recurrences (31.9%) were found by doctors at follow-up, and 64 (68.1%) in the interval between visits, usually by the patient themselves. Melanoma recurrences of all types occurring within one-year were significantly more likely to be found at follow-up visits, and this remained so following adjustment for other factors that could be used to target digital TSSE support.

Conclusions: A digital intervention should be offered to all newly diagnosed patients. This group could benefit most from optimal TSSE practice.

Keywords: Melanoma recurrence, Self-detected, Follow-up, Skin self-examination, Education

Background

Melanoma incidence has risen over the last 50 years, and disproportionately affects younger people [1]. Around three times as many cases were reported in 2000 than in 1970 and it is now the sixth commonest cancer in the UK [2,3]. Scottish guidelines recommend that people treated for cutaneous melanoma receive stuctured follow-up consisting of regular physical examination by a specialist without blood tests or imaging unless subsequently indicated [4]. Follow-up aims to detect melanoma recurrences early and expedite secondary care access if necessary and its delivery is becoming increasingly burdensome to healthcare systems [5-7]. Many recurrences are detected in the interval between structured follow-up visits leading many to question it value [8,9]. On the other hand there is evidence that most early recurrences (within two years) are not self-detected but found at scheduled follow-up appointments [8,10-13]. This is important since there is evidence of superior

* Correspondence: s.hall@abdn.ac.uk
[3]Centre of Academic Primary Care – Division of Applied Health Sciences, University of Aberdeen, Polwarth Building, Foresterhill, Aberdeen AB25 2ZD, UK
Full list of author information is available at the end of the article

Table 1 Melanoma recurrence data sheet

Surname:	DOB:	
Forename(s):	Gender:	
CHI:		
Occupation:	Ethnicity:	
Date of primary melanoma diagnosis:		
Melanoma type:		
Stage of melanoma:		
Tumour thickness (mm):	Breslow depth;	
	Clark level;	
Prognostic features:	Ulceration;	
	Lymph node involvement;	
	Tumour vascularity;	
	lymphovascular invasion;	
	Mitotic rate;	
	Regression;	
	Microsatellites;	
	Tumour-infiltrating lymphocytes;	
	Lactate dehydrogenase serum level;	
Tumour anatomical location:		
Method/Details of treatment:		
Details on how the melanoma was picked up:		
Date of excision biopsies:	Primary biopsy;	
	Secondary biopsy;	
	Punch/Shave biopsy;	
Details of prescribed follow-up program:		
Date of recurrence diagnosis:		
Nature of recurrence: local, regional, distant)		
Melanoma type:		
Melanoma stage:		
Tumour thickness:	Breslow depth;	
	Clark level;	
Prognostic features:		
Tumour anatomical location:		
How was the recurrence detected:		Please Tick
	Self – detected	
	GP	
	Dermatologist	
	Follow-up appointment	
	Other	
If other, please state:		
If self- detected, which of the following apply:		Please Tick:
Recurrence found via;	Routine self-examination	
	Accidental find	
	Aid of partner/Acquaintance	

Table 1 Melanoma recurrence data sheet *(Continued)*

	Experience of related symptoms (e.g. nausea, fatigue, weight loss, pain, shortness of breath etc.)
Route from self-detection to official diagnosis: (e.g. Patient – GP – Hospital)	
Dates of above referrals: (e.g. GP referral, treatment dates etc.)	

survival rates of those who self-detected their recurrence appear to have superior survival, corresponding with with findings that regular total skin self examinations (TSSE) in people treated for primary cutaneous melanoma can reduce mortality rates by as much as 63% [13,14].

Despite this TSSE education and practice appear suboptimal with 70% of American melanoma patients indicating that they had never been advised to do it [15]. There is good reason to suggest that similar statistics would be found in North East Scotland (NES). Where interventions to improve TSSE have been tried, results have been disappointing and those who were educated by brochure or video demonstrations only reported increased TSSE practice for 3–7 months, with overall participation returning to the baseline by 12 months [16-18]. Despite this it is encouraging that educational interventions could achieve 17-50% increases in TSSE practice, albeit in the short-term. Further, stabilisation of mortality in younger patients (aged 25–44), despite increasing incidence, is thought to result from increased public awareness and TSSE promotion [1,16,19,20]. Similarly higher survival and higher TSSE rates are observed in less deprived people [15]. All this supports the view that TSSE is worth doing. Some suggest that digital interventions could promote and sustain TSSE practice [18-20]. Such interventions however, are likely to be expensive to develop and implement so should be targeted at those with the greatest potential to benefit, information which the current studies do not provide.

We are developing a digital intervention to promote and prompt TSSE in Northeast Scotland. We wished to explore patterns of all types of melanoma recurrence within the region over recent years to determine when, and to which patients, this intervention should be targeted.

Methods

Study approval

Formal approval for this study was granted on 10th October 2012 by the Quality, Governance and Risk Unit (Clinical Effectiveness Team) of NHS Grampian (project ID 2483).

Identifying recurrences

A data-base maintained by the Department of Pathology, NHS Grampian was scrutinised to identify melanoma patients from Northeast Scotland potentially diagnosed with any type of recurrence between August 1992 and September 2012.

Data collection

A data collection sheet was constructed (Table 1) and used to abstract data from the secondary care-held medical records of eligible and available cases at the medical records department at Aberdeen Royal Infirmary.

The following data were abstracted (Table 2):

i) Demographics: gender; date of birth; age at diagnosis; age at recurrence; postcode. Postcode was subsequently use to define deprivation and rurality [21,22].
ii) Clinical details of the initial melanoma including: melanoma type; Breslow thickness; anatomical location.
iii) Type of recurrence: local; regional; distant.
iv) Recurrence pathway: time to recurrence; mode of detection (self detected and reported during interval; found at follow-up clinic by clinician; emergency admission during interval; other).

Data were entered handled using a Microsoft Excel worksheet. After scrutiny for errors they were read into SPSS version 20 for further statistical analysis.

Statistical analysis

Demographic and clinical characteristics

Basic descriptive statistics of the sample were prepared. Demographics characteristics, clinical characteristics of the primary melanoma and details of the recurrence and its detection pathway were explored.

Categorising variables

To conduct meaningful univariate analysis on this relatively small sample was challenging. A number of categorical variables were created from the data to address this. After discussion amongst the authors a binary outcome variable was created distinguishing those patients who had their recurrent melanoma detected de-novo at the follow-up clinic versus those in whom the presentation of recurrence had occurred in the interval between scheduled follow-up visits. Arguably, the former group are those who stand most to gain from interventions to promote total skin self examination.

Table 2 Clinicopathological Characteristics; descriptive statistics in relation to frequency within sample of 94 patients

	Frequency:
Demographics:	
Gender;	
Female	37 (39.4%)
Male	57 (60.6%)
Deprivation score;	
1(most deprived)	5 (5.3%)
2	9 (9.6%)
3	22 (23.4%)
4	27 (28.7%)
5(least deprived)	31 (33.0%)
Six-fold rurality score;	
Urban	43 (45.6%)
Rural	51 (54.4%)
Type of recurrence	
Local	21 (22.3%)
Regional	48 (51.1%)
Distant	25 (26.6%)
Details of first primary:	
Age at diagnosis;	
<=50 years	19 (20.2%)
51-70 years	41 (43.6%)
71+ years	33 (35.1%)
Unknown	1 (1.1%)
Melanoma type of first primary;	
Superficial spreading	27 (28.7%)
Nodular malignant	30 (31.9%)
Lentigo maligna	5 (5.3%)
Acral lentiginous	5 (5.3%)
Other	27 (28.7%)
Location of first primary;	
Lower limbs	35 (37.2%)
Trunk	20 (21.3%)
Upper limbs	9 (9.6%)
Head and neck	22 (23.4%)
Mucus membranes	4 (4.3%)
Eye	4 (4.3%)
Breslow thickness of first primary;	
<0.75 mm	1 (1.1%)
0.76-4.00 mm	18 (19.1%)
>4.00 mm	36 (38.3%)
Unknown	27 (28.7%)
	12 (12.8%)
Details of recurrence:	
Age at recurrence;	
<=50 years	14 (14.9%)
51-70 years	40 (42.6%)
71+ years	40 (42.6%)
Time to recurrence;	
0-12 months	27 (28.7%)
13-24 months	28 (29.8%)
25-36	11 (11.7%)
37-48	5 (5.3%)
49-60	7 (7.4%)
5+ years	15 (16.0%)
Unknown	1 (1.1%)
How recurrence was detected;	
Self-detected and reported during interval	45 (48.9%)
New finding at follow-up clinical	30 (31.9%)
Emergency admission with symptoms in interval	11 (11.7%)
Other	5 (5.3%)

Seven predictor variables were then created. These were selected on the basis that there was evidence for, or it seemed plausible that, they could be influential on whether recurrent melanoma was detected at scheduled follow-up or during the interval between scheduled follow-up appointments. Candidates were classified by gender, 5-fold deprivation score and 2-fold rurality score. With reference to recurrent melanoma, variables including age (<65 versus >65 years) time to recurrence (< 1 year versus ≥ 1 year) were considered and details of the initial melanoma (subtype, Breslow thickness (<4 mm; ≥4 mm)) [8].

Univariate analysis

The outcome variable (detected at scheduled follow-up or not) was cross-tabulated with each of the six predictor variables. The chi-squared test was used to ascertain if the six factors were significantly associated with follow-up versus interval detection, with statistical significance being designated as a $p \leq 0.05$. The strength of the relationship between the outcome and each of the six predictor variables was also explored univariately using binary logistic regression to generate odds ratios and 95% CIs.

Multivariate analysis

A multivariate binary logistic regression model was then constructed including all factors found to be significantly predictive of follow-up versus interval recurrence detection, as well as those factors that could conceivably inform targeting of a digital intervention to support

TSSE (Breslow thickness; time to recurrence; age at recurrence; rurality; deprivation score).

Results

Included and excluded cases

149 potential cases of any type of recurrent melanoma were identified (Figure 1). Eighteen people had died and notes were not available and four sets of notes could not be located. Thirty-one people had recurrent melanoma with no record of a prior primary. Two further apparent recurrences proved to be new basal cell carcinomas on review of pathology data. This resulted in 55 exclusions and a final sample of 94 cases for analysis.

Demographic and clinical characteristics

Demographics and characteristics of primary melanomas are shown in Table 2. The sample included 21 (22.3%) local, 48 (51.1%) regional and 25 (26.6%) distant recurrences. Mean age at the time of recurrence was 65 years. Forty-five recurrences (58.5%) had presented within two years of diagnosis. Thirty (31.9%) cases were detected at scheduled melanoma follow-up appointments. The remaining 64 (69.1%) were detected as interval events with 45 (48.9%) being obviously self detected, 11 (11.7%) being emergency admissions to hospital with metastatic disease and five (5.3%) being detected through another route, mostly incidental findings.

Univariate analysis

Those variables deemed most likely to affect whether a recurrence was found at follow-up or self detected in the interval were explored univariately with the chi-squared test (Table 3). The most striking finding was earlier recurrences were significantly more to be detected at structured follow-up. Of recurrences within a year of diagnosis 51.9% were detected at follow-up, while only 23.9% of later recurrences were detected at follow-up. No other potential predictors of recurrence detection location were significant univariately.

Logistic regression

A binary logistic regression of mode of recurrence detection (at follow-up versus interval) was conducted (Table 4). Those who had a recurrence within one year were 3.433 (95% CIs 1.340-8.796) times more likely to be detected at structured follow up than in the interval. Following adjustment for other potential explanatory variables time to recurrence remained the only potentially explanatory variable significantly associated with mode of recurrence detection (OR2.891 (95% CIs 1.082-7.720).

Discussion

Summary of key findings

Approximately one-third of recurrent melanomas in this small sample were detected at a routine scheduled follow-up appointment. Of those presenting in the interval, the majority were detected by the patient themselves. Of potential predictors of mode of melanoma recurrence only time to recurrence was statistically significant, with people being much less likely to detect their own recurrence within the first year since diagnosis.

Context with other literature

In this sample nearly one third of melanoma recurrences were detected at scheduled follow-up appointments. This accords with previous findings that 26-45% of melanoma recurrences are found at scheduled follow-up by a clinician [8,9,13]. Of the remaining two thirds the majority

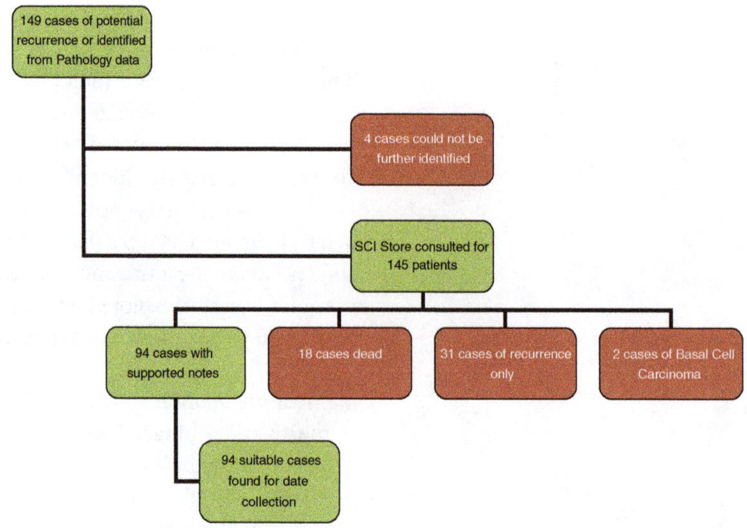

Figure 1 Study flow.

Table 3 Cross tab data analysis; determining the significance of categorised variables on likelihood to present at follow-up or in interval

Descriptive statistic:	Detected at follow-up:	Detected in interval:	p. value:
Gender;			.413
Female	8 (21.6%)	29 (78.4%)	
Male	15 (26.3%)'	42 (73.7%)	
Deprivation score;			.341
1(most deprived)	3 (60.0%)	2 (40.0%)	
2	3 (33.3%)	6 (66.7%)	
3	6 (27.3%)	16 (72.7%)	
4	7 (25.9%)	20 (74.15)	
5(least deprived)	4 (12.9%)	27 (87.1%)	
Rurality;			.571
Urban	14 (32.6%)	29 (67.4%)	
Rural	9 (17.6%)	42 (82.4%)	
Melanoma type;			.964
Superficial spreading	7 (25.9%)	20 (74.1%)	
Nodular malignant	8 (26.7%)	22 (73.3%)	
Lentigo maligna	1 (20.0%)	4 (80.0%)	
Acral lentiginous	1 (20.0%	4 (80.0%)	
Other	6 (22.2%)	21 (77.8%)	
Breslow thickness;			.252
4 mm or less	11 (20.0%)	44 (80.0%)	
>4 mm	12 (30.8%)	27 (69.2%)	
Age at Dx;			.142
Up to 65 years	12 (25.0%)	36 (75%)	
65 years and above	18 (39.1%)	28 (60.9%)	
Time to recurrence;			.008
12 months or less	14 (51.9%)	13 (48.1%)	
Beyond 12 months	16 (23.9%)	51 (76.2%)	

Table 4 Binary logistic regression; odds ratio of having recurrence detected at routine follow-up versus interval, based on key variables and individual factors

	Odds ratio:	95% CI for odds ratio:	
		Lower	Upper
Time to recurrence *(< 1 year)*	**3.433**	**1.340**	**8.796**
Gender *(male)*	1.295	.486	3.449
Age *(>65 years)*	1.351	.518	3.523
Melanoma type			
(Nodular vs. superficial)	.842	.274	2.586
(Lentigo vs. superficial)	.632	.088	4.532
(Acral vs. superficial)	1.684	.162	17.516
(Other vs. superficial)	.842	.267	2.660
Breslow thickness *(Thicker (>4 mm))*	1.667	.694	4.004
Rurality *(Urban)*	1.286	.539	3.067
Deprivation *(Deprived)*	1.750	.548	5.591
Adjusted binary logistic regression:			
Time to recurrence	**2.891**	**1.082**	**7.720**
Age	1.714	.666	4.415
Breslow thickness	1.443	.573	3.635
Rurality	1.377	.527	3.596
Deprivation	1.626	.454	5.816

Adjusted Binary Logistic Regression; adjusted for variables we deemed could influence our values.

were detected by the patients themselves in the interval between follow-up visits. Again, this accords with previous findings which report that between 47-68% of recurrent melanomas are self-detected [8,9]. That almost two thirds of people in this sample, and similar proportions in previous studies, have detected their own recurrence supports the view expressed by some that the resources devoted to melanoma follow-up should be used to educate patients in the practice of TSSE, rather than being spent on blood tests and clinical imaging [8-10,12,23,24]. The 16 patients with emergency or incidental presentation of their melanoma might all represent missed opportunities to self-detect recurrent melanoma with effective TSSE. A digital method to prompting and support TSSE appears timely and warranted [13,14]. Implementing novel technological approaches to cancer can be costly [25]. Our data suggest this cost could be mitigated by targeting those most likely to benefit.

Previous researchers have established that adjusting to a diagnosis of cancer takes time [26]. It is striking that those within a year of diagnosis were less likely to detect their own recurrent melanoma. This finding fits well with the notion of taking time to adjust to melanoma and the practice of TSSE [27]. Perhaps those in the immediate post-diagnostic period have most to gain from intensive support with respect to TSSE. In this context it is reassuring to note that previous interventions to promote TSSE, demonstrate it can be increased by well designed educational interventions [17-20].

Strengths and limitations

Our study contributes knowledge to an under-researched area, the epidemiology of recurrent melanoma. Our study was rigorous and based on high quality clinical databases and medical records. This was not an attempt to fully describe the epidemiology of recurrent melanoma in Northeast Scotland. Instead the authors were able to conduct a pragmatic study which provided invaluable information to inform the further development of a digital intervention to support TSSE in those diagnosed with cutaneous melanoma. The results are broadly in keeping with what has been published on melanoma recurrence before, but the authors were able to identify where such an intervention should be targeted to achieve maximum benefit in a way that previous research has not done.

This sample of patients was small from a relatively small area. The results may not be generalizable. However, two facts mitigate against this limitation. Firstly, in population terms melanoma recurrence is relatively rare and consequently its epidemiology is under-researched. Small studies such as this can signpost the way toward much needed larger studies. Secondly, proportions of follow-up versus self detected melanoma observed here are similar to those previously reported from other regions. This suggests that there is scope for others to add to our findings using similar small samples. A further related limitation is that the sample is dominated by men. Since men are arguably less likely to sustain TSSE this should be borne in mind as a potential confounder for which we have not been adequately able to control. As with all retrospective studies based upon medical records this study was limited by the availability and quality of records. This limitation is, however, common to almost all previous work on the epidemiology of recurrent melanoma, further highlighting the need for larger studies on the epidemiology of melanoma recurrence in future.

Conclusions

Scheduled follow-up is important and effective in detecting recurrent melanoma particularly in the immediate post diagnostic period. Patients who are within one year of being diagnosed with a primary cutaneous melanoma are significantly less likely to detect their own recurrence, potentially placing them at risk of poorer outcomes. A digital intervention to prompt and support TSSE for people diagnosed with cutaneous melanoma should start immediately a patient enters follow-up. Such an intervention should not be viewed as an alternative to current structured follow-up and may become less necessary over time. An immediate research priority is to develop an effective and user friendly digital application to prompt and support TSSE in those newly diagnosed with cutaneous melanoma. Subsequent research should include a randomised trial to ensure that such an intervention can sustain TSSE in the longer term. Further large-scale research on the epidemiology of recurrent melanoma is also required.

Competing interests

All authors declare that they have no competing interests to declare.

Authors' contributions

RA, PW, MN, and PM designed the study. RA and PW collected and managed the data. RA, PW and PM conducted data analysis. RA, PW, SH, MN, PM wrote the manuscript. PM is the guarantor. All authors read and approved the final manuscript.

Acknowledgements

We wish to acknowledge the funders of the research described here which was supported by the award made by the RCUK Digital Economy programme to the dot.rural Digital Economy Hub; award reference: EP/G066051/1. We also wish to acknowledge the University of Aberdeen who acted as sponsors for the study.

Author details

[1]School of Biomedical Sciences, Medical School, Teviot Place, Edinburgh EH8 9AG, UK. [2]Medical School, University of Aberdeen, Polwarth Building, Foresterhill, Aberdeen AB25 2ZD, UK. [3]Centre of Academic Primary Care – Division of Applied Health Sciences, University of Aberdeen, Polwarth Building, Foresterhill, Aberdeen AB25 2ZD, UK. [4]ANCHOR Unit, Aberdeen Royal Infirmary, Foresterhill, Aberdeen AB25 2ZN, UK.

References

1. Erdmann F, Lortet-Tieulent J, Schüz J, Zeeb H, Greinert R, Breitbart BW, Bray F: **International trends in the incidence of malignant melanoma 1953–2008 are recent generations at higher or lower risk?** *Int J Cancer* 2013, **132**:385–400.
2. Garbe C, Leiter U: **Melanoma epidemiology and trends.** *Clin Dermatol* 2009, **27**:3–9.
3. Korner A: **Barriers and facilitators of adherence to medical skin self-examination during melanoma follow-up care.** *BMC Dermatol* 2013, **13**:3.
4. Scottish Intercollegiate Guidelines Network: *Cutaneous Melanoma*, Guideline 72. Edinburgh: SIGN; 2003.
5. Ugurel S, Enk A: **Skin cancer; follow-up, rehabilitation, palliative and supportive care.** *J. Dtsch Dermatol. Ges. IOS* 2008, **6**:492–498.
6. Terushkin V, Halpern AC: **Melanoma early detection.** *Hematol Oncol Clin North Am* 2009, **23**:481–500.
7. Hall SJ, Samuel LM, Murchie P: **Toward shared care for people with cancer: developing the model with patients and GPs.** *Fam Pract* 2011, **28**:554–564.
8. Dicker TJ, Kavanagh GM, Herd RM, Ahmad T, McLaren KM, Chetty U, Hunter JA: **A rational approach to melanoma follow-up in patients with primary cutaneous melanoma.** *Brit J Dermatol* 2009, **140**:249–254.
9. Meyers MO: **Method of detection of initial recurrence of stage II/III cutaneous melanoma: analysis of the utility of follow-up staging.** *Annal Onco* 2009, **16**:941–947.
10. Poo-Hwu WJ, Ariyan S, Lamb L, Papac R, Zelterman D, Hu GL, Brown J, Fischer D, Bolgnia J, Buzaid AC: **Follow up recommendations for patients with American joint committee of cancer stages I-III malignant melanoma.** *Cancer* 1999, **86**:2252–2258.
11. Garbe C: **Prospective evaluation of a follow-up schedule in cutaneous melanoma patients: recommendations for an effective follow-up strategy.** *J Clin Oncol* 2003, **21**:520–529.
12. Kruijff S, Bastiannet E, Surmeijer AJH, Hoekstra HJ: **Detection of melanoma nodal metastases; differences in detection between elderly and young patients do not effect survival.** *Annal Onco* 2010, **17**:3008–3014.
13. Moore-Dalal K, Zhou Q, Panageas KS, Brady MS, Jaques DP, Coit DG: **Methods of detection of first recurrence in patients with stage I/II primary cutaneous melanoma after sentinel lymph node biopsy.** *Annal Onco* 2008, **15**:2206–2214.
14. Hull P, Piemontesi N, Lichtenwald J: **Compliance with self-examination surveillance in patients with melanoma and atypical moles: an anonymous questionnaire study.** *J Cutan Med Surg* 2011, **15**:97–102.
15. Korner A, Coroiu A, Martins C, Wang B: **Predictors of skin self-examination before and after a melanoma diagnosis; the role of medical advice and patient's level of education.** *Int Arch Med* 2013, **6**:8.
16. Janda M, Baade PD, Youl PH, Aitken JF, Whiteman DC, Gordon L, Neale RE: **The skin awareness study: promoting thorough skin self-examination for skin cancer among men 50 years or older.** *Contemp Clin Trials* 2009, **31**:119–130.
17. Janda M, Neale RE, Youl P, Whiteman DC, Gordon L, Baade PD: **Impact of video-based intervention to improve the prevalence of skin self-examinations in men 50 years or older: the randomized skin awareness trial.** *Arch Dermatol* 2011, **147**:799–806.
18. Lee K, Weinstock M, Risica P: **Component of a successful intervention for monthly skin self-examination for early detection of melanoma: the 'check it out' trial.** *J Am Acad Dermatol* 2008, **58**:1006–1012.

19. Oliveria S, Dusza S, Phelan D, Ostroff J, Berwick M, Halpern A: **Patient adherence to skin self-examination; effect of nurse intervention with photographs.** *Am J Prev Med* 2004, **26:**152–155.
20. Weinstock M, Risica P, Martin R, Rakowski W, Dube C, Berwick M, Goldstein MG, Acharyya S, Lasater T: **Melanoma early detection with thorough skin self-examination; The 'Check It Out' Randomized Trial.** *Am J Prev Med* 2007, **32:**517–524.
21. Scottish Government: *Scottish Index of Multiple Deprivation.* 2012. Available: http://www.scotland.gov.uk/Topics/Statistics/SIMD (Accessed 4/9/13).
22. Scottish Government: *Scottish Government 2-Fold Urban Rural Classification.* 2010. Available: http://www.scotland.gov.uk/Topics/Statistics/About/Methodology/UrbanRuralClassification (Accessed 4/9/13).
23. Printz C: **Target melanoma: skin cancer screenings hold promise to reduce mortality rates but usage of widespread screening lags.** *Cancer* 2008, **119:**2359–2360.
24. Leiter U, Marghoob AA, Lasithiotakis K, Eigentler TK, Meier F, Meisner C, Garbe C: **Costs of the detection of metastases and follow-up examinations in cutaneous melanoma.** *Melanoma Res* 2009, **19:**50–57.
25. Beaver K, Hollingworth W, McDonald R, Dunn G, Tysver-Robinson D, Thomson L, Hindley AC, Susnerwala SS, Luker K: **Economic evaluation of a randomized clinical trial of hospital versus telephone follow-up after treatment for breast cancer.** *Brit J Surg* 2009, **96:**1406–1415.
26. Stanton AL, Ganz PA, Rowland JH, Meyerowitz BE, Krupnick JL, Sears SR: **Promoting adjustment after treatment for cancer.** *Cancer* 2005, **104**(11 Suppl):2608–2613.
27. Mackie R, Bray C, Hole D, Morris A, Nicolson M, Evans A, Doherty V, Vestey J: **Incidence of and survival from malignant melanoma in Scotland: an epidemiological study.** *Lancet* 2002, **360:**587–591.

Risk factors for eczema in infants born in Cuba: a population-based cross-sectional study

Ramón Suárez-Medina[1*], Silvia Josefina Venero-Fernández[1], Esperanza de la Mora-Faife[1], Gladys García-García[1], Ileana del Valle-Infante[1], Liem Gómez-Marrero[1], Dania Fabré-Ortiz[2], Hermes Fundora-Hernández[1], Andrea Venn[3], John Britton[3], Andrew W Fogarty[3] and the HINASIC (Historia Natural de la Sibilancia en Cuba/National History of Wheezing in Cuba) Study Group

Abstract

Background: There is a concern that allergic disease in childhood is higher than expected in Cuba. The aim of this study was to determine the risk factors for eczema of infants aged 12–15 months living in Havana.

Methods: We used a cross-sectional epidemiological study design. Data on eczema symptoms and a wide range of lifestyle factors were collected by researcher administered questionnaires.

Results: Data were collected on 1956 children (96% response rate), of whom 672 (34%) were reported as having had eczema. Independent risk factors for eczema included young maternal age (adjusted odds ratio (OR) 0.98 per additional year of age; 95% confidence interval (CI) 0.97-0.99), child's weight (OR 1.13 per additional kg; 95% CI: 1.03-1.25), insect sting allergy (OR 2.11; 95% CI: 1.33-3.35), rodents in the home (OR 1.39; 95% CI: 1.10-1.76), attendance at childcare facilities (OR 1.34: 95% CI: 1.05-1.70) and self-reported mould in the home (OR 1.23; 95% CI: 1.07-1.41). Infant exposure to paracetamol was associated with an increased risk of eczema even after adjustment for wheeze (OR 1.22; 95% CI: 1.03-1.46).

Conclusion: Despite a very different culture and environment, the consistency of these findings with those from more economically developed countries suggests potential causal associations. The association with paracetamol, even after adjustment for wheeze, suggests that intervention studies are required in young infants, to ascertain if this commonly used anti-pyretic medication increases allergic disease.

Keywords: Eczema, Infants, Risk factor, Cuba, Paracetamol

Background

Allergic disease is increasing globally [1], particularly in countries where it was previously relatively rare [2], and is most common in the more affluent, urbanised and economically developed countries. However the aetiological factors responsible remain unknown. It is likely that much of the increase in allergic disease is the result of composite exposures, probably starting *in utero*, which cause disease in susceptible individuals [3]. Hence studies from the early years of childhood are important in identifying risk factors for subsequent development of common allergic diseases such as eczema, which will aid our understanding of the environmental exposures that result in allergic phenotypes.

* Correspondence: ramonsm@inhem.sld.cu
[1]Instituto Nacional de Higiene, Epidemiología y Microbiología, Infanta No 1158 e/ Llinásy Clavel, Código Postal 10300 La Habana, Cuba
Full list of author information is available at the end of the article

One avoidable risk factor of particular interest in the aetiology of allergic disease is use of paracetamol, which has been shown to be associated with eczema in both children and adults [4-7]. However, these associations are potentially confounded by the use of paracetamol to treat symptoms of respiratory infection, which are a common manifestation of childhood asthma. It is therefore important to adjust for this confounding effect, to determine whether paracetamol use and eczema are independently linked.

Cuba has a health care system that delivers infant mortality rates comparable to much richer countries [8], and deals well with common conditions that might be misclassified as eczema. However, as a consequence of the economic embargo on the island imposed by the USA, societal development has been constrained. The combination of good health infrastructure with limited economic growth in recent decades has resulted in a unique environment that provides an ideal setting where risk factors for disease can be studied utilising experienced staff based in the network of policlinics that provide healthcare to the whole population. As the pathogenetic pathways that result in disease are likely to be consistent across human populations, risk factors for allergic disease from Cuba that are consistent with those identified in more affluent countries are more likely to be real and not simply artefacts due to confounding.

In the recent phase three of the International Study of Asthma and Allergies in Childhood (ISAAC), Cuba had one of the highest prevalences of eczema among the countries studied from Latin America [9]. This study concluded that 'environmental risk factors must be evaluated in order to identify potential causes for the differences observed'. To address these issues, we have used a cross-sectional study design to explore the risk factors for eczema in the first year of life for infants born in Havana, Cuba.

Methods

Study population

All children aged between 12–15 months who were living in Havana, Cuba between March 2010 and March 2011 and who attended one of randomly selected 17 policlinics, nested in four municipalities in Havana, Cuba were eligible to be selected to participate in the study (Arroyo Naranjo, Cerro, Habana del Este, La Lisa). Selection of the study population has been described elsewhere [10]. The study protocol was approved by National Institute of Hygiene, Epidemiology and Microbiology, the local Havana Scientific Committee and also by the University of Nottingham Medical School ethics committee. All parents/guardians provided written informed consent for the infants to participate in the study.

Data collection

The baseline data collection consisted of an interviewer administered questionnaire (on-line Additional file 1) that collated the responses from the parent/carer about demographics of the child and mother, and a wide range of prenatal and postnatal exposures of the child including their living environment, the medical history of the family, exposure to medications such as paracetamol, aspirin and antibiotics, and exposure to environmental tobacco smoke. Data on the height and weight at both the time of birth and the interview were also collected. Allergic disease outcomes were collected using the Spanish translation of the ISAAC questionnaire [9,11] which was piloted in the local community. The outcome of interest, eczema, was based on the following question: 'Does your infant have or has had an itchy rash in any of the following places: the folds of the elbows, behind the knees, in front of the ankles, under the buttocks, or around the neck, ears or eyes during the first year of life?' (¿Su bebé tiene o ha tenido erupción con picazón en los siguientes lugares: sitio de flexión del brazo, atrás de las rodillas, en las muñecas, debajo de las nalgas o alrededor del cuello, orejas y ojos durante el primer año de vida?). Data on insect sting allergy were collected using the question "Has your baby been diagnosed with insect sting allergy in the first year of life".

Data analysis

All statistical analyses were carried out in Statav12 (StataCorp, Texas, USA) using the survey commands to allow for the clustered survey design. Univariate analyses were initially performed using logistic regression. Variables that were statistically significant in univariate analysis ($p \leq 0.05$) were then entered into a mutually adjusted multivariable mode and a step-wise modelling procedure followed to obtain a final model of only statistically significant ($p \leq 0.05$) variables. Gender was considered as *a priori* confounder. Associations of the outcome with exposures that were continuous variables were checked for linearity using likelihood ratio tests. The presence of self-reported wheeze was considered in the univariate analyses but omitted from the final model, as this is another manifestation of allergic disease, which would result in overfitting.

Sample size

We aimed to collect data on 2000 children. In the first year of life eczema is a better measure of allergic disease than wheeze and we have used this for the primary power calculation. We anticipate that we will have over 95% power (Epi-info, StatCalc) to detect an increase of the odds ratio of eczema of 1.9 for those who receive any paracetamol in the first year of life compared to those who do not receive paracetamol conservatively assuming a baseline prevalence of eczema of 20% and that 10% of the children in the cohort will receive paracetamol at some point in the first year of life.

Results

Of the 2032 infants who were eligible for inclusion in the study, 1956 provided data giving a 96% response rate. The characteristics of the study participants are presented in Table 1 and the distribution of the risk factors of interest in Table 2. 672 (34%) infants were reported as having had eczema symptoms in the first year of life. This was strongly associated with other allergic disease outcomes measured, including reported wheeze (odds ratio (OR) 2.35, 95% confidence intervals (CI) 1.93, 2.85), asthma diagnosis (OR 1.97, 95% CI: 1.45-2.67) and allergic rhinitis (OR 2.48, 95% CI: 2.00, 3.08).

Table 1 Characteristics of study participants

Variable	Definition of category	Number (%) unless stated otherwise	Prevalence of eczema (%)	Univariate OR for eczema (95% CI) using survey commands
Mean age months, (sd)		13.1 (1.1)	n/a	1.05 (0.91-1.20) per month
Skin colour (%)	White	916 (47)	301 (33)	1
	Mixed	798 (41)	282 (35)	1.12 (0.73-1.70)
	Black	242 (12)	89 (37)	1.19 (0.82-1.73)
Gender (%)	Female	939 (48)	301 (32)	1
	Male	1017 (52)	371 (36)	1.22 (0.90-1.64)
Municipality (%)	Habana del Este	642 (33)	240 (37)	1
	Cerro	374 (19)	81 (22)	0.46 (0.39-0.56)
	La Lisa	282 (14)	109 (39)	1.06 (0.84-1.32)
	Arroyo Naranjo	658 (34)	242 (37)	0.97 (0.80-1.19) $p = 0.06$
Highest educational status of mother (%)	Primary	17 (1)	9 (53)	1
	Secondary	431 (22)	159 (37)	0.52 (0.15-1.83)
	Pre-university	1157 (59)	382 (33)	0.44 (0.10-1.88)
	University	351 (18)	122 (35)	0.47 (0.17-1.31) $p = 0.59$ $p_{(trend)} = 0.18$
Mother with paid work (%)	No	780 (40)	264 (34)	1
	Yes	1176 (60)	408 (35)	1.04 (0.72-1.51)
Household income pesos, (%)	>3000	35 (2)	9 (26)	1
	2000-3000	48 (2)	21 (44)	2.25 (0.69-7.34)
	1001-1999	207 (11)	76 (37)	1.68 (0.41-6.81)
	500-1000	955 (49)	335 (35)	1.56 (0.38-6.41)
	<500	711 (36)	231 (32)	1.39 (0.42-4.55) $p = 0.85$ $p_{(trend)} = 0.44$
Any siblings (%)	No	818 (42)	297 (36)	1
	Yes	1138 (58)	375 (33)	0.86 (0.63-1.18)
Mean age of mother at birth in years (sd)	-	26.7 (6.2)	n/a	0.98 (0.97-0.99) per year
Reported eczema	No	1284 (66)	n/a	
	Yes	672 (34)		

The univariate associations with eczema are shown in Table 1 and Table 2. In the multivariate analysis those variables identified as statistically significant independent risk factors for eczema were young maternal age, increasing child's weight, family history of asthma, insect sting allergy, attendance at childcare facilities, use of antibiotics, use of preparations that contain paracetamol, mould in the home and rodents in the home (Table 3).

The effect of maternal age was such that the risk of eczema decreased by an estimated 2% for every additional year of age of the mother. Similarly, a linear effect of child's weight at the time of the interview was seen, with an estimated 13% increase in eczema risk per additional kg in child's weight; birthweight however was not associated with eczema. To investigate whether the observed relationship between child's paracetamol use and eczema may be confounded by indication (children with eczema more likely to experience respiratory symptoms which may be treated with paracetamol), we adjusted for symptoms of wheeze and this made little change to the association with paracetamol OR (1.22; 95% CI: 1.03, 1.46)). The effect of antibiotics however did weaken when adjusted for wheeze in the first year of life, and was no longer statistically significant (OR 1.24; 95% CI 0.91, 1.69).

Discussion

Cuba is unique, having a high quality health infrastructure despite a weak economy that is limited by political circumstance, which facilitates the delivery of high quality observational epidemiological studies in a relatively poor country. To our knowledge, this is the first large epidemiological study to explore the risk factors for eczema in infants in Cuba in the 21st century, a country that is known to have a very high, unexplained prevalence of symptoms of eczema in children [9]. We have identified that insect sting allergy, family history of

Table 2 Univariate analysis of exposures and risk of eczema since birth

Variable	Definition of category	Number (%) unless stated otherwise	Prevalence of eczema (%)	OR for eczema using survey command (95% CI)
Mother used paracetamol in pregnancy (%)	No	1809 (92)	626 (35)	1
	Yes	147 (8)	46 (31)	0.86 (0.43-1.73)
Mother used aspirin in pregnancy (%)	Never	1778 (91)	596 (34)	1
	Yes	178 (9)	76 (43)	1.48 (0.72-3.05)
Infant's mean birth weight, kg, (sd)		3.34 (0.53)	n/a	0.98 (0.84-1.13) per kg
Infant's mean height at birth cm (sd)*		50.28 (2.38)	n/a	1.02 (0.99-1.06) per cm
Infant's mean weight, kg, (sd)		10.52 (1.56)	n/a	1.14 (1.04-1.26) per kg
Infant's mean height, cm (sd)		74.67 (3.72)	n/a	1.02 (1.00-1.03) per cm
Caesarean birth (%)	No	1163 (59)	394 (34)	1
	Yes	793 (41)	278 (35)	1.05 (0.73-1.52)
Respiratory distress at birth (%)	No	1836 (94%)	620 (34)	1
	Yes	120 (6%)	52 (43)	1.50 (1.04-2.16)
Breastfeeding ≥4 months	No	890 (45)	337 (38)	1
	Yes	1066 (55)	335 (31)	0.75 (0.56-1.01)
Family history of asthma	No	917 (47)	267 (29)	1
	Yes	1039 (53)	405 (39)	1.56 (1.32-1.83)
Insect sting allergy (%)	No	933 (48)	229 (25)	1
	Yes	1022 (52)	443 (43)	2.35 (1.56-3.56)
	Missing	1		
Paracetamol use by infant including kogrip (%)	No	1486 (76)	486 (33)	1
	Yes	470 (24)	186 (40)	1.35 (1.12-1.62)
Antibiotic use by infant	No	1255 (64)	363 (29)	1
	Yes	696 (36)	307 (44)	1.94 (1.40, 2.68)
State of home (%)	Good	1368 (70)	477 (35)	1
	Regular	463 (24)	149 (32)	0.87 (0.77-1.01)
	Poor	125 (6)	46 (37)	1.09 (0.40-2.98) $p = 0.13$ $p_{(trend)} = 0.84$
No. of rooms in house (excluding bathroom and kitchen)	1	246 (13)	91 (37)	1
	2	540 (28)	167 (31)	0.76 (0.38-1.54)
	≥3	1170 (60)	414 (35)	0.93 (0.44-1.99) $p = 0.35$ $p_{(trend)} = 0.83$
Ventilation of home (%)	Good	1535 (78)	524 (34)	1
	Regular	307 (16)	102 (33)	0.96 (0.72-1.28)
	Poor	114 (6)	46 (40)	1.31 (0.70-2.44) $p = 0.62$ $p_{(trend)} = 0.31$
Presence of ornamental plants (%)	No	1405 (72)	484 (34)	1
	Yes	551 (28)	188 (34)	0.99 (0.77-1.26)
Presence of bathroom in home (%)	No	255 (13)	96 (38)	1
	Yes	1701 (87)	576 (34)	0.85 (0.59-1.22)
Mould in home (%)	No	1385 (71)	443 (32)	1
	Yes	571 (29)	229 (40)	1.42 (1.19-1.70)
Child sleeps in cooking area	No	1774 (91)	592 (33)	1
	Yes	182 (9)	80 (44)	1.57 (1.17-2.10)
Cook with gas (%)	No	133 (7)	64 (48)	1
	Yes	1823 (93)	608 (33)	0.54 (0.32-0.90)
Cook with electricity (%)	No	1507 (77)	482 (32)	1
	Yes	449 (23)	190 (449)	1.56 (0.99-2.45)

Table 2 Univariate analysis of exposures and risk of eczema since birth *(Continued)*

Mosquito nets in home (%)	No	728 (37)	240 (33)	1
	Yes	1228 (63)	432 (35)	1.10 (0.83-1.47)
Air conditioning (%)	No	1619 (83)	565 (35)	1
	Yes	337 (17)	107 (32)	0.87 (0.72-1.05)
Infant's room walls painted before birth	No	953 (49)	321 (34)	1
	Yes	1003 (51)	351 (35)	1.06 (0.85-1.32)
Infant's room walls painted after birth	No	1713 (88)	580 (34)	1
	Yes	243 (12)	92 (38)	1.19 (0.66-2.16)
Infant's mattress	Used	1062 (54)	374 (35)	1
	New	894 (46)	298 (33)	0.92 (0.67-1.26)
Infant sleeps alone	No (not alone)	829 (42)	297 (36)	1
	Yes (alone)	1127 (58)	375 (33)	0.89 (0.62-1.30)
Daily use of soap	No	69 (4)	26 (38)	1
	Yes	1887 (96)	646 (34)	0.86 (0.33-2.22)
Use of shampoo	No	615 (31)	209 (34)	1
	Yes	1341 (69)	463 (35)	1.02 (0.69-1.52)
No. of people in household	2	237 (12)	75 (32)	1
	3	485 (25)	170 (35)	1.17 (0.54-2.49)
	4	551 (28)	178 (32)	1.03 (0.50-2.14)
	5	332 (17)	116 (35)	1.16 (0.74-1.83)
	≥6	351 (18)	133 (38)	1.32 (0.63-2.74) $P = 0.80$ $p_{(trend)} = 0.20$
Eats vegetables	No	350 (18)	115 (33)	1
	Yes	1606 (82)	557 (35)	1.08 (0.75-1.57)
Eats fruit	No	184 (9)	65 (35)	1
	Yes	1772 (91)	607 (34)	0.95 (0.49-1.85)
Maternal smoking during pregnancy	No	1779 (91)	609 (34)	1
	Yes	177 (9)	63 (36)	1.06 (0.67-1.67)
Mother currently smokes	No	1557 (80)	513 (33)	1
	Yes	399 (20)	159 (40)	1.35 (0.92-1.97)
Father currently smokes	No	1309 (67)	434 (33)	1
	Yes	647 (33)	238 (37)	1.17 (0.83-1.65)
Number of smokers in home	0	952 (49)	299 (31)	1
	1	494 (25)	176 (36)	1.21 (0.90-1.62)
	2	340 (17)	131 (39)	1.37 (0.86-2.17)
	≥3	170 (9)	66 (39)	1.39 (0.89-2.15) $P = 0.31$ $p_{(trend)} = 0.03$
Any grandparents smoke	No	832 (43)	274 (33)	1
	Yes	1124 (57)	398 (35)	1.12 (0.83-1.50)
Pets in home at time of birth	No	1259 (64)	417 (33)	1
	Yes	697 (36)	255 (37)	1.16 (0.70-1.93)
Pets in home now	No	1239 (63)	419 (34)	1
	Yes	717 (37)	253 (35)	1.07 (0.74-1.52)
Rodents in home	No	1643 (84)	534 (32)	1
	Yes	313 (16)	138 (44)	1.64 (1.33-2.02)
Cockroaches in home	No	1432 (73)	470 (33)	1
	Yes	524 (27)	202 (39)	1.28 (0.77-2.14)

Table 2 Univariate analysis of exposures and risk of eczema since birth *(Continued)*

Air pollution near home	No	1407 (72)	476 (34)	1
	Yes	549 (28)	196 (36)	1.09 (0.57-2.08)
Child attended daycare/nursery	No	1685 (86)	559 (33)	1
	Yes	271 (14)	113 (42)	1.44 (1.14-1.83)
Any parasites**	No	686 (96)	262 (38)	1
	Yes	26 (4)	9 (35)	0.86 (0.23-3.21)
Any wheeze	No	1084 (55)	280 (26)	1
	Yes	872 (45)	392 (45)	2.34 (1.56-3.53)

*5 missing values.
**1244 infants were unable to provide a faeces sample for analysis.

asthma, presence of rodents or mould in the house, day-care attendance, a heavier current weight, having a younger mother as independent risk factors for reported symptoms of eczema in Havana. The association with paracetamol is particularly interesting as it persisted even after adjustment for wheeze, suggesting that this was not simply confounding by association with respiratory infections. It is also of pragmatic importance since exposure to paracetamol in this population, as in developed countries, was common.

Our data have a number of strengths that give us confidence in the integrity of these observed associations. In particular, the relatively large sample of almost 2000 infants with a response rate of 96% is excellent, and a consequence of nesting the data collection within the policlinics minimising inconvenience to the families and staff involved. This reduces the risk of response bias and also permits the associations observed to be generalised to other similar populations. The study questionnaire was developed by local epidemiologists who have much experience of work with these populations and hence allowed consideration of local factors that may be specific to these localities in the analysis. The data were collected by highly trained health professionals who knew the participants, thus enhancing the quality of the information collected.

There are some limitations of our study design, which are unavoidable. Cross-sectional study designs do not allow causality to be attributed, and only associations to be identified. However, the nature of the hypothesis we

Table 3 Multivariate analysis of exposures and risk of eczema in first year of life

Variable	Definition of category	Number	Adjusted OR for any eczema (95% CI)
Gender	Female		1
	Male		1.09 (0.76-1.57)
Infant's mean current weight, per kg*	-	10.52 (1.56)	1.13 (1.03-1.25)
Family history of asthma	No	917 (47)	1
	Yes	1039 (53)	1.34 (1.04-1.73)
Insect sting allergy (%)	No	933 (48)	1
	Yes	1022 (52)	2.11 (1.33-3.35)
Use of paracetamol	No	1486 (24)	1
	Yes	470 (76)	1.22 (1.02-1.46)
Use of antibiotics	No		1
	Yes		1.61 (1.10-2.34)
Age of mother at birth (per year*)	-	26.7 (6.2)	0.98 (0.97-0.99)
Rodents in home	No	1643 (84)	1
	Yes	313 (16)	1.39 (1.10-1.76)
Mould in home (%)	No	1385 (71)	1
	Yes	571 (29)	1.23 (1.07-1.41)
Attended daycare/nursery	No	1685 (86)	1
	Yes	271 (14)	1.34 (1.05-1.70)

1937 individuals provided complete data for analysis.
*linear association.

were testing does not make reverse causality a likely explanation for the relationships that were observed. We were unable to do any detailed measurements when the infants were *in utero*, although we were able to collect data on important exposures related to pregnancy such as maternal smoking in pregnancy, weight and height at birth, the mode of delivery and the duration of breastfeeding. The use of the ISAAC questionnaire definition of eczema allows comparison of our data with other similar studies [11], but it is possible that this practical epidemiological approach to defining the outcome measure may have a degree of imprecision as other causes of itchy rashes in addition of eczema may be included in the outcome measure. We are unable to exclude the possibility of recall bias and residual confounding influencing our data and the associations reported. Finally, we have tested a number of exposures and hence are unable to exclude the possibility that some of the associations we observed are the consequence of chance.

There have been no comparable studies of eczema in infants in Cuba, and so it is difficult to directly compare our data with other study datasets. The third phase of the ISAAC study had a limb in Havana and reported a prevalence of having ever had a eczematous rash of 26%, one of the higher prevalences in Latin America in children aged six to seven years [9] with the data collected in the latter half of the first decade of the 21st century. A rash was reported to have first occurred below the age of two years in 15% of these children, compared to values of less than 1% in centres in Mexico. This is compared to our prevalence of 34% of children having symptoms of eczema in the first year of life in 2010. Obviously these two prevalence estimates are not directly comparable due to differences in definitions and recall bias, but it is possible that eczema prevalence has increased in young infants living in Havana over the first decade of the 21st century.

This is the first study to report an association between paracetamol exposure and eczema after adjustment for symptoms of wheeze in young infants. The only other dataset that studied the impact of paracetamol exposure on incident eczema in 780 children aged between 1 and 3 years living in Ethiopia that adjusted for symptoms of respiratory infections did not observe a similar association [12], although the different ages prevent direct comparison with our population, while the baseline analysis from the same study again did not observe an association with eczema with use of paracetamol [13]. Other studies have reported that paracetamol is a risk factor for eczema using analyses in older children from international datasets [4,6,7,14,15], and also data from a different population of Ethiopian children and adults from the country reported an odds ratio of 1.9 for risk of self-reported eczema in those taking more than three tablets of paracetamol in the past month compared to those who took none [5]. However, although plausible biological mechanisms exist that may possibly explain how paracetamol exposure in early life can result in allergic disease [15], it should be stressed that the role of paracetamol on the aetiology of allergic disease is contentious and the likelihood is that a randomised controlled trial will be required to resolve these issues.

Many of the other risk factors for symptoms of eczema in our dataset have been previously reported and while not novel, these give us confidence in the integrity of the data collected and associations observed. Hence, it is well known that a family history of asthma is a risk factor for allergic diseases such as eczema in children [16] while the presence of mould in the home is also well recognised to be associated with allergic disease [17]. We observed a strong association between a diagnosis of insect sting allergy in the first year of life with eczema symptoms that appears plausible in the light of other studies. One study population from Israel of 13 to 14 year old schoolchildren reported an increased in both rate and severity of allergic reactions to insect stings among those with atopic diseases compared to those who did not have atopic disease [18]. Similarly, a population-based study from the USA reported that people with atopy experienced anaphylaxis, an extreme form of allergic reaction more frequently than people without atopy [19].

To our knowledge, the inverse association between maternal age and risk of eczema has not been reported previously [20-23]. Maternal age is closely related to birth order as older mothers have more children, and this is considered to be a risk factor for allergic disease, with individuals with more elder siblings having less hayfever and eczema [24]. Cord blood IgE is a risk factor for development of atopic disease in childhood, and Scirica reported that older mothers have lower levels of cord blood IgE using data from 874 children from the USA [25], an observation that is compatible with our data. The association between presence of rats in the home and eczema is difficult to explain using the existing literature but we speculate that this could be a surrogate marker for living conditions or other exposures that we were unable to measure.

Conclusion

In conclusion, we report that in infants born in Havana, Cuba, insect sting allergy, family history of asthma, presence of rodents or mould in the house, daycare attendance, a heavier current weight, use of paracetamol, and having a younger mother are all independent risk factors for reported symptoms of eczema. The delivery of high quality observational epidemiological studies in a developing country is challenging for many reasons, but good data from these environments are important as associations that are observed consistently across a range of societies are more likely to be causal and not simply a consequence of confounding, possibly by affluence. Cuba is a unique developing country with excellent public health provision and diagnostic ascertainment, and the consistency of these findings with those from a range of more economically developed countries suggests that the risk factors identified in our study may be important in the development of eczema. The association with paracetamol, even after adjustment for wheeze, suggests that intervention studies are required in young infants, to ascertain if this commonly used anti-pyretic medication increases allergic disease.

Abbreviations

ISAAC: International study of asthma and allergies in childhood; HINASIC: Historia Natural de la Sibilancia en Cuba/National History of Wheezing in Cuba.

Competing interests

There are no competing interests among any of the authors between the reporting of the study findings and financial or non-financial interests that may bias the report.

Authors' contributions

The 8 Cuban authors (SF, RS, EM, GG, IV, LG, DF, HF) came up with the original concept of the study and the study design. AF, AV and JB helped with the study design and obtaining funding. The data were collected by the 8 Cuban authors (SF, RS, EM, GG, IV, LG, DF, HF) and analysed by RS, AF and AV. All authors contributed to the final drafting and approval of the manuscript.

Acknowledgements

We would like to thank all of the participants and their families for making this study possible.
HINASIC study group (Historia Natural de la Sibilancia en Cuba/National History of Wheezing in Cuba) consists of the following individuals:
National Institute of Hygiene, Epidemiology and Microbiology
Menocal-Heredia L, Caraballos-Sánchez Y, Quintana R, Rodríguez-Bertheau AM, Rosado-García FM, Carmen-Hinojosa M, Varona-Pérez P.
Hospital Universitario Pediátrico Docente Centro Habana
Rivero R., Muñoz-Pérez J, González-Morfa C.
Municipality of Arroyo Naranjo
Zaldívar-Ricardo D, Diburt-Amita M, Álvarez-Valdez G, Alfonso-Hernández A, Álvarez-Valdez V, Magaña-Álvarez Y, Figueroa-Barreto Z, Sardiñas-Báez N, Del Toro F, Velásquez-Pérez Y, Felpeto-Fuentes M, Gainza-Bueno Y, Esquivel-Barrios GM, Suárez-Paz M, Magaña-Álvarez BJ, Carménate-Fernández A, Hidalgo-Mederos R, Hidalgo-Mederos L, Silva D, Comas-Fonseca G, Lazaga-Cala DM, Kessel Díaz O.
Municipality of La Lisa
Llopis-Pupo I, Rudy-Colebroork L, Loynaz-González M, Ortiz-Hernández ML, Castillo-Bu M, Betancourt-López M, Gutiérrez-Mendoza ER, Rodríguez-Trujillo N, Pozo-Herrera P, Cruz-Acosta S, Montejo-Guerra VM, Gómez-Suliman V, Vega-Enríquez Y
Municipality of Cerro
Pando CR, Cortina-Mena I, Díaz-Giraldino A, Marrero-Sosa M, Matos-Ramos C, Betancourt-Orue M, Torres Zulueta RM, Alba Monteagudo O, Valle-López M, Ferrer-Ceruto Y, Damas-Martínez A, Peñalver-Pérez M
Municipality of Habana del Este
Castillo- Martínez S, Pérez-Pérez IM, Bravo-Hernández PL, Martínez-Hernández A, Torriente-Barzaga N, Ávila-Rodríguez I, Navarro-Ruiz M, Díaz-Hernández K, Sarduy-Flores R, Sánchez-Díaz E, Zubizarreta-Seguí L, Roque-Pereira G, Corona-Carnero Y, Rafols-Turró M, Cobas-Espino T, Castillo-Hernández N, Tenreiro-Vilda GC, Pulido-Díaz VI, Oropesa-Varona MJ, Luís-Avilés R, Santos-Smith K, Serrano-González T, Vázquez-Lazo B, Pupo-Portal Tania, Torres-Martínez MC, Betancourt-Cabreras I, Cid-Morell Y, Suárez-Quiñones R, García-Pérez K, Griñán-Ramos JA, Calzado-Herrera Y, Rizo-Ramos MN, Verdecia G, García-Sotolongo MB, Del Río-Díaz A, Abreu-Quijano JF, Romeo-Ravelo F.
We also thank all the Municipality Directors and the laboratory workers who have also supported the study.
This work was supported by the Wellcome Trust (090375); Nottingham University Hospital Charitable Trust; the Nottingham Respiratory Biomedical Research Unit and Instituto Nacional de Higiene, Epidemiología y Microbiología, Havana, Cuba.

Author details

[1]Instituto Nacional de Higiene, Epidemiología y Microbiología, Infanta No 1158 e/ Llinásy Clavel, Código Postal 10300 La Habana, Cuba. [2]Hospital Pediátrico Docente "Juan Manuel Márquez", La Habana, Cuba. [3]Nottingham Biomedical Research Unit, Division of Epidemiology and Public Health, University of Nottingham, Clinical Sciences Building, City Hospital, NG5 1 PB Nottingham, UK.

References

1. Asher M, Montefort S, Bjorksten B, Lai C, Strachan D, Weiland S, Williams H, and the ISAAC phase three study group: **Worldwide trends in the prevalence of symptoms of asthma, allergic rhinoconjunctivitis, and eczema in childhood: ISAAC phases one and three repeat multicountry cross-sectional surveys.** *Lancet* 2006, **368:**733–743.
2. Williams H, Stewart A, von Mutius E, Cookson W, Anderson R, and the ISAAC phase one and phase three study groups: **Is eczema really on the increase worldwide?** *J Allergy Clin Immunol* 2008, **121:**947–954.
3. Williams H, Robertson C, Stewart A, Ait-Khaled N, Anabwani G, Anderson R, Asher I, Beasley R, Bjorksten B, Burr M, Clayton T, Crane J, Ellwood P, Keil U, Mallol J, Martinez F, Mitchell E, Montefort S, Pearce N, Shah J, Sibbald B, Strachan D, von Mutius E, Weiland S: **Worldwide variations in the prevalence of symptoms of atopic eczema in the international study of asthma and allergies in childhood.** *J Allergy Clin Immunol* 1999, **103:**125–138.
4. Cohet C, Cheng S, MacDonald C, Baker M, Foliaki S, Huntington N, Douwes J, Pearce N: **Infections, medication use, and the prevalence of symptoms of asthma, rhinitis, and eczema in childhood.** *J Epidemiol Community Health* 2004, **58:**852–857.
5. Davey G, Berhane Y, Duncan P, Aref-Adib G, Britton J, Venn A: **Use of acetaminophen and the risk of self-reported allergic symptoms and skin sensitisation in Butajira, Ethiopia.** *J Allergy Clin Immunol* 2005, **116:**863–868.
6. Beasley R, Clayton T, Crane J, Von Mutius E, Lai C, Monetfort S, Stewart A, Monetfort S, Stewart A, and ISAAC phase three study group: **Association between paracetamol use in infancy and childhood, and risk of asthma, rhinoconjunctivitis, and eczema in children aged 6–7 years: analysis from phase three of the ISAAC programnme.** *Lancet* 2008, **372:**1039–1048.
7. Beasley R, Clayton T, Crane J, Lai C, Montefort S, von Mutius E, Stewart A, and ISAAC phase three study group: **Acetaminophen use and risk of asthma, rhinoconjunctivitis, and eczema in adolescents.** *Am J Respir Crit Care Med* 2011, **183:**171–178.
8. Cooper R, Kennelly J, Ordunez-Garcia P: **Health in Cuba.** *Int J Epidemiol* 2006, **35:**817–824.
9. Sole D, Mallol J, Wandalsen G, Aguirre V, Group LAIPS: **Prevalence of symptoms of eczema in Latin America: results of the international study of asthma and allergies in childhood (ISAAC) phase 3.** *J Investig Allergol Clin Immunol* 2010, **20:**311–323.
10. Venero-Fernandez S, Suarez Medina R, Mora Faife E, García García G, del Valle II, Gomez-Marrero L, Abreu-Suarez G, Gonzalez-Valdez J, Fabro-Ortiz D, Fundora-Hernadez H, Venn A, Britton J, Fogarty AW: **Risk factors for wheezing in infants born in Cuba.** *Q J Med* 2013, **106:**1023–1029.
11. Wordemann M, Polman K, Diaz R, Heredia L, Madurga A-M, Sague K, Gryseels B, Gordea M: **The challenge of diagnosing atopic diseases: outcomes in Cuban children depend on definition and methodology.** *Allergy* 2006, **61:**1125–1131.

12. Amberbir A, Medhin G, Alem A, Britton J, Davey G, Venn A: **The role of acetaminophen and geohelminth infection on the incidence of wheeze and eczema.** *Am J Respir Crit Care Med* 2011, **183:**165–170.
13. Belyhun Y, Amberbir A, Medhin G, Erko B, Hanlon C, Venn A, Britton J, Davey G: **Prevalence of risk factors of wheeze and eczema in 1-year-old children: the Butajira birth cohort, Ethiopia.** *Clin Exp Allergy* 2010, **40:**619–626.
14. Newson R, Shaheen S, Chinn S, Burney P: **Paracetamol sales and atopic disease in children and adults: an ecological analysis.** *Eur Respir J* 2000, **16:**817–823.
15. Holgate S: **The acetaminophen enigma in asthma.** *Am J Respir Crit Care Med* 2011, **183:**147–151.
16. Tattersfield A, Knox A, Britton J, Hall I: **Asthma.** *Lancet* 2002, **360:**1313–1322.
17. Mendell M, Mirer A, Cheung K, Tong M, Douwes J: **Respiratory and allergic health effects of dampness, mold, and dampness-related agents: a review of the epidemiological evidence.** *Environ Health Perspect* 2011, **119:**748–756.
18. Graif Y, Romano-Zelekha O, Livne I, Green M, Shohat T: **Increased rate and greater severity of allergic reactions to insect sting among schoolchildren with atopic diseases.** *Pediatr Allergy Immunol* 2009, **20:**757–762.
19. Yocum M, Butterfield J, Klein J, Volcheck G, Schroeder D, Silverstein M: **Epidemiology of anaphyaxis in Olmsted country: a population-based study.** *J Allergy Clin Immunol* 1999, **104:**452–456.
20. Martinez F, Wright A, Holberg C, Morgan W, Taussig L: **Maternal age as a risk factor for wheezing lower respiratory illnesses in the first year of life.** *Am J Epidemiol* 1992, **136:**1258–1268.
21. Taylor B, Wadsworth J, Golding J, Butler N: **Breast feeding, eczema, asthma, and hayfever.** *J Epidemiol Community Health* 1983, **37:**95–99.
22. Sariachvili M, Droste J, Dom S, Wieringa M, Hagendorens M, Stevens W, van Sprundel M, Desager K, Weyler J: **Early exposure to solid foods and the development of eczema in children up to 4 years of age.** *Pediatr Allergy Immunol* 2010, **21:**74–81.
23. Butland B, Strachan D, Lewis S, Bynner J, Butler N, Britton J: **Investigation into the increase in hay fever and eczema at age 16 observed between the 1958 and 1970 British birth cohorts.** *Brit Med J* 1997, **315:**717–721.
24. Strachan D: **Family size, infection and atopy: the first decade of the "hygiene hypothesis".** *Thorax* 2000, **55:**S2–S10.
25. Scirirca C, Gold D, Ryan L, Abulkerim H, Celedon J, Platts-Mills T, Naccara L, Weiss S, Litonjua A: **Predictors of cord blood IgE levels in children at risk of asthma and atopy.** *J Allergy Clin Immunol* 2007, **119:**81–88.

6

Sentinel lymph node biopsy in melanoma: Our 8-year clinical experience in a single French institute (2002–2009)

Caroline Biver-Dalle[1], Eve Puzenat[1], Marc Puyraveau[2], Delphine Delroeux[3], Hatem Boulahdour[4], Frances Sheppard[2], Fabien Pelletier[1,5], Philippe Humbert[1,5] and François Aubin[1,6,7*]

Abstract

Background: Since the introduction of sentinel lymph node biopsy (SLNB), its use as a standard of care for patients with clinically node-negative cutaneous melanoma remains controversial. We wished to evaluate our experience of SLNB for melanoma.

Methods: A single center observational cohort of 203 melanoma patients with a primary cutaneous melanoma (tumour thickness > 1 mm) and without clinical evidence of metastasis was investigated from 2002 to 2009. Head and neck melanoma were excluded. SLN was identified following preoperative lymphoscintigraphy and intraoperative gamma probe interrogation.

Results: The SLN identification rate was 97%. The SLN was tumor positive in 44 patients (22%). Positive SLN was significantly associated with primary tumor thickness and microscopic ulceration. The median follow-up was 39.5 (5–97) months. Disease progression was significantly more frequent in SLN positive patients (32% vs 13%, $p = 0.002$). Five-year DFS and OS of the entire cohort were 79.6% and 84.6%, respectively, with a statistical significant difference between SLN positive (58.7% and 69.7%) and SLN negative (85% and 90.3%) patients ($p = 0.0006$ and $p = 0.0096$ respectively). Postoperative complications after SLNB were observed in 12% of patients.

Conclusion: Our data confirm previous studies and support the clinical usefulness of SLNB as a reliable and accurate staging method in patients with cutaneous melanoma. However, the benefit of additional CLND in patients with positive SLN remains to be demonstrated.

Keywords: Melanoma, Sentinel lymph node

Background

Since its introduction in 1992 [1], the role of sentinel lymph node biopsy (SLNB) in melanoma care remains controversial and is not included in most guidelines for the management of melanoma in Europe [2]. Its main short term aim is the early identification of patients with occult nodal metastasis, known as micrometastasis, who might benefit from complete lymph node dissection (CLND). The long term aim is to provide a more accurate basis for formulating a prognosis than do standard demographic and histopathological factors. Furthermore, the presence or absence of micrometastases in the sentinel lymph node (SLN) is critical to both accurate AJCC staging[2] and decisions regarding adjuvant therapy and follow-up regimens. The final version of melanoma staging and classification takes into account the results of SLNB [3]. A Cox multivariate analysis of 3,307 stage III patients demonstrated that 5-year survival rates ranged from 70% for patients with micrometastasis (T1-T4N1aM0) to 39% for patients with T1-T4N3M0 CM. However, according to the Multicenter Selective Lymphadenectomy Trial (MSLT) [4], there was no significant difference in disease-specific survival between patients with lymphatic mapping by SLNB (and immediate CLND) and patients with nodal observation. Other

* Correspondence: francois.aubin@univ-fcomte.fr
[1]Department of Dermatology, Besançon University Hospital, Besançon, France
[6]University of Franche Comté, EA3181, SFR FED4234, Besançon, France
Full list of author information is available at the end of the article

retrospective studies have shown similar results and the influence of SLNB and CLND on long term patient survival as well as its therapeutic role are still debated [5].

Despite the fact that SLNB is widely used in France [2], there are no French studies reporting the experience of SLNB. We present our 8-year consecutive clinical experience of performing SLNB for CM. We evaluated the outcome of patients in terms of disease progression and mortality based on the SLNB result.

Methods

Patients

SLNB has been performed at Besançon University Hospital since 2000. Patients who had undergone this technique in the first two years were excluded to allow the medical team to gain experience in guaranteeing reproducibility and reliability of the results [4]. Only patients with a primary cutaneous melanoma (tumour thickness > 1 mm) and without clinical evidence of metastasis who underwent SLNB between January 2002 and December 2009 were included. Furthermore, patients with head and neck CM were also excluded because of the complexity of lymphatic drainage, multi-site drainage and the high number of false negatives [6,7]. Since this retrospective study was conducted in France, it was not eligible for submission to our research ethics committee. Patients were selected and each clinical file obtained from the Cancer Registry of the Besançon University Hospital (authorization from the Privacy and Data Protection National Agency, CNIL number 903417) was re-examined and the following data were collected: epidemiological criteria (sex, age), histological criteria, clinical features, SLN status (positive or negative), results of CLND and evolution criteria (relapse and survival). The epidemiological and histological data were collected from the Cancer Registry, whereas the evolution criteria were gathered from the hospital clinical files or by writing to family practitioners.

SLNB procedure

After information and written consent, preoperative lymphoscintigraphy was performed in all patients by injecting 1 mL of technetium Tc 99 m-labeled sulfur colloid intradermally around the periphery of the primary lesion or biopsy scar in 4-quadrant fashion. Using a gamma camera with a low-energy, high resolution collimator, dynamic and static images were obtained, beginning 15 minutes after injection and continuing every 30 minutes thereafter, until the SLNs were visualized. Surgery took place the following day. A hand-held gamma probe was used to localize the SLN transcutaneously. The SLN was identified intra-operatively using a gamma probe. After SLN harvesting, the radioactive count was measured ex vivo using the gamma probe. Echelon nodes were then harvested if they had a count ≥ 10% of the SLN. The background count of the lymph node basin was then measured to ensure that no further radioactive nodes remained. In addition to preoperative lymphoscintigraphy, 9 patients received an on-table injection of patent Blue V dye (Laboratoire Guerbet, Aulnay-sous-Bois, France) around the biopsy scar. Following completion of SLN dissection, the maximal counts per second *in vivo* and *ex vivo* were recorded to verify that no areas of increased radioactivity remained.

Histopathologic evaluation

Pathological analysis of SLN involved an initial bisection of the node along its hilum after fixation. Then, from each side of the SLN, five serial step sections of 4 mm were cut with 50 mm intervals between different numbers of sections. Finally, all sections were stained with hematoxylin and eosin. All slides were examined histologically, and if melanoma cells were detected immunohistochemistry (S100, HMB45 and MelanA) was then performed for confirmation.

Surgical and adjuvant therapy

Patients with positive SLNs were advised to have CLND of the regional basin. According to French guidelines, all patients with primary CM larger than or equal to 1.5 mm in thickness as well as patients with positive SLN and positive CLND and patients with high-risk primary melanoma (tumor thickness > 4 mm and ulceration) were considered for adjuvant interferon alpha therapy, low-doses and high doses of interferon, respectively. Demographic, clinical and histological characteristics of patients together with primary CM, SLNB and CLND pathological reports, and the lymphoscintigraphy imaging file and surgery report were collected.

Follow-up

Patients were followed up in an outpatient setting by clinical examination one week postoperatively and then on a six monthly basis for the first three years and every year for the next 5 years. In addition, ultrasound analysis of regional lymph nodes was performed in patients with positive SLN. Tumor progression and survival status were gathered from the hospital clinical files or by writing to family practitioners and the observations were censored on December 31st 2010.

Statistical analysis

Statistical analysis was based on chi squared analysis or the exact Fisher test for qualitative data and based on Student test for quantitative data, Kaplan-Meier survival curves and log rank analysis. The significance level was determined at p less than 0.05. The analyses were performed with SAS software, version 9.2 (Sas Institute, Inc, Cary, NC).

Results

From January 2002 to December 2009, 203 patients (100 men and 103 women) with melanoma thickness superior to 1 mm underwent SLNB. The mean age was 56 +/- 16 (16 to 86). Clinical and histological characteristics are shown in Table 1.

Sentinel lymph node biopsy

In all but 6 patients (3%), SLN was identified. A complete failure (absence of reliable scintigraphic imaging and surgical localization) was observed in two patients with truncal melanoma. A surgical failure (i.e. absence of SLN sample) despite scintigraphic localization was reported in two patients with upper limb melanoma. SLN localization and excision could not be carried out in two patients because there was no percutaneous radioactivity on the incision area. The same

Table 1 SLN: sentinel lymph node

	Entire cohort	Patients with positive SLN	Patients with negative SLN	p
Number	203*	44/197* (22%)	153/197* (78%)	
Sex				0.2706
Men	100 (49.3%)	18 (41%)	76 (50%)	
Women	103 (50.7%)	26 (59%)	77 (50%)	
Mean age (+/− SD)	55.8 +/−15.6	52.0 +/−17.4	56.6 +/−15.0	0.0864
Localization				0.1483
Trunk	74 (36.5%)	17 (38.6%)	54 (35.3%)	
Upper limb	39 (19.2%)	3 (6.8%)	33 (21.6%)	
Lower limb	63 (31.0%)	16 (36.4%)	47 (30.7%)	
Hands and feet	27 (13.3%)	8 (18.2%)	19 (12.4%)	
Type				0.6978
Superficial	115 (56.6%)	25 (56.8%)	86 (56.2%)	
Nodular	39 (19.2%)	6 (13.6%)	31 (20.3%)	
Acral	17 (8.4%)	4 (9.1%)	13 (8.5%)	
Other	32 (15.8%)	9 (20.5%)	23 (15.0%)	
Mean tumor thickness (range)	1.88 (0.4 - 10.1)	2.8 (1.2 - 10)	1.6 (0.4 - 10.1)	0.0289
T stage [2]				0.0172
T1	10 (4.9%)	0	10 (6.5%)	
T2	101 (49.7%)	15 (34.1%)	83 (54.3%)	
T3	55 (27.1%)	17 (38.6%)	36 (23.5%)	
T4	33 (16.3%)	11 (25.0%)	21 (13.7%)	
Incalculable[1]	4 (2.0%)	1 (2.3%)	3 (2.0%)	
Clark level				0.3677
I	1 (0.5%)	0	1 (0.7%)	
II	10 (4.9%)	2 (4.5%)	8 (5.2%)	
III	56 (27.6%)	9 (20.5%)	46 (30.1%)	
IV	100 (49.3%)	26 (59.1%)	70 (45.7%)	
V	12 (5.9%)	4 (9.1%)	7 (4.6%)	
Unknown	24 (11.8%)	3 (6.8%)	21 (13.7%)	
Ulceration				0.0080
Yes	60 (29.6%)	21 (47.7%)	37 (24.2%)	
No	131 (64.5%)	20 (45.5%)	107 (69.9%)	
Unknown	12 (5.9%)	3 (6.8%)	9 (5.9%)	

NS: not significant.
*6 complete or partial failures (lymphoscintigraphy and surgery).

level of radioactivity was localized in several axillary lymph nodes in one patient, and CLND was then performed and was negative. The axillary tissue harvested during SLNB procedure did not contain any lymph nodes in one patient. These 6 patients had not undergone blue dye marking.

The SLN identification rate was 97%. The mean number of SLN harvested was 1.5 +/− 1. Only one SLN was harvested in 67% of cases. Nodal basin included unilateral axilla (87 cases), unilateral groin (85 cases), bilateral axillae (11 cases), bilateral groins (1 case), popliteal fossa (2 cases) and epitrochlear (0 case). The drainage area for limb melanomas was always homolateral (data non shown). Drainage to multiple node fields was present in 37 cases (18%) and most of them (57%) originated from dorsal melanomas. Of patients with trunk melanoma, 13 demonstrated interval nodes (17%). Of patients with limbs melanoma, we observed interval nodes, including popliteal (9 patients, 14%), and epitrochlear nodes (2 patients, 5%). Of these 24 patients with interval nodes, 11 had samples taken surgically, demonstrating a melanoma micrometastasis in three patients.

Of the 197 patients in whom a SLN was identified, 44 (22%) were tumor positive. We observed a statistically significant difference between positive and negative SLN patients for tumor thickness ($p = 0.0289$), the presence of ulceration ($p = 0.008$), and T stage ($p = 0.0172$) in primary CM.

Complete lymph node dissection and adjuvant therapy

Of the patients with positive SLN, 95% (42 of 44 patients) underwent additional CLND. One patient had a popliteal positive SLN and refused further surgical intervention and one patient had contraindications for radical lymphadenectomy. None of them relapsed. Eleven patients (25%) had further pathologically positive lymph nodes. Of the patients with positive SLN, 29% were treated with interferon alpha. Eleven patients (7%) with negative SLN but with a high-risk primary melanoma (tumor thickness > 4 mm and ulceration) were treated with interferon.

Recurrence

Patients were followed for a median duration of 39.5 months (range: 5 – 97). Fifteen patients (5 SLN positive patients and 10 SLN negative) were lost to follow-up.

Thirty-four patients (17%) relapsed. Recurrences were significantly more frequent ($p = 0.002$) in SLN positive patients (32%) than in SLN negative patients (13%). The median time for recurrence in our cohort was 12 months (range: 0–58 months), with no significant difference between SLN positive and negative patients (15.2 +/− 15.6 months versus 17.4 +/− 16.6 months, respectively, $p = 0.7107$). The site of initial recurrence is shown in Table 2. There was no significant difference in the type of recurrence between positive and negative SLN patients. The result of CLND in SLN positive patients did not lead to any significant differences in terms of relapse, type of relapse or death (data not shown).

The percentage of false-negative patients in our cohort was 6.5%, as 10 of the 153 SLN negative patients developed regional lymph node relapse. Sensitivity, specificity and the positive and negative predictive values of the SLN status (Table 3) in terms of recurrence were 41%, 81%, 32% and 87% respectively. Sensitivity, specificity and the positive and negative predictive values of the SLN status in terms of mortality were 39%, 80%, 20% and 91% respectively.

Survival analyses

The overall cohort mortality rate was 11.3%. The mortality rate (Figure 1) was significantly higher in the SLN positive group than in the SLN negative group (20.4% versus 7.5%, $p = 0.01$). The 5-year overall survival (OS) rate was 84.6% for all patients, but was significantly higher for SLN negative patients as compared to SLN positive patients (90.3% versus 69.7%; $p = 0.0096$). The

Table 2 Site of initial recurrence by sentinel lymph node status

	Number all patients	SLN positive patients	SLN negative patients	p
SLN status	197	44 (22%)	153 (78%)	
Recurrence:				
Yes	34 (17%)	14 (32%)	20 (13%)	0.002
No	163 (83%)	30 (68%)	133 (87%)	
Site of initial recurrence*:				
Local/in transit	17 (50%)	9 (64%)	8 (40%)	NS
Regional lymph node	16 (47%)	6 (43%)	10 (50%)	NS
Distant metastatic	20 (59%)	8 (57%)	14 (70%)	NS

*Some patients may present multiple sites of recurrence.
SLN: sentinel lymph node.
NS: not significant.

Table 3 SLN status sensitivity, specificity, positive predictive value (PPV) and negative predictive value (NPV) in terms of recurrence and mortality

	SLN +	SLN -	Number of patients
Recurrence	14 (TP)	20 (FN)	34
No recurrence	30 (FP)	133 (TN)	163
Death	9 (TP)	14 (FN)	23
Living	35 (FP)	139 (TN)	174
Number of patients	44	153	197

TP: true-positive; TN: true-negative; FP: false positive; FN: false-negative.

five-year disease-free survival (DFS) rate was 79.6% for all patients, but was significantly higher in SLN negative patients than in SLN positive patients (85.0% versus 58.7%; p = 0.0006) (Figure 2).

Adverse events

Post-operative complications of SLN biopsy (neuropathic pain, infection, seroma, hematoma, lymphedema) were observed in 12% of patients (24/197). Three patients presented with severe complications such as cellulitis (2 patients) and severe invalidating complex regional pain syndrome occurred in one patient after a brachial plexus injury. Post-operative complications of additional CLND were observed in 14% of patients (6/42), including lymphedema (3), hematoma (1) and neuropathic pain (1) and complex regional pain syndrome (1).

Discussion

Despite the small number of patients in our cohort, our results confirm previous studies on SLN analysis in melanoma [3,4,8-11], in terms of SLN identification rate (97%), percentage of SLN positive patients (22%) and percentage of additional positive CLND (25%). We also observed a significant association between positive SLN and primary tumor thickness and microscopic ulceration. Although only one SLN was harvested in 67% of our cases, the mean number of SLN harvested was 1.5 +/− 1 in our study, very similar to those found by previous studies [8,12]. Furthermore, Gershenwald 7. [9] found that among the 343 patients who underwent CLND, the majority (72%) had only one positive SLN as compared to 67% in our study. To our knowledge, there

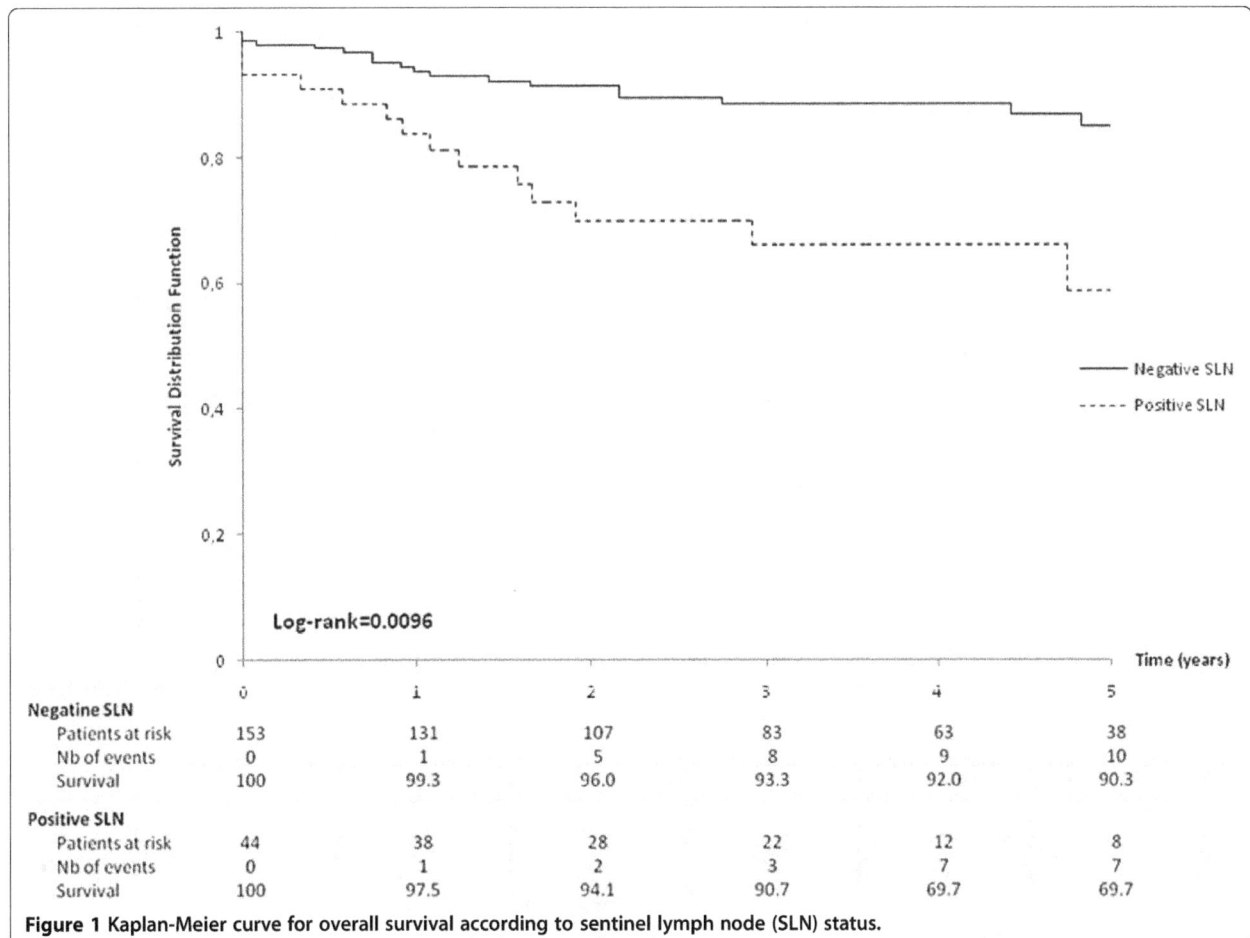

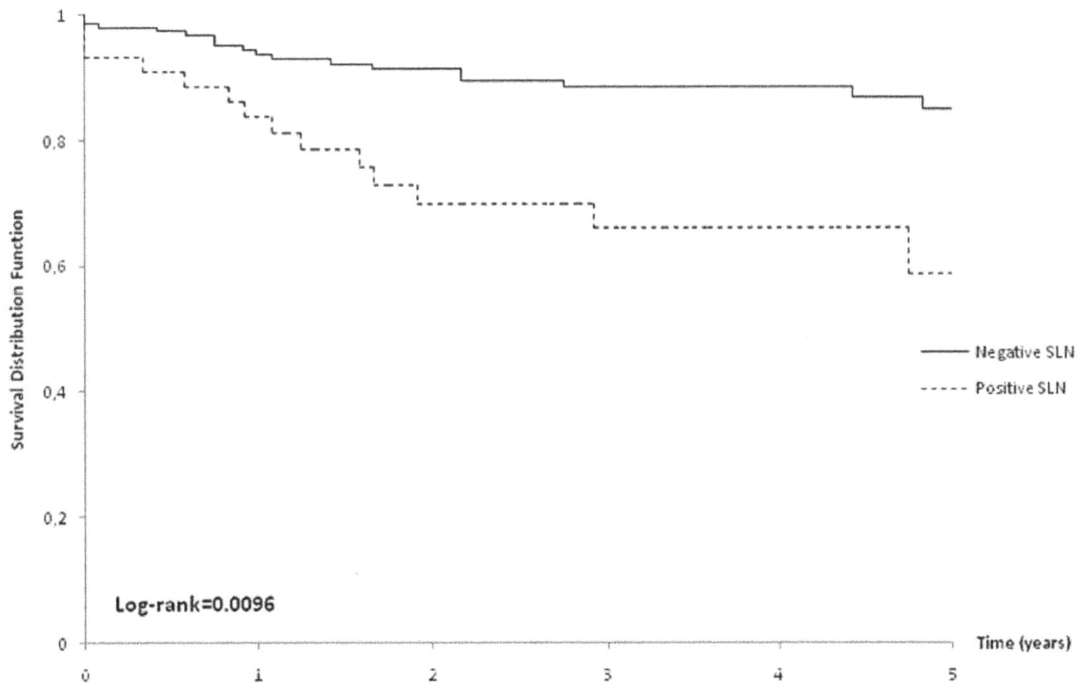

	0	1	2	3	4	5
Negatine SLN						
Patients at risk	153	131	107	83	63	38
Nb of events	0	1	5	8	9	10
Survival	100	99.3	96.0	93.3	92.0	90.3
Positive SLN						
Patients at risk	44	38	28	22	12	8
Nb of events	0	1	2	3	7	7
Survival	100	97.5	94.1	90.7	69.7	69.7

Figure 1 Kaplan-Meier curve for overall survival according to sentinel lymph node (SLN) status.

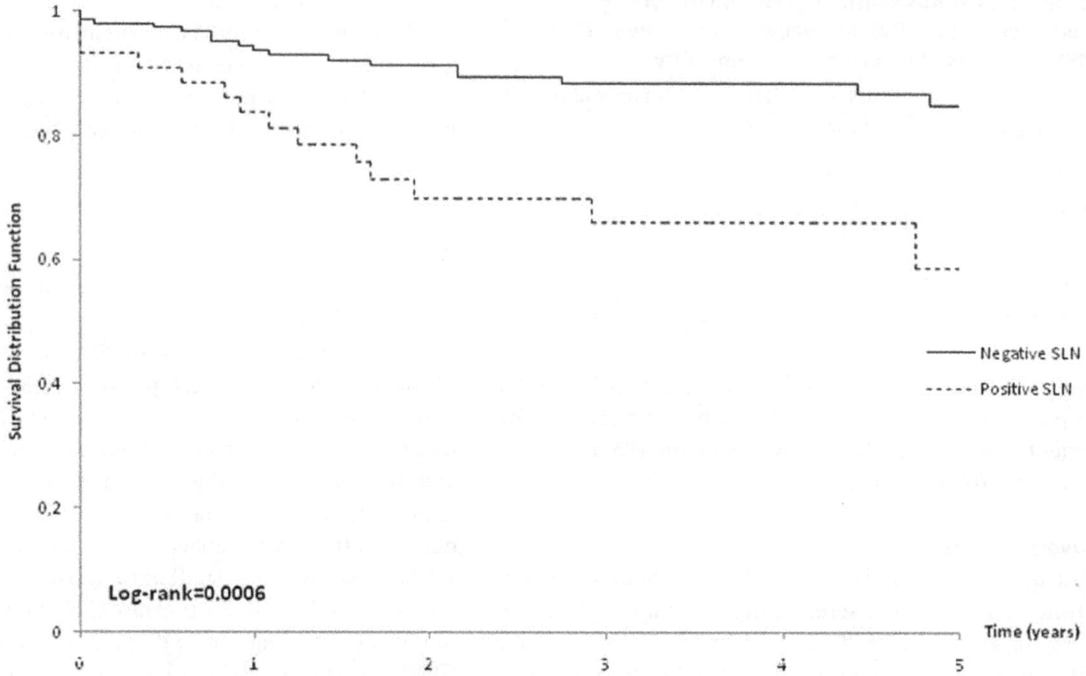

	0	1	2	3	4	5
Negatine SLN						
Patients at risk	153	124	101	77	58	37
Nb of events	0	9	12	15	15	17
Survival	100	93.7	91.3	88.5	88.5	85.0
Positive SLN						
Patients at risk	44	34	23	17	12	7
Nb of events	0	7	12	13	13	14
Survival	100	83.7	69.9	66.0	66.0	58.7

Figure 2 Kaplan-Meier curve for disease-free survival according to sentinel lymph node (SLN) status.

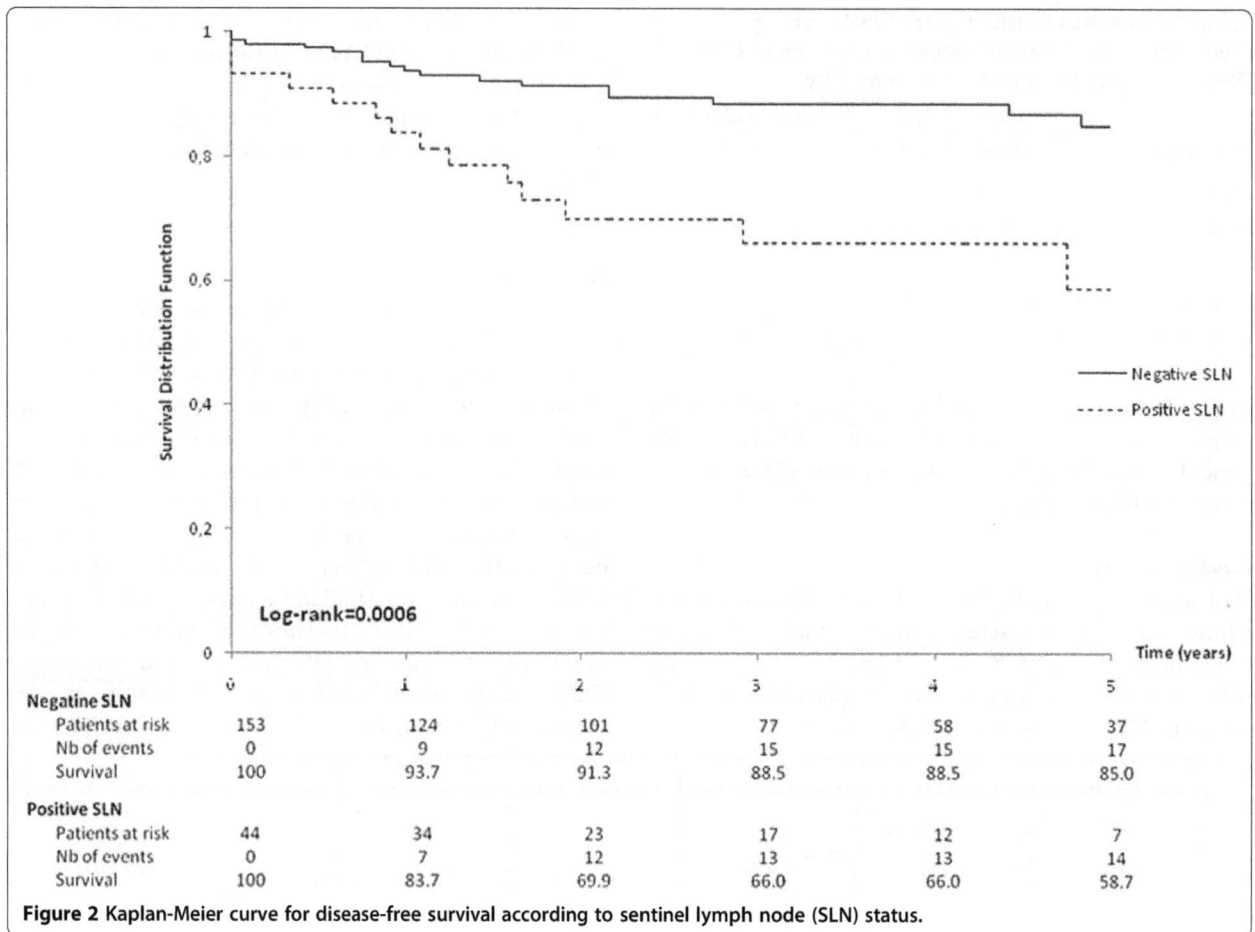

are neither consensus nor recommendations on the minimal or maximal number of SLN that should be harvested during the procedure.

As expected, recurrences were significantly more frequent in SLN positive patients (32%) than in SLN negative patients (13%) suggesting a better regional control of melanoma progression after SLNB and immediate CLND. The rate of locoregional lymph node relapses after lymph node excision in SLN positive patients varied between 0 and 20% [4,13]. Conversely, locoregional relapses after LND of clinically palpable lymph node palpation varied between 20 and 50% [13-15]. It is nonetheless still difficult to know whether better regional lymph node control is related to complementary CLND performed after positive SLN is discovered. Another study [13] retrospectively compared two groups of SLN positive patients from different hospitals, some of whom underwent additional CLND. The authors found no significant difference in terms of survival between the two groups. In our study, relapse and mortality rates in SLN positive patients were not influenced by the result of additional CLND casting further doubt on the benefits of complementary surgery.

The SLNB was considered false-negative if a primary recurrence developed in the regional lymph node basin from which a tumor-free SLN had been removed. In our study, the number of false-negative (10/153 = 6.5%) was similar (3-8%) to other studies [11,16,17]. However, there is ongoing debate on how to correctly calculate the false-negative rate. It should not be expressed as a percentage of the total population, but rather as the number of false-negative results divided by the number of false-negatives and true-positives [18]. In our study, the false negative rate (10/54 = 18.5%) was also similar to the rate calculated in other studies (5.7% to 21%) [14]. Beyond the technical problems associated with the SLN procedure, false negatives may be related to different factors: the time it takes to learn to perform the technique [19], lymphatic drainage disruption related to primary tumour excision, lymphatic obstruction by tumor cell embolism, the presence of a neck SLN [7], inadequate histological analysis and hematogenous dissemination.

The risk factors for recurrence after negative SLN are identical to those observed after positive SLN: presence or absence of macroscopic ulceration and tumoral thickness superior to 4 mm [7]. Analysis of all relapses

(Table 3) according to SLN status (positive or negative) showed a poor sensitivity (41%) and positive predictive value (32%) for SLN analysis but good specificity (81%) and negative predictive value (87%). Although rarely calculated, these values are similar to those found by Saltman *et al.* [6] The same analysis focused on mortality confirmed the good specificity (80%) and negative predictive values (91%), i.e. similar to the findings of Morton *et al.* [4].

Our overall survival rates at 5 years (69.7% and 90.3% for SLN positive and negative patients, respectively) were similar to previous prognostic values of SLN analysis [8,20] when followed by additional CLND. A multivariate analysis of an international cohort of 2313 stage III patients [20] showed that the overall survival rate at 5 years was greater in patients presenting with micrometastases than in patients with palpable lymph node metastases (67% vs 43%). However, there were wide variations (23% to 87%) in patients with micrometastases depending on histological characteristics of primary melanoma (ulceration, mitotic index), its anatomical localization, number of SLN affected and patient age [20]. A bayesian analysis was recently carried out of studies with more than 50 patients undergoing SLN between 1993 and 2010 [11]. The authors focused on the prognostic benefit of the SLN analysis in terms of specific survival for melanoma with tumor thickness between 1 and 4 mm. For these patients, the risk of melanoma-related death varied between 26.2% and 31.6% when SLN was positive versus 9.7% and 15.6% when SLN was negative.

All of these results for relapse and survival involve the combination of two surgical procedures: research and analysis of SLN followed by additional CLND in the event of micrometastases in SLN. At the present time, no advantages of lymph node excision have been shown in terms of regional monitoring of metastatic damage or overall survival [13,15,21]. However, an additional lymph node excision is more often recommended when the SLN is invaded [22].

Many attempts have been made to predict non-SLN (NSLN) metastasis in the additional lymph node excision performed after positive SLN based on demographic, primary tumor, and SN features of patients with melanoma. Previous studies [9,10,23-25] indicate that overall SLN tumor burden, primary tumor thickness, and number of SLN harvested may be useful in identifying a group at low risk for positive NSLN. It is nonetheless interesting that these two parameters are also predictive for SLN micrometastases [20,26]. However, marked variability in the correlation of individual features with NSLN metastases and the degree of this correlation has characterized the literature on this issue to date [27,28]. There is currently no consensus regarding what degree of risk of NSLN involvement indicates that it is safe to forego CLND. Before elimination of CLND can be advocated, prospective clinical trials designed to assess the safety of omitting formal CLND with respect to survival and locoregional control in low-risk groups are needed. The ongoing Multicenter Selective Lymphadenectomy Trial II [29] which compares CLND versus close observation with sonography and clinical examination for patients with a positive SLN, should provide valuable information about which patients might be spared a CLND.

The frequency of post-operative complications (neuropathic pain, infection and lymphocele) observed in our study was similar to other studies in terms of morbidity related to SLN analysis [30].

Conclusions

In conclusion, our retrospective study confirms the results of SLN analysis in patients with melanoma with tumor thickness greater than 1 mm. The main benefit of this analysis was the prognostic value in terms of relapse and survival (as long as additional lymph node excision was performed), and its high predictive negative value. The usefulness of complementary excision is still a subject of debate due to the high percentage of normal results and morbidity. Although already recommended, evaluating the benefit of additional CLND after positive SLN is necessary. New SLN analysis techniques are also under evaluation in order to lower operative morbidity [31].

Competing interests

All authors have significantly contributed to the manuscript and all agree with its contents. All authors have read and approved the manuscript. Authors do not have any relevant financial interests in the findings from this manuscript.

Authors' contributions

CB-D, EP, DD, HB, FP, PH and FA, 1) have made substantial contributions to conception and design and acquisition, analysis and interpretation of data; 2) have been involved in drafting the manuscript or revising it critically for important intellectual content; and 3) have given final approval of the version to be published. MP and FS 1) have made substantial contributions to design and analysis and interpretation of data; 2) have been involved in revising the manuscript critically for important intellectual content; and 3) have given final approval of the version to be published. All authors read and approved the final manuscript.

Author details

[1]Department of Dermatology, Besançon University Hospital, Besançon, France. [2]Clinical Methodology Center, Besançon University Hospital, Besançon, France. [3]Department of Digestive Surgery, Besançon University Hospital, Besançon, France. [4]Department of Nuclear Medicine, Besançon University Hospital, Besançon, France. [5]University of Franche Comté, UMR1098, SFR FED4234, Besançon, France. [6]University of Franche Comté, EA3181, SFR FED4234, Besançon, France. [7]Service de Dermatologie, 2 Place Saint-Jacques, 25030, Besançon, cedex, France.

References

1. Morton DL, Wen DR, Wong JH, Economou JS, Cagle LA, Storm FK, *et al*: **Technical details of intraoperative lymphatic mapping for early stage melanoma.** *Arch Surg* 1992, **127**:392–399.
2. Lourari S, Paul C, Gouraud PA, Tavitian S, Viraben R, Leccia MT, *et al*: **Sentinel lymph node biopsy for melanoma is becoming a consensus: a national survey of French centres involved in melanoma care in 2008.** *J Eur Acad Dermatol Venereol* 2012, **26**:1230–1235.
3. Balch CM, Gershenwald JE, Soong S-J, Thompson JF, Atkins MB, Byrd DR, *et al*: **Final version of 2009 AJCC melanoma staging and classification.** *J Clin Oncol* 2009, **27**:6199–6206.
4. Morton DL, Thompson JF, Cochran AJ, Mozzillo N, Elashoff R, Essner R, *et al*: **Sentinel-node biopsy or nodal observation in melanoma.** *N Engl J Med* 2006, **355**:1307–1317.
5. Thomas JM: **Freedom of expression or protectionism in the debate on sentinel node biopsy in melanoma.** *J Am Acad Dermatol* 2009, **61**:1079.
6. Saltman BE, Ganly I, Patel SG, Coit DG, Brady MS, Wong RJ, *et al*: **Prognostic implication of sentinel lymph node biopsy in cutaneous head and neck melanoma.** *Head Neck* 2010, **32**:1686–1692.
7. Savoia P, Fava P, Caliendo V, Osella-Abate S, Ribero S, Quaglino P, Macripò G, Bernengo MG: **Disease progression in melanoma patients with negative sentinel lymph node: does false-negative specimens entirely account for this phenomenon?** *J Eur Acad Dermatol Venereol* 2012, **26**:242–248.
8. Gershenwald JE, Thompson W, Mansfield PF, Lee JE, Colome MI, Tseng CH, *et al*: **Multi-institutional melanoma lymphatic mapping experience: the prognostic value of sentinel lymph node status in 612 stage I or II melanoma patients.** *J Clin Oncol* 1999, **17**:976–983.
9. Gershenwald JE, Andtbacka RHI, Prieto VG, Johnson MM, Diwan AH, Lee JE, *et al*: **Microscopic tumor burden in sentinel lymph nodes predicts synchronous nonsentinel lymph node involvement in patients with melanoma.** *J Clin Oncol* 2008, **26**:4296–4303.
10. Kunte C, Geimer T, Baumert J, Konz B, Volkenandt M, Flaig M, *et al*: **Analysis of predictive factors for the outcome of complete lymph node dissection in melanoma patients with metastatic sentinel lymph nodes.** *J Am Acad Dermatol* 2011, **64**:655–662. quiz 637.
11. Rhodes AR: **Prognostic usefulness of sentinel lymph node biopsy for patients who have clinically node negative, localized, primary invasive cutaneous melanoma: a Bayesian analysis using informative published reports.** *Arch Dermatol* 2011, **147**:408–415.
12. Testori A, De Salvo GL, Montesco MC, Trifirò G, Mocellin S, Landi G, *et al*: **Clinical considerations on sentinel node biopsy in melanoma from an Italian multicentric study on 1,313 patients (SOLISM-IMI).** *Ann Surg Oncol* 2009, **16**:2018–2027.
13. Wong SL, Morton DL, Thompson JF, Gershenwald JE, Leong SPL, Reintgen DS, *et al*: **Melanoma patients with positive sentinel nodes who did not undergo completion lymphadenectomy: a multi-institutional study.** *Ann Surg Oncol* 2006, **13**:809–816.
14. Kretschmer L, Neumann C, Marsch WC, Lee RJ, *et al*: **Nodal basin recurrence following lymph node dissection for melanoma: implications for adjuvant radiotherapy.** *Int J Radiat Oncol Biol Phys* 2000, **46**:467–474. Int J Radiat Oncol Biol Phys 2000, 48: 1267–1268.
15. Pasquali S, Mocellin S, Campana LG, Bonandini E, Montesco MC, Tregnaghi A, *et al*: **Early (sentinel lymph node biopsy-guided) versus delayed lymphadenectomy in melanoma patients with lymph node metastases: personal experience and literature meta-analysis.** *Cancer* 2010, **116**:1201–1209.
16. Gershenwald JE, Colome MI, Lee JE, Mansfield PF, Tseng C, Lee JJ, *et al*: **Patterns of recurrence following a negative sentinel lymph node biopsy in 243 patients with stage I or II melanoma.** *J Clin Oncol* 1998, **16**:2253–2260.
17. van Akkooi AC, Voit CA, Verhoef C, Eggermont AM: **New developments in sentinel node staging in melanoma: controversies and alternatives.** *Curr Opin Oncol* 2010, **22**:169–177.
18. Nieweg OE, Estourgie SH: **What is a sentinel node and what is a false-negative sentinel node?** *Ann Surg Oncol* 2004, **11**(3 Suppl):169S–173S.
19. Veenstra HJ, Wouters MJWM, Kroon BBR, Olmos RAV, Nieweg OE: **Less false-negative sentinel node procedures in melanoma patients with experience and proper collaboration.** *J Surg Oncol* 2011, **104**:454–457.
20. Balch CM, Gershenwald JE, Soong S-J, Thompson JF, Ding S, Byrd DR, *et al*: **Multivariate analysis of prognostic factors among 2,313 patients with stage III melanoma: comparison of nodal micrometastases versus macrometastases.** *J Clin Oncol* 2010, **28**:2452–2459.
21. Kingham TP, Panageas KS, Ariyan CE, Busam KJ, Brady MS, Coit DG: **Outcome of patients with a positive sentinel lymph node who do not undergo completion lymphadenectomy.** *Ann Surg Oncol* 2010, **17**:514–520.
22. Moroi Y: **Significance of sentinel lymph node biopsy in malignant melanoma: overview of international data.** *Int J Clin Oncol* 2009, **14**:485–489.
23. van Akkooi ACJ, Nowecki ZI, Voit C, Schäfer-Hesterberg G, Michej W, de Wilt JHW, *et al*: **Sentinel node tumor burden according to the Rotterdam criteria is the most important prognostic factor for survival in melanoma patients: a multicenter study in 388 patients with positive sentinel nodes.** *Ann Surg* 2008, **248**:949–955.
24. van der Ploeg APT, van Akkooi ACJ, Rutkowski P, Nowecki ZI, Michej W, Mitra A, *et al*: **Prognosis in patients with sentinel node-positive melanoma is accurately defined by the combined Rotterdam tumor load and Dewar topography criteria.** *J Clin Oncol* 2011, **29**:2206–2214.
25. Cadili A, Scolyer RA, Brown PT, Dabbs K, Thompson JF: **Total sentinel lymph node tumor size predicts nonsentinel node metastasis and survival in patients with melanoma.** *Ann Surg Oncol* 2010, **17**:3015–3020.
26. White RL Jr, Ayers GD, Stell VH, Ding S, Gershenwald JE, Salo JC, *et al*: **Factors predictive of the status of sentinel lymph nodes in melanoma patients from a large multicenter database.** *Ann Surg Oncol* 2011, **18**:3593–3600.
27. Scolyer RA, Li LX, McCarthy SW, Shaw HM, Stretch JR, Sharma R, *et al*: **Immunohistochemical stains fail to increase the detection rate of micrometastatic melanoma in completion regional lymph node dissection specimens.** *Melanoma Res* 2004, **14**:263–268.
28. Debarbieux S, Duru G, Dalle S, Béatrix O, Balme B, Thomas L: **Sentinel lymph node biopsy in melanoma: a micromorphometric study relating to prognosis and completion lymph node dissection.** *Br J Dermatol* 2007, **157**:58–67.
29. Morton DL: **Sentinel node mapping and an International Sentinel Node Society: Current issues and future directions.** *Ann Surg Oncol* 2004, **11**:137S–143S.
30. Kretschmer L, Thoms K-M, Peeters S, Haenssle H, Bertsch H-P, Emmert S: **Postoperative morbidity of lymph node excision for cutaneous melanoma-sentinel lymphonodectomy versus complete regional lymph node dissection.** *Melanoma Res* 2008, **18**:16–21.
31. Voit CA, van Akkooi AJC, Schäfer-Hesterberg G, Sterry W, Eggermont AMM: **Multimodality approach to the sentinel node: an algorithm for the use of presentinel lymph node biopsy ultrasound (after lymphoscintigraphy) in conjunction with presentinel lymph node biopsy fine needle aspiration cytology.** *Melanoma Res* 2011, **21**:450–456.

7

Employment is maintained and sick days decreased in psoriasis/psoriatic arthritis patients with etanercept treatment

Robert L Boggs[1*], Sarolta Kárpáti[2], Wenzhi Li[1], Theresa Williams[3], Ronald Pedersen[3], Lotus Mallbris[3] and Robert Gniadecki[4]

Abstract

Background: Psoriasis and psoriatic arthritis (PsA) impair quality of life, including reduction in employment or job duties. The PRESTA (Psoriasis Randomized Etanercept STudy in Patients with Psoriatic Arthritis) study, a randomized, double-blind, two-dose trial, examined the efficacy of etanercept treatment in patients with moderate-to-severe plaque psoriasis and PsA and the main results have been presented previously. This analysis examined employment status, job duties and sick days, pre-defined endpoints in PRESTA, among this patient population.

Methods: Participants (N = 752) were randomized to receive etanercept 50 mg twice weekly (BIW; n = 379) or 50 mg once weekly (QW; n = 373) for 12 weeks by subcutaneous injection. All participants then received open-label etanercept 50 mg QW for 12 additional weeks, while remaining blinded to the randomization. A pharmacoeconomic questionnaire was administered at baseline, week 12 and week 24 of treatment. The questionnaire included employment status and changing job responsibilities and sick time taken due to psoriasis or PsA. The statistical methods included analysis of covariance, *t*-test, Fisher's exact test and McNemar's test. Last-observation-carried-forward imputation was used for missing data.

Results: Employment was at least maintained from baseline to week 24 in both dose groups (56% [BIW/QW] and 60% [QW/QW] at baseline, 61% and 60%, respectively, at week 24). Among employed participants, the proportion of patients whose job responsibilities changed due to PsA decreased significantly from baseline to week 24 (17–23% to 5–8%; $p < 0.01$). Similar results were seen with job responsibility changes due to psoriasis (11–14% to 4%; $p < 0.01$). The number of monthly sick days also decreased from baseline to week 24 (2.4 days for both treatment groups to 0.7 (BIW/QW) and 1.1 (QW/QW); $p \leq 0.03$ for each). No significant differences between the treatment groups were observed for any economic endpoint at any time point.

Conclusions: For patients with moderate-to-severe plaque psoriasis and PsA, etanercept treatment resulted in reducing job responsibility changes due to disease and in reducing sick time. Effective treatment of psoriasis and PsA may reduce missed work days.

Keywords: Psoriasis, Psoriatic arthritis, Pharmacoeconomics, Etanercept, Employment, Sick days

Background

The prevalence of psoriatic arthritis (PsA) in patients with psoriasis is estimated to be as high as 30%, in contrast with a prevalence of <1% in the general population [1-3]. Both psoriasis and PsA negatively affect quality of life. Even patients with only mild psoriasis have reported problems in everyday life [4], including an inability to work [5,6]. PsA has been implicated in absences from work and career activities in previous studies [7,8]. However, more information is needed regarding employment, absenteeism and productivity in patients with PsA. A validated employment and productivity questionnaire that is specific for PsA is not currently available.

Etanercept, a fully human tumor necrosis factor-soluble receptor, is approved for the treatment of both PsA and

* Correspondence: bobboggs.nc@gmail.com
[1]Formerly of Pfizer Inc., 3921 Glenlake Garden Drive, Raleigh, NC 27612, USA
Full list of author information is available at the end of the article

moderate-to-severe plaque psoriasis based on demonstrated efficacy in treating both joint and skin symptoms.

In the PRESTA (Psoriasis Randomized Etanercept STudy in Patients with Psoriatic Arthritis) study [9-11], the efficacy, safety and patient-reported outcomes of two etanercept regimens were examined in patients with both moderate-to-severe psoriasis and PsA. Employment status and absenteeism were pre-defined outcomes of PRESTA and were determined via a pharmacoeconomic questionnaire.

The objective of this analysis is to examine the data from the pharmacoeconomic questionnaire to assess the impact of psoriasis plus PsA on working for pay and missed work days of patients who were treated with etanercept during the PRESTA study.

Methods

The PRESTA study was conducted between December 2005 and March 2008, primarily in Europe and included sites in the Middle East, Asia-Pacific, Central America and South America [9]. Participants were enrolled from dermatology clinics based on having moderate/severe psoriasis and active PsA (with PsA evaluated by a rheumatologist or trained arthritis evaluator). In this multicenter, randomized study, patients received either etanercept 50 mg twice weekly (BIW) or 50 mg once weekly (QW) during the initial 12-week, double-blind period, followed by 50 mg QW during the subsequent 12-week, open-label period (initial randomization remained blinded; Figure 1).

Patients in the PRESTA study were aged at least 18 years, had clinically stable, moderate-to-severe plaque psoriasis with a body surface area involvement of ≥10% and had a Physician Global Assessment (PGA) of psoriasis ≥3 on a scale of 0 to 5 (0 = clear to 5 = severe). All patients had been diagnosed with PsA that included two or more swollen joints and two or more painful joints at screening and baseline, patient-reported joint pain for ≥3 months before screening and negative serum rheumatoid factor within 6 months of screening. Efficacy, safety and patient-reported outcomes for the PRESTA study have been published in detail [9-11].

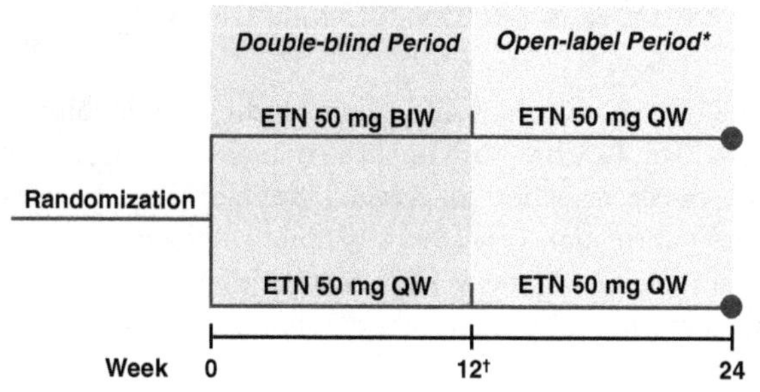

Figure 1 Study design. *Patients/physicians remained blinded to initial randomized treatment groups until end of open-label period. †Primary endpoint was percent of patients achieving clear or almost clear status on PGA of psoriasis at week 12. BIW: twice weekly; ETN: etanercept; PGA: Physician Global Assessment; QW: once weekly.

Pharmacoeconomic outcomes

A pharmacoeconomic questionnaire was used to assess the impact of PsA on employment, which included the following questions:

1. Are you currently employed (working for pay)?
2. Have you changed job responsibilities in the previous month because?
    i. Your arthritis prevented you from continuing your old duties?
    ii. Your psoriasis prevented you from continuing your old duties?
3. How many hours per week were you paid to work in the previous month?
4. How many sick days have you taken off from work in the previous month?

Patients were asked the same questions at baseline, week 12 and week 24. Sick leave was counted as number of days and was not adjusted for expected/planned number of working hours.

Statistical analysis

All patients who completed the pharmacoeconomic questionnaire were included in the employment analyses. Only patients who were working for pay at baseline were included in the analyses of job changes and sick days. Statistical tests were two-tailed with an alpha of 0.05. Last-observation-carried-forward was used for imputation of missing values. Within-group changes from baseline in proportions were tested using McNemar's test; changes from baseline for continuous endpoints were tested using t-tests. Between-group comparisons of proportions were tested using the Cochran-Mantel-Haenszel test; ANCOVA was used for between-group comparisons of continuous endpoints.

Stepwise logistic regression or linear regression analyses were conducted on predictors of employment outcomes at weeks 12 and 24. Separate models were run for those employed and not employed at baseline because follow-up questions about employment characteristics were only asked if the patient indicated that they were employed. The following parameters were included in models used for patients employed at baseline: age, gender, duration of psoriasis, duration of arthritis, treatment, baseline change of job responsibilities (yes or no) for psoriasis, baseline change of job responsibilities (yes or no) for arthritis, baseline sick days, baseline weekly hours worked. For those not in employment at baseline, only age, gender, duration of psoriasis, and duration of arthritis were included as the other information was not available.

The PRESTA study was designed and performed according to the guidelines for Good Clinical Practice and according to the version of the Declaration of Helsinki that was in place during the time the study was conducted.

The protocol and its amendments received independent ethics committee or institutional review board approval and regulatory review and approval before site initiation and recruitment of patients (Additional file 1). All participants signed and dated an approved informed consent form (ICF); the pharmacoeconomic questionnaire was referenced within the ICF.

Results

A total of 752 patients were included in the modified intent-to-treat (mITT) population (n = 379, etanercept 50 mg BIW/QW; n = 373, etanercept 50 mg QW/QW). Baseline demographics and clinical characteristics for the overall mITT population have been described previously; no significant differences were observed between treatment groups, with the exceptions of prior methotrexate use and prior topical steroid use [9-11].

Most patients in this study who were of traditional working age (<65 years old) were employed for pay (61.0%). The proportion of male patients working for pay (68.1%) was higher than female patients (40.3%). Overall employment across the European, Latin American and Asian regions were similar (57.9%, 59.4% and 54.9%, respectively).

Baseline demographics and disease characteristics differed significantly between patients who were employed and those who were not (Table 1). Those with more severe disease and poorer quality of life were less likely to be employed.

The proportion of patients employed increased significantly in the 50 mg BIW/QW group from baseline (56%) to weeks 12 (60%) and 24 (61%; $p \leq 0.003$), but not in the 50 mg QW/QW group (60%, 58% and 60%, respectively; Figure 2). However, differences between groups were not significant at any of the three time intervals, including baseline. The number of hours paid to work per week was 38.3 (BIW/QW group) and 39.2 (QW/QW group) at baseline, and remained steady at 39.5 and 41.8, respectively, by week 24 (p value was not significant between treatment groups).

Significantly higher percentages of patients reported job changes due to arthritis (50 mg BIW/QW: 16.5%; 50 mg QW/QW: 23.0%) than due to psoriasis (10.9% and 13.5%, respectively, $p < 0.0001$ for pooled treatments) at baseline. The proportion of patients who reported having to change job responsibilities due to arthritis or psoriasis decreased significantly from baseline to weeks 12 and 24 in each group ($p < 0.01$; Figure 2). No significant differences were observed between groups at baseline or post-baseline in the proportion of patients who changed job responsibilities because of arthritis or psoriasis symptoms ($p \geq 0.336$).

At baseline, the mean number of monthly sick days taken was 2.4 in both treatment groups; these numbers

Table 1 Baseline demographics and clinical characteristics for employed vs. not employed patients (patient subpopulation <65 years old)

	Employed (n = 431)	Not employed (n = 276)	Total (n = 707)
Age, years	43.6 (9.4)*	47.4 (10.9)	45.1 (10.2)
Gender, male, n (%)	321 (74.5)†	133 (48.2)	454 (64.2)
Race, White, n (%)	386 (89.6)	238 (86.2)	624 (88.3)
Body mass index	27.7 (5.2)	28.3 (5.9)	28.0 (5.5)
Psoriasis disease duration, years	18.0 (10.2)	19.1 (12.6)	18.4 (11.2)
PsA disease duration, years	6.7 (6.7)	7.5 (7.5)	7.0 (7.0)
Physician Psoriasis Assessment (scale: 0–5; higher scores = worse psoriasis)	3.6 (0.6)*	3.7 (0.7)	3.6 (0.7)
PASI (scale: 0–72; higher scores = worse psoriasis)	18.5 (9.5)*	21.4 (11.1)	19.6 (10.3)
BSA affected, %	28.7 (21.4)*	34.7 (23.6)	31.0 (22.5)
PGA of arthritis (scale: 0–100; higher scores = worse arthritis)	48.9 (20.4)*	53.2 (21.5)	50.6 (20.9)
Swollen joints (0–68)	11.4 (13.9)*	14.5 (16.8)	12.6 (15.2)
Tender joints (0–72)	17.6 (16.8)*	22.0 (19.1)	19.4 (17.9)
DLQI, total (scale: 0–30; higher scores = worse dermatology-related quality of life)	11.6 (7.3)*	13.8 (7.7)	12.5 (7.3)
EQ-5D Utility (scale: 0–1; higher scores = better quality of life), mean	0.55 (0.28)*	0.38 (0.35)	0.48 (0.32)
EQ-5D VAS (scale: 1–100; higher scores = better health), mean	58.0 (20.7)*	51.9 (20.6)	55.6 (20.9)
HAQ DI (scale: 0–3; higher scores = more disability), mean	0.72 (0.59)*	1.20 (0.75)	0.91 (0.69)

*$p < 0.01$, for employed vs. not employed, one-way analysis of variance; †$p < 0.01$, for employed vs. not employed, Fisher's Exact Test p-value (2-tail).
Mean (SD), unless otherwise noted.

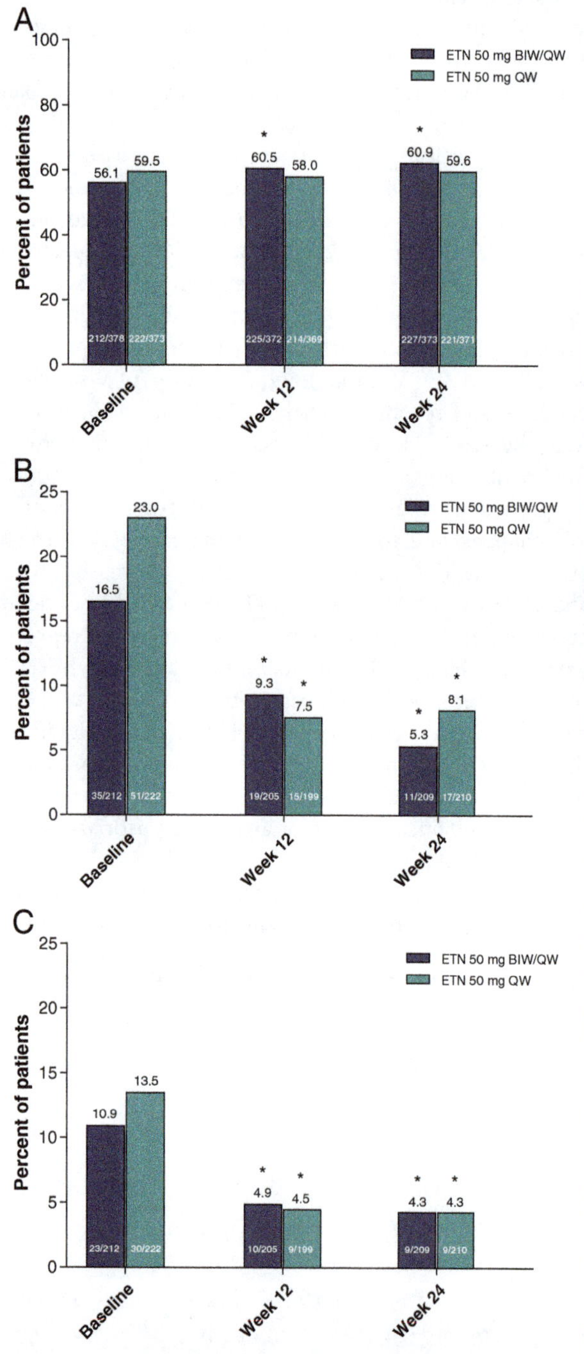

Figure 2 Percent of patients employed and who changed job responsibilities due to arthritis symptoms or psoriasis symptoms. **A**: Percent of patients employed. *$p < 0.003$ for within-group comparisons to baseline (McNemar's test); $p > 0.05$ for between-group comparisons (Cochran-Mantel-Haenszel test). **B**: Percent of patients employed who changed job responsibilities in the previous month due to arthritis symptoms. *$p < 0.004$ for within-group comparisons to baseline (McNemar's test); $p > 0.05$ for between-group comparisons (Cochran-Mantel-Haenszel test). **C**: Percent of patients employed who changed job responsibilities in the previous month due to psoriasis symptoms. *$p < 0.009$ for within-group comparisons to baseline (McNemar's test); $p > 0.05$ for between-group comparisons (Cochran-Mantel-Haenszel test). BIW: twice weekly; ETN: etanercept; QW: once weekly.

declined from baseline to week 24 significantly in both groups (BIW/QW: 68.4%; QW/QW: 47.0%; $p \leq 0.031$), without significant differences between the groups ($p \geq 0.268$; Figure 3).

In those patients who were employed at baseline, treatment with etanercept 50 mg BIW/QW remained a significant predictor of post-baseline employment following adjustment for predictive baseline characteristics (Table 2) (week 12: $p = 0.001$; week 24: $p = 0.02$). Treatment group was not a significant predictor of other post-baseline outcomes (hours worked, sick days, or post-baseline changes in employment due to arthritis or psoriasis), or of becoming employed in those patients not employed at baseline.

In patients employed at baseline, the probability of continued employment was also positively associated at week 12 with the number of hours worked at baseline ($p < 0.0001$) and negatively associated at week 24 with the number of sick days at baseline ($p < 0.001$). Female gender ($p = 0.03$) and fewer weekly hours worked ($p = 0.02$) at baseline were predictors of changing job responsibilities due to psoriasis at week 12 and week 24, respectively; neither was predictive of changing job responsibilities due to PsA at either post-baseline observation. The probability of changing job responsibilities due to PsA was negatively associated with baseline hours worked at week 12 ($p = 0.005$) and week 24 ($p < 0.001$) and also positively associated with older age at week 24 ($p < 0.001$). Baseline sick days and fewer weekly hours worked at baseline were predictive of more sick days recorded at week 12 and week 24 (all $p < 0.01$). In patients not employed at baseline, the probability of becoming employed at weeks 12 and 24 was lower for older patients and females. Duration of psoriasis and duration of psoriatic arthritis

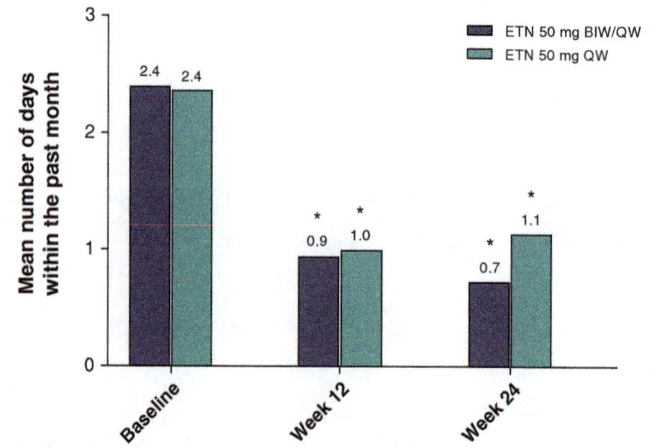

Figure 3 Mean number of sick days taken during the past month. *$p < 0.001$ for within-group comparisons to baseline in BIW/QW group (paired *t*-test); *$p \leq 0.031$ for within-group comparisons to baseline in QW/QW group (paired *t*-test); $p > 0.05$ for between-group comparisons (ANCOVA). ANCOVA: analysis of covariance; BIW: twice weekly; ETN: etanercept; QW: once weekly.

were not predictive of employment, changing job responsibilities or sick days at either week 12 or 24.

Discussion

In the PRESTA trial, treatment of psoriasis and PsA patients with etanercept over 24 weeks resulted in maintenance of employment in both treatment groups. Patients in the higher dose group had statistically significant improvements in the proportions employed, but the baseline proportions of employed patients were lower than in the 50 mg QW/QW dose group. In addition to the percentage of patients remaining employed, the number of hours worked each week improved slightly but not significantly. The majority of senior patients (aged ≥65 years) were not employed, suggesting they were retired and not seeking work. Among the working age patients (aged <65 years) the group who were not employed had more severe disease relative to the employed group. The percentage of employed patients from Europe who were <65 years old in this study (61.2%, 95% CI: 57.2% – 65.1%) is slightly less than the percentage employed in the overall population in the European area who were aged 15 to 64 at the end of 2006 (65%) and 2007 (66%) [12].

One of the strengths of this study is that the pharmacoeconomic questionnaire could distinguish between employment changes due to skin disease symptoms versus arthritis symptoms. In both treatment groups, a larger proportion of patients reported changing job responsibilities due to arthritis symptoms than due to psoriasis symptoms. The proportion of patients who had to change jobs for either reason decreased significantly from baseline to the end of the study.

There was a >47% reduction in sick days after 12 weeks of treatment. These data are comparable with a previous study that looked at treatment of active PsA with etanercept over 24 months [13]. Unlike the current study, those investigators observed a nonsignificant decline in missed work days (absenteeism for any reason) from 0.7 days per 2 weeks at baseline to 0.3 days per month after 2 years of treatment ($p = 0.3436$).

Previous studies have shown that patients with PsA have an elevated rate of work disability relative to normal populations, consistent with our findings at baseline [14]. In addition, etanercept treatment of PsA has been seen to result in impediments to labor (paid or unpaid) declining significantly over 2 years ($p < 0.001$) [13]. Our study did not look specifically at impediments to work, but the data indirectly support the previous research.

Limitations

The PRESTA study was not designed to specifically study employment. Furthermore, the pharmacoeconomic questionnaire used in the PRESTA study has not been validated in other clinical trials. At the time this study was conducted, work productivity questionnaires, including the Work Productivity and Activity Index for psoriasis [15] and for rheumatoid arthritis [16] were not widely used. Although the pharmacoeconomic questionnaire has not undergone extensive validation, the results are similar to other work productivity instruments [13,14]. The pharmacoeconomic questionnaire can also be viewed

Table 2 Predictive ability of baseline characteristics on employment outcomes

Independent variables (X variables used as predictors)	Dependent variables (Y variable being predicted)							
	Employed		Job responsibility change due to psoriasis		Job responsibility change due to PsA		Sick days	
	Week 12	Week 24	Week 12	Week 24	Week 12	Week 24	Week 12	Week 24
Age	NS	NS	1.05 (1.00, 1.11)	NS	NS	1.04 (1.00, 1.09)	NS	NS
Female	NS	NS	3.1 (1.1, 9.0)	NS	NS	NS	NS	NS
Duration of psoriasis	NS	NS	NS	NS	NS	NS	NS	NS
Duration of PsA	NS	NS	NS	NS	NS	NS	NS	NS
ETN BIW/QW	5.2 (1.7, 15.7)	3.0 (1.1, 8.0)	NS	NS	NS	NS	NS	NS
Baseline job change due to psoriasis	NS	NS	22.9 (7.9, 66.3)	10.9 (4.0, 29.9)	3.1 (1.2, 8.6)	NS	2.6 (1.4, 3.8)	3.4 (1.8, 5.0)
Baseline job change due to PsA	NS	NS	NS	NS	4.9 (1.8, 12.9)	6.3 (2.7, 14.6)	NS	-1.7 (-3.0, -0.4)
Baseline sick days*	NS	0.94 (0.90, 0.99)	NS	NS	NS	NS	0.17 (0.11, 0.24)	0.15 (0.08, 0.22)
Baseline hours worked†	1.05 (1.02, 1.08)	NS	NS	0.96 (0.93, 0.99)	0.96 (0.94, 0.98)	0.95 (0.92, 0.97)	-0.04 (-0.06, -0.01)	-0.04 (-0.07, -0.01)

NS = Not significant.

Data for all dependent variables are odds ratio (95% confidence intervals) except Sick days which show slope (95% confidence intervals). *Odds are for a one-day increase in baseline sick days. †Odds are for a one-hour increase in baseline hours worked.

as having face validity – the quality of prompting patients to provide the appropriate information. Both arms of PRESTA involved treatment with etanercept, thus comparisons with placebo were not available. However, one might expect employment to decline slowly for patients with PsA given the cumulative damage to joints that can occur. The lack of a placebo arm in PRESTA raises the possibility that some of the improvement observed with etanercept treatment could be due to regression to the mean although the lack of association between disease duration and employment outcomes reduces the likelihood that this problem was the primary determinant of these results.

Conclusions

For patients with moderate to severe psoriasis and PsA, etanercept provides economic value, in part, by reducing changes in job responsibilities and missed work days.

Abbreviations

BIW: Twice weekly; DLQI: Dermatology Life Quality Index; EQ-5D Utility: EuroQol – 5 Dimension Utility index; EQ-5D VAS: EuroQol – 5 Dimension visual analog scale; HAQ DI: Health Assessment Questionnaire Disability Index; mITT: Modified intent-to-treat; PASI: Psoriasis Area and Severity Index; PsA: Psoriatic arthritis; QW: Once weekly; SD: Standard deviation.

Competing interests

RLB, TW, LM, and RP were employees of Pfizer Inc during the PRESTA study and subsequent analyses. RG has been a paid lecturer and investigator for Pfizer, MSD, Abbvie, Janssen, Celgene and Actelion, and is a member of the Danish National Advisory Boards for MSD, Janssen and Abbvie. SK has been a principal investigator for Abbvie, Janssen, Actelion, Pfizer and a National Advisory Board member for Janssen. WL was an employee of Quintiles Inc. and a paid contractor to Pfizer Inc during the PRESTA study and development of this manuscript.

Authors' contributions

RLB and TW were involved in the design and implementation of the PRESTA study and provided data interpretation. RG and SK were investigators in the PRESTA study and provided data interpretation. WL and RP provided statistical analyses. LM provided valuable clinical insight and data interpretation. All authors provided reviews of each draft of the manuscript and approved the final draft for submission.

Acknowledgment

The PRESTA study was funded by Wyeth, which was acquired by Pfizer Inc in 2009. We would like to thank Tapani Tuominiranta (Hatanpää City Hospital, Tampere, Finland), Bruce Freundlich, Charles Molta and Deborah Robertson (employees of Wyeth during the PRESTA study) for significant contributions to this analysis. Medical writing support was provided by Patricia McChesney and John Bilbruck of Engage Scientific Solutions and was funded by Pfizer.

Author details

[1]Formerly of Pfizer Inc., 3921 Glenlake Garden Drive, Raleigh, NC 27612, USA. [2]Semmelweis University, Budapest, Hungary. [3]Pfizer Inc, Collegeville, PA, USA. [4]University of Copenhagen, Copenhagen, Denmark.

References

1. Gladman DD: **Psoriatic arthritis.** *Dermatol Ther* 2004, **17**:350–363.
2. Gottlieb AB, Chao C, Dann F: **Psoriasis comorbidities.** *J Dermatol Treat* 2008, **19**:5–21.
3. Mease P: **Management of psoriatic arthritis: the therapeutic interface between rheumatology and dermatology.** *Curr Rheumatol Rep* 2006, **8**:348–354.
4. Stern RS, Nijsten T, Feldman SR, Margolis DJ, Rolstad T: **Psoriasis is common, carries a substantial burden even when not extensive, and is associated with widespread treatment dissatisfaction.** *J Investig Dermatol Symp Proc* 2004, **9**:136–139.
5. Dubertret L, Mrowietz U, Ranki A, van de Kerkhof PC, Chimenti S, Lotti T, Schäfer G: **European patient perspectives on the impact of psoriasis: the EUROPSO patient membership survey.** *Br J Dermatol* 2006, **155**:729–736.
6. Gelfand JM, Feldman SR, Stern RS, Thomas J, Rolstad T, Margolis DJ: **Determinants of quality of life in patients with psoriasis: a study from the US population.** *J Am Acad Dermatol* 2004, **51**:704–708.
7. Zachariae H, Zachariae R, Blomqvist K, Davidsson S, Molin L, Mørk C, Sigurgeirsson B: **Quality of life and prevalence of arthritis reported by 5,795 members of the Nordic Psoriasis Associations. Data from the Nordic Quality of Life Study.** *Acta Derm Venereol* 2002, **82**:108–113.
8. Radtke MA, Reich K, Blome C, Rustenbach S, Augustin M: **Prevalence and clinical features of psoriatic arthritis and joint complaints in 2009 patients with psoriasis: results of a German national survey.** *J Eur Acad Dermatol Venereol* 2009, **23**:683–691.
9. Sterry W, Ortonne JP, Kirkham B, Brocq O, Robertson D, Pedersen RD, Estojak J, Molta CT, Freundlich B: **Comparison of two etanercept regimens for treatment of psoriasis and psoriatic arthritis: PRESTA randomised double blind multicentre trial.** *BMJ* 2010, **340**:c147.
10. Gniadecki R, Robertson D, Molta CT, Freundlich B, Pedersen R, Li W, Boggs R, Zbrozek AS: **Self-reported health outcomes in patients with psoriasis and psoriatic arthritis randomized to two etanercept regimens.** *J Eur Acad Dermatol Venereol* 2012, **26**:1436–1443.
11. Prinz JC, Fitzgerald O, Boggs RI, Foehl J, Robertson D, Pedersen R, Molta CT, Freundlich B: **Combination of skin, joint and quality of life outcomes with etanercept in psoriasis and psoriatic arthritis in the PRESTA trial.** *J Eur Acad Dermatol Venereol* 2011, **25**:559–564.
12. **Short-Term Labour Market Statistics: Employment Rate.** http://stats.oecd.org/Index.aspx?QueryId=38900.
13. Gladman DD, Bombardier C, Thorne C, Haraoui B, Khraishi M, Rahman P, Bensen W, Syrotuik J, Poulin-Costello M: **Effectiveness and safety of etanercept in patients with psoriatic arthritis in a Canadian clinical practice setting: the REPArE trial.** *J Rheumatol* 2011, **38**:1355–1362.
14. Wallenius M, Skomsvoll JF, Koldingsnes W, Rødevand E, Mikkelsen K, Kaufmann C, Kvien TK: **Work disability and health-related quality of life in males and females with psoriatic arthritis.** *Ann Rheum Dis* 2009, **68**:685–689.
15. Pearce DJ, Singh S, Balkrishnan R, Kulkarni A, Fleischer AB, Feldman SR: **The negative impact of psoriasis on the workplace.** *J Dermatol Treat* 2006, **17**:24–28.
16. Zhang W, Bansback N, Boonen A, Young A, Singh A, Anis AH: **Validity of the work productivity and activity impairment questionnaire–general health version in patients with rheumatoid arthritis.** *Arthritis Res Ther* 2010, **12**:R177.

8

A laboratory-based study on patients with Parkinson's disease and seborrheic dermatitis: the presence and density of *Malassezia* yeasts, their different species and enzymes production

Valentina S Arsic Arsenijevic[1*], Danica Milobratovic[2], Aleksandra M Barac[1], Berislav Vekic[3], Jelena Marinkovic[4] and Vladimir S Kostic[5]

Abstract

Background: Seborrheic dermatitis (SD) and Parkinson's disease (PD) are frequently associated conditions. Aims of this study were: to determine severity of SD, presence of different species and density of *Malassezia* yeasts; to assess yeast lipases and phosphatases production *in vitro* and to compare these results between SD patients with and without PD.

Methods: This case–control prospective study was conducted at the Dermatology and Neurology Units, Clinical Centre of Serbia and at the National Medical Mycology Reference Laboratory, University of Belgrade Medical School, Serbia. A total of 90 patients and 70 healthy controls (HC) were investigated: 60 patients with SD (SDN) and 30 patients with SD and PD (SDP). Culture-based mycological examination was carried out on lesional skin (LS) and non-lesional skin (NLS). A yeasts density was determined by counting the *Malassezia* colony forming units per tape (CFU/tape). Enzymes production by isolated *Malassezia* was investigated.

Results: The most patients with SD were male (76.7%; SDP and 63.3%; SDN) and the intensity of SD was dominantly severe or moderate (76.7%; SDP and 75%; SDN). The presence of *Malassezia* was high on LS in both groups (87.3%; SDP and 86.7%; SDN) (p=0.667).
The highest yeasts density (mean CFU/tape=67.8) was detected on LS in 53% of SDP group and in 21.7% of SDN group (mean CFU/tape=31.9) ($p < 0.01$). The presence of negative cultures was lower in SDP group (13.3%) in comparison to HC and SDN groups (37% and 31.7%, respectively). *Malassezia* density on NLS in SDP group (mean CFU/tape=44.3) was significantly higher in comparison to SDN and HC (p=0.018). *M. globosa* was the most abundant species identified amongst isolates from the SDP group (42.3%) and exhibited high production of phosphatase and lipase *in vitro*.

Conclusion: From this laboratory-based study a positive correlation between SD, PD, *M. globosa* incidence, high yeast density and high phosphatase and lipase activity was established. Our data lead to conclusion that local skin performance of PD patient's characterized with increased sebum excretion ratio play a role in SD by stimulation of yeasts replication and enzyme production.

Keywords: Seborrheic dermatitis, Parkinson's disease, *Malassezia* species, Colony forming units, Enzymes

* Correspondence: mikomedlab@yahoo.com
[1]Institute of Microbiology and Immunology, University of Belgrade Medical School, Dr Subotica 1, Belgrade, Serbia
Full list of author information is available at the end of the article

Background

Parkinson's disease (PD) is the second most common neurodegenerative disorder which affects approximately seven million people globally and one million people in the United States [1]. The prevalence of PD is about 0.3% of the whole population in industrialized countries, 1% in the elderly over 60 years of age and 4% of the population over 80 years [2]. "Young-onset PD" appears between ages 21 and 40 years with greater probability for developing various adverse effects of treatment, and deterioration of the quality of life [3].

Patients with PD, in addition to motor system disorders, often suffer from non-motile symptoms, which can include decreased facial skin motility resulting in a characteristic hypomimic facial expression, which has an impact on their quality of life [4]. This condition is associated with seborrheic dermatitis (SD) and increased sebum excretion ratio (SER) in almost 60% of the cases most likely due to the parasympathetic system hyperactivity as well as to the systemic effect of Melanocyte-stimulating hormone (MSH) [4,5].

SD is chronic skin disease presented with typical sharply demarcated red patches and plaques with greasy scales in areas with increased density of sebaceous glands, namely the scalp, face, hairline, eyebrow, glabella, nasolabial folds, ears, upper trunk and flexures. SD affects approximately 3-5% of the population [6]. The intensity of symptoms, including inflammation and itching, varies with more severe clinical presentation occurring in predisposed groups. SD prevalence was found to be higher in some medical conditions including HIV positive and AIDS patients (34-83%) [7] and PD patients (52-59%) [8]. Endogenous and exogenous conditions, such as hormones (androgens), increased SER, altered immune response and neurological factors [9,10] were found to play an important role in the pathogenesis of SD, but the exact mechanisms are still to be elucidated.

Evident is recent increased research interest in lipophilic *Malassezia* yeasts. Genus *Malassezia* now contains 14 species, among which 7 are well characterized culturally and biochemically [11]. Members of this genus are part of normal human flora, however they are also thought to be exacerbating factor in a number of skin conditions, such as pityriasis versicolor, *Malassezia* folliculitis, SD, atopic dermatitis and even some life threatening nosocomial bloodstream infections [12,10]. *Malassezia* species and their skin density vary in different populations [13], countries, age groups and genders, as well as between normal, non-lesional skin (NLS) and lesional skin (LS) [14,11]. For currently unknown reason, these yeasts can change their saprophytic state and invade stratum corneum of the skin as pathogens.

Although SD is a multifactorial disease, there are two major factors in developing SD: the increased production of host sebum and the presence and increased reproduction of *Malassezia* yeasts. The presence and density of *Malassezia* yeasts, different species and production of enzymes in PD patients have not been investigated yet, thus the aim of this study was to determine the following: (I) the severity of SD in study group, (II) the presence and density of *Malassezia* and (III) enzyme production in isolated species in patients with SD and PD.

Methods

Source population

PD and SD patients treated at the Neurology and the Dermatology Units, Clinical Centre of Serbia from January to June 2011 were included in this study.

Study population

There were 90 patients with SD, 21 to 82 years old, (61 men, 29 women; mean age 54 ± 17.5 years), among those 30 patients suffered from PD and SD at the same time (SDP group, 23 men, 7 women; mean age 67 ± 7 years) while 60 patients had SD only (SDN group, 38 men, 22 women; mean age 48 ± 18 years). Healthy control (HC) group were persons without SD ($n = 60$) randomly selected and matched by age and sex (44 men, 26 women; mean age 49 ± 19.5 years). HC had apparently normal facial skin, without any evidence of dermatitis. None of these patients had received topical or systemic antifungal therapy or corticosteroids for at least 4 weeks prior to sampling. All patients signed informed consents.

Study design

This was a prospective case–control study which was conducted at the National Reference Medical Mycology Laboratory, Faculty of Medicine, University of Belgrade (laboratory-based investigation) and at Neurology and the Dermatology Units, Clinical Center of Serbia (clinically-based investigation). Determination of SD severity and laboratory-based investigation was done in order to determine the *Malassezia* yeast presence and their density, type and enzymes production.

Determination of SD severity

A clinical assessment of SD was carried out and scored. The overall SD score was calculated by scoring the severity of SD (from 1 to 12) and the facial skin area affected (from 1 to 5). The severity of SD was evaluated according to the presence of: erythema, scale, infiltration and pustule. A four-point score was used for each parameter (0–absent, 1–mild, 2–moderate, 3–severe). The second scale was based on the percentage of the affected skin area: less than 10% (1 point), 10-30% (2 points), 30-50% (3 points), 50-70% (4 points) and over 70% (5 points). The result was obtained by multiplying the scores of both scales giving an overall score: mild SD (5 or less);

moderate SD (6 to 11) and severe SD (from 12 to 60). Severity of SD has been described as: mild (the total score ≤5); moderate (the total score between 6 and 11); and severe (the total score between 12 and 60) [15].

Sampling procedure, isolation and quantification of *Malassezia* yeast

Three skin samples were taken from SD patients' foreheads, from LS and NLS, as well as from normal-looking skin from the foreheads of HC. The sampling was done by stripping 4 cm^2 tape (Superabsorb® F, Lohmann Rauscher) [16]. Each tape was transferred to Dixon and Leeming-Notman agar (LNA) in order to isolate *Malassezia* lipophilic yeast and to Sabouraud agar in order to isolate non-lipophilic yeasts *M. pachydermatis* or *Candida*. Plates were incubated at 32°C for 10 days and observed daily. The cultures were considered positive for *Malassezia* if there was growth on Dixon and LNA. Yeasts isolates were quantified and identified using morphological and biochemical tests. The number of *Malassezia* colonies was counted and the growth densities were expressed as the mean number of colony forming units per tape (mean CFU/tape). The *Malassezia* density (CFU/tape) was performed of Dixon and LNA media and ranked into three levels: low (CFU/tape 1 ≤ 19), medium (CFU/tape =20-40) and high (CFU/tape > 40) [13]. Production of enzymes from the protease, lipase, phosphatase and glycosidase classes was determined for selected isolates.

Identification of Malassezia yeasts

Seven lipophylic *Malassezia* species were identified: *M. globosa, M. furfur, M. slooffiae M. sympodialis, M. restricta, M. obtusa* and *M. japonica* based on microscopic characteristics, presence of catalase and the ability of each isolate to utilize different Tweens [17]. The presence of catalase was determined by applying a drop of 10% hydrogen peroxide on a culture smeared on a glass slide. The production of gas bubbles indicated a positive reaction. The ability to utilize different Tween substrate was assessed on the agar plates, by spreading fresh yeast suspension onto plates. Tween 20, 40, 60 and 80 (5 µl) were added in 4 wells (2 mm diameter) in each plate. The plates were incubated at 32°C for one week and the growth of yeast around individual wells contain different Tween was recorded and *Malassezia* were identified (Figure 1).

Determination of *Malassezia* yeasts enzyme production by ApiZym assay

The activity of 19 different enzymes produced by *Malassezia* was tested using the API Zym assay (bioMerieux, Marcy l'Etoile, France). A total of 26 *Malassezia* isolates from SD groups were tested for: proteases (n = 5), lipases (n = 3), phosphatases (n = 3), glycosidases (n = 8). Results were expressed semi-quantitatively, ranging from no activity to maximum enzymatic activity.

Data collection

All subjects had a complete history, physical examinations and necessary procedures from skin were done to confirm the diagnosis. Trained mycologists carried out laboratory analysis and were engaged in data collection and data entry.

Data analysis

Statistical analysis was done using the Statistical Package for Social Science (SPSS) program version 15.0. T-test was used to analyze the differences between severity of disease and demographic data; Mann–Whitney and Kruskal Wallis tests were used to analyze the median number of *Malassezia* CFU/tape within the same groups on LS and NLS and the median number of *Malassezia* CFU/tape from all patients with SD and HC. Chi-square tests were performed to determine the differences in: (I) the prevalence of different species of *Malassezia* in SDN and SDP groups, (II) the prevalence of different species of *Malassezia* in all patients with SD and HC. The relationship between study groups and culture-based mycological findings was determined by logistic regression analyses adjusted on sex and age.

The study was approved by the Ethical Board of the School of Medicine, University of Belgrade, and the Clinical Center of Serbia (No 5030/5). The anonymity of individuals was preserved during the study.

Results

Patient's demographic data and determination of SD severity

Most SD patients were male (77%; SDP and 63%; SDN) ($p < 0.01$) and intensity of SD was dominantly in severe or moderate form (76.7%; SDP and 75%; SDN). Taking into account SD categories, there was no statistically significant difference between SDP and SDN groups in terms of SD severity: mild (23.3%; SDP and 25%; SDN); moderate (60%; SDP and 45%; SDN); severe (17%; SDP and 30%; SDN) ($p = 0.175$) (Table 1). However, when SD was measured by scale there was a significant difference between SDP and SDN patients (OR 0.81; 95%CI = 0.66-0.99; $p = 0.043$).

The correlation between presence and growth density of *Malassezia* yeasts on LS and NLS

Comparison of *Malassezia* counts (CFU/tape) on LS and NLS between studied groups was carried out. The correlation between negative cultures and growth density of *Malassezia* yeasts on LS and NLS is shown on Table 2. The presence of *Malassezia* was high in LS in both groups (87.3%; SDP and 86.7%; SDN) ($p = 0.667$). The highest yeasts density (mean CFU/tape = 67.8) was detected on

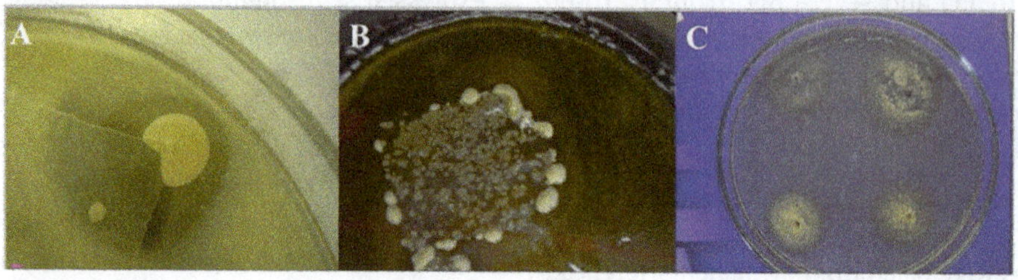

Figure 1 Pictures of isolated *Malassezia* on culture. Colony forming unit's per tape (CFU/tape) expressed low density of *Malassezia* yeasts isolated on Leeming-Notman agar (LNA) from non-lesional skin (NLS) in healthy controls (HC) **(A)**; high density of *Malassezia* yeasts isolated on Dixon agar from lesional skin (LS) in Parkinson disease (PD) **(B)** and identification of *Malassezia* by Tween assimilation test **(C)**.

LS in 53% of SDP group and in 21.7% of SDN group (mean CFU/tape = 31.9) (p < 0.01). The mean CFU/tape on NLS was the highest in the SDP (mean CFU/tape = 44.3) followed by SDN (mean CFU/tape = 19.8) and HC (mean CFU/tape = 17.4) (p < 0.01). Correlation between studied groups in *Malassezia* CFU/tape on NLS highlighting significantly higher *Malassezia* density in SDP group (p = 0.018) (Table 2).

The prevalence of different *Malassezia* species and their enzyme production

The prevalence of different *Malassezia* isolated from NLS and LS in studied groups is shown in Figure 2. The most prevalent species in SDP/LS was *M. globosa* 11/26 (42.3%), followed by *M. furfur* 7/26 (26.9%) and *M. obtusa* 4/26 (15.4%). In SDN/LS the most prevalent species was *M. slooffiae* 14/53 (26. 5%), followed by *M. sympodialis* 9/53 (17%) and *M. globosa* 9/53 (17%) (p = 0.023). The differences were noted only for *M. globosa* (42.3%; SDP/LS) and *M. sloffiae* (26.4%; SDN/LS) (p < 0.05).

On NLS the most common species were: *M. slooffiae* (22%) in SDN group; *M. globosa* (25%) in HC and *M. globosa* (42.3%) in PD group. In SDP group the most prevalent species (*M. globosa, M. furfur* and *M. obtusa*) were the same on LS and NLS. The observed difference between isolated *Malassezia* on LS vs. NLS was not statistically significant for SDN and HC groups (SDN; p = 0.933), (HC; p = 0.541) (Figure 2).

The observed data suggest a significant role of infection, presence of different *Malassezia* species and yeast density in ethiopathogenesis of SD. Therefore, we evaluated the hypothesis that *Malassezia* yeasts replication and lipases production on the host skin may be important for pathogenesis of SD. Thus we tested (selection of isolates, n = 26) for production of different enzyme classes *in vitro*. All phosphatase and lipase enzymes were produced in significant amount from all tested *Malassezia* isolates. High rate of β–glucuronidase and leucine arylamidase activity was detected at *M. furfur* isolates only (Table 3).

Correlation between study groups and culture-based mycological findings

The correlation between studied groups and culture-based mycological findings performed by logistic regression analysis for sex and age showed significant higher intensity of SD in SDN group (OR 0.81; 95% CI = 0.66-0.99; p = 0.043) (Table 4). Our data demonstrated predominant male sex in patients with SD and moderate or severe form of SD in both studied groups. There was no difference between studied groups in SD severity regarding categories, but when SD was measured by scale SD severity was a

Table 1 Demographics and description of SD

Variables	Healthy Control (HC) n = 70	SDN n = 60	SDP n = 30	Total n = 160	p
Demographics					
Sex M/F (%)	26/44 (37.1)	38/22(63.3)	23/7 (76.7)	87/73 (54.4)	0.000
Age	48.7 ± 19.9	48.3 ± 17.9	66.6 ± 6.3*	51.9 ± 18.7	0.000
Description of SD					
Intensity	-	8.65 ± 6.7	6.9 ± 2.7	8.1 ± 5.7	0.175
Intensity in categories					0.314
Mild (≤5)	-	15 (25)	7 (23.3)	22 (24.2)	
Moderate (>5 and < 12)	-	27 (45)	18 (60)	45 (50)	
Sever (≥ 12)	-	18 (30)	5 (16.7)	23 (25.6)	

Abbreviations: *HC*, Healthy controls; *SD*, Seborrheic dermatitis; *SDN*, Seborrheic dermatitis in patients without Parkinson disease; *SDP*, Seborrheic dermatitis in patients with Parkinson disease; *M*, Male; *F*, Female; *p<0.05.

Table 2 Comparison of *Malassezia* colonies number (CFU/tape) on lesional and non-lesional skin between studied groups

The characteristics of experiment					
LS	**HC n = 70**	**SDN n = 60**	**SDP n = 30**	**Total n = 160**	**p**
Number of colonies (CFU/tape)	-	31.9 ± 38.1	67.8 ± 51.7	43.9 ± 46.1	0.006
Number of colonies in categories	-				
None	-	7 (11.7)	4 (13.3)	11 (12.2)	
Low CFU/tape (≤20)		30 (50)	3 (10)	33 (20.6)	
Medium CFU/tape (20–49)	-	10 (16.7)	7 (23.3)	17 (10,6)	
High CFU/tape (≥ 50)	-	13 (21.7)	16 (53.3)	29 (18.1)	
NLS					
Number of colonies (CFU/tape)	17.4 ± 30.1	19.8 ± 31.1	44.3 ± 44.7**	23.4 ± 34.9	0.018
Number of colonies in categories					
None	26 (37.1)	19 (31.7)	4*** (13.3)	49 (30.6)	
Low CFU/tape (≤20)	27 (38.6)	23 (38.3)	11 (36.7)	61 (38.1)	
Medium CFU/tape (20–49)	9 (12.9)	9 (15)	4 (13.3)	22 (13.7)	
High CFU/tape (≥ 50)	8 (11.4)	9 (15.0)	11 (36.7)	28 (17.5)	

Abbreviations: *HC*, Healthy controls; *SDN*, Seborrheic dermatitis in patients without Parkinson disease; *SDP*, seborrheic dermatitis in patients with Parkinson disease; *LS*, Lesional skin; *NLS*, Non-lesional skin; *CFU*, Colony forming units; **p < 0.05; ***p <0.01.

significantly higher in SDN group (logistic regression analyses for sex and age) (Table 4). Therefore, a positive correlation between SD, PD, *M. globosa*, high yeast density and high phosphatase and lipase activity of *Malassezia* yeasts was observed. This may suggest the possible role of the skin SER in PD patients for yeasts replication and lipases enzyme production.

Discussion

The concept of skin as a mirror of Parkinsonism dates back to the beginning of the last century. Since then, a good deal of evidence has been accumulated in support of the causal association between the neurological disturbance and changes detectable on areas of the integument with the richest sebaceous gland supply. SD is a common

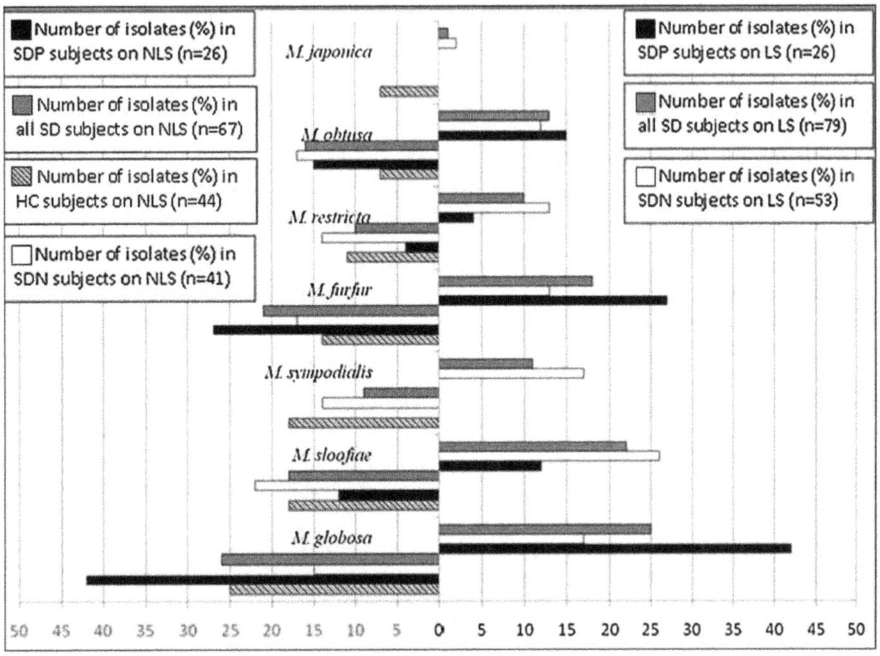

Figure 2 Quantitative graphical presentation of different *Malassezia* species. Graphical presentation based on the percent of total positive culture on LNA and Dixon media, isolated from non lesional skin (NLS) and lesional skin (LS) on the: (i) all patients with SD; (ii) patients with SD and without Parkinson's disease (SDN); (iii) patients with SD and Parkinson's disease (SDP) and (iv) healthy controls (HC).

Table 3 Enzymatic activity of different *Malassezia* species determined by the Api Zym assay

Class of enzymes	Type of enzymes	All strains n = 26 (%)	*M. furfur* n = 9 (%)	*M. globosa* n = 7 (%)	*M. slooffiae* n = 4 (%)	*M. obtusa* n = 6 (%)
Proteases	Leucine arylamidase	11 (42)	7 (78)	2 (29)	1 (25)	1 (17)
	Valine arylamidase	ø	ø	ø	ø	ø
	Cystine arylamidase	ø	ø	ø	ø	ø
	Trypsin	ø	ø	ø	ø	ø
	α - Chymotrypsin	ø	ø	ø	ø	ø
Lipases	Lipase (C14)	14 (54)	6 (67)	4 (57)	3 (75)	2 (33)
	Esterase lipase (C8)	25 (96)	9 (100)	7 (100)	4 (100)	5 (83)
	Esterase (C4)	25 (96)	6 (67)	4 (57)	3 (75)	2 (33)
Phosphatases	Acid phosphatase	26 (100)	7 (100)	7 (100)	4 (100)	6 (100)
	Alkaline phosphatase	18 (69)	7 (78)	4 (57)	3 (75)	3 (50)
	Naphthol-AS-BI- phosphohydrolase	23 (89)	8 (89)	7 (100)	4 (100)	5 (83)
Glycosidase	β – Glucuronidase	9 (35)	3 (33)	2 (29)	2 (50)	2 (33)
	α - Galactosidase	ø	ø	ø	ø	ø
	β - Galactosidase	ø	ø	ø	ø	ø
	N -acetil-β-glucosaminadase	ø	ø	ø	ø	ø
	α - Glucosidase	ø	ø	ø	ø	ø
	β - Glucosidase	ø	ø	ø	ø	ø
	α - Mannosidase	ø	ø	ø	ø	ø
	α - Fucosidase	ø	ø	ø	ø	ø

Data showed all type of enzymes from lipase and phosphate classes detected in a high percentage from the tested species isolated in this study.

chronic and relapsing inflammatory skin disorder which primarily affects sebum rich areas. The prevalence of SD is 11.6% in USA [6] but can be higher in elderly people (over 80%) [5] and in Parkinsonism (52–59.5%) [8]. In recent years, a few studies concerning SD and PD have been published [18-20]. To our best knowledge, this is the first culture-based epidemiology study performed on patients with SD and PD. In the present study male SDP was dominant and this was in agreement with the study carried out by Gupta who explained the observed result by stronger action of androgens in the male SD patients [20], as well as with the study by Wooten who found a male to female ratio in PD of 1.49 [21]. Mean age of our SDP patients was 67 ± 7 years (Table 1) which was in agreement with studies restricted to individuals 65 years or above, confirming that the median incidence rate of PD was considerably higher in group above 60 year old [22].

The severity of SD depends on medical conditions and underlying diseases [13,11]. Accordingly, we observed a high

Table 4 Correlation between study groups and culture-based mycological findings expressed as number and presence of *Malassezia* colonies on lesional and non-lesional skin

Variables/potential classificatory of selected groups	Logistic regression analysis adjusted on age and sex (OR; 95% CI; p)		
	SDN vs. SDP	HC vs. SDN	HC vs. SDP
Intensity of SD	0.81; 0.66-0.99; 0.043*	-	-
Intensity of SD in categories	0.46; 0.20-1.04; 0.063	-	-
Number of colonies (CFU/tape) on LS	1.01; 0.99-1.02; 0.110	-	-
Number of colonies (CFU/tape) on LS by categories	1.51; 0.62-3.64; 0.363	-	-
Number of colonies (CFU/tape) on NLS	1.01; 0.99-1.02; 0.398	0.99; 0.98-1.01; 0.786	1.01; 0.99-1.02; 0.288
Number of colonies (CFU/tape) on NLS by categories	1.35; 0.56-3.29; 0.504	0.98; 0.54-1.78; 0.954	1.60; 0.75-3.42; 0.225
Presence of *Malassezia* on LS	0.89; 0.17-4.68; 0.898	-	-
Presence of *Malassezia* on NLS	1.89; 0.45-8.02; 0.387	0.97; 0.44-2.12; 0.933	2.32; 0.63-8.53; 0.206

Abbreviations: *OR*, Odds ratio; *CI*, Confidence interval; *SD*, Seborrheic dermatitis; *SDN*, Seborrheic dermatitis in patients without Parkinson disease; *SDP*, Seborrheic dermatitis in patients with Parkinson disease; *HC*, Healthy controls; *LS*, Lesional skin; *NLS*, Non-lesional skin; *CFU*, Colony forming units; *p<0.05.

number of SDP with moderate or severe SD form and a high number of positive cultures (Table 2). Our data could be explained by predominant male gender and an increased level of SER and MSH secretion in PD patients [23].

Our culture-based study demonstrated six different *Malassezia* isolated in SDP patients, with *M. globosa* (42.3%) as the most dominant species (Figure 1). Several studies identified *M. globosa* as the most prevalent species in SD, suggesting its principal role in SD [24] but data for patients with PD have not been reported yet. By comparing the severity of SD and *Malassezia* presence on LS we did not find a significant difference between studied groups. By contrast, using the laboratory based quantitative test for *Malassezia* yeasts density (expressed as CFU/tape) we found more than twice higher CFU/tape for SDP/LS than SDN/LS group. Literature data are controversial; some studies showed that the density increases with the intensity of skin lesions, while other studies were unable to confirm this result [10]. However, the reduction of *Malassezia* yeast density always results in SD outcome improvement [14].

The effects of the anti-Parkinson's agent L-dopa on SD have been reportedly evaluated in Parkinson's and data showed that treatment with L-dopa restores MHC-inhibiting factor synthesis and reduces sebum secretion in Parkinson's [25]. Our patients were treated with L-dopa during the course of this study so this can be reason for the similarity in the clinical findings between different groups, even high SD intensity in SDN group (Table 4). However, other factors contribute to SD development such as facial immobility ("mask-like face") which may lead to an increased sebum accumulation.

The pathogenesis of SD is still not completely understood but some clinical studies indicated that *Malassezia* presence and replication plays a pivotal role. Positive clinical response of SD to antifungals (i.e., azoles, ciclopirox) could be explained by their role in reduction of *Malassezia* yeast proliferation, again confirming an important role of *Malassezia* density and infection in pathogenesis of SD.

Malassezia requires exogenous specific lipids for growth, therefore tends to appear on skin around the time of puberty, when there is an increase in androgens and consequently an elevation in sebum production [12]. In patients with SD triglycerides and cholesterol are usually elevated but squalene and free fatty acids were significantly decreased compared to normal controls. Free fatty acids are formed from triglycerides through the action of bacterial lipases such as *Propionibacterium acnes*. This suggests that an imbalance of microbial flora and alterations in the composition of skin surface lipids may be involved [26].

Malassezia represents a part of human flora normally colonizing the skin surface but in some conditions it can change its saprophytic state and invade stratum corneum. Some culture-based laboratory studies identified differences between NLS and LS in the percentage of negative culture or in the presence and density of *Malassezia* [13]. We did not find significant difference in the absence of *Malassezia* on NLS between HC and SDN, but very low number of negative *Malassezia* cultures was detected on NLS in SDP. It may suggest an important role of the host environment such as the SER in PD group which may provide favorable conditions for expressing higher virulence capacity of *Malassezia*. Recent study showed a possible role of lipase in the host environment to produce free fatty acids, which are important for enhancing the *Malassezia* virulence [27]. The mechanisms of the *Malassezia* transition from commensal to pathogen are not clear yet, but this evidence is important for further studies due to the fact that lipases are further involved in the release of arachidonic acid, which can be important in cutaneous inflammation and disease [28].

It is well known that the development of infections depends on microbe's replication while the severity of disease may depend of microbe's enzyme production. In pathogenicity of SD phosphatase and lipase yeasts enzymes can initiate inflammatory response by releasing oleic and arahidonic acids from the sebum lipids [12,28]. Fatty acids have direct irritant and desquamative effects on keratinocytes, while arahidonic acid metabolized by cyclooxigenase serves as a source of pro-inflammatory eicosanoides and leads to inflammation and damage to stratum corneum. Our strains tested for different enzymes classes' expressed all type of phosphatase and lipase enzymes manly at a high level (Table 4). These findings suggest that the infection, yeasts replication and density are key pathogenic mechanisms in SD and can contribute to the development of *Malassezia*-driven pathogenic "vicious circle", which closes due to the fact that saturated fatty acids, released by *Malassezia* lipase, are used as a "proliferative fuel" for these yeasts. *M. globosa* showed the highest lipase activity, suggesting that lipase could be a pathogenic factor in the skin diseases associated with different *Malassezia* and providing an explanation about *M. globosa* as the most important pathogenic species in PD patients with SD [29].

Literature data suggest the role of another mechanism in pathogenicity of SD. Beside infection the allergy host reaction to *Malassezia* antigens can be involved in SD. In atopic patients, some enzymes from protease and glycosidase classes, such as β–glucuronidase and leucine arylamidase, may act as antigens. Thus, genetic predisposition, as well as *Malassezia* antigens can lead to the local skin immune response and immunopathology and to development of SD [12,29,30]. In our study we clearly demonstrated very low impact of enzymes which may act as *Malassezia* antigens (Table 3).

Conclusions

This is the first culture-based epidemiology study performed on patients with SD and PD. The data demonstrated a positive correlation between SD, PD and *Malassezia* presence and density. Our findings that SDP group had high yeast density and associated high phosphatase and lipase activity *in vitro* may lead to conclusion that infection is the key mechanism of SD in PD patients. Future better understanding of the interactions between different *Malassezia* and PD host may provide new opportunities for improved SD control in PD. The appropriate antifungal treatment can be useful for PD patients. Antifungals may reduce *Malassezia* growth and their enzymes production overall improving patients well-being and quality of life. Correlation between reduction of *Malassezia* density, positive outcome of SD and the reduction of the non-motile symptoms in PD patients need to be further investigated.

Abbreviations

SD: Seborrheic dermatitis; PD: Parkinson's disease; SDP: Patients with SD and PD; SDN: Patients with SD without PD; HC: Healthy controls; LS: Lesional skin; NLS: Non-lesional skin; CFU/tape: Colony forming units per tape; SER: Sebum excretion ratio; MSH: Melanocyte-stimulating hormone.

Competing interests

The authors declare that they have no competing interests.

Authors' contributions

VAA and DM were involved in study design, data collection, and analysis and results interpretation. DM and AB had done laboratory tests and data presentation. BV and JM were involved in data correlation and interpretation. VAA and VK were responsible for laboratory and clinical part of the study, had advisory and supervisory role and were responsible for important intellectual content. All authors drafted the manuscript and made substantial contributions to the revised manuscript. All authors read and approved the final manuscript.

Acknowledgment

The paper has been published with the supports of the Projects of Ministry of Education, Science and Technology of the Republic of Serbia (grants No OI 175034 and No OI 175033) and Pfizer H.C.P. Corporation, Serbia. We thank Dr Milena Radulović (University of Belgrade School of Dental Medicine, Belgrade, Serbia), Dr Jasmina Nikodinović Runić (Laboratory of Molecular Genetics and Microbial Ecology, University of Belgrade Institute of Molecular Genetics and Genetic Engineering) and Smiljka Surla (London, UK) for correction of English language in the manuscript.

Author details

[1]Institute of Microbiology and Immunology, University of Belgrade Medical School, Dr Subotica 1, Belgrade, Serbia. [2]Department of Dermatology, Dermatology Unit, Clinical Center of Serbia; Military Medical Centre, Belgrade, Serbia. [3]Management School, Alfa University, Belgrade, Serbia. [4]Institutes for Statistics and Medical Informatics, University of Belgrade School of Medicine, Belgrade, Serbia. [5]Institute of Neurology Clinical Centre of Serbia, University of Belgrade, School of Medicine, Belgrade, Serbia.

References

1. Yao SC, Hart AD, Terzella MJ: **An evidence-based osteopathic approach to Parkinson disease.** *Osteopath Fam Physician* 2013, **5:**96–101.
2. de Lau LM, Breteler MM: **Epidemiology of Parkinson's disease.** *Lancet Neurol* 2006, **5:**525–535.
3. Kostić VS: **Treatment of young-onset Parkinson's disease: role of dopamine receptor agonists.** *Parkinsonism Relat Disord* 2009, **15:**71–75.
4. Shuster S, Thody AJ, Goolamali SK, Burton JL, Plummer N, Bates D: **Melanocyte-stimulating hormone and parkinsonism.** *Lancet* 1973, **3:**463–464.
5. Binder RL, Jonelis FJ: **Seborrheic dermatitis in neuroleptic induced Parkinsonism.** *Arch Dermatol* 1983, **119:**473–475.
6. Naldi L, Rebora A: **Clinical practice: seborrheic dermatitis.** *N Engl J Med* 2009, **360:**387–396.
7. Marino CT, McDonald E, Romano JF: **Seborrheic dermatitis in acquired immunodeficiency syndrome.** *Cutis* 1991, **50:**217–218.
8. Braak H, del Tredici K: **Non-dopaminergic pathology in Parkinson's disease.** In *The Non-Motor and Non-Dopaminergic Features of Parkinson's Disease.* Edited by Olanow CW, Stocchi F, Lang AE. Oxford: Blackwell Publishing Ltd; 2011:40–41.
9. Mastrolonardo M: **Seborrheic dermatitis, increased sebum excretion and Parkinson's disease: a survey of (im)possible links.** *Med Hypotheses* 2003, **60:**907–911.
10. Ashbee HR, Evans EGV: **Immunology of disease associated with *Malassezia* species.** *Clin Microbiol Rev* 2002, **15:**21–57.
11. Gaitanis G, Magiatis P, Hantschke M, Bassukas ID, Velegraki A: **The Malassezia genus in skin and systemic diseases.** *Clin Microbiol Rev* 2012, **25:**106–141.
12. Gupta AK, Batra R, Bluhm R, Boekhout T, Dawson TL Jr: **Skin diseases associated with *Malassezia* species.** *J Am Acad Dermatol* 2004, **51:**785–798.
13. Gupta AK, Kohli Y, Summerbell RC, Faergemann J: **Quantitative culture of Malassezia species from different body sites of individuals with or without dermatoses.** *Med Mycol* 2001, **39:**243–251.
14. Pechère M, Krischer J, Remondat C, Bertrand C, Trellu L, Saurat JH: ***Malassezia* spp. carriage in patients with seborrheic dermatitis.** *J Dermatol* 1999, **26:**558–561.
15. Koca R, Altinyazar HC, Esturk E: **Is topical metronidazole effective in seborrheic dermatitis? A double blind study.** *Int J Dermatol* 2003, **42:**632–635.
16. Pechère M, Remondat C, Bertrand C, Didierjean L, Saurat JH: **A simple quantitative culture of Malassezia spp. in HIV-positive persons.** *Dermatology* 1995, **191:**348–349.
17. Guillot J, Guého E, Lesourd M, Midgley G, Chevrier G, Dupont B: **Identification of *Malassezia* species.** *J Mycol Med* 1996, **6:**103–110.
18. Aubin F, Blanc D, Guinchard C, Agache P: **Absence of minocycline in sebum?** *J Dermatol* 1989, **16:**369–373.
19. Villares JC, Carlini EA: **Sebum secretion in idiopathic Parkinson's disease: effect of anticholinergic and dopaminergic drugs.** *Acta Neurol Scand* 1989, **80:**57–63.
20. Gupta AK, Kohli Y: **Prevalence of *Malassezia* species on various body sites in clinically healthy subjects representing different age groups.** *Med Mycol* 2004, **42:**35–42.
21. Wooten GF, Currie LJ, Bovbjerg VE, Lee JK, Patrie J: **Are men at greater risk for Parkinson's disease than women?** *J Neurol Neurosurg Psychiatry* 2004, **75:**637–639.
22. Hirtz D, Thurman DJ, Gwinn-Hardy K, Mohamed M, Chaudhuri AR, Zalutsky R: **How common are the "common" neurologic disorders?** *Neurology* 2007, **68:**326–337.
23. Martignoni E, Godi L, Pacchetti C, Berardesca E, Vignoli GP, Albani G, Mancini F, Nappi G: **Is seborrhea a sign of autonomic impairment in Parkinson's disease?** *J Neural Transm* 1997, **104:**1295–1304.
24. Rincon S, Celis A, Sopo L, Motta A, Cepero de Garcia MC: ***Malassezia* yeast species isolated from patients with dermatologic lesions.** *Biomedica* 2005, **25:**189–195.
25. Milani M, di Molfetta SA, Gramazio R, Fiorella C, Frisario C, Fuzio E, Marzocca V, Zurilli M, di Turi G, Felice G: **Efficacy of betamethasone valerate 0.1% thermophobic foam in seborrhoeic dermatitis of the scalp: an open-label, multicentre, prospective trial on 180 patients.** *Curr Med Res Opin* 2003, **19:**342–345.
26. Bolognia JL: **Dermatology.** In *Dermatology: 3e Expert Consult Premium Edition.* Edited by Bolognia JL, Jorizzo JL, Schaffer JV. Spain: Elsevier; 2012:75–77.
27. Lee YW, Lee SY, Jung WH: **Evaluation of expression of Lipases and Phospholipases of Malassezia in Patient with Seborrheic Dermatitis.** *Ann Dermatol* 2013, **25:**310–314.
28. Juntachai W, Oura T, Kajiwara S: **Purification and characterization of a secretory lipolytic enzyme, MgLIP2, from *Malassezia globosa*.** *Microbiology* 2011, **157:**3492–3499.

29. Juntachai W, Oura T, Murayama SY, Kajiwara S: **The lipolytic enzymes activities of *Malassezia* species.** *Med Mycology* 2009, **47**:477–484.
30. de Angelis YM, Gemmer CM, Kaczvinsky JR, Kenneally DC, Schwartz JR, Dawson TL Jr: **Three etiologic facets of dandruff and seborrheic dermatitis: *Malassezia* fungi, sebaceous lipids and individual sensitivity.** *J Investig Dermatol Symp Proc* 2005, **10**:295–297.

Exploring the association between Morgellons disease and Lyme disease: identification of *Borrelia burgdorferi* in Morgellons disease patients

Marianne J Middelveen[1], Cheryl Bandoski[2], Jennie Burke[3], Eva Sapi[2], Katherine R Filush[2], Yean Wang[3], Agustin Franco[3], Peter J Mayne[1] and Raphael B Stricker[1,4*]

Abstract

Background: Morgellons disease (MD) is a complex skin disorder characterized by ulcerating lesions that have protruding or embedded filaments. Many clinicians refer to this condition as delusional parasitosis or delusional infestation and consider the filaments to be introduced textile fibers. In contrast, recent studies indicate that MD is a true somatic illness associated with tickborne infection, that the filaments are keratin and collagen in composition and that they result from proliferation and activation of keratinocytes and fibroblasts in the skin. Previously, spirochetes have been detected in the dermatological specimens from four MD patients, thus providing evidence of an infectious process.

Methods & Results: Based on culture, histology, immunohistochemistry, electron microscopy and molecular testing, we present corroborating evidence of spirochetal infection in a larger group of 25 MD patients. Irrespective of Lyme serological reactivity, all patients in our study group demonstrated histological evidence of epithelial spirochetal infection. Strength of evidence based on other testing varied among patients. Spirochetes identified as *Borrelia* strains by polymerase chain reaction (PCR) and/or in-situ DNA hybridization were detected in 24/25 of our study patients. Skin cultures containing *Borrelia* spirochetes were obtained from four patients, thus demonstrating that the organisms present in dermatological specimens were viable. Spirochetes identified by PCR as *Borrelia burgdorferi* were cultured from blood in seven patients and from vaginal secretions in three patients, demonstrating systemic infection. Based on these observations, a clinical classification system for MD is proposed.

Conclusions: Our study using multiple detection methods confirms that MD is a true somatic illness associated with *Borrelia* spirochetes that cause Lyme disease. Further studies are needed to determine the optimal treatment for this spirochete-associated dermopathy.

Keywords: Morgellons disease, Lyme disease, *Borrelia burgdorferi*, Spirochetes, Dermopathy

Background

Morgellons disease (MD) is a complex dermopathy characterized by the spontaneous appearance of slowly-healing skin lesions that contain multicolored filaments either lying under, embedded in, or projecting from skin (Figure 1A-C) [1-9]. Patients may also exhibit constitutional, musculoskeletal and neurocognitive symptoms that are associated with Lyme disease (LD) and tickborne coinfections. The presence of these symptoms suggests an infectious etiology of the dermopathy and possible vectoring by ticks [4,7,8].

Previous studies found that MD patients demonstrate seroreactivity to *Borrelia burgdorferi* (Bb) antigens and multisystemic symptoms consistent with LD, suggesting a spirochetal etiology [4,7,8]. In addition, histological, electron microscopic and PCR studies of dermatological tissue containing filamentous inclusions from four MD patients confirmed the presence of *Bb sensu stricto* spirochetes [6,7]. Successful bacterial culture of motile spirochetes in BSK-H medium inoculated with MD dermatological tissue

* Correspondence: rstricker@usmamed.com
[1]International Lyme and Associated Diseases Society, Bethesda, MD, USA
[4]450 Sutter Street, Suite 1504, San Francisco, CA 94108, USA
Full list of author information is available at the end of the article

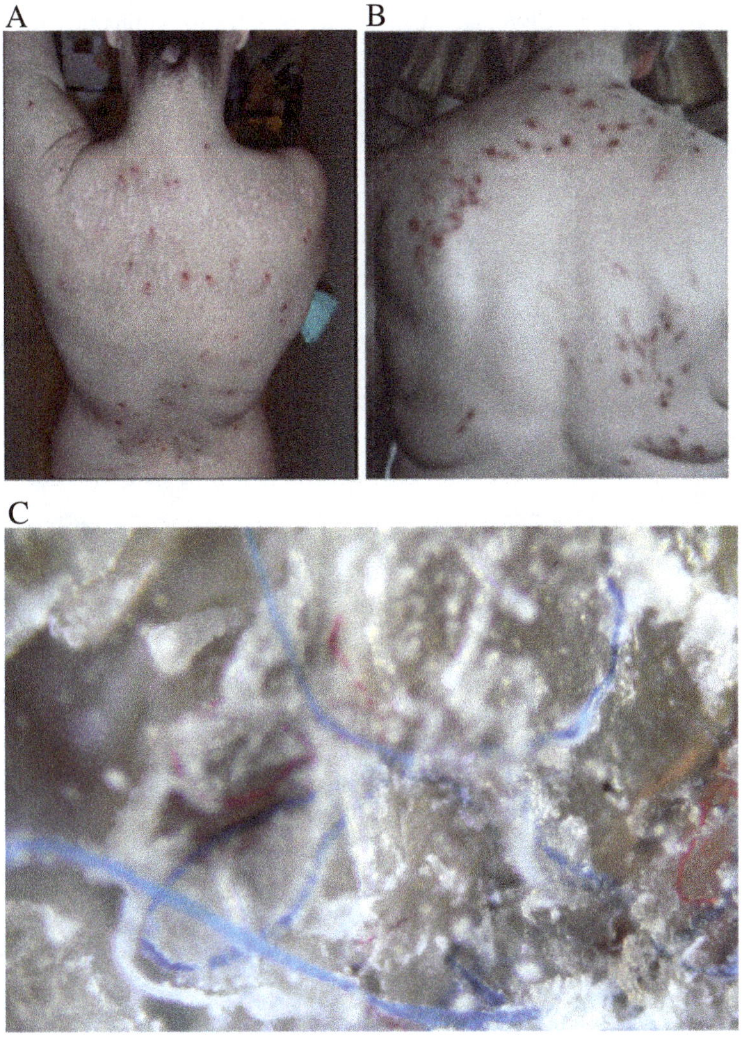

Figure 1 Clinical features of Morgellons disease. A, MD patient back showing lesions covering entire surface, including areas out of patient's reach. **B**, Back of patient with scratching-induced lesions showing distribution limited to patient's reach. **C**, Multicolored fibers embedded in skin callus from MD Patient 2 (100x). **B** reproduced from Reference 19, used with permission of the publisher.

demonstrated the viability of spirochetes in two of these patients, and one culture was confirmed as *Bb sensu stricto* by PCR analysis [7]. A case study of an MD patient in Australia reported that endpoint PCR and Basic Local Alignment Search Tool (BLAST) analysis resulted in the detection and identification of *Borrelia garinii* [8]. These preliminary studies suggest that MD may be a particular manifestation of LD and that strains of *Bb sensu stricto* and *Bb sensu lato* are implicated as etiologic agents [7,8].

In light of the preliminary studies indicating an association of Lyme spirochetes with MD, we undertook a histological, electron microscopic and DNA study of North American MD patients to investigate the presence of borrelial spirochetes systemically and in dermatological specimens. Culture was also undertaken to establish if spirochetes detected in MD tissue were viable organisms and to determine whether *Borrelia* infection in these patients is systemic.

Methods

Patient selection

All patients included in this study met the key diagnostic criterion documented by a healthcare provider: the presence of fibers that were visible underneath unbroken skin or that were embedded in or projecting from skin. Patients were selected from across Canada and the USA, and they were included in the chronological order in which they volunteered. No patients were excluded from study participation provided that they had sample material that was suitable for study and provided that they met the diagnostic criterion. Written informed consent for participation in the study was obtained from all participants.

Approval for sample collection was obtained from the Western Institutional Review Board, Olympia, WA. Further approval for sample testing was obtained from the Institutional Review Board of the University of New Haven, West Haven, CT.

A diagnosis of Lyme disease or positive Lyme serologic testing prior to study participation was not a requirement. Some patients had a prior Lyme diagnosis or serologic testing for Lyme disease while others did not, as shown in Table 1. Those who were not tested with Lyme serology prior to the study were encouraged to be tested, but did so after samples for the study had been collected. Some patients declined to have Lyme serologic testing performed. Some of the subjects had received antibiotic therapy for Lyme disease but were not receiving treatment during the time of sample collection. Two subjects, 1 and 12, were currently taking antibiotics during the time of sample collection.

A total of 25 patients were included in the study. Patients 1-5 were previously presented as case studies [6,7,9]. Clinical patient data is shown in Table 1. All patient samples were deidentified and coded, and all laboratory testing was performed in a blinded fashion.

Cultures

Borrelia culture medium was prepared using Barbour–Stoner–Kelly H (BSK-H) complete medium with 6% rabbit serum (Sigma Aldrich, #B8291) and the following antibiotics: phosphomycin (0.02 mg/ml) (Sigma Aldrich), rifampicin (0.05 mg/ml) (Sigma Aldrich), and amphotericin

Table 1 Clinical data for study patients

Patient #	Age	Gender	Lyme serology	Coinfecting tickborne diseases	Antibiotic treatment
1	86	Female	Positive	*Babesia microti, Bartonella henselae*	Treated at time of sampling
2	52	Female	Positive	*Ehrlichia chaffeensis,Anaplasma phagocytophilum*	Previous treatment, but off at time of study
3	56	Female	*Positive	Not tested	Never treated
4	75	Female	*Positive	Not tested	Not treated at time of study
5	50	Male	Equivocal	Not tested	Never treated
6	41	Male	Positive	Spotted fever group and typhus fever group	Began treatment after start of study
7	51	Female	*Positive	Not tested	Never treated
8	53	Female	Positive	Not tested	Previous treatment, but off at time of study
9	35	Female	Not tested	Not tested	Never treated
10	63	Female	Positive	Spotted fever group and Mycoplasma spp. (Labcorp)	Not treated at time of study
11	47	Female	*Positive	Not tested	Not treated at time of study
12	38	Male	Positive	None	On antibiotic therapy during study
13	43	Female	Positive	*Babesia* spp.	Treated but off antibiotics during study
14	53	Female	*Positive	Not tested	Never treated
15	48	Female	Clinical diagnosis, not tested	Not tested	Not treated at time of study
16	56	Female	Not tested	Not tested	Never treated
17	62	Female	*Positive	Not tested	Not treated at time of study
18	51	Female	Not tested	Not tested	Never treated
19	75	Female	**Positive	Not tested	Had 2 weeks treatment for Lyme but no treatment after
20	60	Female	**Positive	Not tested	Had 3 weeks erythromycin after EM rash and + serology, no treatment after
21	37	Female	Positive	Not tested	Not treated at time of study
22	53	Female	Not tested	Not tested	Not treated at time of study
23	68	Female	Not tested	Not tested	Never treated
24	73	Female	Not tested	Not tested	Never treated
25	58	Female	***Positive	Not tested	Never treated

All Lyme serology except that of patients 19, 20, and 25 tested and interpreted by IGeneX Reference Laboratories, Palo Alto, CA [10].
*Tested for *B. burgdorferi* after skin sampling was taken for study.
**Positive by 2-tiered CDC surveillance criteria.
***Tested by Spectracell Laboratories, Houston, TX.

B (2.5 μg/ml) (Sigma-Aldrich), as described previously [11]. Inocula for blood cultures were prepared as follows: Ten milliliters of whole blood were collected by venipuncture and left at room temperature for 10 to 15 minutes to allow clotting, followed by low speed centrifugation to separate red blood cells. Serum and some blood cells just below the serum layer were used as inocula. The serum/blood cell preparation was inoculated into the BSK medium.

For other cultures, whole scabs removed from the patient, skin scrapings from small lesions removed by a scalpel blade, or vaginal samples collected by swabbing inside the vagina with a sterile cotton-tipped swab were inoculated into the BSK medium. Cultures were incubated in an Oxoid anaerobic jar (Thermo Scientific) containing an AnaeroGen sachet (Thermo Scientific) to provide an anaerobic environment at 32°C. Culture fluid samples were examined by bright-field and/or dark-field microscopy for visible motile spirochetes weekly for up to 4 weeks. Cultures were processed for imaging and PCR by centrifuging the fluid at 15,000 g for 20 minutes to concentrate spirochetes, retaining the pellet and discarding the supernatant.

Dieterle and anti-Bb immunostaining

Dermatological specimens and/or culture pellets from patients were processed for specialized staining at either McClain Laboratories LLC, Smithtown, NY; Interscope Laboratories, Interscope Pathology Medical Group, Canoga Park, CA; or the University of New Haven, West Haven, CT. Dieterle silver-nitrate staining was performed at either Interscope Laboratories or McClain Laboratories. Anti-Bb immunostaining was performed at McClain Laboratories or the University of New Haven.

For those samples submitted to McClain Laboratories for anti-Bb immunostaining, the following protocol was used: formalin-fixed, paraffin-embedded dermatological tissue and culture pellets were sectioned and immunostained using an unconjugated rabbit anti-Bb polyclonal antibody (Abcam ab20950) and then incubated with an alkaline phosphatase probe (Biocare Medical #UP536L) followed by a chromogen substrate (Biocare Medical #FR805CHC) and counterstained with hematoxylin. Positive and negative controls of both Dieterle and anti-Bb immunostains were prepared for comparison purposes using liver sections from uninfected mice and mice experimentally inoculated with Bb, as previously described [12]. Staining was titrated to define optimal antibody dilutions. For comparison purposes, controls of culture pellets from mixed Gram-positive bacteria and mixed Gram-negative bacteria, and sections of normal human skin were also examined to determine possible cross-reactivity with commonly encountered dermatological microorganisms.

For those samples submitted to the University of New Haven, anti-Bb immunofluorescent staining was performed as follows: formalin-fixed paraffin-embedded MD sections were processed for staining and imaging as previously described [13]. Dermatological specimens were formalin-fixed, blocked in paraffin and sectioned by McClain Laboratories. Culture fluid was fixed with acetone at -20°C onto SuperFrost™ slides (Thermo Fisher Scientific, Waltham, MA). Fixed specimens, both dermatological sections and fixed culture fluid, were pre-incubated with 10% normal goat serum (Thermo Fisher Scientific) in PBS containing 0.5% bovine serum albumin (BSA) (Sigma-Aldrich, St. Louis, MO) for 30 minutes to block non-specific binding of the secondary antibody. The slides were then washed with PBS containing 0.5% BSA and then incubated for 1 hour with fluorescein isothiocyanate (FITC)-labeled *Borrelia*-specific polyclonal antibody (Thermo Fisher Scientific, #73005) at a 1:50 dilution in PBS containing 1% BSA pH 7.4 followed by washing and then counterstained with 4', 6-diamidino-2-phenylindole (DAPI) for 10 minutes. For the negative control samples, anti-specifically targeted antibody was replaced with normal rabbit IgG (Vector Laboratories, Burlingame, CA, #I–1000). Images were obtained using fluorescent microscopy.

Electron microscopy

Samples for scanning electron microscopy (SEM) and transmission electron microscopy (TEM) were forwarded to the Electron Microscopy Facility, Department of Materials Science and Engineering, Clemson University, Anderson, South Carolina. Procedures were performed as previously described [6,7].

For SEM, culture pellets, fixed in buffered 2.5% glutaraldehyde were washed in buffer and dehydrated in a graded series of ethanol concentrations, followed by immersion in hexamethyldisilazane for 5–15 minutes and then air-dried at room temperature. Dry samples were mounted on Al mounts and were not coated but placed into a Hitachi TM3000 microscope (Tokyo, Japan) and imaged in the variable pressure mode.

For TEM, glutaraldehyde-fixed samples were washed in buffer and dehydrated in a graded series of ethanol concentrations. Samples were immersed in a 50:50 mixture of LR White embedding resin and 100% ethanol for 30 minutes, followed by pure LR White resin until they settled on the bottom of the vial. Resin-immersed samples were placed into pure resin in beam capsules and polymerized at 60°C overnight. Sections were cut on an Ultracut E microtome (Leica Microsystems, Wetzlar, Germany) producing sections 60–90 nm thick, and were placed onto copper grids then stained in uranyl acetate for 20 minutes. Imaging was performed using a Hitachi 7600 microscope.

Molecular testing

PCR - University of New Haven

DNA was extracted from culture pellets and/or dermatological tissue by lysing overnight in 180 µl tissue lysis buffer (Qiagen) and 20 µl Proteinase K (Qiagen) at 56°C in a shaking water bath and phenol:chloroform extraction the following day. DNA was resuspended in 50-100 µl 1X TE buffer.

A published TaqMan assay targeting a 139-bp fragment of the gene encoding the *Borrelia* 16S rRNA was used for the detection of *Borrelia* in DNA extracted from patient samples [14]. Reactions were carried out in a final volume of 20 µl and consisted of 900 nM of each primer, 200 nM of probe, and 10 µl of 2X TaqMan Universal PCR Master Mix (Applied Biosystems). Amplifications were carried out on a CFX96 Real-Time System (Bio-Rad) and cycling conditions consisted of 50°C for 2 minutes, 95°C for 10 minutes, followed by 40 cycles of 95°C for 15 seconds and 60°C for 60 seconds. Fluorescent signals were recorded using CFX96 Real-Time software and Cq threshold was set automatically. Reactions were performed in triplicate. Positive and negative controls were run simultaneously. The positive control was *Bb sensu stricto* strain B-31. Four negative controls were used: water, normal human foreskin, normal skin from two Lyme patients, and normal skin from one Morgellons patient. *Borrelia* DNA was not detected in any of the negative controls.

Nested PCR primers for the 16S rRNA, flagellin (Fla), OspC, uvrA and pyrG genes were used as previously described [15-17]. Reactions were carried out in a final volume of 50 µl using 10 µl template DNA. Final concentrations were 2X Buffer B (Promega), 2 mM MgCl2, 0.4 mM dNTP mix, 2 µM of each primer, and 2.5 U Taq polymerase (Invitrogen). "Outer" primers were used in the first reaction. "Inner" primers were used for the nested reaction, in which 1 µl of PCR product from the first reaction was used as template for the second. Cycling parameters were as follows: 94°C for 5 minutes followed by 40 cycles of denaturation at 94°C for 1 minute, annealing for 1 minute (temperature based on the primer set used), and extension at 72°C for 1 minute, with a final extension step at 72°C for 5 minutes. PCR products were visualized on 1-2% agarose gels.

Sanger sequencing was used for gene analysis. PCR products were extracted from the agarose gels using the QIAquick Gel Extraction kit (Qiagen) according to the manufacturer's instructions. The eluates from each sample were sequenced in both directions using the primers that generated the products. Obtained sequences were compared by searching the GenBank database (National Center for Biotechnology Information) using BLAST analysis. Sequence alignment (Clustel W) and neighbor-joining phylogenetic analyses were conducted using MEGA version 5. Tree support was evaluated by bootstrapping with 500 replications.

PCR - Australian biologics

Dermatological specimens and/or culture pellets were concentrated by centrifugation and stabilized with AL buffer (Qiagen). Samples were forwarded to Australian Biologics for *Borrelia* detection by real-time PCR targeting the 16S rRNA gene and endpoint PCR targeting the rpoC gene, as previously described [8,18]. The Eco™ Real-Time PCR system with software version 3.0.16.0 was used. DNA was extracted from the dermatological specimens and the culture pellets using the QIAamp DNA Mini Kit (Qiagen). Samples were analyzed in duplicate with positive and negative controls using primers for the *Borrelia* 16S rRNA and rpoC gene targets, as previously described [8,18]. Thermal profiles for all analyses were performed with incubation for 2 minutes at 50°C, polymerase activation for 10 minutes at 95°C then PCR cycling for 40 cycles of 10 secs at 95°C dropping to 60°C sustained for 45 secs. The magnitude of the PCR signal generated (ΔR) for each sample was interpreted as either positive or negative as compared to positive and negative controls.

PCR products were visualized on 1-2% agarose gels and extracted from the gels using the QIAquick Gel Extraction kit (Qiagen) according to the manufacturer's instructions. Sanger sequencing was used for gene analysis, as described previously [18].

Bb molecular beacons

Dr. Alan MacDonald designed the DNA sequences and generously donated the Bb molecular beacon DNA probes. Probe FlaB, a sequence of 23 nucleotides, was derived from the Bb open reading frame (ORF) BB0147 of the flagellin B gene that contains more than 1000 nucleotides. A nucleotide BLAST search of the 23 nucleotide probe sequence disclosed no matches other than that of Bb BB0147. Probe 740 was derived from the Bb ORF BB740 representing a Bb inner cell membrane protein, and a nucleotide BLAST search disclosed no matches other than that of the Bb ORF BB740.

Bb DNA staining and detection with molecular beacons was performed by the following protocol, as previously described [12]. Paraffin sections of dermatological specimens and culture pellets were completely dewaxed by baking at 60°C then immersed in serial 100% xylene baths, followed by serial immersion through 100% ethanol, 90% ethanol, 80% ethanol and distilled H_2O, then air-dried. Fixed sections were immersed in 20 µl of working DNA beacon solution. Sectioned specimens were covered with plastic cut from a Ziploc® freezer bag then were heated at 90°C for 10 minutes to denature all DNA and RNA. Heat was reduced to 80°C for 10 minutes, then samples cooled gradually to room temperature. The stained slides were washed in PBS, and covered with 30% glycerol and a glass coverslip, then examined under an EPI Fluor microscope. Staining of research specimens was performed alongside staining of positive and negative controls. Positive controls consisted of a known Bb strain embedded in agarose, formalin-fixed and sectioned, as well as experimentally Bb-infected mouse liver sections. The negative control consisted of uninfected mouse liver sections.

Results

Histological examination – dermatological specimens

All patients were clinically diagnosed with MD by a healthcare provider based on the presence of skin lesions and/or skin crawling sensations with intradermal filaments that were visible with a hand-held microscope, as described in previous publications [4-9]. The dermatological material that met our diagnostic criterion was mainly in the form of calluses embedded with filaments, many of which were blue or red. MD calluses were easily removed from patients as they were composed of thickened skin that has separated from the dermis at the stratum basale. Histological examination of cross sections revealed epidermal layers from the stratum basale to the stratum corneum. In MD calluses, collagen and keratin filaments could be seen distributed throughout the epidermal tissue or projecting down from the stratum basale towards the dermis.

Dermatological specimens consisting of callus material from the following patients were submitted for histological sectioning and examination: 1-4, 8, 10-13, 15, 16, 18-20, 22, 23, 25. Biopsy sections were submitted for histological examination for patient 24. Sections of hair follicular bulbs and attached follicular sheaths rather than sectioned calluses were submitted for patient 5. Samples from patients 6, 7, 9, 14, 17 and 21 were used for culture and/or PCR detection only.

All histological sections were examined at 400X and 1000X magnification. In slides stained with Dieterle silver nitrate stain and/or anti-Bb antibodies, sectioned filaments embedded in epithelial cells were observed in samples of all callus material and in the biopsy material from patient 24. All filaments demonstrated the same morphology: a hollow medulla surrounded by a solid cortex. Filamentous material demonstrated no characteristics consistent with fungal elements such as hyphae, or any characteristics of known parasites such as microfilariae.

Dieterle silver nitrate staining revealed bacteria morphologically consistent with *Borrelia* spirochetes in 17/19 patients (Table 2). Positively-stained spirochetes were observed in dermatological sections from the specimens submitted for patients 1-4, 8, 10-13, 15, 16, 18, 19, 20, 22 and 23 (Figure 2A). No spirochetes were observed for patients 5 or 24. Patient 5 had only sectioned follicular bulbs and sheaths submitted and patient 24 had biopsy sections submitted. These biopsy sections demonstrated bacterial forms consistent with cystic variants of Bb.

Anti-Bb immunohistochemical staining was reactive in all the histological sections of dermatological specimens submitted including the follicles and follicular sheaths from patient 5 and the two biopsy sections from patients 24 and 25 (100%). Individual spirochetes were discernible in many of these specimens (Figure 2B). Staining of Bb spirochetes was positive in infected mouse liver samples. There was no significant Bb immunostaining of the Bb-negative mouse liver control, the mixed Gram-positive bacterial pellet or normal human skin. Staining of sections of mixed Gram-negative bacteria from the Gram-negative culture pellet showed only weak background staining. In control studies of the anti-Bb immunostaining performed at the University of New Haven, the antibody reacted with Bb but not with *Treponema denticola*.

Bb spirochetes in a callus specimen from patient 2 were detected by SEM and on sectioned calluses from patients 1 and 2 by TEM as previously reported [6].

Culture – general observations

Cultures were performed on skin, blood and/or vaginal specimens taken directly from patients 3, 4, 6-9, 13, 14, 17, 21 and 24. Motile viable organisms were observed in all cultures at 4 weeks of incubation except for the skin culture taken from patient number 6. Motile organisms displayed morphological variation, ranging from spherules to longer helical-shaped bacteria. None of the specimens could be subcultured onto blood agar, even in anaerobic conditions, and there was no contamination by commonly encountered aerobic Gram-positive bacteria. Some of the cultures had very few organisms, and documentation of growth by photography was difficult because of morphological variation. Some cultures were therefore concentrated by centrifugation and stained with Dieterle silver nitrate stain and anti-Bb immunostain for further characterization.

Skin culture

Dermatological specimens were submitted for culture from patients 3, 4, 6, 9, 13 and 21. Examination of culture fluid at 4 weeks incubation revealed motile spirochetes, except for the culture from patient 6. The culture from patient 9 revealed little growth, but one long motile spirochete was observed. Dieterle silver nitrate staining of skin cultures was performed on specimens from patients 3, 6, and 13. These specimens demonstrated positive staining of both spherules and spirochetes consistent with morphological forms of *Borrelia*. All specimens demonstrated strongly positive Bb polyclonal immunostaining of the bacteria present as well as the surrounding cellular debris. This may have been due to secreted exoantigens, antigens released by lysed Bb, or the presence of Bb intracellular infection. Data is summarized in Table 3.

Table 2 Microscopic examination of dermatological tissue sections with Dieterle or Warthin Starry silver nitrate stain and anti-Bb polyclonal immunostain

Patient #	Dieterle	Bb-polyclonal immunostain	Filaments morphologically consistent with MD
1	Spirochetes observed	*Positive	Detected
2	Spirochetes observed	*Positive	Detected
3	Spirochetes observed	*Positive	Detected
4	Spirochetes observed	*Positive	Detected
5	Spirochetes not observed	**Positive	Detected
8	Spirochetes observed	Positive	Detected
10	Spirochetes observed	Positive	Detected
11	Spirochetes observed	Positive	Detected
12	Spirochetes observed	Positive	Detected
13	Spirochetes observed	Positive	Detected
15	Spirochetes observed	Positive	Detected
16	Spirochetes observed	Positive	Detected
18	Spirochetes observed	Positive	Detected
19	Spirochetes observed	Positive	Detected
20	Spirochetes observed	Positive	Detected
22	Spirochetes observed	Positive	Detected
23	Spirochetes observed	Positive	Detected
24	Spherules consistent with Bb morphological variants observed	Positive	Detected
25	Spirochetes observed	Positive	Detected

Dieterle and or Warthin-Starry silver nitrate staining performed at Interscope Laboratories, Los Angeles, CA, and or McClain Laboratories, Smithtown, NY.
Bb polyclonal immunostaining performed at McClain Laboratories.
*Polyclonal Bb immunostaining performed at University of New Haven, West Haven, CT and McClain Laboratories.
**Sectioned specimen consisted of hair follicular bulbs with attached root sheaths rather than skin. Polyclonal Bb immunostaining performed at the University of New Haven.

The culture fluid from patient 6 did not reveal motile spirochetes, so to ascertain the presence of spirochetes a centrifuged culture pellet was submitted for SEM. SEM revealed that spirochetes with morphological features consistent with Bb were present in the culture pellet (Figure 2C).

Blood culture

Blood specimens for culture were taken from patients 3, 4, 7, 8, 13, 14, 17 and 24. Motile bacteria with spirochetal morphology were observed in culture fluid from the eight patients. Dieterle silver nitrate staining and anti-Bb immunostaining was performed on blood cultures concentrated by centrifugation from these patients. Patients 3, 7, 8, 13 and 17 demonstrated positive staining of both spirochetes and spherules consistent with morphological forms of *Borrelia* with Dieterle silver nitrate staining. These patients also demonstrated strongly positive Bb immunostaining of the bacteria in the samples as well as the surrounding cellular debris, as described above. Data is summarized in Table 3.

Vaginal culture

Swabs of vaginal secretions were submitted for culture from patients 8, 14, 21 and 24. Motile bacteria were visible in culture fluid from all four patients. Staining of vaginal cultures concentrated by centrifugation followed by Dieterle silver nitrate staining and anti-Bb immunostaining was performed for specimens taken from patients 8 and 21. Both specimens demonstrated positive staining of both spherules and spirochetes consistent with morphological forms of *Borrelia* with Dieterle silver nitrate stain. Both specimens demonstrated strongly positive Bb immunostaining of the bacteria in the samples as well as the surrounding cellular debris, as described above. Data is summarized in Table 3.

Molecular testing

A. PCR Detection of Borrelia

Various sample types from 20 patients were submitted for PCR detection of *Borrelia* at three independent laboratories. These samples included whole dermatological calluses, histological skin sections, skin culture, blood culture, vaginal cultures, and one specimen of intestinal

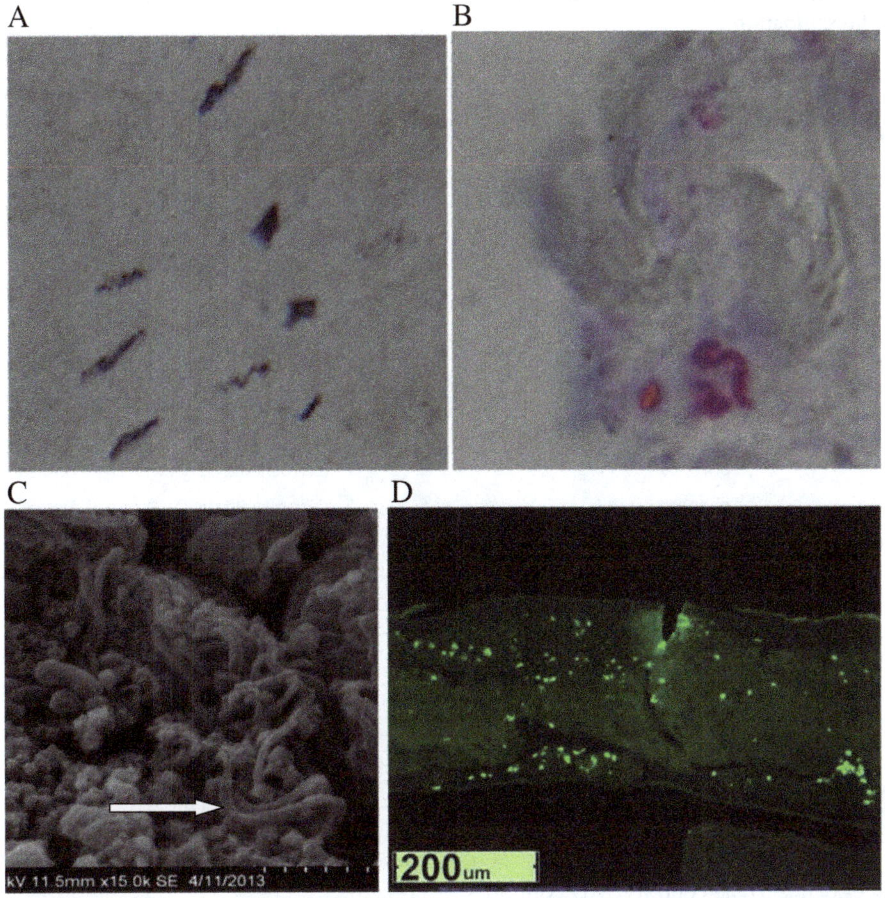

Figure 2 Evaluation of skin samples from Morgellons disease patients. **A**, Dieterle silver stain of skin sample from MD Patient 15 showing dark-staining spirochetes (1000x). **B**, Immunostaining of spirochete with anti-Bb antibody in skin sample from MD Patient 4 (1000x). **C**, Scanning electron micrograph of skin culture sample from MD Patient 6 showing wavy spirochetes (arrows). **D**, Hybridization of Bb-specific molecular beacon FlaB with spirochetes in skin sample from MD Patient 3 (400x).

epithelial tissue that had sloughed off in the patient's feces during an intestinal cleanse. *Borrelia* genes were detected in 18 of the patients whose samples were submitted, and results were equivocal for 2 patients. Amplicon sequences consistent with *Borrelia* DNA were obtained for the PCR products from 14 patients. *Bb sensu stricto* sequence was confirmed in 12 patients, while patient 23 was found to have an amplicon sequence consistent with *B. miyamotoi* and patient 24 had a sequence consistent with *B. garinii*. The latter patient had contracted Lyme disease in Europe. Positive PCR results are summarized in Table 4.

Skin cultures from patients 6, 9, 13 and 21 were subjected to PCR testing, and three of the four samples tested positive, confirming the presence of *Borrelia* in the cultures. The fourth culture sample (patient 21) had equivocal PCR testing using the 16S rRNA probe but tested positive using the FlaB molecular probe (see below). Thus molecular testing confirmed the presence of viable *Borrelia* spirochetes in all four skin culture samples.

Treponema denticola was detected in 5/16 scab/callus samples sent to Australian Biologics. *T. denticola* was not detected in any blood, skin or vaginal cultures (data not shown).

B. In-situ DNA hybridization

Bb DNA was detected by staining with the fluorescent molecular probes FlaB and 740. Histological sections of callus material from patients 2, 3, 10, 11, 13, 15, 19, 20, 22 and sections of skin and/or vaginal culture pellets from patients 21 and 24 were stained with the FlaB probe. All these specimens were positively stained (Figure 2D). Histological sections of callus material from patients 1-4, 8, 10-13, 15, 16, and 18-20, and sections of the skin culture from patient 6 and blood culture from patient 7 were stained with probe 740. All of these specimens were positively stained. The results are summarized in Table 5.

Table 3 Microscopic examination of sectioned culture pellets with Dieterle or Warthin Starry silver nitrate stain and anti-Bb polyclonal immunostain

Patient #	Inoculum type	Culture fluid	Dieterle	Bb polyclonal immunostain*
3	Skin	Motile spirochetes	Spirochetes	Positive**
3	Blood	Motile bacteria	Spirochetes	Positive
4	Skin	Motile spirochetes	Not submitted	Not submitted
4	Blood	Motile bacteria	Not submitted	Not submitted
6	Skin***	Little growth observed	Spirochetes	Positive
7	Blood	Spherules	Spherules	Positive
8	Blood	Spherules	Spirochetes	Positive
8	Vaginal	Motile spherules	Spherules	Positive
9	Skin	Little growth, single long motile spirochete	Not submitted	Not submitted
13	Skin	Spherules/motile elongated bacteria	Spirochetes/ spherules	Positive
13	Blood	Spherules	Spirochetes/ spherules	Positive
14	Blood	Spherules	Not submitted	Not submitted
14	Vaginal	Motile spirochetes	Not submitted	Not submitted
17	Blood	Spherules	Spirochetes/ spherules	Positive
21	Skin	Spherules/ spirochetes	Not submitted	Not submitted
21	Vaginal	Motile spherules	Spherules	Positive
24	Blood	Spherules/ Motile bacteria	Not submitted	Not submitted
24	Vaginal	Motile spirochetes	Not submitted	Not submitted

*Anti-Bb immunostaining performed at McClain Laboratory, Smithtown, NY, except for the skin culture from patient 3.
**Anti-Bb immunostaining performed at the University of New Haven, West Haven, CT.
***SEM revealed well-defined spirochetes with periplasmic flagella.

Discussion

Despite compelling evidence to the contrary, MD continues to be attributed to delusions of parasitosis or delusional infestation [19-23]. The earlier studies demonstrating *Borrelia* spirochetes in MD dermatological specimens have involved only a small number of study subjects, and therefore a study involving a larger number of subjects was needed.

A major strength of our study is that MD patients were identified based on the presence of multicolored fibers within skin lesions or detectable under unbroken skin. Some of our patients did suffer from neuropsychiatric symptoms, and we do not deny that primary delusional infestation can occur in rare cases [1-4]. By selecting only MD patients meeting our dermopathy criterion, however, we have presumably excluded primary delusional infestation patients from our study. Although some MD patients suffering from neuropsychiatric symptoms with *Borrelia*-associated intradermal filaments may claim to have worms, parasites or the like, the skin crawling and stinging sensations that these patients feel coupled with visible skin lesions, anxiety and anthropomorphic thinking may result in complaints that are misinterpreted by clinicians as a primary delusional disorder. Other MD patients in our study had no neuropsychiatric symptoms and yet had the same *Borrelia*-associated dermopathy, so it appears that in our well-defined MD patient cohort these symptoms, when they occurred, were the result rather than the cause of the infectious dermopathy, as previously described [1-4,23].

We have provided evidence linking *Borrelia* infection with MD in a study group consisting of 25 patients. We detected *Borrelia* DNA by PCR and/or staining with Bb-specific DNA probes in 24/25 patients. We were able to demonstrate the presence of *Borrelia* in dermatological tissue and we were able to culture viable Bb spirochetes from skin, blood and vaginal secretions in some patients. The presence of spirochetes was confirmed by numerous testing methodologies, including culture, histology, anti-Bb immunostaining, electron microscopy, PCR and *in situ* Bb DNA hybridization. Laboratory testing methodologies were performed at five independent laboratories. Histological staining and electron microscopy of Morgellons dermatological tissue and cultures was performed at three different laboratories, while molecular testing for *Borrelia* was performed at three different laboratories using real-time PCR, nested PCR and *in situ* Bb DNA hybridization. Furthermore, *Borrelia* DNA amplicon sequencing was conducted at two different laboratories. We have thus provided corroborating evidence of *Borrelia* infection in MD patients that should be difficult to refute.

Recent studies reported similarities between MD and bovine digital dermatitis (BDD), a disease that is common in dairy herds [5,9]. BDD is characterized by skin lesions that commonly occur on and directly above the

Table 4 Detection of *Borrelia* DNA by PCR in samples derived from Morgellons patients

#	Specimen	PCR University of New Haven	PCR Australian Biologics	Sequencing
1	Whole callus	pyrG, fla, ospC	16S rRNA	pyrG, fla, ospC
2	Whole callus	pyrG, fla, 16S rRNA	16S rRNA	pyrG
3	Whole callus	fla, pyrG, 16S rRNA, uvrA, ospC	16S rRNA	16S RNA, pyrG, fla, uvrA, ospC
3	Blood culture	fla		
4	Callus section	16S rRNA		
4	Blood culture	fla		
5	Whole callus	pyrG	16S rRNA	pyrG
6	Skin culture	16S rRNA		
7	Blood culture	fla		
8	Whole callus	pyrG, 16S rRNA, fla		pyrG, fla,
8	Blood culture	fla, pyrG		fla
9	Skin culture	fla		fla
10	Whole callus	16S rRNA, pyrG, fla	16S rRNA	16S rRNA, pyrG
10	Intestinal specimen		16S rRNA	
11	Whole callus	fla+/- indeterminate	Inhibited	
13	Whole callus	uvrA		uvrA
13	Blood culture	pyrG	16S rRNA	
13	Skin culture	pyrG		
14	Blood culture	fla	16S rRNA	fla
14	Vaginal culture	fla	16S rRNA	fla
15	Whole callus		16S rRNA	
16	Whole callus		rpoC	rpoC
17	Whole callus	pyrG, uvrA	16S rRNA	pyrG, uvrA
17	Blood culture	Real-time 16S rRNA +/- equivocal		
18	Whole callus	fla	16S rRNA	fla
21	Skin culture		16S rRNA +/- equivocal	
23	Whole callus		16S rRNA	rpoC*
24	Blood culture	fla	16S rRNA	
24	Vaginal culture		16S rRNA	rpoC**

*Sequence consistent with *B. miyamotoi.*
**Sequence consistent with *B. garinii.*
Amplicon sequences from all patients were consistent with *Bb sensu stricto* except for sequence from patient 23, which was consistent with *B. miyamotoi*, and patient 24, which was consistent with *B. garinii.*

heel bulb of the hind feet of cattle [24,25]. Chronic BDD lesions demonstrate proliferative keratin filaments, and histological examination of diseased tissue reveals spirochetes identified as *Treponema* spp. dispersed among enlarged keratinocytes throughout the stratum spinosum and dermal papillae [26-30]. Though spirochetes are consistently detected in tissue from lesions, coinvolvement of other bacterial pathogens has been proposed as a contributing etiologic factor [27,28,31,32]. Treponemal spirochetes were confirmed as the primary etiologic agents when the condition was duplicated via experimental infection with pure cultured treponemes [33,34].

As with BDD, MD filaments are not textile fibers. MD fibers are biofilaments of human cellular origin produced by epithelial cells and stemming from deeper layers of the epidermis and the root sheath of hair follicles [5,9]. Immunohistochemical and histological staining has demonstrated that these multicolored filaments are composed of collagen and keratin [6,9]. They are nucleated at the base of attachment to adjacent epithelial cells, and the cells at the filament base are continuous in appearance with the surrounding skin cells [6]. Although the cause of coloration of red fibers has not been defined, the blue coloration is the result of melanin pigmentation rather than a dye, as shown by Fontana Masson histological staining [6]. There are no known textile fibers that are collagen in composition, nucleated at their base of attachment, or pigmented blue with melanin. Thus the

Table 5 Detection of Bb DNA by *in situ* hybridization with Bb-specific DNA probes in samples derived from Morgellons patients

Patient #	Specimen	Probe FlaB	Probe 740
1	Callus	Not performed	Positive
2	Callus	Positive	Positive
3	Callus	Positive	Positive
4	Callus	Not performed	Positive
6	Skin culture	Not performed	Positive
7	Blood culture	Not performed	Positive
8	Callus	Not performed	Positive
10	Callus	Positive	Positive
11	Callus	Positive	Positive
12	Callus	Not performed	Positive
13	Callus	Positive	Positive
15	Callus	Positive	Positive
16	Callus	Not performed	Positive
18	Callus	Not performed	Positive
19	Callus	Positive	Positive
20	Callus	Positive	Positive
21	Skin culture	Positive	Not performed
21	Vaginal culture	Positive	Not performed
22	Callus	Positive	Not performed
24	Biopsy	Positive	Not performed

characteristic fibers in MD are clearly distinct from textile fibers [6].

Histological sections of MD dermatological tissue reacted with anti-Bb immunostain in 19/19 of the dermatological specimens submitted for histological examination. Motile *Borrelia* spirochetes were cultured in medium inoculated with skin scrapings from 4 patients, thus demonstrating that *Borrelia* spirochetes in MD lesions are viable. *Borrelia* spirochetes were also detected in blood cultures from some MD patients in our study, confirming systemic Lyme borreliosis. Spirochetes characterized as strains of *Borrelia* were detected by PCR and/or in situ DNA hybridization in tissue or culture specimens from 24/25 patients; 15 of these patients had *Borrelia* gene products detected in dermatological specimens and/or skin cultures taken from MD lesions, and DNA amplicons from 14 patients were sequenced and confirmed to be *Borrelia* strains. Vaginal secretions from four patients were cultured, and three isolates were identified as *Borrelia* strains by PCR and in situ DNA hybridization.

Lyme borreliosis is a systemic infection that is commonly associated with dermatological manifestations [35]. Given that most MD patients are serologically reactive to Bb antigens, the presence of Lyme spirochetes in MD dermatological lesions is predictable and supports an etiologic role of the spirochetal disease. *Bb sensu stricto* and *Bb sensu lato* have been associated with numerous dermatological manifestations including erythema migrans, borrelial lymphocytoma, acrodermatitis chronica atrophicans, morphea, lichen sclerosus, cutaneous B-cell lymphoma, scleroderma, lymphadenosis cutis and prurigo pigmentosa [35-38]. Likewise it appears that MD is associated with Lyme disease in a subgroup of patients with this spirochetal illness [6-8]. It is possible that spirochetes other than *Bb sensu stricto* and the *Bb sensu lato* complex, such as the agent of syphilis, *Treponema pallidum,* could be responsible for similar manifestations in other patients. In support of this supposition, Ekbom's original 1945 description of delusions of parasitosis reported that many of the patients in that study were diagnosed with syphilis, thus linking treponemal infection with pruritus, crawling sensations and belief of infestation [39]. Furthermore, treponemal spirochetes have been shown to induce the formation of filamentous lesions in animal models [26-30].

The mechanism of filament formation in MD is not yet elucidated. The filaments are composed of keratin and collagen and arise from proliferative keratinocytes and fibroblasts in human epithelial tissue [6,9]. Bb appears to have a predilection for fibroblasts and keratinocytes, and invasion of these cells by *Borrelia* spirochetes has been reported [40-42]. Bb appears to attach to fibroblasts followed by engulfment of the spirochetes, formation of vacuoles and intracellular replication [42]. Intracellular sequestration of Bb in skin fibroblasts and keratinocytes may protect the spirochetes from host defense mechanisms [40,41]. It is therefore reasonable to hypothesize that Bb intracellular infection of keratinocytes and fibroblasts may alter keratin and collagen expression and that the presence of *Borrelia* spirochetes in dermatological tissue is a primary etiologic factor in the evolution of MD lesions.

Viable Bb spirochetes have been isolated from lysates of fibroblast and keratinocyte monolayers treated with antibiotics [40,41]. Therefore, in addition to protection from host defenses, sequestration within fibroblasts and keratinocytes may protect Bb from antibiotic therapy. Spirochetes in MD dermatological tissue from Patients 1 and 12 were reactive to anti-Bb immunostains and we detected *Borrelia* DNA in dermatological tissue taken from these two patients. These patients were receiving aggressive antibiotic therapy at the time of this study. Patients 2, 8, 13, 19 and 20 had previously received antibiotic therapy for Lyme disease, yet still had detectable spirochetal infection. Persistent infection refractory to antibiotic treatment may therefore result from sequestration of *Borrelia* spirochetes within keratinocytes and fibroblasts in MD patients.

Although spirochetes appear to be the primary etiologic agents of MD, evidence suggests that the etiology is multifactorial. Secondary etiologic factors, such as female predominance, immune dysfunction, and other tickborne coinfections appear to play a role in the development of this dermopathy [1-5]. As noted in Table 1, we found serological evidence of tickborne coinfections including *Babesia, Anaplasma, Ehrlichia, Bartonella and Rickettsia* spp. in five of six patients who were tested. The role of these coinfections in MD remains undefined. Although we demonstrated the presence of *Borrelia* spirochetes in all of the patients in our study group, *T. denticola* was detected in dermatological specimens from five patients. The role of these commonly occurring oral spirochetes in the evolution of MD dermatological lesions and subsequent filament formation is uncertain, and we speculate that coinvolvement of these and perhaps other pathogens could be contributing or exacerbating factors in MD.

A study from the Centers for Disease Control and Prevention (CDC) concluded that pathogens were not involved in MD [22]. The search for spirochetal pathogens in that study was limited to Warthin-Starry staining on a small number of tissue samples and commercial two-tiered serological Lyme disease testing as interpreted by the CDC Lyme surveillance criteria [22]. It should be noted that only two of the patients in our study group were positive for Lyme disease based on the CDC Lyme surveillance criteria and yet *Borrelia* spirochetes were readily detectable in this group of 25 MD patients.

The diagnosis of Lyme disease is a controversial topic in the medical literature. Serological tests for Lyme disease lack sensitivity, and seronegativity has been demonstrated in patients with Bb infection [43,44]. PCR detection is not standardized, and sensitivity and specificity of testing therefore varies from laboratory to laboratory [45,46]. We detected *Borrelia* strains using different primers and different methodologies, and our findings show that primer hybridization differed between samples. Likewise *Borrelia* antigen detection may be unreliable, and immunostaining may lack sensitivity or specificity [46,47]. Although our dermatological and culture pellet sections were consistently reactive with anti-Bb polyclonal antibodies, we were not certain of the specificity of our testing. We wish to emphasize, however, that repeated detection of *Borrelia* spirochetes using a combination of diverse laboratory methods makes false-positive testing highly unlikely in these MD patients.

Borrelia culture is not available in many laboratories and can be challenging because of fastidious growth requirements and spirochetal pleomorphism [48,49]. The formation of spherical forms, truncated forms, straight forms, wavy forms and the like could result in positive cultures being overlooked. Our cultures demonstrated significant pleomorphism, and cystic or truncated variants were present, more so in blood cultures than skin cultures. In our experience histological identification is complicated because pleomorphism occurs in vivo as well as in vitro [50,51]. Sensitivity and specificity differences between laboratory methodologies to detect *Borrelia* spirochetes necessitate the use of several different methodologies to confirm the presence of *Borrelia* infection. If MD is determined to be pathognomonic for Lyme borreliosis it will aid in the diagnosis of Lyme disease in this group of patients. A recent study from Australia found MD in 6% of patients diagnosed with Lyme disease on that continent [52].

We achieved a high degree of success in detecting Bb and closely-related spirochetes from MD dermatological tissue. We attribute our success to several key factors. First, as stated previously we had a clear diagnostic criterion that allowed us to select the appropriate clinical cohort. Second, in contrast to *T. pallidum*, the treponemal agent of syphilis, *Borrelia* spp. can be cultured, thereby magnifying their numbers *in vitro* and increasing the opportunity for detection. Third, unlike secondary and tertiary syphilitic skin lesions where treponemes are seldom detected, we observed that MD lesions carry a high spirochetal load that allows for relatively easy detection, similar to lesions seen in cattle with BDD. Finally, we used a variety of sensitive microscopic and molecular methodologies to detect *Borrelia* spp., including molecular hybridization and PCR techniques that can detect spirochetal DNA in the picogram range.

The detection of *Borrelia* spirochetes in dermatological samples from a larger group of MD patients further validates the infectious nature of this dermopathy. As noted above, *T. pallidum* spirochetes are seldom detected in secondary and tertiary syphilitic skin lesions, even when sensitive molecular techniques such as PCR are performed, yet syphilis spirochetes are acknowledged to be the causative agent of these lesions [53-55]. The use of a clinical classification system for syphilis has helped with diagnosis and treatment of this systemic treponemal infection. In contrast to syphilis, we were able to consistently isolate and/or detect *Borrelia* spirochetes from MD dermatological specimens. Also in contrast to syphilis, no clinical classification system exists for MD.

Based on our experience with several hundred MD patients, we propose a clinical classification scheme that reflects the duration and location of MD lesions, as follows:

1. Early localized: lesions/fibers present for less than three (3) months and localized to one area of the body (head, trunk, extremities).
2. Early disseminated: lesions/fibers present for less than three (3) months and involving more than one area of the body (head, trunk, extremities).
3. Late localized: lesions/fibers present for more than six (6) months and localized to one area of the body (head, trunk, extremities).

4. Late disseminated: lesions/fibers present for more than six (6) months and involving more than one area of the body (head, trunk, extremities).

The classification scheme provides a medical framework that should help to validate and standardize the diagnosis of MD. Further studies are needed to determine whether this classification will have therapeutic and prognostic significance for MD patients.

Conclusions

We undertook a detailed microscopic and molecular study of North American MD patients to investigate the presence of borrelial spirochetes systemically and in dermatological specimens. Based on culture, histology, immunohistochemistry, electron microscopy and molecular testing, we present extensive evidence for spirochetal infection in MD patients. Our study confirms that MD is a true somatic illness associated with Lyme disease. The proposed clinical classification scheme for MD should aid in the diagnosis and treatment of this complex illness.

Competing interests

MJM, PJM and RBS serve without compensation on the scientific advisory panel of the Charles E. Holman Morgellons Disease Foundation. The other authors have no competing interests to declare.

Authors' contributions

MJM participated in the study design and coordination, performed culture, histology and immunohistochemistry experiments and drafted the manuscript. CB, JB, ES, KRF, YW and AF performed PCR tesing, in situ hybridization and DNA sequencing experiments. PJM participated in the study design and edited the manuscript. RBS participated in the study design and coordination and edited the manuscript. All authors read and approved the final manuscript.

Acknowledgements

The authors thank Drs. Stewart Adams, Robert Allan, Gordon Atkins, Robert Bransfield, George Chaconas, Douglas Demetrick, Dorte Dopfer, Christopher Hardy, Doug Kahn, Alan MacDonald, Steve McClain, Elizabeth Rasmussen, Ginger Savely and Janet Sperling for helpful discussion. We thank Joel Israel for technical support and Lorraine Johnson for manuscript review, and we are grateful to Cindy Casey and the Charles E. Holman Morgellons Disease Foundation for funding support.

Funding source

Partial funding for this study was provided by the Charles E. Holman Morgellons Disease Foundation, Austin, TX, USA. The Foundation provided funds for analytical reagents and for publishing fees. The Foundation had no role in any of the following: the study design, the collection, analysis, and interpretation of data, writing of the manuscript, or the decision to submit the manuscript for publication.

Author details

[1]International Lyme and Associated Diseases Society, Bethesda, MD, USA. [2]Department of Biology and Environmental Science, University of New Haven, West Haven, CT, USA. [3]Australian Biologics, Sydney, NSW, Australia. [4]450 Sutter Street, Suite 1504, San Francisco, CA 94108, USA.

References

1. Savely VR, Leitao MM, Stricker RB. The mystery of Morgellons disease: Infection or delusion? Am J Clin Dermatol. 2006;7:1–5.
2. Savely G, Leitao MM. Skin lesions and crawling sensation: disease or delusion? Adv Nurse Pract. 2005;13:16–7.
3. Savely VR, Stricker RB. Morgellons disease: the mystery unfolds. Expert Rev Dermatol. 2007;2:585–91.
4. Savely VR, Stricker RB. Morgellons disease: analysis of a population with clinically confirmed microscopic subcutaneous fibers of unknown etiology. Clin Cosmet Investig Dermatol. 2010;3:67–78.
5. Middelveen MJ, Stricker RB. Filament formation associated with spirochetal infection: A comparative approach to Morgellons disease. Clin Cosmet Investig Dermatol. 2011;4:167–77.
6. Middelveen MJ, Mayne PJ, Kahn DG, Stricker RB. Characterization and evolution of dermal filaments from patients with Morgellons disease. Clin Cosmet Investig Dermatol. 2013;6:1–21.
7. Middelveen MJ, Burugu D, Poruri A, Burke J, Mayne PJ, Sapi E, et al. Association of spirochetal infection with Morgellons disease. F1000 Res. 2013;2:25.
8. Mayne P, English JS, Kilbane EJ, Burke JM, Middelveen MJ, Stricker RB. Morgellons: a novel dermatological perspective as the multisystem infective disease borreliosis. F1000 Res. 2013;2:118.
9. Middelveen MJ, Rasmussen EH, Kahn DG, Stricker RB. Morgellons disease: A chemical and light microscopic study. J Clin Exp Dermatol Res. 2012;3:140.
10. Shah JS, Du Cruz I, Narciso W, Lo W, Harris NS. Improved sensitivity of Lyme disease Western blots prepared with a mixture of *Borrelia burgdorferi* strains 297 and B31. Chronic Dis Int. 2014;1:7.
11. Bankhead T, Chaconas G. The role of VlsE antigenic variation in the Lyme disease spirochete: persistence through a mechanism that differs from other pathogens. Mol Microbiol. 2007;65:1547–58.
12. Middelveen MJ, McClain SA, Bandoski C, Israel JR, Burke J, MacDonald AB, et al. Granulomatous hepatitis associated with chronic *Borrelia burgdorferi* infection: a case report. Research Open Access. 2014;1:875.
13. Sapi E, Kaur N, Anyanwu S, Luecke DF, Datar A, Patel S, et al. Evaluation of in-vitro antibiotic susceptibility of different morphological forms of *Borrelia burgdorferi*. Infect Drug Resist. 2011;4:97–113.
14. O'Rourke M, Traweger A, Lusa L, Stupica D, Maraspin V, Barrett PN, et al. Quantitative detection of *Borrelia burgdorferi* sensu lato in erythema migrans skin lesions using internally controlled duplex real time PCR. PLoS One. 2013;8:e63968.
15. Margos G, Hojgaard A, Lane RS, Cornet M, Fingerle V, Rudenko N, et al. Multilocus sequence analysis of *Borrelia bissettii* strains from North America reveals a new Borrelia species. Borrelia kurtenbachii Ticks Tick Borne Dis. 2010;1:151–8.
16. Sapi E, Pabbati N, Datar A, Davies EM, Rattelle A, Kuo BA. Improved culture conditions for the growth and detection of Borrelia from human serum. Int J Med Sci. 2013;10:362–76.
17. Clark KL, Leydet B, Hartman S. Lyme borreliosis in human patients in Florida and Georgia. USA Int J Med Sci. 2013;10:915–31.
18. Mayne PJ. Investigations of *Borrelia burgdorferi* genotypes in Australia obtained from erythema migrans tissue. Clin Investig Dermatol Res. 2012;5:69–78.
19. Lorenzo CR, Koo J. Pimozide in dermatologic practice: A comprehensive review. Am J Clin Dermatol. 2004;5:339–49.
20. Freudenmann RW, Lepping P. Delusional infestation. Clin Microbiol Rev. 2009;22:690–732.
21. Hylwa SA, Bury JE, Davis MD, Pittelkow M, Bostwick JM. Delusional infestation, including delusions of parasitosis: Results of histologic examination of skin biopsy and patient-provided skin specimens. Arch Dermatol. 2011;147(9):1041–5.
22. Pearson ML, Selby JV, Katz KA, Cantrell V, Braden CR, Parise ME, et al. Clinical, epidemiologic, histopathologic and molecular features of an unexplained dermopathy. PLoS One. 2012;7(1):e29908.
23. Stricker RB, Middelveen MJ. Morgellons disease: More questions than answers. Psychosomatics. 2012;53(5):504–5.
24. Cheli R, Mortellaro CM. Digital dermatitis in cattle. *Proc 8th Int Meet Dis Cattle* Milan. Italy. 1974;8:208–13.
25. Blowey RW, Sharp MW. Digital dermatitis in dairy cattle. Vet Rec. 1988;122:505–8.
26. Read DH, Walker RL, Castro AE, Sundberg JP, Thurmond JC. An invasive spirochaete associated with interdigital papillomatosis of dairy cattle. Vet Rec. 1992;130:59–60.
27. Borgmann JE, Bailey J, Clark EG. Spirochete-associated bovine digital dermatitis. Can Vet J. 1996;37:35–37.
28. Döpfer D, Koopmans A, Meijer FA, Szaskall I, Schukken WH, Klee W, et al. Histological and bacteriological evaluation of digital dermatitis in cattle,

with special reference to spirochaetes and Campylobacter faecalis. Vet Rec. 1997;140:620–3.
29. Read DH, Walker RL. Papillomatous digital dermatitis (footwarts) in California dairy cattle: clinical and gross pathologic findings. J Vet Diagn Invest. 1998;10:67–76.
30. Vink WD, Jones G, Johnson WO, Brown J, Demirkan I, Carter SD, et al. Diagnostic assessment without cut-offs: application of serology for the modeling of bovine digital dermatitis infection. Prev Vet Med. 2009;92:235–48.
31. Grund S, Nattermann H, Horsch F. Electron microscopic detection of spirochetes in digital dermatitis of cattle. Zentralbl Veterinarmed B. 1995;42:533–42.
32. Demirkan I, Carter SD, Murray RD, Blowey RW, Woodward MJ. The frequent detection of a treponeme in bovine digital dermatitis by immunohistochemistry and polymerase chain reaction. Vet Microbiol. 1998;60:285–92.
33. Berry SL, Read DH, Famula TR, Mongini A, Döpfer D. Long-term observations on the dynamics of bovine digital dermatitis lesions on a California dairy after topical treatment with lincomycin HCl. Vet J. 2012;193:654–8.
34. Döpfer D, Anklam K, Mikheil D, Ladell P. Growth curves and morphology of three Treponema subtypes isolated from digital dermatitis in cattle. Vet J. 2012;193:685–93.
35. Malane MS, Grant-Kels JM, Feder Jr HM, Luger SW. Diagnosis of Lyme disease based on dermatologic manifestations. Ann Intern Med. 1991;114:490–8.
36. Afa G, Caprilli F, Crescimbeni E, Morrone A, Progano G, Fazio M. Anti-*Borrelia burgdorferi* antibodies in chronic erythema migrans, benign lymphadenosis cutis, scleroderma and scleratrophic lichen. G Ital Dermatol Venereol. 1990;125:369–73.
37. Chao LL, Lu CF, Shih CM. Molecular detection and genetic identification of *Borrelia garini* and *Borrelia afzelii* from patients presenting a rare skin manifestation of prurigo pigmentosa in Taiwan. Int J Infect Dis. 2013;17:1141–7.
38. Vasudevan B, Chatterjee M. Lyme borreliosis and skin. Indian J Dermatol. 2013;58:167–74.
39. Ekbom KA, Yorston G, Miesch M, Pleasance M, Rubbert S. The pre-senile delusion of infestation. 1945. Translation: Hist Psychiatry. 2003;14(54 Pt2):229–56.
40. Georgilis K, Peacock M, Klempner MS. Fibroblasts protect the Lyme disease spirochete, *Borrelia burgdorferi*, from ceftriaxone in vitro. J Infect Dis. 1992;166:440–4.
41. Klempner MS, Rogers RA, Noring R. Invasion of fibroblasts by the Lyme spirochete *Borrelia burgdorferi*. J Infect Dis. 1993;167:1074–81.
42. Chmielewski T, Tylewska-Wierzbanowska S. Interactions between *Borrelia burgdorferi* and mouse fibroblasts. Pol J Microbiol. 2010;59:157–60.
43. Stricker RB, Johnson L. Serologic tests for Lyme disease: more smoke and mirrors. Clin Infect Dis. 2008;47:1111–2.
44. Dattwyler RJ, Volkman DJ, Luft BJ, Halperin JJ, Thomas J, Golightly MG. Seronegative Lyme disease. N Engl J Med. 1988;319:1441–6.
45. Schmidt BL. PCR in laboratory diagnosis of human *Borrelia burgdorferi* infections. Cin Microbiol Rev. 1997;10:185–201.
46. Lange R, Seyyedi S. Evidence of a Lyme borreliosis infection from the viewpoint of laboratory medicine. Int J Med Microbiol. 2002;291 Suppl 33:120–4.
47. Péter O, Bretz AG, Bee D. Occurrence of different genospecies of *Borrelia burgdorferi* sensu lato in ixodid ticks of Valais. Switzerland Eur J Epidemiol. 1995;11:463–7.
48. Mursic VP, Wanner G, Reinhardt S, Wilske B, Busch U, Marget W. Formation and cultivation of *Borrelia burgdorferi* spheroplast-L-form variants. Infection. 1996;4:218–26.
49. Brorson O, Brorson SH. An in vitro study of the susceptibility of mobile and cystic forms of *Borrelia burgdorferi* to tinidazole. Int Microbiol. 2004;7:139–42.
50. Embers ME, Barthold SW, Borda JT, Bowers L, Doyle L, Hodzic E, et al. Persistence of *Borrelia burgdorferi* in rhesus macaques following antibiotic treatment of disseminated infection. PLoS One. 2012;7:e29914.
51. Meriläinen L, Herranen A, Schwarzbach A, Gilbert L. Morphological and biochemical features of *Borrelia burgdorferi* pleomorphic forms. *Microbiology.* published ahead of print January 6, 2015, doi:10.1099/mic.0.000027
52. Mayne PJ. Clinical determinants of Lyme borreliosis, babesiosis, bartonellosis, anaplasmosis, and ehrlichiosis in an Australian cohort. Int J Gen Med. 2015;8:15–26.
53. Alessi E, Innocenti M, Ragusa G. Secondary syphilis: Clinical morphology and histopathology. Am J Dermatopathol. 1983;5(1):11–7.
54. Zoechiling N, Schluepen EM, Soyer HP, Kerl H, Volkenandt M. Molecular detection of *Treponema pallidum* in secondary and tertiary syphilis. Br J Dermatol. 1997;136:683–6.
55. Pereira TM, Fernandes JC, Viera AP, Basto AS. Tertiary syphilis. Int J Dermatol. 2007;46:1192–5.

Metabolic changes in psoriatic skin under topical corticosteroid treatment

Beathe Sitter[1*], Margareta Karin Johnsson[2,3], Jostein Halgunset[4,5] and Tone Frost Bathen[6]

Abstract

Background: MR spectroscopy of intact biopsies can provide a metabolic snapshot of the investigated tissue. The aim of the present study was to explore the metabolic pattern of uninvolved skin, psoriatic skin and corticosteroid treated psoriatic skin.

Methods: The three types of skin biopsy samples were excised from patients with psoriasis (N = 10). Lesions were evaluated clinically, and tissue biopsies were excised and analyzed by one-dimensional ^{1}H MR spectroscopy. Relative levels were calculated for nine tissue metabolites. Subsequently, relative amounts of epidermis, dermis and subcutaneous tissue were scored by histopathological evaluation of HES stained sections.

Results: Seven out of 10 patients experienced at least 40% reduction in clinical score after corticosteroid treatment. Tissue biopsies from psoriatic skin contained lower levels of the metabolites *myo*-inositol and glucose, and higher levels of choline and taurine compared to uninvolved skin. In corticosteroid treated psoriatic skin, tissue levels of glucose, *myo*-inositol, GPC and glycine were increased, whereas choline was reduced, in patients with good therapeutic effect. These tissue levels are becoming more similar to metabolite levels in uninvolved skin.

Conclusion: This MR method demonstrates that metabolism in psoriatic skin becomes similar to that of uninvolved skin after effective corticosteroid treatment. MR profiling of skin lesions reflect metabolic alterations related to pathogenesis and treatment effects.

Keywords: Tissue, Metabolites, Corticosteroids, Psoriasis treatment, MR spectroscopy

Background

Psoriasis is a common immune-mediated disease that affects the skin and joints. The cause of the disease remains unknown. Many patients have a genetic predisposition. The disease affects around 2–3% of the population worldwide. Clinically, psoriatic plaques are characterized by sharply demarcated erythematous lesions with thick silvery scales, often distributed in a symmetrical pattern. Histopathologically there is hyperproliferation of epidermal cells and an inflammatory cell infiltrate [1]. There is increasing awareness that psoriasis is a multisystem affection with substantial comorbidity, particularly of cardiovascular diseases and metabolic syndrome [2]. The course is that of a chronic, relapsing disease which requires long term treatment. Various topical and systemic treatment options exist for psoriatic lesions. Topical corticosteroids remain the cornerstone, either used as monotherapy or in combination with other treatment modalities. These agents exert anti-inflammatory and immunosuppressive effects by stimulation or inhibition of the genes involved in inflammatory pathways, including inhibition of cytokine production and reduction of such mediators of inflammation as prostaglandins and leucotrienes, inhibition of T-cell proliferation and T-cell dependent immunity, and suppression of fibroblast and endothelial cell functions [3,4]. Corticosteroids also have anti-proliferative effects, by delaying the onset of DNA synthesis and decreasing the mitotic rate [5].

Molecular studies of outbreak and healing of psoriatic lesions can provide insight in the underlying biological processes. Genome wide association scans (GWAS) have identified genetic susceptibility factors [6], and molecular analysis have revealed associations of psoriasis with specific molecular pathways [7,8]. Detailed molecular characterization of autoimmune diseases can provide

* Correspondence: beathe.sitter@hist.no
[1]Department of Technology, Sør Trøndelag University College, 7004 Trondheim, Norway
Full list of author information is available at the end of the article

information about mechanisms involved in disease progression and action of drugs, and also provide biomarkers to predict and monitor disease course. Cellular enzymatic processes involve small molecular metabolites as substrates, intermediates and end products, and such metabolites are crucial in energy turnover and membrane synthesis. Metabolic studies have been applied in numerous biomedical settings [9], and for instance metabolic characterization of cancerous tissue is expected to contribute to a more detailed tumor portrait by defining specific fingerprints reflecting diagnostic status or predicting therapeutic response [10]. Magnetic resonance spectroscopy (MRS) analysis of intact tissue specimens can provide a detailed description of the biochemical composition of the tissue, using so-called high resolution (HR) magic angle spinning (MAS) MRS. This technology requires a minimum of preparation of samples, and detailed biochemical information can be obtained from small specimens (typically 20 mg). Multiple cellular metabolites can be measured simultaneously, and the sample is kept intact for subsequent analysis by other techniques.

The purposes of the present study were to characterize the metabolic patterns of intact uninvolved and affected skin in psoriasis patients and to monitor the biochemical changes in psoriatic skin accompanying corticosteroid treatment. Ten patients were included, three biopsy samples being excised from each: uninvolved skin, psoriatic skin, and corticosteroid treated psoriatic skin, respectively. All biopsy samples were investigated by MAS MRS, and the resulting spectra were further analyzed by peak area calculations to obtain relative measures of tissue metabolite contents.

Methods

Subjects

Ten patients with stable light to moderate plaque psoriasis volunteered to participate in the study. Eight of the patients were men and two were women (not pregnant or nursing) with a median age of 52 (range 28–75) years. None of the patients used systemic treatment for psoriasis. Three patients were on systemic medication for non-dermatological reasons: irbesartan (hypertension) and terbinafine (tinea unguium), aspirin and pravastatin (hypercholesterolemia) and amlodipine (hypertension). The Regional Committee for Medical and Health Research Ethics, Central Norway approved the study protocol, and all patients signed a written informed consent form.

Study design

Two symmetrical psoriatic lesions were chosen for each patient. The psoriatic lesions were localized at elbows (n = 3), knees (n = 3), upper back (n = 1), hips (n = 1), flanks (n = 1) and buttocks (n = 1). After at least two weeks of treatment with only emollient (Locobase®, Yamanouchi), one plaque was assigned for continued treatment with emollient. The other chosen psoriatic lesion was treated once daily (evening time) with the very potent corticosteroid clobetasol propionate ointment 0,05% (Dermovate®, GlaxoSmtihKline). In addition, the emollient was used both on the lesion treated with corticosteroid and the control lesion according to needs. Both psoriatic lesions were evaluated clinically before the start of the treatment and after four weeks of treatment. The severity of scaling, erythema and infiltration of the lesions was scored on a scale from 0–4 for each parameter (0 absent and 4 severe). After four weeks, three punch biopsies (4 mm) were taken after local anaesthesia with lidocaine with epinephrine: from uninvolved skin, from psoriatic skin and from corticosteroid treated psoriatic skin in the same body area.

Sample treatment

The punch biopsy samples were put in a cryo-tube and frozen in liquid nitrogen (-195.8°C) within one minute after tissue resection, and further stored in liquid nitrogen until MR analysis. Samples weighed 21.9 mg on average (range from 11.6 to 35.7 mg).

MR spectroscopy

The MR experiments were performed as previously described [11]. Briefly, samples were thawed on an ice-block to provide a cold environment, and transferred to a 4 mm MAS rotor (total sample volume 50 μL) containing 40 μL phosphate buffered saline with TSP (1 mM). The rotor was thereafter placed in a Bruker AVANCE DRX600 spectrometer equipped with a $^{1}H/^{13}C$ MAS probe with gradients (Bruker BioSpin GmbH, Germany). During signal acquisition, which started within 42 minutes in average after sample thawing (maximum 1 hour and 35 minutes), the samples were spun at 5 kHz and kept at 4°C. One-dimensional ^{1}H spectra were recorded, using a spin-echo sequence which suppresses broad peaks and the water signal. The resulting spectra are highly resolved, with relatively enhanced signals from small metabolites. Spectral assignments were performed based on metabolite appearances in previously recorded MR spectra of intact human tissue [12,13] and in MR spectra of extracts from skin tissue [14]. Totally 17 metabolites were assigned.

Analysis of MR spectra

The spectral region 4.7 to 3.0 ppm was used for peak area calculations, which was performed using the curve fitting program PeakFit version 4 (SeaSolve Inc, USA (MA)), by combined Lorenzian and Gaussian functions (Voigt area) for curve area estimation. Areas were calculated for the nine peaks arising from glucose, lactate, *myo*-inositol, glycine, taurine, glycerophosphocholine (GPC), phosphocholine (PCho), choline and creatine. The program uses a least squares function to optimize the fit to the real spectrum, and the correlation factor which describes the goodness of fit was better than 0.95 for all area calculations. To obtain a semi-quantitative measure for each metabolite, its peak area was normalized to the total peak area of all nine metabolites for every spectrum. Kruskal-Wallis multiple sample analysis was applied for paired comparisons of metabolite content in the three types of skin samples. Differences in tissue metabolites between corticosteroid treated and untreated psoriatic skin were calculated for all patients. Metabolic changes ascribed to corticosteroid treatment were compared between the group with poor ($N = 3$) and good ($N = 7$) clinical effect using Mann–Whitney significance test. Statistical analyses were performed using SPSS (SPSS 16, SPSS Inc.).

Histopathology

Tissue samples were stored in liquid nitrogen for 20 months after MAS MRS analysis. For histological evaluation, samples were thawed and immersed in 4% buffered formaldehyde fixative solution for 24 hours, followed by embedment in paraffin. From each block, one 5 μm tissue section was cut and stained with haematoxilin, erythrosine and saffron (HES). The microscopic sections were photographed with a digital camera, and the relative amounts of epidermis, dermis and subcutaneous tissue were determined by point counting [15]. Briefly, the micrographs were overlaid with a randomly positioned point grid, and the number of points falling on each of the three tissue components was counted, considering the stratum corneum as part of the epidermis. The relative number of points falling on one particular component was taken as an estimate of the section area occupied by the respective tissue element. The area fraction thus obtained is an unbiased estimate of the corresponding volume fraction in the tissue sample, provided the section is chosen randomly.

Results

Patients

All patients experienced a reduced degree of psoriatic affection after four weeks of treatment with corticosteroid ointment. Seven of the patients experienced at least 40% reduction of the clinical score of the skin, of which four patients had almost complete normalization of the skin (score grade 1 for erythema and infiltration, no scaling). Three patients had 40% or less reduction of clinical skin scoring, and were considered to have poor effect of the corticosteroid treatment. Concerning the untreated psoriatic lesions, five of the patients showed no change over four weeks, three experienced less scaling after application of emollient whereas in two patients a worsening was noted.

Histology

All samples could be evaluated with respect to tissue composition after MR analysis and long-term storage in liquid nitrogen. Epidermis was thicker in psoriasis lesions, and comprised a significantly larger fraction of the biopsies both in untreated (12%) and corticosteroid treated (9%) skin than in the uninvolved skin (3%) ($p < 0.05$, ANOVA). All patients but one had lower epidermal fraction in corticosteroid treated than in untreated psoriatic skin, with about 40% reduction in epithelial thickness. The one patient with an increased thickness of epidermis after corticosteroid treatment was also clinically scored as showing poor response to treatment.

Metabolites

The MR spectra of the skin samples showed signals from numerous small molecular weight metabolites and lipids (Figure 1). The nine metabolites were detectable in all spectra, and were identified as cell building blocks (amino acids and choline compounds), osmolytes (taurine) and metabolites involved in energy consumption (glucose and lactate). Peak areas of the nine selected metabolites could be calculated for all samples. In addition, the anesthetic lidocaine contributed significantly to most spectra, giving rise to a total of seven peaks. Statistical analysis showed that the tissue content of glucose, *myo*-inositol, taurine, GPC and choline were different in the three types of sample ($p < 0.05$, Kruskal-Walis) (Figure 2). The levels of *myo*-inositol and glucose were highest in uninvolved skin and lowest in psoriatic skin, whereas those of taurine and choline were highest in psoriatic skin and lowest in uninvolved skin. The levels of GPC were highest in corticosteroid treated skin and lowest in psoriatic skin. We observed no differences in the tissue levels of creatine, glycine, lactate or phosphocholine between the three types of sample.

Seven of the patients showed a good clinical effect of topical corticosteroid treatment (at least 40% reduction of clinical score), whereas three patients had poor effect (less than 40% reduction of clinical score). We found metabolic changes that were different in these two patient groups for five of the metabolites ($p < 0.05$, Mann–Whitney) (Figure 3). In skin samples from patients with good treatment results, glucose, *myo*-inositol, GPC and glycine increased with treatment, whereas choline decreased.

Discussion

Four weeks of anti-psoriatic treatment with topical corticosteroids led to clinical improvements, as expected. This was recorded as reductions in the clinical score for

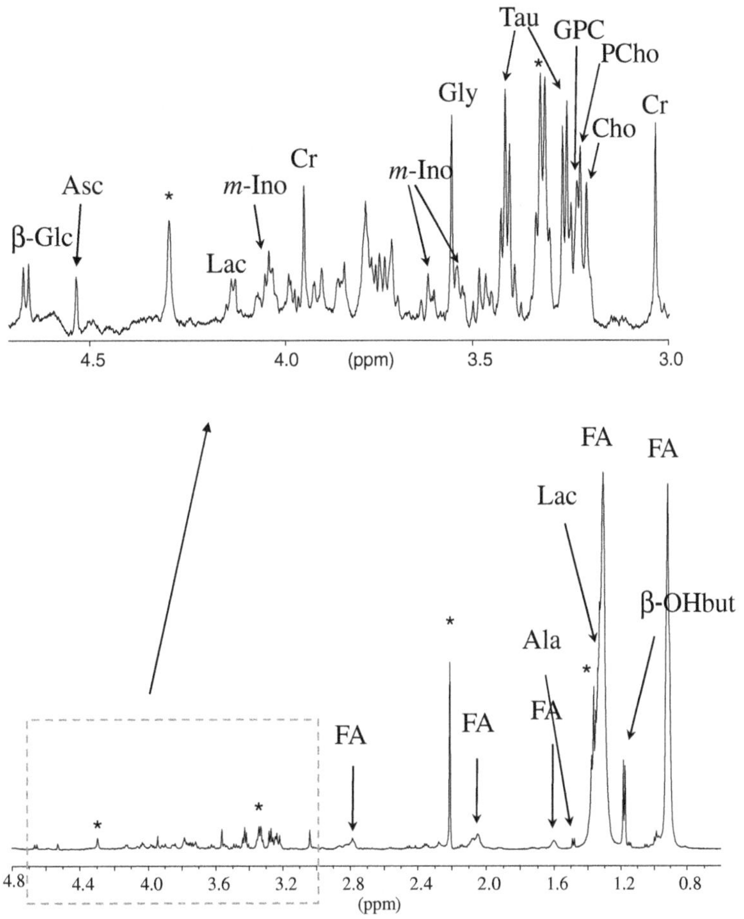

Figure 1 HR MAS spectrum of psoriatic skin biopsy (not treated). The spectral region 4.8 to 0.3 ppm is shown (lower part) with the expanded region 4.8 to 3.0 ppm above. Abbreviations used: β-Glc: β-Glucose, Asc: Ascorbate, Lac: Lactate, m-Ino: *myo*-Inositol, Cr: Creatine, Gly: Glycine, Tau: Taurine, GPC: Glycerophosphocholine, PCho: Phosphocholine, Cho: Choline FA: Fatty Acids, Ala: Alanine and βOH-But: β-hydroxybutyrate. *: Denotes signals from lidocaine.

erythema, infiltration and scaling. We also observed by histopathology that the relative thickness of the epidermis was reduced in nine out of 10 patients as an effect of corticosteroid treatment.

The spectral quality was partly influenced by the heterogeneity of the skin biopsies and by signals from the local anesthetic. MR spectroscopy of intact skin biopsies provided semi-quantitative information about tissue metabolites. It was not possible to perform absolute quantification, as this would require T2 measurements to allow for T2 correction. The MR acquisition protocol could thus not provide an absolute quantification of tissue metabolites, but the relative quantification enabled inter-sample comparisons.

We found that psoriatic skin had significantly lower levels of *myo*-inositol and glucose, and higher levels of choline than uninvolved skin. These differences between affected and healthy tissue of psoriatic patients are analogous to the differences found between affected and healthy tissue in cancer patients [10]. Both psoriasis and cancer are characterized by high cellular proliferation rates. Similarities in metabolic profiles are thus expected, in particular higher availability of nutrients for the synthesis of new biomass. Lower levels of glucose are presumably due to high glucose turnover in rapidly proliferating cells, whereas increased choline levels are associated with the need of cellular building blocks [10]. In a previous study by Kim *et al.* [14], perchloric acid extracts of skin biopsy samples from psoriasis plaques, malignant melanomas and control skin were analyzed with MR spectroscopy and GC/MS. Several metabolic ratios and concentrations were altered in psoriasis plaques compared to uninvolved psoriatic skin. The majority of metabolite concentrations were higher in psoriasis plaque. For metabolites analyzed in our study, Kim *et al.* [14] reported higher creatine-to-glycine ratio, higher lactate and lower glycine in psoriatic plaque than in non-involved psoriatic skin. The reduced glycine in steroid treated skin from responders (Figure 3) resembles the lower glycine in non-involved skin reported by Kim *et al.*

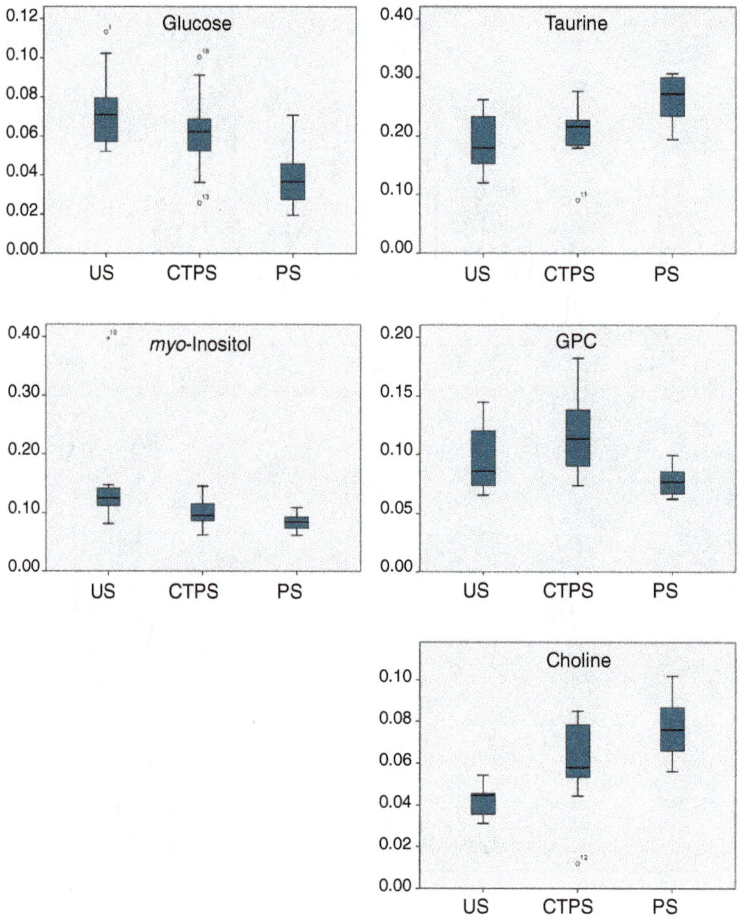

Figure 2 Box-plot of relative levels of tissue metabolites in uninvolved skin (US), corticosteroid treated psoriatic skin (CTPS) and psoriatic skin (PS). Only metabolites found to be differently expressed in different types of samples by statistical analysis ($p < 0.05$, Kruskal-Wallis) are shown: glucose, *myo*-inositol, taurine, glycerophosphocholine and choline.

No other similar metabolic findings were observed, possibly due to different approaches in metabolite analysis.

We observed increased levels of glucose and *myo*-inositol, and decreased levels of choline in steroid treated skin from responders, which indicate that the metabolic profile approaches that of uninvolved skin when treatment is effective. This metabolic change probably reflects the anti-proliferative effect of steroids, which leads to a decreased demand of nutrients for biomass synthesis. The decreased choline levels can also reflect the anti-inflammatory effect of corticosteroid treatment, as choline is known to accumulate in inflammatory processes [16]. Thus, the metabolic profile of tissue can be a molecular indicator of treatment effects and provide insight into specific pathways of drug action. There is an increased understanding of changes in molecular and cellular processes in psoriasis, and the roles and functions of several macromolecules are established. The method applied in this study can portray the small organic molecules that are substrates, intermediates and end products in cellular processes. Their function and role in psoriasis is not established. In order to understand how drugs affect metabolic pathways, tissue metabolic analysis should be combined with molecular profiling [17].

This study was performed on a small number of patients ($N = 10$), where three of the patients were receiving systematic treatment for other conditions. These ongoing, systematic treatments are unlikely to influence the observed metabolic patterns and alterations in the skin. However, a larger population without patients receiving systematic treatments will rule out possible biasing and provide more robust data. This study demonstrates the potential value of metabolic profiling as a provider of information complementary to clinical and molecular evaluation, including information which may shed new light on the changes occurring with treatment. By modifying the experimental procedures we may obtain absolute quantitative measures of tissue metabolites

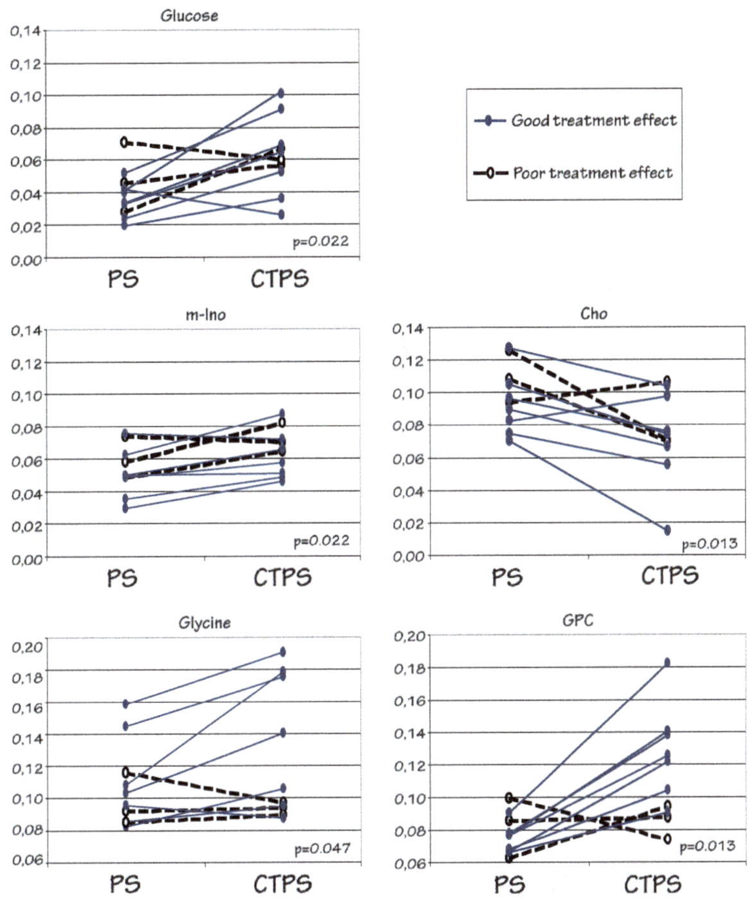

Figure 3 Differences in tissue metabolic levels of glucose, myo-inositol, glycine, GPC and choline between psoriatic skin (PS) and corticosteroid treated psoriatic skin (CTPS), discriminating patients with good effect of corticosteroid treatment (n = 7) and patients with poor effect of corticosteroid treatment (n = 3).

[18]. Furthermore, metabolic profiling can be combined with subsequent analysis of gene expression profiles [17,19], thus enabling detailed and complex information on several molecular levels. Although demonstrated for topical corticosteroid treatment, metabolic profiling of psoriatic lesions can also be applied in a diverse range of psoriasis treatment regimens, providing increased understanding of the processes of pathogenesis and their reversal due to treatment. MR spectroscopy of skin biopsies may also be utilized to obtain metabolic status of other skin conditions.

Conclusion

This study demonstrated detectable differences in tissue metabolites between uninvolved skin, psoriatic skin and corticosteroid treated psoriatic skin. We also found that metabolic differences induced by corticosteroid treatment were related to the actual therapeutic effect. The application of MR spectroscopy in dermatological research provides information about tissue metabolites, thus presenting a novel approach for studies of pathogenesis and treatment effects in the skin.

Competing interests

None of the authors have any financial or non-financial competing interests in the findings from this manuscript.

Authors' contributions

All authors have significantly contributed to the manuscript. All read and approved the final manuscript. BS and MKJ have designed the study. BS, MKJ and JH have conducted acquisition of data. BS and TFB have performed data analysis and interpretation. BS, MKJ, JH and TFB have all been involved in drafting the manuscript and revising it critically for important intellectual content.

Acknowledgements

Financial support has been granted from the Norwegian Psoriasis Association and from Sintef Unimed Forskningsfond.

Author details

[1]Department of Technology, Sør Trøndelag University College, 7004 Trondheim, Norway. [2]Department of Dermatology, St. Olavs Hospital HF, Trondheim University Hospital, Trondheim, Norway. [3]Department of Cancer Research and Molecular Medicine, Norwegian University of Science and Technology, Trondheim, Norway. [4]Department of Laboratory Medicine, Children's and Women's Health (LKB), Norwegian University of Science and Technology, Trondheim, Norway. [5]Department of Pathology and Medical

Genetics, St. Olavs Hospital HF, Trondheim University Hospital, Trondheim, Norway. [6]Department of Circulation and Medical Imaging, Norwegian University of Science and Technology, Trondheim, Norway.

References

1. Nestle FO, Kaplan DH, Barker J: **Psoriasis.** *N Engl J Med* 2009, **361**:496–509.
2. Gottlieb AB, Dann F: **Comorbidities in patients with psoriasis.** *Am J Med* 2009, **122**:1150–1159.
3. Hughes J, Rustin M: **Corticosteroids.** *Clin Dermatol* 1997, **15**:715–721.
4. Reich K, Bewley A: **What is new in topical therapy for psoriasis?** *J Eur Acad Dermatol Venereol* 2011, **25**(Suppl 4):15–20.
5. Millikan LE: *Drug therapy in dermatology.* New York: Dekker; 2000.
6. Bowes J, Barton A: **The genetics of psoriatic arthritis: lessons from genome-wide association studies.** *Discov Med* 2010, **10**:177–183.
7. Caruso R, Botti E, Sarra M, Esposito M, Stolfi C, Diluvio L, Giustizieri ML, Pacciani V, Mazzotta A, Campione E, Macdonald TT, Chimenti S, Pallone F, Costanzo A, Monteleone G: **Involvement of interleukin-21 in the epidermal hyperplasia of psoriasis.** *Nat Med* 2009, **15**:1013–1015.
8. Liu Y, Krueger JG, Bowcock AM: **Psoriasis: genetic associations and immune system changes.** *Genes Immun* 2007, **8**:1–12.
9. Lindon JC, Beckonert OP, Holmes E, Nicholson JK: **High-resolution magic angle spinning NMR spectroscopy: application to biomedical studies.** *Prog Nucl Magn Reson Spectrosc* 2009, **55**:79–100.
10. Bathen TF, Sitter B, Sjobakk TE, Tessem MB, Gribbestad IS: **Magnetic resonance metabolomics of intact tissue: a biotechnological tool in cancer diagnostics and treatment evaluation.** *Cancer Res* 2010, **70**:6692–6696.
11. Sitter B, Lundgren S, Bathen TF, Halgunset J, Fjosne HE, Gribbestad IS: **Comparison of HR MAS MR spectroscopic profiles of breast cancer tissue with clinical parameters.** *NMR Biomed* 2006, **19**:30–40.
12. Sitter B, Sonnewald U, Spraul M, Fjosne HE, Gribbestad IS: **High-resolution magic angle spinning MRS of breast cancer tissue.** *NMR in Biomedicine* 2002, **15**:327–337.
13. Martinez-Bisbal MC, Marti-Bonmati L, Piquer J, Revert A, Ferrer P, Llacer JL, Piotto M, Assemat O, Celda B: **1H and 13C HR-MAS spectroscopy of intact biopsy samples ex vivo and in vivo 1H MRS study of human high grade gliomas.** *NMR Biomed* 2004, **17**:191–205.
14. Kim YH, Orenberg EK, Faull KF, Wade-Jardetzky NG, Jardetzky O: **^{1}H NMR spectroscopy: an approach to evaluation of diseased skin in vivo.** *J Invest Dermatol* 1989, **92**(2):210–216.
15. Weibel ER, Kistler GS, Scherle WF: **Practical stereological methods for morphometric cytology.** *J Cell Biol* 1966, **30**:23–38.
16. van Waarde A, Elsinga PH: **Proliferation markers for the differential diagnosis of tumor and inflammation.** *Curr Pharm Des* 2008, **14**:3326–3339.
17. Borgan E, Sitter B, Lingjaerde OC, Johnsen H, Lundgren S, Bathen TF, Sorlie T, Borresen-Dale AL, Gribbestad IS: **Merging transcriptomics and metabolomics–advances in breast cancer profiling.** *BMC Cancer* 2010, **10**:628.
18. Sitter B, Bathen TF, Singstad TE, Fjosne HE, Lundgren S, Halgunset J, Gribbestad IS: **Quantification of metabolites in breast cancer patients with different clinical prognosis using HR MAS MR spectroscopy.** *NMR Biomed* 2010, **23**:424–431.
19. Cuperlovic-Culf M, Chute IC, Culf AS, Touaibia M, Ghosh A, Griffiths S, Tulpan D, Leger S, Belkaid A, Surette ME, Ouellette RJ: **(1)H NMR metabolomics combined with gene expression analysis for the determination of major metabolic differences between subtypes of breast cell lines.** *Chem Sci* 2011, **2**:2263–2270.

11

Experiences with Surgical treatment of chronic lower limb ulcers at a Tertiary hospital in northwestern Tanzania: A prospective review of 300 cases

Fidelis Mbunda[1†], Mabula D Mchembe[2], Phillipo L Chalya[1*], Peter Rambau[3†], Stephen E Mshana[4†], Benson R Kidenya[5] and Japhet M Gilyoma[1]

Abstract

Background: Chronic lower limb ulcers constitute a major public health problem of great important all over the world and contribute significantly to high morbidity and long-term disabilities. There is paucity of information regarding chronic lower limb ulcers in our setting; therefore it was necessary to conduct this study to establish the patterns and outcome of chronic lower limb ulcers and to identify predictors of outcome in our local setting.

Methods: This was a descriptive prospective study of patients with chronic lower limb ulcers conducted at Bugando Medical Centre between November 2010 and April 2012. Ethical approval to conduct the study was sought from relevant authorities. Statistical data analysis was done using SPSS version 17.0 and STATA version 11.0.

Results: A total of 300 patients were studied. Their ages ranged from 3 months to 85 years (median 32 years). The male to female ratio was 2:1. The median duration of illness was 44 days. Traumatic ulcer was the most frequent type of ulcer accounting for 60.3% of patients. The median duration of illness was 44 days. The leg was commonly affected in 33.7% of cases and the right side (48.7%) was frequently involved. Out of 300 patients, 212 (70.7%) had positive aerobic bacterial growth within 48 hours of incubation. *Pseudomonas aeruginosa* (25.5%) was the most frequent gram negative bacteria isolated, whereas gram positive bacteria commonly isolated was *Staphylococcus aureus* (13.7%). Twenty (6.7%) patients were HIV positive with a median CD4+ count of 350 cells/μl. Mycological investigation was not performed. Bony involvement was radiologically reported in 83.0% of cases. Histopathological examination performed in 56 patients revealed malignancy in 20 (35.7%) patients, of which malignant melanoma (45.0%) was the most common histopathological type. The vast majority of patients, 270 (90.0%) were treated surgically, and surgical debridement was the most common surgical procedure performed in 24.1% of cases. Limb amputation rate was 8.7%. Postoperative complication rate was 58.3% of which surgical site infection (77.5%) was the most common post-operative complications. The median length of hospital stay was 23 days. Mortality rate was 4.3%. Out of the two hundred and eighty-seven (95.7%) survivors, 253 (91.6%) were treated successfully and discharged well (healed). After discharge, only 35.5% of cases were available for follow up at the end of study period.

(Continued on next page)

* Correspondence: drphillipoleo@yahoo.com
†Equal contributors
[1]Department of Surgery, Catholic University of Health and Allied Sciences-Bugando, Mwanza, Tanzania
Full list of author information is available at the end of the article

(Continued from previous page)

Conclusion: Chronic lower limb ulcers remain a major public health problem in this part of Tanzania. The majority of patients in our environment present late when the disease is already in advanced stages. Early recognition and aggressive treatment of the acute phase of chronic lower limb ulcers at the peripheral hospitals and close follow-up are urgently needed to improve outcomes of these patients in our environment.

Keywords: Chronic lower limb ulcers, Patterns, Treatment outcome, Predictors of outcome, Tanzania

Background

Chronic ulceration of the lower limb constitutes a major public health problem of great important all over the world and contributes significantly to high morbidity and long-term disabilities [1]. It is a stressful disease to those affected as well as their family and the community in general, and its impact on hospital resources is great due to prolonged hospitalization, high cost of health care, loss of productivity and reduced quality of life [1-3]. Lower limb ulceration presenting late may end up being treated by limb amputation and is associated with increased risk of recurrence and malignant change [3].

Globally, the prevalence of chronic lower limb ulcers in the community has been reported in literature to range from 1.9 to 13.1% [1-3]. In developed countries, chronic ulceration of the lower limb affects approximately 2% of the population [4]. In the United Kingdom, the prevalence of chronic lower limb ulcers in the adult population is 1% and the prevalence in the more than 65 years age group is 3–5% [4,5]. In the United States of America, approximately 6,000,000 new lower limb ulcer cases are reported each year and in Sweden, 4–5% of the population over the age of 80 years presents with this pathology. The annual cost for treating chronic lower limb ulceration patients globally is estimated at some $25 million [6,7].

In Tanzania, chronic lower limb ulceration continues to be one of the leading causes of morbidity and long term disabilities. The disease tends to affect the young, reproductive age group. Observation at Bugando Medical Centre shows; chronic lower extremity ulceration is the single commonest indication for admission reported in the surgical wards and the majority of patients present late with advanced disease [8]. The etiological patterns of lower extremity ulceration in most developing countries have been reported to differ from that in developed countries. While, most of lower limb ulceration in the Western population is related to vascular diseases such as venous and arterial disease; trauma, malignancies, diabetes mellitus and infections are the most common causes in developing countries [2,9,10].

The effective treatment and outcome of lower limb ulceration is highly dependent upon establishing the etiology of the ulceration and the identification of other associated conditions that may have an adverse effect on healing [11].

The majority of chronic lower limb ulcers are preventable and have a multifactorial etiology, therefore understanding the etiological pattern of this condition in our local setting will provides information that is important for accurate diagnosis, prediction of outcome and may help in hospital resource allocations and establishment of prevention strategies as well as treatment protocols [12].

The aim of this study was to describe the patterns and treatment outcome of chronic lower limb ulcers in our local setting and to identify factors predicting the outcome. The study provides basis for establishment of treatment guidelines as well as prevention strategies.

Methods

Study design and setting

This was a descriptive prospective hospital-based study of patients with chronic lower limb ulcers carried out at Bugando Medical Centre (BMC) in Northwestern Tanzania between November 2010 and February 2012. BMC is located in Mwanza city along the shore of Lake Victoria in the northwestern part of Tanzania. It is a tertiary care and teaching hospital for the Catholic University of Health and Allied Sciences- Bugando (CUHAS-Bugando) and other paramedics and has a bed capacity of 1000. BMC is one of the four largest referral hospitals in the country and serves as a referral centre for tertiary specialist care for a catchment population of approximately 13 million people from Mwanza, Mara, Kagera, Shinyanga, Tabora and Kigoma regions.

Study subjects and procedures

The study included all patients with chronic lower limb ulcers of all age groups and both genders seen in the surgical wards and surgical outpatient clinics of BMC during the study period. Patients who failed to consent for the study, treatment (e.g. limb amputation) and HIV testing were excluded from the study.

Recruitment of patients to participate in the study was done at the Accident and Emergency department, surgical outpatient clinic and in the surgical wards. Patients were screened for inclusion criteria and those who met the inclusion criteria were offered explanations about the study and requested to consent before being enrolled into the study. Convenience sampling of patients who met the inclusion criteria was performed until the sample size was reached. The diagnosis of chronic lower limb ulcers was made by clinical history and physical examination and chronic lower limb ulcers was defined as defect in the skin on the lower extremities that remains unhealed for at least four or more weeks. Pus or pus swabs were obtained from the ulcer and transported to the laboratory within an hour of collection. In the laboratory, the specimens were registered in the log books and processed as per standard operative procedures. Bacterial identification was done using an in house biochemical panel [13]. Antibacterial susceptibility testing to various antibiotics was performed using disc diffusion methods as previously described [14,15]. In addition, blood was taken from all patients for random blood sugar testing and CD4 enumeration in HIV positive patients. HIV test was done using national algorithm of rapid test. Mycological investigation was not performed due to logistic problems. Biopsies from chronic lower limb ulcers were taken under sterile technique and specimens were transported in a formalin solution to the histopathology laboratory for processing.

All recruited patients were managed accordingly. The authors ensured that the study patients were receiving the appropriate treatment and supportive care as prescribed by the surgeon. Patients were followed up until discharge or death. After discharge patients were followed up at our surgical outpatient clinic for up to six months.

Data were collected using a pre-tested coded questionnaire. Data administered in the questionnaire included; patients characteristics (e.g. age, sex, premorbid illness, history of smoking and use of immunosuppressive drugs), causes of chronic lower limb ulcers, clinical pattern, investigations, treatment modalities and postoperative complications. Length of hospital stay (LOS) and mortality were recorded at the end of study period.

Statistical data analysis

Statistical data analysis was done using SPSS software version 17.0 (SPSS, Inc, Chicago, IL) and STATA version 11.0. Data was summarized in form of proportions and frequent tables for categorical variables. Continuous variables were summarized using means, median, mode and standard deviation. P-values were computed for categorical variables using Chi – square (χ^2) test and Fisher's exact test depending on the size of the data set. Independent student t-test was used for continuous variables. Multivariate logistic regression analysis was used to determine predictor variables that are associated with outcome. Post-operative complications were entered into univariate and multivariate analysis after been categorized into presence or absence of post-operative complications. LOS was arbitrarily categorized as ≤14 and > 14 days. A p-value of less than 0.05 was considered to constitute a statistically significant difference.

Ethical consideration

Ethical approval to conduct the study was obtained from the CUHAS-Bugando/BMC joint institutional ethic review committee before the commencement of the study. Informed consent was sought from each patient before being enrolled into the study.

Results

During the period under study, a total of 312 patients with chronic lower limb ulcers were managed at Bugando Medical Centre. Of these, 12 patients were excluded from the study due failure to meet the inclusion criteria. Thus, 300 patients were studied. The ages of the study population ranged from 3 months to 85 years with a median of 32 years. The modal age group was 21–30 years. Out of 300 patients recruited into the study, two hundred (66.7%) were males and 100 (33.3%) were females. The male to female ratio was 2:1 with a male predominance in each age group (Figure 1).

Fifty-four (18.0%) patients presented with history of premorbid illness such as diabetes mellitus in 32 (59.3%), chronic pulmonary diseases in 8 (14.8%), hypertension in 6 (11.1%), peripheral vascular diseases in 4 (7.4%) and congenital cardiac diseases and obstructive jaundice in 2 (3.7%) patients each respectively. In this study, sixty-eight (22.7%) patients had history of cigarette smoking. There was no history of immunosuppressive drugs use or radiotherapy.

The median duration of illness was 44 days (range 31 to 3218 days). Traumatic ulcers were the most frequent type of ulcer accounting for 60.3% of patients. Road traffic accidents (RTAs) were the most common cause of traumatic ulcers accounting for 122 (67.4%) patients (Table 1). Seventy-three (59.8%) of RTAs were related to motorcycle injuries. Other causes of traumatic ulcers included burn in 45 (24.9%), falls in 8 (4.4%), gunshot injuries in 3(1.7%0, hit by falling object and sport injuries

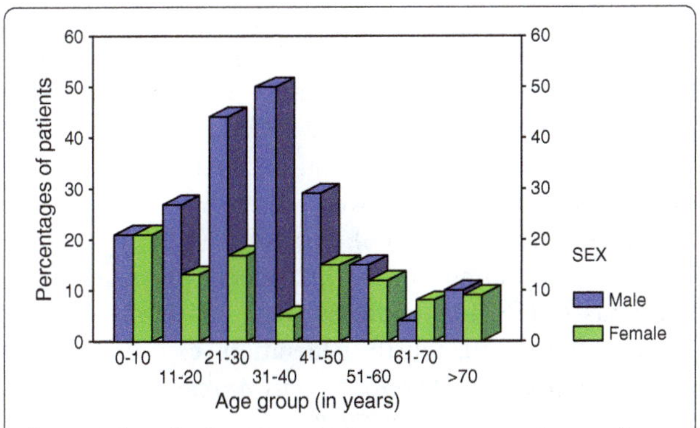

Figure 1 Sex distribution according to age group (In years).

Table 1 Distribution of study population according to the type of ulcers

Type of ulcers	Frequency	Percentage
Traumatic ulcers	**181**	**60.3**
· Mechanical trauma	131	72.4
· Burns	50	27.6
Infective ulcers	**43**	**14.3**
· Osteomyelitis	30	69.8
· Tropical ulcer	6	13.9
· Cellulitis	5	11.6
· Others	2	4.7
Metabolic ulcers	**35**	**11.7**
· Diabetic ulcer	32	91.4
· Pellagra	3	8.6
Neoplastic/malignant ulcers	**20**	**6.7**
· Malignant melanoma	9	45.0
· Kaposi's sarcoma	5	25.0
· Squamous cell carcinoma	4	20.0
· Others	2	10.0
Vascular ulcers	**11**	**3.7**
· Arterial ulcers	5	45.5
· Venous ulcers	4	36.4
· Mixed ulcers	2	18.2
Neuropathic ulcers	**8**	**2.7**
· Pressure sores	6	75.0
· Others	2	25.0
Ulcerating skin lesions e.g. Pyogenic Granulomatous	**2**	**0.7**

in 2(1.1%) and 1(0.6%) respectively. Table 1 shows distribution of study population according to the type of ulcers.

The leg was commonly affected in 33.7% of cases (Figure 2) and the right, left and both limbs were involved in 146 (48.7%), 126 (42.0%) and 28 (9.3%) patients respectively. The size ulcers ranged from 2 to 30 cm with a median of 5 cm.

Out of 300 patients with CLLUs, 212 (70.7%) had positive aerobic bacterial growth within 48 hours of incubation. Of these, 10 (4.7%) patents had polymicrobial growth. *Pseudomonas spp.* (25.5%) and *Proteus spp.* (21.2%) were the most common bacteria isolated, while the least isolated bacteria were *Enterobacter spp* (2.8%) and *Enterococcus spp* (1.4%). Forty-one (19.3%) bacterial isolates were found to be Extended Spectrum Beta-Lactamases (ESBL) producers (i.e. resistant to first, second, third and fourth generation cephalosporins). Methicilin Resistant *Staphylococcus aureus* (MRSA) was detected in 23 out of 29 (79.3%) *Staphylococcus aureus* isolates.

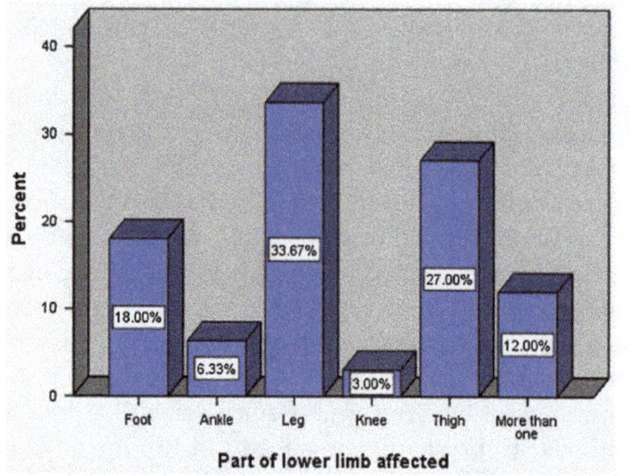

Figure 2 Part of lower limb affected.

In this study, twenty (6.7%) patients were HIV positive. Of these, 6 (30.0%) patients were known cases on antretroviral therapy (ARV) and the remaining 14 (70.0%) patients were newly diagnosed patients. Their CD 4+ count, available in 15 patients, ranged from 180 to 480 cells/μl (median = 350cells/μl). A total of two HIV patients (13.3%) had CD4+ count below 200 cells/μl and the remaining 13 patients (86.7%) had CD4+ count of ≥200 cells/μ.

Plain x-rays of the affected limbs were performed in 235 (78.3%) patients. Of these, 195 (83.0%) patients had abnormal x-ray findings including associated fractures, chronic osteomyelitis, bone tumors and others in 144 (73.9%), 47 (24.1%), 3 (1.5%) and 1 (0.5%) patients respectively.

Doppler ultrasound of the affected limbs was done in 203 (67.7%) patients. Of these, only seventeen (8.4%) patients had abnormal Doppler ultrasound findings.

A total of 56 histopathological examinations were performed. Of these, 20 (35.7%) had a histopathologically proven malignancy, of which malignant melanoma was the most common histopathological type in 9 (45.0%) patients. This was followed by Kaposi's sarcoma in 5 (25.0%), squamous cell carcinoma in 4 (20.0%), neurofibrosarcoma and liposarcoma in 1 (5.0%) patient each respectively.

A total of 287 (95.7%) patients were treated as inpatients and the remaining 13 (4.3%) patients were treated as outpatients. The vast majority of patients, 270 (90.0%) were treated surgically (Figure 3). The remaining 30 (10.0%) patients were treated conservatively (non-surgical approach) with daily dressing, antimicrobial agents, compression bandage, antibiotics.

A total of 178 post-operative complications were recorded in 175 (58.3%) patients. Of these, surgical site infection (77.5%) was the most common post-operative complications (Figure 4). Table 2 shows predictors of postoperative complications among patients with

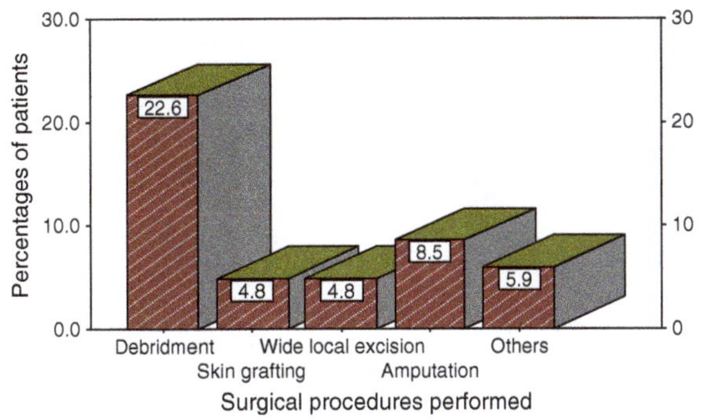

Figure 3 Distribution of patients according to surgical procedure performed.

chronic lower limb ulcers according to univariate and multivariate logistic regression analysis

The overall length of hospital stay (LOS) ranged from 1 day to 180 days with a median of 23 days. The LOS for non-survivors ranged from 1 day and 42 days (median = 10 days). Table 3 shows predictors of LOS among patients with chronic lower limb ulcers according to univariate and multivariate logistic regression analysis

In this study, thirteen patients died giving a mortality rate of 4.3%. The causes of death were complications of diabetes mellitus (5 patients), HIV infection (4 patients) and advanced malignancy (2 patients). The cause of death was not established in 2 patients.

Out of the two hundred and eighty-seven (95.7%) survivors, 253 (91.6%) were treated successfully and discharged well (healed). Thirteen (4.5%) patients were discharged with permanent disabilities resulting from lower limb amputation and the remaining six (2.1%) patients were discharged home advised to continue with daily dressing at their nearby health facilities. Thirteen (4.5%) patients were treated as outpatients and two (0.7%) patients discharged themselves against medical advice.

Discussion

In this review, chronic lower limb ulcers were in the third decade of life and tended to affect more males than

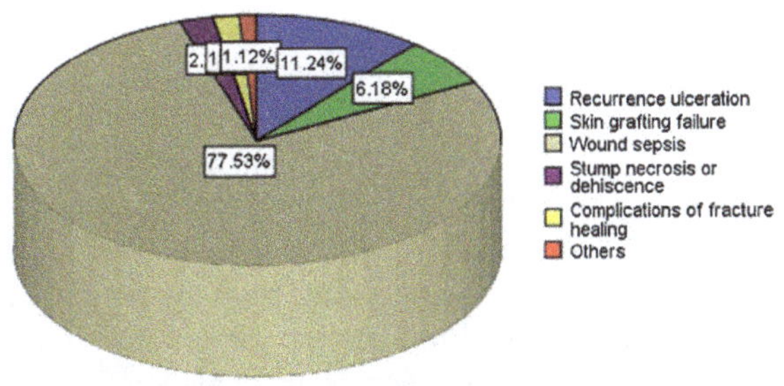

Figure 4 Distribution of patients according to postoperative complications.

females, with a male to female ratio of 2:1 which is comparable with other studies in developing countries [16,17]. Our demographic profile is in sharp contrast to what is reported in developed countries where the majority of the patients are in the sixth decade and above [17-19]. Male predominance in this age group may be due to their increased susceptibility to trauma which was found to be the major etiological agent of chronic lower limb ulcers in this study.

The presence of pre-morbid illness, such as diabetes mellitus, chronic obstructive pulmonary disease, arteriosclerosis, peripheral vascular disease, heart disease, and any conditions leading to hypotension, hypovolaemia, edema, and anemia has been reported elsewhere to have an effect on the outcome of patients with chronic lower limb ulcers [20,21]. Pre-morbid illnesses influence the healing process as a result of their influence on a number of bodily functions [20-23]. In the presence study, diabetes mellitus was the most common premorbid illness accounting for 59.3% of cases which is agreement with other studies in developing countries [21,22,24]. Diabetes mellitus is associated with delayed cellular response to injury, compromised cellular function at the site of injury, defects in collagen synthesis, and reduced wound tensile strength after healing. Diabetes-related peripheral neuropathy, reducing the ability to feel pressure or pain, contributes to a tendency to ignore pressure points and avoid pressure relief strategies [25].

In the present study, cigarette smoking was reported in 22.7% of cases which is in keeping with other studies [26,27]. Cigarette smoking has been reported to have an impact on wound healing through impairment of tissue oxygenation and local hypoxia via vasoconstriction [28]. Tobacco smoke has high concentration of carbon monoxide, which binds hemoglobin, forming carboxyhemoglobin. Carboxyhemoglobin binds to oxygen with high affinity and thereby interferes with normal oxygen delivery to hypoxic tissues [29].

The etiological pattern of chronic lower limb ulcers have been reported in literature to vary from one part of the world to another depending on the prevailing sociodemographic and environmental factors [2,9]. In Western societies, most chronic lower limb ulcers are due to vascular diseases, whereas in developing countries, trauma, infections, malignancies and poorly controlled diabetes remain the most common causes of chronic lower limb ulceration [2,9,10]. In the present study, traumatic ulcers secondary to road traffic accidents were the most common type of chronic lower limb ulcers accounting for more than sixty percent of cases, which is in keeping with other studies done in developing countries [9,10,20,21]. High incidence of traumatic ulcers secondary to road traffic accidents may be attributed to recklessness and negligence of the driver, poor

Table 2 Predictors of Postoperative complications according to univariate and multivariate logistic regression analysis

Predictor (Independent) variables	Post operative complications n (%)		Univariate analysis			Multivariate analysis		
	Absent	Present	OR	95% CI	P value	OR	CI	P value
Age								
≤20	39(48.8)	41(51.3)						
>20	83(37.7)	137(62.3)	1.6	0.9-2.6	0.087	3.0	1.4-6.3	**0.004**
Sex								
Male	102(51.0)	98(49.0)						
Female	20(20.0)	80(80.0)	4.2	2.4-7.3	<0.001	4.3	2.1-8.7	**<0.001**
HIV status								
Positive	4(20.0)	16(80.0)						
Negative	118(42.1)	162(57.9)	2.9	0.9-8.9	0.062			
CD4 count								
<200 cells/μl	1(50.0)	1(50.0)						
≥200 cells/μl	3(23.1)	10(76.9)	1.3	0.2-2.7	0.082			
Pre-morbid illness								
Absent	11(20.4)	43(79.6)						
Present	111(45.1)	135(54.9)	3.2	1.6-6.5	0.001	0.4	0.2-1.0	**0.041**
Tobacco smoking								
Yes	30(44.1)	38(55.9)						
No	92(39.7)	140(60.3)	1.9	0.4- 5.4	0.897			
Duration of illness								
1/12-3/12	115(48.7)	121(51.3)						
3/12-1 year	3(7.1)	39(92.9)	12.4	3.7-41.1	<0.001	8.0	2.1-30.0	**0.002**
>1 year	4(18.2)	18(81.8)	4.3	1.4-13.0	0.010			
Type of ulcer								
Traumatic ulcer	107(59.1)	74(40.9)						
Vascular ulcer	4(36.4)	7(63.6)	2.5	0.7-9.0	0.150			
Neoplastic ulcer	4(20.0)	16(80.0)	5.8	1.9-18.0	0.002			
Infective ulcer	3(7.0)	40(93.0)	19.3	5.7-64.7	<0.001	17.6	4.7-66.0	**<0.001**
Metabolic ulcer	2(5.7)	33(94.3)	23.9	5.6-102.5	<0.001	8.4	1.8-39.4	**0.007**
Neuropathic ulcer	2(25.0)	6(75.0)	4.3	0.9-22.1	0.077			
Ulcerating skin disease	0(0.0)	2(100)	-	-	-			
Ulcer size in cm								
≤5	90(47.9)	98(52.1)						
>5-10	28(31.8)	60(68.2)	2.0	1.2-3.4	0.013			
>10	4(16.7)	20(83.3)	4.6	1.5-13.9	0.007			
Mode of treatment								
Conservative	14(36.8)	24(63.2)						
Surgical	108(41.2)	154(58.8)	0.8	0.4-1.7	0.608			

maintenance of vehicles, driving under the influence of alcohol or drugs and complete disregard of traffic laws.

In agreement with other studies in developing countries [3,24], the majority of patients in the present study presented late to hospital with advanced and complicated chronic lower limb ulcers which may end up being treated by limb amputation with increased risk of recurrence and malignant change. Late presentation in this study may be attributed to poor economic capabilities in cost shared healthcare systems, inadequate knowledge of self-care and socio-cultural reasons. Other contributing factors for late presentation include attempts at home

Table 3 Predictors of length of hospital stay (LOS) among patients with chronic lower limb ulcers according to univariate and multivariate logistic regression analysis

Predictor (Independent) variables	LOS n (%)		Univariate analysis			Multivariate analysis		
	≤14	>14	OR	95% CI	P- value	OR	CI	P-value
Age								
<20	14(17.5)	66(82.5)	1					
>20	45(20.4)	175(79.6)	1.1	0.4-1.6	0.570			
Sex								
Male	42(21.0)	158(79.0)	1					
Female	17(17.0)	83(83.0)	1.3	0.7-2.4	0.412			
HIV status								
Positive	2(10.0)	18(90.0)	1					
Negative	57(20.4)	223(79.6)	2.3	0.5-10.2	0.273			
Pre-morbid illness								
Absent	51(20.7)	195(79.3)	1					
Present	8(14.8)	46(85.2)	1.5	0.7-3.4	0.324			
Duration of illness								
1/12-3/12	47(19.9)	189(80.1)	1					
3/12-1 year	7(16.7)	35(83.3)	1.2	0.5-3.0	0.624			
>1 year	5(22.7)	17(77.3)	0.8	0.3-2.4	0.753			
Type of ulcer								
Traumatic ulcer	42(23.2)	139(76.8)	1					
Vascular ulcer	2(18.2)	9(81.8)	1.4	0.3-6.5	0.701			
Neoplastic ulcer	4(20.0)	16(80.0)	1.2	0.4-3.8	0.746			
Infective ulcer	6(14.0)	37(86.1)	1.9	0.7-4.7	0.189			
Metabolic ulcer	3(8.6)	32(91.4)	3.2	0.9-11.1	0.063	3.5	1.0-12.5	**0.056**
Neuropathic ulcer	1(12.5)	7(87.5)	2.1	0.3-17.7	0.489			
Ulcerating skin disease	1(50.0)	1(50.0)	0.3	0.01-4.9	0.401			
Ulcer size in cm								
<5	38(20.2)	150(79.8)	1					
>5-10	17(19.3)	71(80.7)	1.1	0.6-2.0	0.862			
>10	4(16.7)	20(83.3)	1.3	0.4-3.9	0.682			
Mode of treatment								
Conservative	13(34.2)	25(65.8)	1					
Surgical	46(17.6)	216(82.4)	2.4	1.2-5.1	0.018	3.2	1.4-7.1	**0.005**
Postoperative complications								
Absent	26(21.3)	96(78.7)	1					
Present	33(18.5)	145(81.5)	1.2	0.7-2.1	0.553			

surgery, trust in faith healers, poor management of acute lower limb ulcers and delayed referral in most health centers and peripheral hospitals.

As reported in other studies [30,31], the leg was the most frequent anatomical site affected in our series and the right side was frequently involved. We could not find the reasons for this anatomical site distribution.

The microbiological profile of chronic ulcers of the lower limbs has application to general principles of treatment as well as institution-specific guidelines for management [32]. In the present study, *Pseudomonas aeruginosa* was the most frequent gram negative bacteria isolated, whereas gram positive bacteria commonly isolated was *Staphylococcus aureus*. Similar bacterial profile was reported by Lim *et al.* [32]. The study also found that most of the pathogens were multiply resistant to the commonly prescribed antibiotics such as Ampicillin, Augmentin, Cotrimoxazole, Tetracycline, gentamicin, erythromycin, and Ceftriaxone. Similar antimicrobial susceptibility pattern has been reported previously [33]. These findings reflect the widespread and indiscriminate use of antibiotics, coupled with poor patient compliance and self treatment without prescription among African patients [32,33]. The majority of gram negative isolates were sensitive to Meropenem while gram positive being sensitive to Vancomycin; this could be explained by the fact that these antibiotics are relatively rare in the hospital and are more expensive so they are rarely misused.

The prevalence of HIV infection in the present study was 6.7% that is relatively similar to that in the general population in Tanzania (6.5%) [34]. High HIV seroprevalence among patients with CLLUs was reported in a Zimbabwean study [35]. HIV seropositive patients have been reported to have a higher risk of developing postoperative complications and have a greater risk of prolonged hospital stay and mortality [16,18]. HIV infection has been reported to increase the risk of wound sepsis and poor healing [35]. However, in the present study, there were no significant differences in the outcome between patients who are HIV infected and those who are non-HIV infected.

Fungal infections have been reported to be common in chronic lower limb ulcers with the prevalence ranging from 4.5%–50% and [36,37], are also responsible for some chronic lower limb ulcers e.g. Madura foot [38,39]. In the present study, fungal infection was not investigated due to logistic problems. This calls for other authors to investigate on this.

Histopathological examination remains the most important definitive diagnostic procedure, and it should be performed on any suspicious lesion or any chronic nonhealing ulcers, especially those with any recent change in appearance or considerable drainage [40]. In the present study, malignant ulcers were histopathologically proven in 8.4% of cases, a figure closely to 10.4% reported by Senet *et al.* [41]. In our study, malignant melanoma was the most frequent histopathological type as previously reported by Chalya *et al.* [42] at the same centre, but at variant with Senet *et al.* [41] who reported squamous cell carcinoma as most common histopathological type. This difference in histopathological type reflects geographic differences in exposure to risk factors for developing malignant ulcers. While solar radiation has been suggested as a major cause of malignant melanoma among Caucasians, many of malignant melanoma among black Africans has been reported to be unrelated to solar exposure since they occur on the unexposed plantar of the foot [43-51]. Higher incidence of malignant melanoma in our study may be attributed to repeated trauma and constant pressure on the weight bearing areas of the foot as shoe-wearing is less frequent among people especially those from rural areas [42,52]. In the present study, Kaposi's sarcoma ranked third after squamous cell carcinoma. Since the emergence of HIV infection, there has been a steady increase in the prevalence of KS worldwide [53,54]. The rate of HIV infection among patients with Kaposi's sarcoma in our study was 60%, a figure slightly lower than that reported by Chalya *et al.* [42]. Thus it is obvious that successful HIV control will go a long way to reduce the incidence of this vascular malignancy.

The treatment of chronic lower limb ulcers requires multidisciplinary approach [54,55]. The treatment modalities of chronic lower limb ulcers include surgical treatment (such as wound debridement, wide local excision, split thickness skin graft (STSG) or flap cover, block dissection of the regional nodes and limb amputation in advanced lesions) and non-surgical treatment such daily dressing, compressive bandages and antimicrobial agents bases on drug sensitivity pattern [54,56-58]. In the present study, wound debridement with or without STSG or flap cover was the most common surgical procedure performed which is in keeping with studies done elsewhere [55].

The presence of complications has an impact on the final outcome of patients presenting with chronic lower limb ulcers [21]. Most complications are related to late presentation to hospital following ignorance, treatment at home, cost, poverty, advanced malignancy, premorbid conditions like diabetes mellitus, hypertension, and the treatment choices made and the procedures performed. In the present study a total of 178 complications were recorded in 175 (58.3%) patients, mostly being post operative complications. Of these, surgical site infections (77.5%) was the most common post operative complication followed by recurrent ulceration (11.2%) and skin grafting failure (6.2%). Callam *et al.* [21] reported a similar observation.

The length of hospital stay is an important measure of morbidity in which estimates of length of hospital stay are important for financial matters and accurate early estimates so as to facilitate better financial planning by the payers since it takes long for the chronic lower limb ulcers to heal so increasing the costs as well as seen in other studies as well [16,18]. In this study, the overall mean length of hospital stay was 28.9 days, a figure which is higher than that reported in other studies [59,60]. A mean length of hospital stay of 38.2 days was also reported in Nigerian study [16]. A mean of 36.2 days and 64.2 days were reported in Tanzanian and Nigerian studies respectively [16,24]. Prolonged LOS in our study was observed in patients with diabetic foot ulcers and in patients who required surgical treatment.

In this study, the mortality rate was 4.3% which is relatively lower than that reported in other studies [16]. Mortality rate in the present study was attributed to complications of diabetes mellitus, hypertension, HIV infection and advanced malignancy. The causes of death in our study is at variant with a Nigerian study which reported anemic heart failure, septicemia and multiple organ failure as causes of death [16]. Addressing these factors responsible for mortality in our patients is mandatory to be able to reduce mortality associated with chronic lower limb ulcers.

In this study, complete healing at discharge from the hospital was achieved in more than 90% of the patients, which is comparable with other studies [16,61]. This is satisfactorily acceptable to both the patient and the surgical team.

Self discharge by patient against medical advice is a recognized problem in our setting and this is rampant, especially amongst patients with chronic lower limb ulcers [62]. In the present study discharge against medical advice was noted in 0.7% of cases. Discharge against medical advice in our study is attributed to patients feeling well enough to leave and dissatisfaction with treatment received.

Poor follow up visits after discharge from hospitals remain a cause for concern in most developing countries [63]. These issues are often the results of poverty, long distance from the hospitals and ignorance. In the present study, only 33.1% of patients were available for follow up at three months, the reasons for low follow up rate at our study may be attributed to long distance from the hospital, lack of funds for transport and feeling of being cured.

Delay in getting histopathological results was the major limitation in this study and this might have affected the treatment outcome of patients who needed this confirmatory diagnostic investigation for definitive treatment.

Conclusion

Chronic lower limb ulceration remains a major public health problem in this part of Tanzania. Traumatic ulcers are the most common type of chronic lower limb ulcers. The majority of patients in our environment present late when the disease is already in advanced stages predisposing them to increased risk of recurrence, malignant change and limb amputation. Early recognition and aggressive treatment of the acute phase of chronic lower limb ulcers at the peripheral hospitals and close follow-up are urgently needed to improve outcomes of these patients in this environment. Further study looking at the factors associated with late presentation to tertiary health facilities is highly recommended. A population based study is highly needed to be able to assess the better picture of the magnitude of the problem in this region.

Competing interests

The authors declare that they have no competing interests.

Authors' contributions

FM conceived the study and did the literature search, participated in data analysis, writing of the manuscript and editing. MDM and BBK participated in the literature search, writing of the manuscript and editing. SEM participated in writing of the manuscript, editing and performed the microbiological analysis. PFR participated in writing of the manuscript, editing and performed the pathological work up. PLC participated in writing of the manuscript, editing, data analysis and submission of the manuscript. JMG coordinated the write-up, editing and supervised the study. All the authors read and approved the final manuscript.

Acknowledgements

The authors would like to thank all those who participated in the preparation of this manuscript.

Author details

[1]Department of Surgery, Catholic University of Health and Allied Sciences-Bugando, Mwanza, Tanzania. [2]Department of Surgery, Muhimbili University of Health and Allied Sciences, Dar Es Salaam, Tanzania. [3]Department of Pathology, Catholic University of Health and Allied Sciences- Bugando, Mwanza, Tanzania. [4]Department of Microbiology, Catholic University of Health and Allied Sciences- Bugando, Mwanza, Tanzania. [5]Department of Biochemistry and Molecular Biology, Catholic University of Health and Allied Sciences- Bugando, Mwanza, Tanzania.

References

1. Lees TA, Lambert D: **Prevalence of lower limb ulceration in an urban health district.** *Br J Surg* 1992, **79**(10):1032–1034.
2. Barclay KL, Granby T, Elton PJ: **The prevalence of leg ulcers in Hospitals.** *Hosp Med* 1998, **59**(11):8.
3. Bricksson SV, Lundeberg T, Malm MA: **Placebo-controlled trial of ultrasound therapy in chronic leg ulceration.** *Scandinavian J Rehabilitation Med* 1991, **23**(4):211–213.
4. Shaw JE, Boulton AJ: **The pathogenesis of diabetic foot problems: an overview.** *Diabetes* 1997, **46**(Suppl. 2):58–61.
5. Baker SR, Stacey MC, Jopp-McKay AG: **Epidemiology of chronic venous ulcers.** *Br J Surg* 1991, **78:**864–867.
6. Phillips TJ: **Chronic cutaneous ulcers etiology and epidemiology.** *J Invest Dermatol* 1994, **102**(Suppl):38–41.
7. Dormandy JA, Stock G: *Critical leg ischaemia its pathophysiology and management*. Berlin: Springer Verlag; 1990:7–16.
8. Bugando Medical Centre database: *Medical record database.*; 2008.
9. London NJ, Donnely R: **ABC of arterial and venous disease Ulcerated lower limb.** *Br Med J* 2000, **320:**1589–1591.
10. Cleverland TJ, Gaines P: **Stenting in peripheral vascular disease.** *Hosp Med* 1999, **60:**630–632.
11. Valencia IC, Falabella A, Kirsner RS, Eaglstein WH: **Chronic venous insufficiency and venous leg ulceration.** *J Am Acad Dermatol* 2001, **44:**401–421.
12. Frykberg RG: **Epidemiology of the diabetic foot: ulcerations and amputations.** *Adv Wound Care* 1999, **12:**139–141.
13. Windsor AC KA, Somers SS: **Manipulation of local and systemic host defence in the prevention of perioperative sepsis.** *Br J Surg* 1995, **82:**1460–1467.
14. Kaizer AB, Jacobs JK: **Cefoxitin versus erythromicin, neomycin and cefozolin in colorectal operation. Importance of duration of surgical procedure.** *Ann Surg* 1983, **198:**525–530.
15. Holzheimer RGHW, Thidel A: **The challenge of post operative infection; does the surgeon make a difference.** *Infection Control Epidemol* 1997, **18:**449–456.
16. Adegbehingbe LMO OO, Olabanji JK, Alatise OI: **Chronic leg ulcer presenting through emergency surgical unit.** *Internet J Surg* 2007, **9**(1). doi:10.5580/1051.
17. Chalya PL, Mabula JB, Rambau P, Mchembe MD, Kahima KJ, Chandika AB, Giiti G, Masalu N, Ssentongo R, Gilyoma JM: **Marjolin's ulcers at a university**

teaching hospitalin Northwestern Tanzania: a retrospective review of 56 cases. *World J Surg Oncol* 2012, **10**:38.
18. Meckkes JR, Loots MA, AC VDw, Bos JD: **Causes, Investigation, and treatment of Leg Ulceration.** *Br J Dermatol* 2003, **148**(3):388–401.
19. Jull W, Walker N, Hackett N, Jones M, Rodgers A, Birchall N, Norton R, Macmahon S: **Leg ulceration and perceived health: a population based case–control study.** *Brit Geriatr Soc* 2004, **33**:236–241.
20. Liedberg E, Persson BM: **Increased incidence of lower limb amputation for arterial occlusive disease.** *Acta Orthop Scand* 1983, **54**:230–234.
21. Margolis DJ, Bilker W, Santanna J, Baumgarten M: **Venous leg ulcer: incidence and prevalence in the elderly.** *J Am Acad Dermatol* 2002, **46**:381–386.
22. De Silva TES: **Surgical options in the management of intransigent leg ulcers.** *Wounds* 2012, **8**(1):18.
23. Grey EJHK, Enoch S: **ABC ofwound healing: venous and arterial leg ulcers.** *Br Med J* 2006, **332**(7537):347–350.
24. Chalya PL, Mabula JB, Das RM, Kabangila R, Jaka H, Mchembe DM, Kataraihya JB, Mbelenge N, Gilyoma JM: **Sugical management of Diabetic foot ulcers: A Tanzanian University teaching hospital experience.** *BMC Research Notes* 2011, **4**:365.
25. American Diabetes Association: **consensus development conference on diabetic foot wound care.** *Diabetes Care* 1999, **22**:1354–1360.
26. US Department of Health and Human Services: In *Women and Tobacco.* Edited by Sheet F; 2009.
27. US Department of Health and Human Services: *Tobacco-Related Mortality.* 2009.
28. Jone SK, Tripleff RG: **The relationship of cigarette smoking to impaired intra-oral wound healing: a review evidence and implication for patient care.** *J oral Maxillo Surg* 1992, **50**:237–240.
29. Nagachinta T, Stephens M, Reitz B, Polk BF: **Risk factors for surgical wound infection. Muisory cardiac surgery.** *S Inf Dis* 1987, **156**:967–973.
30. Georgios SNL: **The evaluation of lower-extremity ulcers.** *Semin Intervent Radiol* 2009, **26**(4):286–295.
31. Snyder RJ: **Treatment of nonhealing ulcers with allografts.** *Clin Dermatol* 2005, **23**(4):388–395.
32. Tao S, Lim, Bibombe PM, Ronan M, Kishore S, Manzoor A, Donna A: **Microbiological profile of chronic ulcers of the lower limb: A prospective observational study cohort study.** *ANZ J Surg* 2006, **76**(8):688–692.
33. Mawalla BM, Mshana SE, Chalya PL, Imirzalioglu C, Mahalu W: **Predictors of surgical site infections among patients undergoing major surgery at Bugando Medical Centre in Northwestern Tanzania.** *BMC Surg* 2011, **11**:21.
34. Samaila SA MOA: **A histopathological analysis of cutaneous malignancies in a tropical African population.** *Niger J Surg Res* 2005, **7**(3–4):300–304.
35. Sibanda M, Sibanda E, Jönsson K: **A prospective evaluation of lower extremity ulcers in a Zimbabwean population.** *Int Wound J* 2009, **6** (5):361–366.
36. English MP, Harman RR: **The fungal flora of ulcerated legs.** *Dermatol Br J* 1971, **84**(6):567–581.
37. Hansson CF, Swanbeck G: **Fungal infections occurring under bandages in leg ulcer patients.** *Acta Derm Venereol* 1987, **67**(4):341–345.
38. Lipsky BA: **Osteomyelitis of the foot in diabetic patients.** *Clin Infect Dis* 1997, **25**:1318–1366.
39. Carrascosa JM, Ribera M, Bielsa I: **Bacillary angiomatosis presenting as a malleolar ulcer.** *Arch Dermatol* 1995, **131**:963–964.
40. Julius S, Luiz Felipe B, Mello M, Norberto C: **Malignancy in chronic ulcers and scars of the leg.** *Skeletal Radiol* 2001, **6**:331–337.
41. Sene P, Combemale P, Debure C, Baudot N, Machet L, Aout M, Vicaut E, Lok C: *Malignancy and Chronic Leg Ulcers The Value of Systematic Wound Biopsies: A Prospective, Multicenter.* Arch Dermatol: Cross-sectional Study; 2012 [Epub ahead of print].
42. Chalya PL, Gilyoma JM, Kanumba ES, Mawala B, Masalu N, Kahima KM, Rambau P: **Dermatological malignancies at a University Teaching Hospital in north-western Tanzania: a retrospective review of 154 cases.** *Tanzan J Health Res* 2012, **14**:1.
43. Filamer DK, Lisa CK, Geanina P, Constantin AD, Doru TA: **Malignant melanoma in African-Americans.** *Dermatol Online J* 2009, **15**(2):3.
44. Bellows CF, Fortgang IS, Beech DJ: **Melanoma in African-Americans: trends in biological behavior and clinical characteristics over two decades.** *J Surg Oncol* 2001, **78**:10–16.
45. Cormier JN, Ding M, Lee JE, Mansfield PF, Gershenwald JE, Ross MI, Du XL: **Ethnic differences among patients with cutaneous melanoma.** *Arch Intern Med* 2006, **166**:1907–1914.
46. Cress RD, Holly EA: **Incidence of cutaneous melanoma among non-Hispanic whites, Hispanics, Asians, and blacks: an analysis of california cancer registry data, 1988-93.** *Cancer Cause Control* 1997, **8**(2):246–252.
47. Swan MC: **Malignant melanoma in South Africans of mixed ancestry: a retrospective analysis.** *Melanoma Res* 2003, **13**:415–419.
48. Byrd KM, Hoyler SS, Peck GL: **Advanced presentation of melanoma in African Americans.** *J Am Acad Dermatol* 2004, **50**:21–24.
49. Giraud RM, Rippey JJ: **Malignant melanoma of the skin in Black Africans.** *S Afr Med J* 1975, **49**:665–668.
50. Reintgen DS, Cox E, Seigler HF: **Malignant melanoma in the American black.** *Curr Surg* 1983, **40**:215–217.
51. Camain RTA, Sarrat H, Quenum C, Faye I: **Cutaneous cancer in Dakar.** *J Natl Cancer Inst* 1972, **48**:33–49.
52. Oettle AG: **Epidemiology of melanoma in South Africa.** In *Structure and control of melanocyte.* Edited by Della P, Mulbock GE. Berlin: Springer; 1966:292.
53. Mandong BM, Chirdan LB, Anyebe AO, Mannaseh AN: **Histopathological study of Kaposi's sarcoma in Jos: A 16 year review.** *Ann Afr Med* 2004, **3**:174–176.
54. Ruckley CV: **Caring for patients with chronic leg ulcer.** *BMJ* 1998, **316**:407–408.
55. Rahman IA, Fadeyi A: **Epidemiology, etiology, and treatment of chronic leg ulcer: Experience with sixty patients.** *Ann Afr Med* 2010, **9**(1):1–4.
56. Oluwatosin OM, Oluwatosin OA, Shokunbi MT: **Management of pressure ulceration using fenestrated foam and honey.** *Quarterly J Hosp Med* 1998, **8**:264–266.
57. Akinyanju OA: **Leg ulceration in sickle cell disease in Nigeria.** *Trop Geogr Med* 1979, **31**:87.
58. Durosinmi MA, Esan GJ: **Chronic leg ulcers in sickle cell disease.** *Afr J Med Sci* 1991, **20**:11–14.
59. Ashry HR LL, Armstrong DG, Lavery DC, van Houtum WH: **Cost of diabetes-related amputations in minorities.** *J Foot Ankle Surg* 1998, **37**(3):186–190.
60. Payne BC: **Diabetes-related lower-limb amputations in Australia.** *MJA* 2000, **173**(7):352–354.
61. Rahman GA AI, Fadeyi A: **Epidemiology, etiology, and treatment of chronic leg ulcer: Experience with sixty patients.** *Ann Afr Med* 2010, **9**:1–4.
62. Saitz R: **Discharges against medical advice: time to address the causes.** *CMAJ* 2002, **167**(6):647–648.
63. Stephen W, Hwang JL, Gupta R, Chien V, Rochelle EM: **What happens to patients who leave hospital against medical advice.** *CMAJ* 2003, **168**(4):417–420.

12

Validation of the global resource of eczema trials (GREAT database)

Helen Nankervis[1*], Alison Devine[2], Hywel C Williams[1], John R Ingram[3], Elizabeth Doney[4], Finola Delamere[4], Sherie Smith[1] and Kim S Thomas[1]

Abstract

Background: Eczema (syn. Atopic Eczema or Atopic Dermatitis) is a chronic, relapsing, itchy skin condition which probably results from a combination of genetic and environmental factors. The Global Resource of EczemA Trials (GREAT) is a collection of records of randomised controlled trials (RCTs) for eczema treatment produced from a highly sensitive search of six reference databases. We sought to assess the sensitivity of the GREAT database as a tool to save future researchers repeating extensive bibliographic searches.

Methods: All Cochrane systematic review on treatments for eczema and five non-Cochrane systematic reviews on eczema were identified as a reference set to assess the utility of the GREAT database in identifying randomised controlled trials (RCTs). RCTs included in the systematic reviews were checked for inclusion in the GREAT database by two independent authors. A third author resolved any disagreements.

Results: Five Cochrane and six non-Cochrane systematic reviews containing a total of 105 RCTs of eczema treatments were included. Of these, 95 fitted the inclusion criteria for the GREAT database and 88 were published from 2000 onwards. Of the 88 eligible studies, 92% were found in the GREAT database. Seven trials were not included in the GREAT database - two of these were reported within a review paper and one as an abstract with no trial results.

Conclusions: The sensitivity of the GREAT database for trials from 2000 onwards was high (75/88 trials, 94%). Sensitivity for the period prior to 2000 was less sensitive, due to differences in how the trials were identified prior to this time. 'Dual' filtering for new records has recently become part of the GREAT database methodology and should further improve the sensitivity of the database in time. The GREAT database can be considered as a primary source for future systematic reviews including randomised controlled trials of eczema treatments, but searches should be supplemented by checking reference lists for eligible trials, searching trial registries and contacting pharmaceutical companies for unpublished studies.

Keywords: Validation, Database, Randomised controlled trials, Eczema, Atopic dermatitis

Background

Eczema is a chronic, relapsing, itchy skin condition (syn. Atopic Eczema or Atopic Dermatitis) which is the result of a combination of genetic and environmental factors [1].

Searching for published reports of randomised controlled trials (RCTs) can be time consuming and complex. In order to facilitate the speedy identification of RCTs of eczema treatments, the Global Resource of EczemA Trials database (GREAT) was created. This free, publicly accessible database (www.greatdatabase.org.uk) contains summary details of published randomised controlled trials (RCTs) on the treatment of eczema. Trials are identified using a highly sensitive search of six databases [2]. The aim of the GREAT database is to save research time by: 1) creating only one database to search for trials of eczema treatment; and 2) providing enough pertinent information about each trial to allow systematic reviewers and guideline writers to decide whether the trial fits their inclusion criteria without having to obtain and scrutinise the full papers for all possible trials themselves.

If potential users of the GREAT database are not convinced that it will provide a comprehensive list of all

* Correspondence: helen.nankervis@nottingham.ac.uk
[1]Centre of Evidence Based Dermatology, School of Medicine, University of Nottingham, Nottingham, UK
Full list of author information is available at the end of the article

eczema RCTs, then they are far less likely to use it as their main database to search and will conduct their own searches. This will not save research time or help to prevent research wastage as was the original intention.

The objective of this study was to evaluate the sensitivity of the GREAT database by comparing those studies found in systematic reviews with those in the GREAT database. Sensitivity was defined as the number of relevant RCTs identified in the GREAT database, divided by the total number of relevant RCTs in the included systematic reviews.

Methods

All methods described below were undertaken by two authors independently, with any discrepancies being resolved by another author acting as an arbiter.

As there is no obvious 'gold standard' resource of trials of eczema treatments, systematic reviews were considered the 'gold standard' and the GREAT database was the 'comparator'.

It was decided, a priori, to restrict the comparison of the GREAT database to all published Cochrane reviews of eczema treatments, and five non-Cochrane reviews of eczema treatments. The latter were those with the most recent search end dates. Reviews also had to have a full list of citations for the included studies and sufficient details of the review's inclusion criteria to allow a fair comparison with the GREAT database. The validation only compared included RCTs, as the GREAT database only includes RCTs.

Results of this study are presented as being for the period from 2000 onwards and pre-2000 due to differences in the way that the searches were conducted during these periods. RCTs published prior to 2000 were identified from a previously published systematic review of eczema treatments [3], whereas RCTs published from 2000 onwards were identified prospectively as the GREAT database was developed.

Identifying systematic reviews of eczema treatments

The mapping of systematic reviews of atopic eczema project developed by the Centre of Evidence Based Dermatology [4,5] has records of systematic reviews from 2000 onwards (including both Cochrane and non-Cochrane reviews). This map of systematic reviews was mined independently by two authors for all Cochrane systematic reviews and five non-Cochrane reviews involving eczema treatments. Any disagreements about which systematic reviews to include as per the pre-specified inclusion criteria were resolved by the arbiter before the list was finalised.

Identifying included and excluded trials from systematic reviews

Two authors independently scrutinised the included systematic reviews to obtain the list of citations of included RCTs studies (other included studies depending on the nature of the review). Any disagreements between the two authors about the included and excluded studies were resolved by the arbiter. Excluded studies were defined as those described as such in the review text or a table(s). Any trials not in English and not in GREAT had the appropriate data extracted by a researcher with the required language skills, if further information was required.

Identifying trials from the GREAT database

Two authors independently attempted to find all the included and excluded trials identified from the systematic reviews, using the search facility and exploration of the GREAT database via the browse and filter facilities. Where an included or excluded trial was not found in the GREAT database, the reasons for this were explored and recorded.

The reported inclusion criteria for each systematic review were used to identify any additional RCTs in the GREAT database which could have been eligible for inclusion in the review, but were not in the list of included studies of that review. Where an RCT was identified in the GREAT database that was not in the included studies list of one or more of the systematic reviews, the reasons for this were explored, consulting the full trial paper and GREAT if necessary. Any disagreements between the two author's results were resolved by the independent arbiter before the results were analysed.

Results

Summary of results

A search of the mapping of eczema systematic reviews [4] revealed 59 eczema treatment systematic reviews published since 2000. Of these, six were Cochrane reviews [6-11] and were included in this validation study. Five non-Cochrane systematic reviews [12-16] with the most recent search end dates and which matched all other inclusion criteria were included in the study.

The six Cochrane reviews included 72 randomised controlled trials (RCTs) on eczema treatments and no other types of studies. All of the reviews searched The Cochrane Library, MEDLINE, and Embase; three searched the Allied and Complementary Medicine Database (AMED) [7,9,11]; one searched the Cumulative Index to Nursing and Allied Health Literature (CINAHL) [11]; two searched the Latin American and Caribbean Health Sciences database (LILACS) [7,9]; three searched PsycINFO® [7,9,10]; and two searched the ISI Web of Science [7,9]. Four [6,8,10,11] of the six Cochrane reviews searched various other databases and repositories such as trials databases, the Food and Drug Administration (FDA) website, European Medicines Agency (EMEA) website, and Chinese databases. The Cochrane reviews included in this study covered topical calcineurin inhibitors, antibacterials, dietary interventions,

Chinese herbal medicine, psychological and educational interventions and probiotics.

The five non- Cochrane reviews included 33 RCTs on eczema treatments that could be included in this validation study. In addition, 52 other studies included in the non-Cochrane reviews were excluded from the validation study as they were either controlled clinical trials, cohort studies, or RCTs involving other dermatoses.

Four reviews searched the Cochrane Library [12-14,16],, four searched MEDLINE [12,14,15], three searched Embase [12-14]; one searched Current Contents [15], one searched HomInform [15], and two searched PubMed [13,15]. Four [12,14-16] out of five of the reviews undertook manual searching of the reference lists of included trials, reviews and other sources such as textbooks and guidelines. The non-Cochrane reviews included in this study covered homeopathy, azathioprine, topical calcineurin inhibitors, topical corticosteroids.

Assessment of trials published from 2000 onwards in the GREAT database

Trials missing from GREAT but found in systematic reviews

The GREAT database did not contain all the included RCTs for four [6,8,9,14] of the eleven included systematic reviews. There were 13 out of 88 trials in total (see *Table* 1) that were not found in the GREAT database. The reasons for this are discussed below.

Trial missing with reason

One of the trials [17], was included in a Cochrane review but did not fulfil the GREAT inclusion criteria as it assessed changes in bacterial numbers rather than clinical outcomes.

Five trials [18-22] were included in a Cochrane review, but had been identified through a pharmaceutical company trials database [23] and did not contain enough information in the trial records provided to be certain whether these trials appear in the GREAT database or not (see *Table* 2).

Trials missing in error

Seven trials 7/88 (8%) were identified from systematic reviews and fitted the GREAT inclusion criteria, but were not present in the GREAT database (see *Table* 2). Two of these trials [24,25], were additional citations for a trial that was already included in the GREAT database. Of the remaining five trials two were reported only within a review paper [26-28] and one [29] was published as a conference abstract and did not report trial results.

Potential implications of trials missing from GREAT

One Cochrane review from which one of the missing in error trials was included may possibly not have drawn such strong conclusions about the level of problems with adverse event if the trial had not been included. The other two Cochrane reviews and two non-Cochrane reviews from which one of the missing in error trials were included would have been very unlikely to have drawn different conclusions if the trials had not been included.

Trials published from 2000 onwards found in the GREAT database that potentially should have been included in systematic reviews

For one of the included Cochrane reviews on anti-staphylococcal interventions [8], three trials [30-32] were identified using the GREAT database that were not included in the review. We believe from the trial reports and the reported inclusion criteria of the review, that these three trials should have been included in this review. It is possible that the review authors managed to gather additional information about these trials which resulted in them being excluded; however, as the trials are not listed as excluded studies when they would have been so close to inclusion, this is less likely.

Assessment of pre 2000 trials missing from the GREAT database

As trials published before 2000 were added to GREAT directly from a systematic review [3], a strict validation comparison was not performed for trials before 2000.

Four trials [33-36] published before 2000 and included in one Cochrane review [8], were not present in the GREAT database. All four trials were returned in the search strategy for the Cochrane systematic review [8] and so they were not found exclusively through hand searching.

It is most likely that the four trials [33-36] were not selected for inclusion in the overarching systematic review that provided the source for pre-2000 RCTs due to errors in the filtering process; or possibly the trials were excluded as they did not match the systematic review [3] inclusion criteria.

Discussion

The GREAT database is free to use and has been specifically designed to be quick and easy to access by all potential users, including guideline writers, patient information developers, methodologists, healthcare practitioners, and patients. The GREAT database offers much more than a standard bibliographic database; which provides citations and abstracts of articles only. Researchers identifying references from other databases would be well advised to cross-check them in the GREAT database, in order to take advantage of the additional data extraction and analysis available there.

In this validation study, the GREAT database was found to include 92% of the RCTs identified in published systematic reviews, and was also able to identify an additional three trials that had not been included in published reviews.

Table 1 Summary of results for trials from 2000 onwards

Review	Number of RCTs included in the review	Proportion of included eczema RCTs found in GREAT	Reasons for RCTs missing from GREAT	Sensitivity of the GREAT database (all missing RCTs)	Sensitivity of GREAT (RCTs missing in error)
Cochrane reviews					
Ashcroft et al. 2007 [6]	31	23/31	Unpublished trial records obtained from a pharmaceutical company (n = 5) A report of the same trial was present in GREAT, but the citation for the included study was not (n = 2). One trial not included in GREAT in error (n = 1).	(23/31) 74%	(28/31) 87%
Bath-Hextall et al. 2008 [7]	2	2/2	No trials missing from the GREAT database	100%	100%
Birnie et al. 2008 [8]	7	6/7	Trial was not aiming to 'treat' the eczema, only reduce bacterial numbers (n = 1).	(6/7) 91%	100%
Boyle et al. 2008 [9]	11	10/11	Filtered incorrectly in error, should have been an included trial (n = 1)	(10/11) 91%	(10/11) 91%
Ersser et al. 2007 [9]	4	4/4	No trials missing from the GREAT database	100%	100%
Zhang et al. 2005 [11]	1	1/1	No trials missing from the GREAT database	100%	100%
Totals for Cochrane reviews	**56 included RCTs**	**46/56 RCTs included in the GREAT database**	**10 trials missing from the GREAT database**	**(46/56) 82%**	**(52/56) 93%**
Non Cochrane Reviews					
Schram et al. 2011 [12]	2	2/2	No trials missing from the GREAT database	100%	100%
Yin et al. 2011 [13]	4	4/4	No trials missing from the GREAT database	100%	100%
Svensson et al. 2007 [14]	17	14/17	Abstract which did not present information about results (n = 1). Two Japanese phase II RCTs which fit GREAT inclusion criteria reported only within a review, omitted from GREAT in error.(n = 2)	(14/17) 82%	(14/17) 82%
Simonart et al. 2011 [15]	1	1/1	No trials missing from the GREAT database	100%	100%
Schmitt et al. 2011 [16]	8	8/8	No trials missing from the GREAT database	100%	100%
Totals for non-Cochrane Reviews	**32 included RCTs**	**29/ 32 RCTs included in the GREAT database**	**3/32 trials missing from the GREAT database**	**(29/32) 91%**	**(29/32) 91%**
Totals for Cochrane and Non-Cochrane reviews	**88 included RCTs**	**75/88 RCTs included in the GREAT database**	**13/88 trials missing from the GREAT database**	**(13/88) 85%**	**(81/88) 92%**

Footnote: Totals in bold.

Table 2 Summary of the sensitivity of the GREAT database

Proportion of trials missing from the GREAT database	**13/88 (15%)**
Proportion of trials missing in error from the GREAT database (two of these were included, but under a different citation)	7/88 (8%)
Proportion of trials truly missing from the GREAT database in error (two of these were only cited in a review paper, one as abstract only with no results provided)*	5/88 (6%)

*These five citations have now been added to the GREAT database.

Two trial reports were counted as missing where the trial itself was reported in the GREAT database, but not the particular citations used in the systematic review. This is something that could helpfully be addressed in the future by linking all reports and abstracts from the same trial to the same trial record in the GREAT database. This would prevent bias being introduced by multiple reporting of the same trial.

Although the GREAT database is comprehensive, if conducting a comprehensive systematic review, other methods of identifying trials may be required, such as searching trials databases, as well as hand-searching and contacting of trial authors. In addition, reviews including studies other than RCTs will require additional searches of bibliographic databases to search for observational and non-randomised studies.

Conclusions

Strengths and weaknesses

Although using published systematic reviews as the gold standard for validation of the GREAT database is a useful tool for establishing coverage of the database, direct comparison can be challenging due to differences in eligibility criteria for reviews compared to the GREAT database. This can lead to an apparent lowering of the sensitivity of the database if different eligibility criteria have been applied.

Many treatments that the GREAT database covers have not been assessed in this validation study, as only a selection of systematic reviews were used. Sensitivity of the database may differ depending on the treatment being reviewed and so ongoing validation of the GREAT database is required.

Reviewing the GREAT database against all of the Cochrane systematic reviews of eczema treatments has ensured a complete comparison has been made using a very rigorous search methodology. The main weakness with this comparison is that authors of Cochrane reviews are expected to contact trial authors for information not present in the trial report. The GREAT database methodology does not include this due to time and resource constraints.

One review included RCTs that were identified from a trials database in which most trials were reported to be unpublished. Unfortunately it is impossible to be sure if five of the missing trials are in the GREAT database or not, as insufficient information is available in the public domain. For all eczema trials to be included in GREAT they must be published. Efforts to get all clinical trials registered and published, such as the AllTrials campaign [37], are helping to achieve this.

Implications for the future development of the GREAT database

One area for improvement of the GREAT database is dual filtering of references in order to reduce errors of omission of potentially eligible RCTs. Dual filtering involves two authors independently assessing the search results to determine eligibility of the included studies, with disagreements being resolved by a third party as necessary. Dual filtering has recently become part of the GREAT database methodology and should further improve the sensitivity of the database. It is our intention to apply dual-filtering retrospectively in order to ensure complete coverage of the GREAT database, but in the meantime, additional searches of bibliographic databases may be required, especially for RCTs published prior to 2000.

Other possible sources for trials to add to the GREAT database could be the interrogation of unpublished trials databases, searching of additional specialist databases such as PsycINFO® or Chinese databases, or adding all citations found for a particular trial (including conference abstracts). Whether or not to widen the inclusion criteria of the GREAT database beyond its current scope requires careful consideration as to its feasibility, impact and resource implications.

The GREAT database is sufficiently sensitive for most users, and is a resource that is quick and simple to interrogate; particularly for those looking for the best evidence for specific treatments that have not yet been included in a full systematic review, or for people looking for new trial evidence published after a systematic review's search end date. The more the GREAT database is used and added to on an iterative basis, the better it will be.

Although there are other databases, such as for transfusion [38], as far as the authors are aware there are no other databases similar to GREAT for any other dermatological condition. It is therefore particularly important that the impact of the GREAT database on eczema research is assessed in order to enhance its potential to improve patient care and methodology of clinical trials in dermatology research. Over the next 5–10 years, similar databases for other common skin diseases such as psoriasis, acne, hand eczema and skin cancer might be developed with the aim of facilitating more effective mobilisation of evidence for clinical and research uses. The resources required to develop and maintain databases such as GREAT for the public good should not be underestimated. Collating the evidence and designing and testing the database required 20 months of researcher time, specialist IT input and hosting costs. Ongoing updates now require around 2 weeks of researcher time per month.

Competing interests

Helen Nankervis - lead the creation of the GREAT database as part of her work on an NIHR funded Programme Grant (RP-PG-0407-10177).
John Ingram – current co-investigator of an eczema trial funded by Atopix Therapeutics Ltd. He has not received any reimbursements, fees, funding, or salary from involvement in the trial.
Kim Thomas – co-applicant for the NIHR funded Programme Grant (RP-PG-0407-10177) that supported this work.
Hywel Williams – co-applicant for the NIHR funded Programme Grant (RP-PG-0407-10177) that supported this work.
Alison Devine - No competing interests.
Elizabeth Doney – No competing interests.
Sherie Smith – No competing interests.
Finola Delamere – No competing interests.

Authors' contributions

HN contributed to the design of the study, extracted data, coordinated data extraction, comparison and arbitration, drafted the first draft of the manuscript and revised the manuscript according to co-author comments. AD extracted data and commented on the final manuscript. HCW contributed to the design of the study and commented on the manuscript, JRI compared data extraction data and arbitrated where the data did not agree, ED contributed to the design of the study, extracted data and commented on the manuscript, FD contributed to the design of the study and commented on the manuscript, SS contributed to the design of the study and commented on the manuscript, KST contributed to the design of the study and commented on the manuscript. All authors read and approved the final manuscript.

Acknowledgements

This publication presents independent research funded by the National Institute for Health Research (NIHR) under its Programme Grants for Applied Research Programme (RP-PG-0407-10177). The views expressed in this publication are those of the author(s) and not necessarily those of the NHS, the NIHR or the Department of Health.

Author details

[1]Centre of Evidence Based Dermatology, School of Medicine, University of Nottingham, Nottingham, UK. [2]Glan Clwyd Hospital, Betsi Cadwaladr University Health Board, Bodelwyddan, Rhyl, UK. [3]Department of Dermatology & Wound Healing, Institute of Infection & Immunity, Cardiff University, Cardiff, Wales. [4]Cochrane Skin Group, Centre of Evidence Based Dermatology, University of Nottingham, Nottingham, UK.

References

1. Williams HC, Wuthrich B. In: Williams HC, editor. Atopic Dermatits, vol. 1. Cambridge: Cambridge University Press; 2000.
2. Nankervis H, Maplethorpe A, Williams HC. Mapping randomized controlled trials of treatments for eczema–the GREAT database (the Global Resource of EczemA Trials: a collection of key data on randomized controlled trials of treatments for eczema from 2000 to 2010). BMC Dermatol. 2011;11:10.
3. Hoare C, Li Wan Po A, Williams H. Systematic review of treatments for atopic eczema. Health Technol Assess. 2000;4(37):1–191.
4. Mapping of systematic reviews of atopic eczema. [http://www.nottingham.ac.uk/research/groups/cebd/documents/methodological-resources/maponaewebsitefeb2013.pdf]
5. Futamura M, Thomas KS, Grindlay DJC, Doney EJ, Torley D, Williams HC. Mapping systematic reviews on atopic eczema—an essential resource for dermatology professionals and researchers. PLoS ONE. 2013;8(3):e58484.
6. Ashcroft DM, Chen LC, Garside R, Stein K, Williams HC. Topical pimecrolimus for eczema. Cochrane Database Syst Rev. 2007;4:CD005500.
7. Bath-Hextall F, Delamere FM, Williams HC. Dietary exclusions for established atopic eczema. Cochrane Database Syst Rev. 2008;1:CD005203.
8. Birnie AJ, Bath-Hextall FJ, Ravenscroft JC, Williams HC. Interventions to reduce Staphylococcus aureus in the management of atopic eczema. Cochrane Database Syst Rev. 2008;3:CD003871.
9. Boyle RJ, Bath-Hextall FJ, Leonardi-Bee J, Murrell DF, Tang ML. Probiotics for treating eczema. Cochrane Database Syst Rev. 2008;4:CD006135.
10. Ersser SJ, Latter S, Sibley A, Satherley PA, Welbourne S. Psychological and educational interventions for atopic eczema in children. Cochrane Database Syst Rev. 2007;3:CD004054.
11. Zhang W, Leonard T, Bath-Hextall F, Chambers CA, Lee C, Humphreys R, et al. Chinese herbal medicine for atopic eczema. Cochrane Database Syst Rev. 2005;2:CD002291.
12. Schram ME, Borgonjen RJ, Bik CM, van der Schroeff JG, van Everdingen JJ, Spuls PI. Off-label use of azathioprine in dermatology: a systematic review. Arch Dermatol. 2011;147(4):474–88.
13. Yin Z, Xu J, Luo D. Efficacy and tolerance of tacrolimus and pimecrolimus for atopic dermatitis: A meta-analysis. J Biomed Res. 2011;25(6):385–91.
14. Svensson A, Chambers C, Ganemo A, Mitchell SA. A systematic review of tacrolimus ointment compared with corticosteroids in the treatment of atopic dermatitis. Curr Med Res Opin. 2011;27(7):1395–406.
15. Simonart T, Kabagabo C, De Maertelaer V. Homoeopathic remedies in dermatology: a systematic review of controlled clinical trials. Br J Dermatol. 2011;165(4):897–905.
16. Schmitt J, von Kobyletzki L, Svensson A, Apfelbacher C. Efficacy and tolerability of proactive treatment with topical corticosteroids and calcineurin inhibitors for atopic eczema: systematic review and meta-analysis of randomized controlled trials. Br J Dermatol. 2011;164(2):415–28.
17. Boguniewicz M, Sampson H, Leung SB, Harbeck R, Leung DY. Effects of cefuroxime axetil on Staphylococcus aureus colonization and superantigen production in atopic dermatitis. J Aller Clin Immunol. 2001;108(4):651–2.
18. Novartis. A 4-week, randomized, multicenter, double-blind, vehicle-controlled, parallel-group clinical trial to evaluate the efficacy and safety of pimecrolimus cream 1% in the short-term treatment of patients with mild to moderate Atopic Dermatitis (Eczema). In: Novartis Trials Database. 2005.
19. Novartis. A 6-month, randomized, multicenter, parallel-group, double-blind, vehicle-controlled study to evaluate the efficacy and safety of pimecrolimus 1% cream twice daily vs. standard of care in the management of mild to severe atopic dermatitis in adults.In: Novartis Trials Database. 2005.
20. Novartis. A 12 week multicenter study consisting of a 6 week double blind, randomized, vehicle controlled, parallel group phase, followed by a 6 week open label phase, to assess the safety and efficacy of pimecrolimus cream 1% in mild to moderate head and neck atopic dermatitis of patients intolerant of topical corticosteroid. In: Novartis Trials Database; 2006.
21. Novartis. Confirmatory study in pediatric patients with atopic dermatitis-multicenter, randomized, double-blind, parallel-group, vehicle-controlled study with a 26-weeks treatment phase to determine the efficacy, safety of pimecrolimus cream for long-term treatment of pediatric patients with atopic dermatitis. In: Novartis Trials Database. 2005.
22. Novartis. A multicenter, 5-week, randomized, double-blind, placebo controlled, parallel group study exploring the effects of pimecrolimus cream 1% (twice daily application) vs. placebo control (twice daily application) on the molecular and cellular profile of adult male patients with atopic dermatitis. In: Novartis Trials Database. 2006.
23. Clinical Trials Results database. [http://www.novctrd.com/ctrdWebApp/clinicaltrialrepository/public/login.jsp]
24. Staab D, Kaufmann R, Brautigam M, Wahn U, Group CAC-S. Treatment of infants with atopic eczema with pimecrolimus cream 1% improves parents' quality of life: a multicenter, randomized trial. Pediatr Allergy Immunol. 2005;16(6):527–33.
25. Thaci DF-HR, Foelster-Holst R, Hoger P, Kaufmann R, Brautigam M, Weidinger G, et al. Pimecrolimus cream 1% is effective in the treatment of atopic eczema in infants irrespective of clinical score. J Eur Acad Dermatol Venereol. 2003;17 Suppl 3:2.37.
26. Kirjavainen PV, Salminen SJ, Isolauri E. Probiotic bacteria in the management of atopic disease: underscoring the importance of viability. J Pediatr Gastroenterol Nutr. 2003;36(2):223–7.
27. Nakagawa H. Comparison of the efficacy and safety of 0.1% tacrolimus ointment with topical corticosteroids in adult patients with atopic

dermatitis: review of randomised, double-blind clinical studies conducted in Japan. Clin Drug Investig. 2006;26(5):235–46.
28. Siegfried EKN, Molina C, Kianifard F, Abrams K. Safety and efficacy of early intervention with pimecrolimus cream 1% combined with corticosteroids for major flares in infants and children with atopic dermatitis Safety and efficacy of early intervention with pimecrolimus cream 1% combined with corticosteroids for major flares in infants and children with atopic dermatitis. J Dermatol Treat. 2006;17(3):143–50.
29. Breneman D, Fleischer Jr A, Abramovits W, Farber H. Tacrolimus ointment with and without topical steroids in patients with moderate to severe atopic dermatitis. J Am Acad Dermatol. 2006;54(3, Suppl 1 AB88):832. Abstract.
30. Hung SH, Lin YT, Chu CY, Lee CC, Liang TC, Yang YH, et al. Staphylococcus colonization in atopic dermatitis treated with fluticasone or tacrolimus with or without antibiotics. Ann Allergy Asthma Immunol. 2007;98(1):51–6.
31. Larsen FS, Simonsen L, Melgaard A, Wendicke K, Henriksen AS. An efficient new formulation of fusidic acid and betamethasone 17-valerate (fucicort lipid cream) for treatment of clinically infected atopic dermatitis. Acta Derm Venereol. 2007;87(1):62–8.
32. Ravenscroft JC, Layton AM, Eady EA, Murtagh MS, Coates P, Walker M, et al. Short-term effects of topical fusidic acid or mupirocin on the prevalence of fusidic acid resistant (FusR) Staphylococcus aureus in atopic eczema. Br J Dermatol. 2003;148(5):1010–7.
33. Polano MK, De Vries HR. Analysis of the results obtained in the treatment of atopic dermatitis with corticosteroid and neomycin containing ointments. Dermatologica. 1960;120:191–9.
34. Nilsson EJ, Henning CG, Magnusson J. Topical corticosteroids and Staphylococcus aureus in atopic dermatitis. J Am Acad Dermatol. 1992;27(1):29–34.
35. Leyden JJ, Marples RR, Kligman AM. Staphylococcus aureus in the lesions of atopic dermatitis. Br J Dermatol. 1974;90(5):525–30.
36. Fattah AA, El-Shiemy S, Faris R, Tadros SS. A comparative clinical evaluation of a new topical steroid 'halcinonide' and hydrocortisone in steroid-responsive dermatoses. J Int Med Res. 1976;4(4):228–31.
37. Alltrials. [http://www.alltrials.net/]
38. Transfusion evidence library. [http://evidentiapublishing.com/transfusion-evidence-library/]

13

Distribution of *Malassezia* species on the skin of patients with atopic dermatitis, psoriasis, and healthy volunteers assessed by conventional and molecular identification methods

Tomasz Jagielski[1*], Elżbieta Rup[2], Aleksandra Ziółkowska[1], Katarzyna Roeske[1], Anna B Macura[2] and Jacek Bielecki[1]

Abstract

Background: The *Malassezia* yeasts which belong to the physiological microflora of human skin have also been implicated in several dermatological disorders, including pityriasis versicolor (PV), atopic dermatitis (AD), and psoriasis (PS). The *Malassezia* genus has repeatedly been revised and it now accommodates 14 species, all but one being lipid-dependent species. The traditional, phenotype-based identification schemes of *Malassezia* species are fraught with interpretative ambiguities and inconsistencies, and are thus increasingly being supplemented or replaced by DNA typing methods. The aim of this study was to explore the species composition of *Malassezia* microflora on the skin of healthy volunteers and patients with AD and PS.

Methods: Species characterization was performed by conventional, culture-based methods and subsequently molecular techniques: PCR-RFLP and sequencing of the internal transcribed spacer (ITS) 1/2 regions and the D1/D2 domains of the 26S rRNA gene. The Chi-square test and Fisher's exact test were used for statistical analysis.

Results: *Malassezia sympodialis* was the predominant species, having been cultured from 29 (82.9%) skin samples collected from 17 out of 18 subjects under the study. Whereas AD patients yielded exclusively *M. sympodialis* isolates, *M. furfur* isolates were observed only in PS patients. The isolation of *M. sympodialis* was statistically more frequent among AD patients and healthy volunteers than among PS patients ($P < 0.03$). Whether this mirrors any predilection of particular *Malassezia* species for certain clinical conditions needs to be further evaluated. The overall concordance between phenotypic and molecular methods was quite high (65%), with the discordant results being rather due to the presence of multiple species in a single culture (co-colonization) than true misidentification. All *Malassezia* isolates were susceptible to cyclopiroxolamine and azole drugs, with *M. furfur* isolates being somewhat more drug tolerant than other *Malassezia* species.

Conclusions: This study provides an important insight into the species composition of *Malassezia* microbiota in human skin. The predominance of *M. sympodialis* in both normal and pathologic skin, contrasts with other European countries, reporting *M. globosa* and *M. restricta* as the most frequently isolated *Malassezia* species.

Keywords: Identification, *Malassezia* spp, PCR-RFLP, Sequence analysis, Drug susceptibility

* Correspondence: t.jagielski@biol.uw.edu.pl
[1]Department of Applied Microbiology, Institute of Microbiology, Faculty of Biology, University of Warsaw, I. Miecznikowa 1, 02-096 Warsaw, Poland
Full list of author information is available at the end of the article

Background

The fungi of the *Malassezia* genus, whose first description dates back to the middle of the XIX century, have only recently gained considerable attention of the dermatological community. This is because those basidiomycetous yeasts, being components of the microbiota of human and animal skin and constituting up to 80% of the total skin fungal population [1] are now increasingly recognized as opportunistic pathogens resulting in different dermatological pathologies. *Malassezia* yeasts are the causative agents of pityriasis versicolor (PV), which is one of the commonest superficial mycoses in human population worldwide [2]. *Malassezia* species are also involved in the pathogenesis of various dermatoses with global distribution, such as seborrheic dermatitis (SD), atopic dermatitis (AD), and, more recently, psoriasis (PS) [3-6]. A growing number of reports demonstrate the implication of *Malassezia* yeasts in other skin disorders, including folliculitis, onychomycosis, confluent and reticulated papillomatosis, and neonatal cephalic pustulosis [7-10]. Finally, *Malassezia* yeasts have been associated with systemic infections and outbreaks in neonatal and immunocompromised adults intensive care units [11,12].

The species content of the *Malassezia* genus has repeatedly been revised over the last two decades. In the early 1990s the genus *Malassezia* contained only three species, namely *M. furfur*, *M. pachydermatis*, and *M. sympodialis*. In 1996, four other species (i. e. *M. globosa*, *M. obtusa*, *M. restricta*, and *M. slooffiae*) were identified within the genus, through a comparative sequence analysis of nuclear ribosomal DNA (rDNA) operons [13]. Since 2002 seven more new species have been described, on the basis of molecular data: *M. dermatis*, *M. equina*, *M. japonica*, *M. nana*, *M. yamatoensis*, *M. caprae*, and *M. cuniculi* [14-19]. Overall, the genus *Malassezia* now accommodates 14 species, all but one (*M. pachydermatis*) being lipid-dependent species.

Among the *Malassezia* species, one of the most frequently isolated is *M. sympodialis*, which has been considered to be associated with AD. One of the clearest indications to support this is the fact that almost half of the adult patients suffering from AD are sensitized to *M. sympodialis*, as evidenced by allergen-specific IgE and/or T-cell reactivity to the yeast, and that such reactivity is rarely observed in other allergic diseases [20,21].

The identification of most of *Malassezia* species can be achieved by using a combination of morphological, biochemical, and physiological characteristics. The currently used protocol, based on the phenotypic criteria, includes the examination of colony and cell morphology, determination of urease, catalase, and β-glucosidase activities, growth at 37°C and 40°C, and the capacity to grow with different polyoxyethylene sorbate compounds (Tween 20, 40, 60, 80) and polyoxyethylene castor oil (Cremophor EL), as the sole lipid source [22].

With the advent of molecular biology tools, several new, DNA-targeted methods have been developed and tested for species identification within the *Malassezia* taxon. These include pulsed-field gel electrophoresis (PFGE) [23,24], randomly amplified polymorphic DNA (RAPD) analysis [23,25], amplified fragment length polymorphism (AFLP) analysis [25,26], denaturing gradient gel electrophoresis (DGGE) [25], multilocus enzyme electrophoresis (MEE) [27], PCR-based single strand confirmation polymorphism (PCR-SSCP), PCR-based restriction fragment length polymorphism (PCR-RFLP) [7,28-34], nested PCR [32,35-37], real-time (RT) PCR [35,38], and direct sequencing of various genetic loci, such as rDNA and internal transcribed spacer (ITS) 1 and 2 regions in particular, the chitin synthase (*CHS2*) gene, and the RNA polymerase subunit 1 (*RPB1*) gene [18,26,39-41].

The purpose of this study was to explore the species composition of *Malassezia* microflora on the skin of healthy volunteers and patients with AD and PS. Species determination was performed by using both conventional, culture-based methods and molecular techniques, that is PCR-RFLP and direct sequencing targeting the rDNA cluster of the *Malassezia* genome.

Methods

Subjects

The study group comprised of 18 subjects (8 (44.4%) males and 10 (55.6%) females, aged from 22–70 years; mean age: 34.8 years; median age: 30 years), all being Polish and living in the Lesser Poland province. The subjects were split into three, equally sized groups (i.e. six subjects per each group), consisting of healthy volunteers (i) and patients diagnosed with either atopic dermatitis (ii) or psoriasis (iii). Both AD and PS patients were recruited from the routine dermatology outpatient clinic at the Collegium Medicum of the Jagiellonian University in Kraków, where they were assessed clinically and received treatment during a 3-year period (2008–2010). The diagnosis of AD was made according to the Hanifin-Rajka criteria [42], and the severity of the disease was categorized based on the Severity Scoring of Atopic Dermatitis (SCORAD) index [43]. The diagnosis of PS was based on clinical features and confirmed by histopathological analysis. The severity of psoriatic lesions was evaluated using the Body Surface Area (BSA) and Psoriasis Area and Severity (PASI) indexes [44,45].

Information on demographic characteristics and clinical aspects of the disease were collected in a standardized questionnaire by reviewing the medical records and analysed (Table 1).

Table 1 Characteristics of 18 subjects under the study and microbiological details of 35 isolated *Malassezia* species

	Patient[a]	Subject group[b]	Collection site	Sex[c]	Age	Lesion severity[d]	Episode[e]	Duration of disease [yrs]	Treatment[f]	Family history of disease	Other diseases[g]	Strain no.	Species identifiction[h]
1.	TK	AD	Head	M	24	37	R	24	Topical; sys: antihistaminics	Positive	No	40.10.I.	*M. sympodialis*
2.			Face									40.10.II.	*M. sympodialis*
3.			Back									40.10.IV.	*M. sympodialis*
4.	MP		Head	F	28	31	R	23	Topical; sys: antihistaminics	Positive	Rhinoconjunctivitis	8.11.I.	*M. sympodialis*
5.			Chest									8.11.III.	*M. sympodialis* + *C. d.**
6.			Back									8.11.IV.	*M. sympodialis*
7.	DJ		Chest	M	29	34.6	R	29	Topical; sys: antihistaminics	Positive	Rhinoconjunctivitis	27.10.III.	*M. sympodialis*
8.			Back									27.10.IV.	*M. sympodialis*
9.	JW		Chest	F	22	10.2	R	22	Topical; sys: antihistaminics	Positive	No	7.11.III.	*M. sympodialis*
10.			Back									7.11.IV.	*M. sympodialis*
11.	MB		Back	M	22	39.4	R	22	Topical; sys: antihistaminics	Negative		25.10.IV.	*M. sympodialis*
12.	EP		Back	F	31	10.2	R	31	Topical; sys: antihistaminics	Negative	Vitiligo	17.10.IV.	*M. sympodialis*
13.	BT	PS	Head	F	50	8.2	R	20	Topical; sys: CyA	Positive	No	10.11.I.	*M. sympodialis*
14.			Face									10.11.II.	*M. sympodialis* + *A. p.***
15.			Chest									10.11. IIIA.	*M. furfur*
16.			Back									10.11.IV.	*M. sympodialis*
17.	BH		Face	F	44	10	R	15	Topical	Negative	No	45.08.II.	*M. furfur*
18.			Chest									45.08.III.	*M. furfur* + *M. sympodialis*
19.	SK		Back	M	38	3.6	R	5	Topical; sys: CS	Negative	No	20.09.IV.	*M. furfur* + *M. sympodialis*
20.	EN		Back	F	31	6.6	R	5	Topical	Negative	No	17.09.IV.	*M. sympodialis*
21.	KK		Face	M	23	11.2	R	12	Topical; sys: CyA	Positive	No	43.08.II.	*M. furfur*
22.	MB		Back	F	29	5.7	R	15	Topical	Positive	No	6.11.IV.	*M. sympodialis*
23.	MT	Control	Head	F	31						No	1.11.IA.	*M. globosa*
24.			Face									1.11.II.	*M. globosa* + *M. restricta*
25.			Chest									1.11.IIIA.	*M. sympodialis*
26.			Back									1.11.IVA.	*M. sympodialis*
27.	CM		Chest	M	70						No	69.09.III.	*M. slooffiae*

Table 1 Characteristics of 18 subjects under the study and microbiological details of 35 isolated *Malassezia* species *(Continued)*

28.		Back				69.09.IV.	*M. slooffiae + M. sympodialis*
29.	BP	Chest	M	69	No	67.09.III.	*M. sympodialis*
30.		Back				67.09.IV.	*M. sympodialis*
31.	PK	Chest	M	27	No	68.09.III.	*M. sympodialis*
32.		Back				68.09.IV.	*M. sympodialis*
33.	MS	Chest	F	28	No	2.11.III.	*M. sympodialis*
34.		Back				2.11.IV.	*M. sympodialis*
35.	JP	Back	F	31	No	12.09.IV.	*M. sympodialis*

[a]Patient initials.
[b]Three subject groups under investigation: (i) patients with atopic dermatitis (AD) (ii) patients with psoriasis (PS), and (iii) healthy volunteers (control).
[c]M, male; F, female.
[d]The numbers represent the SCORAD index values in AD patients, or the PASI index values in psoriatic patients.
[e]R, recurrent.
[f]Topic treatment for AD patients included emolients, corticosteroids, tacrolimus, pimecrolimus, antibiotics, whereas topic treatment for psoriatic patients included corticosteroids, calcipotriol, tacrolimus, pimecrolimus, emollients; CS, corticosteroids; CyA: Cyclosporine A; sys., systemic.
[g]Based on direct interviewing of the patients.
[h]Final species identification results, based upon integration of conventional and molecular data. *C. d., *Cryptococcus diffluens*; **A. p., *Aureobasidium pullulans*.

Sample collection

From each patient, four samples originating from four different anatomical sites of the body, that is the scalp, face, chest (interclavicle region) and back (interscapular region) were collected by a standard swab method. A sterile cotton swab soaked with sterile saline was used to rub against the skin surface, with continuous rotation of the swab and over at least 15 seconds, and immediately streaked evenly onto modified Dixon's agar (mDA) medium.

Culture conditions and yeast strains

The yeasts were cultured on mDA plates at 32°C, with growth being monitored every day for two weeks. The suspected colonies of *Malassezia* sp. were subcultured, by streaking onto mDA slants, and subjected to the identification procedures described hereafter. The cultures were maintained by weekly passaging on fresh mDA slants.

Apart from the *Malassezia* sp. strains isolated from clinical samples, six reference strains representing as many *Malassezia* species (*Malassezia furfur* CBS 6001; *M. globosa* CBS 7966; *M. obtusa* CBS 7876; *M. slooffiae* CBS 7956; *M. restricta* CBS 7877; *M. sympodialis* CBS 7222) and purchased from the CBS (Centraalbureau voor Schimmelcultures, Utrecht, The Netherlands) culture collection were included in the study.

Drug susceptibility testing

In vitro susceptibility testing was performed by using commercially available Neo-Sensitabs diffusion assays (Neo-Sensitabs, Rosco Diagnostica, Denmark), according to the instructions provided by the manufacturer and following the Clinical and Laboratory Standards Institute (CLSI) guidelines [46] with some modifications. Colonies from a seven-day yeast culture, grown on mDA, were scraped off and suspended in sterile saline with sterile glass beads. The suspension was mixed vigorously for 30 seconds in a vortex mixer, and adjusted to a turbidity equivalent of a 5.0 McFarland standard. The so prepared inoculum was swabbed over the mDA plates. After allowing the plates to dry completely, Neo-Sensitabs tablets containing 50 μg of ciclopirox (CPO), 25 μg of fluconazole (FLZ), 15 μg of ketoconazole (KTZ), 10 μg of econazole (ECZ), 10 μg of miconazole (MNZ), and 8 μg of itraconazole (ITZ) were applied onto the surface and the plates were incubated at 32°C, with reading taken after 48 and 72 h. The zones of inhibition were measured at a point in which either there was prominent reduction of growth or no visible growth occurred. Since the interpretation of antifungal resistant/susceptible categories among the *Malassezia* species has not yet been established, interpretive criteria for the yeasts reported by the CLSI [46] and provided by the manufacturer of the Neo-Sensitabs were employed. Accordingly, resistance was assumed if the inhibition zone was less than 10 mm for ITZ, less than or equal to 11 mm for CPO, ECZ, and MNZ, less than or equal to 14 mm for FLZ, and less than or equal to 22 mm for KTZ.

To validate the performance of the Neo-Sensitabs drug susceptibility testing, two quality control (QC) strains were used: *Pichia kudriavzevii* (teleomorph *of Candida krusei*) DBVPG 7235 (corresponding to ATCC 6258) and *Candida parapsilosis* DBVPG 6150 (corresponding to ATCC 22019), from the Industrial Yeasts Collection DBVPG (Perugia, Italy).

All *Malassezia* strains were tested in duplicate. Also, the QC strains were assayed twice.

DNA isolation

Genomic DNA extraction was done from pure cultures. Briefly, a few yeast colonies were suspended in 200 μL of TE buffer (10 mM Tris–HCl [pH 8.0], 1 mM EDTA) and subjected to 3 rounds of sonication (three sonication cycles of 15 s each separated by 15 s intervals) in ice water bath, at 20% amplitude in a Vibra Cell sonicator (Sonics & Materials Inc., USA). The obtained homogenate was further processed with the Genomic Mini AX Yeast kit (A&A Biotechnology, Poland) following the manufacturer's instructions.

Species identification

Identification by phenotypic methods

All yeast cultures were identified to species level by using conventional mycological methods, including examination of colonial and microscopic morphologies (i.e. colonies' shape, texture, and colour, and cell size, shape and budding characteristics) as well as physiological and biochemical tests, including assimilation of Tween 20, 40, 60, and 80, assimilation of Cremophor EL, catalase reaction, cleavage of esculin, and growth at 37°C. Phenotypic feature testing was performed essentially as described elsewhere [47], and the characteristics table of *Malassezia* spp. provided by Ashbee and Evans [48] served as the species identification key.

Molecular analysis

Molecular identification involved PCR-RFLP analysis along with sequence analysis of different nuclear loci within the rDNA operon of *Malassezia* spp., including the ITS1 and ITS2 regions and the D1 and D2 domains of the 26S rRNA gene.

PCR-RFLP analysis

Two PCR-RFLP assays, targeting the ITS2 region and partial 26S rRNA gene, were performed, as described previously [28,29], with slight modifications. Briefly, primers ITS3 (5′-GCATCGATGAAGAACGCAGC-3′) and ITS4 (5′-TCCTCCGCTTATTGATATGC-3′) were used to amplify the ITS2 region, whereas primers Malup (5′-AGCGGAGGAAAAGAAACT-3′) and Maldown (5′-GCGCGAAGGTGTCCGAAG-3′) were used to amplify the 26S rRNA gene fragment (Figure 1). PCR mixtures were prepared by using the TopTaq Master Mix kit (QIAGEN, Germany) in a total volume of 25 μL, containing 2× TopTaq Master Mix (final conc. 1×; the mix contains 1.25 U of *Taq* DNA polymerase, 200 μM each deoxyucleoside triphosphate, and 1× PCR buffer with 1.5 mM $MgCl_2$), 0.4 μM each primer, and 1 μL (*ca.* 10–20 ng) of template DNA. The PCR conditions were as follows: 94°C for 3 min, 30 cycles at 94°C for 30 s, 50°C for 30 s, and 72°C for either 30 s (ITS2) or 50 s (26S rDNA), and a final step at 72°C for 10 min. After confirmation of the presence of the amplicons of correct sizes with gel electrophoresis, the purified PCR products of the ITS2 and 26S rDNA regions were subjected to RFLP analysis with *Alu*I and *Hae*II enzymes, respectively. Restriction reactions were carried out in 20 μL volumes containing 8 μL (*ca.* 200 ng) of PCR product and 1 U of the restriction enzyme together with the appropriate reaction buffer (final conc. 1×) at 37°C for 45 min (FastDigest restriction enzymes; Fermentas UAB, Lithuania). Restriction patterns were compared with those of reference *Malassezia* strains and virtual, species-specific patterns established in the original publications [28,29].

PCR-sequencing

Sequencing of the ITS1 and ITS2 regions and the D1/D2 domains of the 26S rRNA gene was performed, as reported earlier [26]. In short, primers V9 (5′-TGCGTTGATTACGTCCCTGC-3′) and RLR3R (5′-GGTCCGTGTTTCAAGAC-3′) amplified a fragment encompassing ITS1, the 5.8S rRNA gene, ITS2, and partial regions of the 18S and 26S rDNA (Figure 1).

The PCR was carried out in a 25-μL reaction volume containing 2× TopTaq Master Mix (final conc. 1×) (QIAGEN, Germany), 0.5 μM each primer, and 1 μL (*ca.* 20 ng) of template DNA. The thermal cycling profile was 94°C for 5 min, 30 cycles at 94°C for 45 s, 56°C for 30 s, and 72°C for 1.5 min, and a final step at 72°C for 10 min. The resulting amplicons were electrophoresed to verify the presence of a single product of the correct size, purified, and sequenced either directly or after cloning into a plasmid vector using the pGEM-T Easy Vector system (Promega, USA), according to the vendor's protocol, when initial sequence information showed the possible presence of two (or more) different species.

The primers used in the sequence reaction were ITS4 (5′-TCCTCCGCTTATTGATATGC-3′) and ITS5 (5′-GGAAGTAAAAGTCGTAACAAGG-3′) for analysis of the ITS1/ITS2, and NL1 (5′-GCATATCAATAAGCGGAGGAAAAG-3′) and RLR3R for analysis of the D1/D2 domains of the 26S rRNA gene (Figure 1).

Forward and reverse sequences were assembled and edited with ChromasPro ver. 1.7.1 (Technelysium, Australia) and the resulting consensus sequences were searched against the GenBank database of the National Center for Biotechnology Information (NCBI) using the BLASTN algorithm (http://blast.ncbi.nlm.nih.gov/).

Distance scores of up to 1.00% (99% match) were used as a proxy for species identity, and the species giving the closest match was considered the correct identification.

The nucleotide sequences determined in the study were deposited in the GenBank database (NCBI) under the accession numbers listed in Table 2.

Statistical analysis

The Chi-square test and Fisher's exact test were used to evaluate the differences in the frequency and distribution of *Malassezia* species between the AD patients, PS patients, and healthy subjects. A P value < 0.05 was considered statistically significant.

Ethics

The study was approved by the Ethics Committee of the Jagiellonian University in Kraków. All the patients gave informed consent to participate in the study.

Results

A total of 35 *Malassezia* sp. cultures were obtained from clinical samples, with back being the most frequent site of isolation (16 cultures; 45.7% of all *Malassezia* cultures), followed by chest (10; 28.6%), face (5; 14.3%), and head (4; 11.4%). Of 24 skin samples collected from each of the three subject groups, 13 (54.2%), 12 (50%), and 10 (41.7%) gave positive culture in the control group, AD group, and PS group, respectively. The overall positive culture rate of the *Malassezia* yeasts from 4 different body sites of 18 patients under the study was 48.6% (35 positive samples out of 72 samples tested).

Phenotypic identification

Based on conventional, phenotypic methods, all 35 yeast cultures were initially separated into 5 different *Malassezia* species. There were recognized 19 (54.3%) *M. sympodialis*, 7 (20%) *M. furfur*, 5 (14.3%) *M. slooffiae*, 2 (5.7%) *M. globosa*, and 2 (5.7%) *M. obtusa* isolates. Among the isolates from AD patients and healthy volunteers, *M. sympodialis* predominated and accounted for 66.7% (8/12) and 46.1% (6/13) of the isolates, respectively. In both these groups there were isolates of other four (control group) or three (all but *M. globosa*) species (AD group). In psoriatic patient group, only two species, equally abundant, were identified, namely *M. sympodialis* and *M. furfur*.

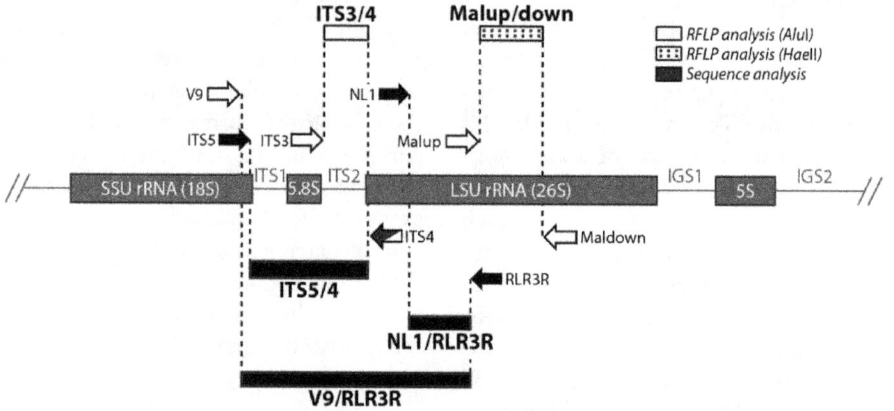

Figure 1 Schematic representation of the rDNA operon in *Malassezia* yeasts. The loci under analysis are depicted. Major rRNA genes are shown as grey boxes. Primers used for PCR amplification of the target DNA sequences and those used for sequencing are indicated as white and black block arrows, respectively. Loci analysed by PCR-RFLP or direct sequencing are shown as black or white rectangles, respectively, and are designated after the primers used for their amplification (or sequencing). LSU, large subunit (rRNA); SSU, small subunit (rRNA); IGS, intergenic spacer region; ITS, internal transcribed spacer.

PCR-RFLP analysis

PCR amplification of the partial 26S rRNA gene produced, for all isolates, a single amplicon of the expected size of *ca.* 550 bp. Upon digestion of the amplified products with the *Hae*II restriction enzyme 4 different restriction patterns could be distinguished. Three of them matched exactly the *Hae*II restriction patterns predicted for *M. sympodialis* (26 isolates; 74.3% of all isolates), *M. furfur* or *M. slooffiae* (6; 17.1%), and *M. globosa* or *M. restricta* (2; 5.7%). For one isolate (20.09.IV.) a mixed *Hae*II restriction pattern was obtained, corresponding to *M. sympodialis* and *M. furfur* or *M. slooffiae.*

A single amplicon of *ca.* 400–500 bp in size was generated by PCR amplification of the ITS2 region for all *Malassezia* isolates except one (20.09.IV.), for which two PCR products were visualized (one of *ca.* 400 bp and another of *ca.* 500 bp). When the PCR products were digested with the *Alu*I restriction enzyme 6 different restriction patterns were demonstrated, 4 of which corresponded to those expected for *M. sympodialis* (24 isolates; 68.6% of all isolates), *M. furfur* (4; 11.4%), *M. slooffiae* (2; 5.7%), and *M. globosa* (1; 2.9%). The restriction pattern of one isolate (1.11.II.) was a combination of those for *M. globosa* and *M. restricta.* The restriction patterns of 2 isolates (10.11.II.; 8.11.III.) contained a fragment characteristic of *M. sympodialis*, along with two additional fragments whose sizes did not correlate with the sizes of the *Alu*I restriction fragments previously reported for *Malassezia* species. In case of one isolate, for which two PCR products were obtained, they were both purified by gel extraction and subjected to *Alu*I digestion separately (20.09.IV.A/B). This resulted in 2 single restriction profiles, conforming to that of *M. sympodialis* and of *M. furfur.*

Based on the results from two PCR-RFLP assays, 31 (88.6%) of the isolates tested could be separated into 4 distinct *Malassezia* species, namely, *M. sympodialis* (24 isolates; 68.6% of all isolates), *M. furfur* (4; 11.4%), *M. slooffiae* (2; 5.7%), and *M. globosa* (1; 2.9%). Two isolates were identified as a mixture of two different *Malassezia* species, that is *M. sympodialis* and *M. furfur* (20.09.IV.) and *M. globosa* and *M. restricta* (1.11.II.). Finally, 2 isolates (10.11.II.; 8.11.III.) appeared to represent *M. sympodialis* mixed with another unknown fungal species.

PCR-sequence analysis

The rDNA region containing the ITS1/ITS2 sequences and D1/D2 domains of the 26S rRNA was successfully amplified, for all isolates tested, resulting in a sole product of *ca.* 1,500 bp. The purified PCR products were used as templates in two independent sequencing reactions, targeting the ITS and D1/D2 loci, respectively. Upon ITS1/ITS2 sequence analysis, 33 (94.3%) of the isolates tested, could be unambiguously identified at the species level. The consensus ITS sequences of those isolates shared ≥99% similarity with the sequences of previously characterized fungal species, as evidenced by the BLAST search of the GenBank database. Twenty-four (68.6% of all isolates) isolates had a 100% similarity with the sequence of *M. sympodialis.* Four (11.4%) isolates showed 100% sequence identity with *M. furfur*, and 2 (5.7%) isolates showed 99% sequence similarity with *M. slooffiae.* The ITS1/ITS2 sequences of 2 isolates designated 8.11.III and 10.11.II., formerly identified as *M. sympodialis* (on PCR-RFLP analysis) showed a complete match (100% identity) to the ITS1/ITS2 sequences of *Cryptococcus diffluens* and *Aureobasidium proteae/pullulans*), respectively. The results for those two isolates were consistent, even if sequencing was performed on PCR products from different PCR runs using DNA from three different isolations. Sequence analysis of the ITS

Table 2 Species identification results obtained upon phenotypic testing and molecular typing of 35 *Malassezia* cultures

	Strain no.	Species identification by means of								Final species identification[d]
		Phenotypic methods[a]	Molecular methods							
			PCR-RFLP[b]	PCR sequencing[c]						
				ITS accession no.	Similarity with ITS of [%]:		D1/D2 accession no.	Similarity with D1/ D2 of [%]:		
1.	40.10.I.	*M. slooffiae*	*M. sympodialis*	KC141968	*M. sympodialis* MA 73	100%	KC415092	*M. sympodialis* IFM 48109	100%	*M. sympodialis*
2.	40.10.II.	*M. slooffiae*	*M. sympodialis*	KC141969	*M. sympodialis* CBS 7222	100%	KC415093	*M. sympodialis* IFM 48109	100%	*M. sympodialis*
3.	40.10.IV.	*M. sympodialis*	*M. sympodialis*	KC141970	*M. sympodialis* CBS 7222	100%	KC415094	*M. sympodialis* IFM 48109	100%	*M. sympodialis*
4.	8.11.I.	*M. obtusa*	*M. sympodialis*	KC152895	*M. sympodialis* CBS 7222	100%	KC415085	*M. sympodialis* IFM 48109	100%	*M. sympodialis*
5.	8.11.III.	*M. furfur*	*M. sympodialis*	KC152904	*C. diffluens* CBS 160	100%	KC241877	*C. diffluens* CBS 6436	100%	*M. sympodialis + C. d.*[*]
6.	8.11.IV.	*M. sympodialis*	*M. sympodialis*	KC152896	*M. sympodialis* CBS 7222	100%	KC415086	*M. sympodialis* IFM 48109	100%	*M. sympodialis*
7.	27.10.III.	*M. sympodialis*	*M. sympodialis*	KC141966	*M. sympodialis* MA 73	100%	KC415095	*M. sympodialis* IFM 48109	100%	*M. sympodialis*
8.	27.10.IV.	*M. sympodialis*	*M. sympodialis*	KC141967	*M. sympodialis* MA 73	100%	KC415096	*M. sympodialis* IFM 48109	100%	*M. sympodialis*
9.	7.11.III.	*M. sympodialis*	*M. sympodialis*	KC152893	*M. sympodialis* CBS 7222	100%	KC415083	*M. sympodialis* IFM 48109	100%	*M. sympodialis*
10.	7.11.IV.	*M. sympodialis*	*M. sympodialis*	KC152894	*M. sympodialis* MA 73	100%	KC415084	*M. sympodialis* IFM 48109	100%	*M. sympodialis*
11.	25.10.IV.	*M. sympodialis*	*M. sympodialis*	KC119577	*M. sympodialis* CBS 7222	100%	KC415097	*M. sympodialis* IFM 48109	100%	*M. sympodialis*
12.	17.10.IV.	*M. sympodialis*	*M. sympodialis*	KC119576	*M. sympodialis* CBS 7222	100%	KC415098	*M. sympodialis* IFM 48109	100%	*M. sympodialis*
13.	10.11.I.	*M. sympodialis*	*M. sympodialis*	KC152897	*M. sympodialis* CBS 7222	100%	KC415087	*M. sympodialis* IFM 48109	100%	*M. sympodialis*
14.	10.11.II.	*M. sympodialis*	*M. sympodialis*	KC152905	*A. pullulans* CPC 13701	100%	KC241878	*A. pullulans* RA406	100%	*M. sympodialis + A. p.*[**]
15.	10.11.IIIA.	*M. furfur*	*M. furfur*	KC152897	*M. furfur* M235	100%	KC415088	*M. furfur* VG Ig 02	99%	*M. furfur*
16.	10.11.IV.	*M. sympodialis*	*M. sympodialis*	KC152901	*M. sympodialis* CBS 7222	100%	KC415091	*M. sympodialis* IFM 48109	100%	*M. sympodialis*
17.	45.08.II.	*M. furfur*	*M. furfur*	KC141972	*M. furfur* M235	100%	KC415099	*M. furfur* VG Ig 02	100%	*M. furfur*
18.	45.08.III.	*M. furfur*	*M. furfur*	KC141973	*M. sympodialis* CBS 7222	100%	KC415100	*M. sympodialis* IFM 48109	99%	*M. furfur + M. sympodialis*
19.	20.09.IV.	*M. furfur*	*M. furfur + M. sympodialis*	KC141965	*M furfur* M235	100%	KC415101	*M. furfur* VG Ig 02	99%	*M. furfur + M. sympodialis*
20.	17.09.IV.	*M. sympodialis*	*M. sympodialis*	KC109788	*M. sympodialis* MA 73	100%	KC415102	*M. sympodialis* IFM 48109	100%	*M. sympodialis*
21.	43.08.II.	*M. furfur*	*M. furfur*	KC141971	*M. furfur* M235	100%	KC415103	*M. furfur* VG Ig 02	100%	*M. furfur*
22.	6.11.IV.	*M. sympodialis*	*M. sympodialis*	KC152892	*M. sympodialis* MA 73	100%	KC415082	*M. sympodialis* IFM 48109	100%	*M. sympodialis*
23.	1.11.IA.	*M. globosa*	*M. globosa*	KC152884	*M. globosa* CBS 7966	96%	KC415074	*M. sympodialis* IFM 48109	100%	*M. globosa*
24.	1.11.II.	*M. globosa*	*M. globosa + M. restricta*	KC152885	*M. restricta* MRE28	99%	KC415075	*M. sympodialis* IFM 48109	100%	*M. globosa + M. restricta*

Table 2 Species identification results obtained upon phenotypic testing and molecular typing of 35 *Malassezia* cultures *(Continued)*

25.	1.11.IIIA.	*M. sympodialis*	*M. sympodialis*	KC152886	*M. sympodialis* MA 73	100%	KC415076	*M. sympodialis* IFM 48109	100%	*M. sympodialis*
26.	1.11.IVA.	*M. furfur*	*M. sympodialis*	KC152888	*M. sympodialis* MA 73	100%	KC415078	*M. sympodialis* IFM 48109	100%	*M. sympodialis*
27.	69.09.III.	*M. slooffiae*	*M. slooffiae*	KC141978	*M. slooffiae* CBS 7956	99%	KC415104	*M. slooffiae* sc7LG	99%	*M. slooffiae*
28.	69.09.IV.	*M. slooffiae*	*M. slooffiae*	KC141979	*M. slooffiae* CBS 7956	99%	KC415105	*M. sympodialis* IFM 48109	100%	*M. slooffiae* + *M. sympodialis*
29.	67.09.III.	*M. sympodialis*	*M. sympodialis*	KC141974	*M. sympodialis* CBS 7222	100%	KC415106	*M. sympodialis* IFM 48109	100%	*M. sympodialis*
30.	67.09.IV.	*M. slooffiae*	*M. sympodialis*	KC141975	*M. sympodialis* CBS 7222	100%	KC415107	*M. sympodialis* IFM 48109	100%	*M. sympodialis*
31.	68.09.III.	*M. sympodialis*	*M. sympodialis*	KC141976	*M. sympodialis* CBS 7222	100%	KC415108	*M. sympodialis* IFM 48109	100%	*M. sympodialis*
32.	68.09.IV.	*M. sympodialis*	*M. sympodialis*	KC141977	*M. sympodialis* CBS 7222	100%	KC415109	*M. sympodialis* IFM 48109	100%	*M. sympodialis*
33.	2.11.III.	*M. sympodialis*	*M. sympodialis*	KC152890	*M. sympodialis* MA 73	100%	KC415080	*M. sympodialis* IFM 48109	100%	*M. sympodialis*
34.	2.11.IV.	*M. obtusa*	*M. sympodialis*	KC152891	*M. sympodialis* MA 73	100%	KC415081	*M. sympodialis* IFM 48109	100%	*M. sympodialis*
35.	12.09.IV.	*M. sympodialis*	*M. sympodialis*	JX915741	*M. sympodialis* MA 73	100%	KC415110	*M. sympodialis* IFM 48109	100%	*M. sympodialis*

[a]Identification algorithm included macro- and microscopic examination of fungal colonies along with biochemical tests, as described in the Materials and Methods section.
[b]Based on two PCR-RFLP assays (i. e. with *AluI* and *HaeII* restriction endonucleases).
[c]Results of BLAST search of GenBank (http://blast.ncbi.nlm.nih.gov/); The ITS and D1/D2 accession numbers are those under which the respective sequences determined in this study can be found in the GenBank; Percentage similarities with ITS or D1/D2 sequences deposited in the GenBank are given.
[d]Based on combined molecular methods results; [*]*C. d., Cryptococcus diffluens*; [**]*A. p., Aureobasidium pullulans.*

regions from one isolate (1.11.II.), identified as a mixture of *M. globosa* and *M. restricta* by PCR-RFLP analysis, was informative only after subcloning of the PCR product into the pGEM-T plasmid. Although several recombinants were examined, each time the ITS sequence homologous (99% identity) to that of *M. restricta* was resolved. Interestingly, when applying the same procedure (i. e. sequence analysis from the pGEM-T vector) to the second isolate (20.09.IV.) that was identified as consisting of two different *Malassezia* species (*M. furfur* and *M. sympodialis*), only a sequence with 100% similarity with that of *M. furfur* could be revealed. Two isolates designated 2.11.III. and 1.11.IA. yielded ITS1/ITS2 sequences with <99% similarity with the closest sequence in the GenBank database; the former gave the closest sequence match to *M. sympodialis*, whereas the latter – to *M. globosa*, at a similarity level of 97% and 96%, respectively (Table 2).

Sequence analysis of partial 26S rRNA gene allowed clear species discrimination of all isolates tested. The sequences of 33 (94.3%) isolates displayed ≥99% sequence identity to 4 *Malassezia* species strains, namely *M. sympodialis* (26 isolates; 74.3% of all isolates), *M. furfur* (4; 11.4%), *M. globosa* (2; 5.7%), and *M. slooffiae* (1; 2.9%). Finally, two isolates had a perfect match (100% sequence identity), one for *C. diffluens*, and the other for *A. pullulans*.

The results from the sequence analysis of the D1/D2 and ITS loci were almost entirely concordant, with the concordance rate, calculated as percent agreement between paired results, of 94.3% (33/35 cases). The only discrepant results were from 2 isolates designated 69.09.IV. and 1.11.II., identified by D1/D2 sequencing as *M. sympodialis* and *M. globosa*, respectively. Whereas the former isolate had previously been identified (both by PCR-RFLP analysis and ITS sequencing) as *M. slooffiae*, the latter had initially been recognized as a mixture of *M. globosa* and *M. restricta* (upon PCR-RFLP analysis), with the presence of only *M. restricta* confirmed by ITS sequencing. Based on the combined ITS and D1/D2 sequence analysis, those 2 isolates were considered to represent mixtures of two *Malassezia* species, that is *M. slooffiae* and *M. sympodialis* (69.09.IV.) and *M. globosa* and *M. restricta* (1.11.II.).

Comparison of PCR-RFLP analysis and PCR-sequencing analysis

Concordance of the species identification results by using PCR-RFLP analysis and PCR-sequencing analysis was 85.7% (30/35 cases). Two isolates identified, upon

PCR-RFLP analysis, as *M. sympodialis* (8.11.III.; 10.11.II.), were identified as *C. diffluens* (8.11.III.) and *A. pullulans* (10.11.II.) with PCR-sequencing. Another 2 isolates initially recognized as *M. furfur* (45.08.III.) and *M. slooffiae* (69.09.IV.) were re-identified as *M. sympodialis* and a mixture of *M. slooffiae* and *M. sympodialis*, accordingly. For one isolate (20.09.IV.) being a mixture of *M. furfur* and *M. sympodialis*, as demonstrated by PCR-RFLP, only the presence of *M. furfur* was confirmed by sequence analysis.

Comparison of phenotypic and molecular methods

The results of phenotypic and molecular identification methods showed a concordance rate of 65.7% (23/35 cases). Twelve (34.3%) isolates produced discrepant results. These included 6 *M. sympodialis* isolates, which by phenotypic methods had initially been identified as *M. slooffiae* (in 3 cases), *M. obtusa* (2 cases), and *M. furfur* (one case), as well as 6 mixed-species isolates. Of the latter, morphological and biochemical tests correctly identified one of 2 co-occurring species in 5 cases. One isolate recognized as a mixture of *M. sympodialis* and *C. diffluens* had previously been identified as *M. furfur*, based on the physiological testing.

Overall, among the isolates under investigation, 29 (82.9%) were identified as homogenous species, namely *M. sympodialis* (24; 68.6%), *M. furfur* (3; 8.6%), *M. globosa* (1; 2.9%), and *M. slooffiae* (1; 2.9%). The remaining 6 (17.1%) isolates were demonstrated heterogeneous, being mixtures of two species; 2 isolates consisted of *M. furfur* and *M. sympodialis*, (20.09.IV.; 45.08.III.), one isolate contained *M. sympodialis* and *M. slooffiae* (69.09.IV.), and the other one *M. globosa* and *M. restricta* (1.11.II.). Two isolates were mixtures of *M. sympodialis* and a non-*Malassezia* species, that is either *C. diffluens* (8.11.III.) or *A. pullulans* (10.11.II.).

Drug susceptibility testing

Evaluation of drug susceptibility of *Malassezia* spp. to 6 antifungal drugs was conducted on 19 isolates representing all *Malassezia* isolates cultured from 4 patients with AD, 4 patients with PS, and 4 healthy volunteers, randomly selected within each subject groups. All isolates examined were found susceptible to all 6 antifungals tested (Table 3). Six (31.6%) isolates showed intermediate susceptibility to at least one drug; 2 isolates (one of *M. furfur* (45.08.II.) and the other of *M. sympodialis* (12.09.IV.)) were intermediately susceptible to ECZ; one isolate, identified as a mixture of *M. slooffiae* and *M. sympodialis* (69.09.IV.) was intermediately susceptible to MNZ. Two isolates, identified as mixtures of *M. furfur* and *M. sympodialis*, and designated 45.08.III. and 20.09.IV. were intermediately susceptible to 2 (KTZ + ECZ) and 3 (KTZ + ECZ + MNZ) drugs, respectively. A three-drug intermediate susceptible pattern (KTZ + ECZ + MNZ) was also observed in one *M. furfur* isolate (43.08.II.). Overall, based on the inhibition zone diameter values, the more susceptible isolates included *M. slooffiae* and most of the *M. sympodialis* isolates, whereas the least susceptible isolates were represented by *M. furfur* and *M. furfur* co-cultured with *M. sympodialis* (Table 3).

Distribution of *Malassezia* species

The final species identification, based on the molecular data, was used to determine the frequency distribution of *Malassezia* species among different subject groups. Of the culture-positive samples from AD patients, all yielded *M. sympodialis* isolates. These were homogeneous cultures in all cases, except one, where a mixed culture of *M. sympodialis* and *C. diffluens* was obtained. Among the PS patients, 2 *Malassezia* species were identified, with *M. sympodialis* having been isolated from 7 (out of 9) samples of 5 (out of 6) patients, and *M. furfur* – from 5 samples of 4 patients. Those 2 species co-occurred in 2 samples from 2 different patients. A specimen from one psoriatic patient yielded a co-culture of *M. sympodialis* and *A. pullulans*. In the control group *M. sympodialis* was the most frequently observed, having been isolated from a total of 10 (out of 13) skin samples of all healthy subjects, including every sample of 4 of them. *Malassezia globosa* and *M. slooffiae* were isolated from 2 samples of single subjects either alone or in combination with *M. restricta* and *M. sympodialis*, respectively.

Overall, *M. sympodialis* was the predominant species in all 3 subject groups, having been cultured from a total of 29 (82.9%) skin samples collected from all subjects under the study except one PS patient. The second most common species was *M. furfur*, recovered from 5 specimens of 4 PS patients. *Malassezia globosa* and *M. slooffiae* were isolated from 2 samples, each, originating from 2 normal individuals. Two non-*Malassezia* species, namely *C. diffluens* and *A. pullulans* , both co-occurring with *M. sympodialis*, were recovered from a patient with AD and a patient with PS, respectively.

Statistical analysis of the data showed that the only significant association was that isolation of *M. sympodialis* alone was more frequent among AD patients and healthy volunteers, as opposed to PS patients, for whom isolation of other *Malassezia* and non-*Malassezia* species, either alone or mixed (also with *M. sympodialis*) was reported ($P < 0.03$).

Discussion

Although several *Malassezia* species have been associated with various dermatological diseases, the exact pathological role of individual species remains obscured. An essential and still open question is whether there

Table 3 Results of drug susceptibility testing of 19 *Malassezia* sp. isolates, as determined by Neo-Sensitabs assay

Malassezia sp. (no.)	Antifungal drug[a]											
	CPO		FLZ		KTZ		ITZ		ECZ		MNZ	
	Zone [mm][b]	Cat. (no.)[c]	Zone [mm]	Cat. (no.)	Zone [mm]	Cat. (no.)	Zone [mm]	Cat. (no.)	Zone [mm]	Cat. (no.)	Zone [mm]	Cat. (no.)
M. sympodialis (13)	28	S (13)	43	S (13)	33.9	S (13)	36.5	S (13)	24.5	S (12)	26.5	S (13)
									17	I (1)		
M. furfur (2)	23	S (2)	36	S (2)	30	S (1)	29	S (2)	15.5	I (2)	20	S (1)
					25	I (1)					17	I (1)
M. furfur + *M. sympodialis* (2)	22.5	S (2)	39	S (2)	25.5	I (2)	28.5	S (2)	14.5	I (2)	20	S (1)
											15	I (1)
M. slooffiae (1)	30	S (1)	45	S (1)	35	S (1)	45	S (1)	30	S (1)	20	S (1)
M. slooffiae + *M. sympodialis* (1)	30	S (1)	40	S (1)	40	S (1)	40	S (1)	30	S (1)	16.5	I (1)

[a]CPO, ciclopirox; FLZ, fluconazole; KTZ, ketoconazole; ITZ, itraconazole; ECZ, econazole; MNZ, miconazole; number of isolates are given in brackets.
[b]Inhibition zone diameter mean value [mm] (each isolated was tested twice).
[c]Susceptibility categorization (S, susceptible; I, intermediate; R, resistant) based on the following criteria: CPO, ECZ, MNZ: S, ≥ 20; I, 12–19; R, ≤ 11; FLZ: S, ≥ 22; I, 15–21; R, ≤ 14; ITZ: S, ≥ 16; I, 10–15; R, < 10; KTZ: S, ≥ 30; I, 23–29; R, ≤ 22.

exists a relationship between particular *Malassezia* species and various skin disorders. Other clinical questions to be resolved include whether any of the *Malassezia* species preferentially occupies certain sites of the body, whether there are any differences in the distribution of the yeasts between lesioned and normal-appearing skin of patients, between adult and children, or between patients and healthy individuals, and finally whether there is variation in the prevalence of *Malassezia* species depending on gender, age, or geographical origin of the human host. There are now a growing number of works addressing these issues. For instance, studies of the *Malassezia* microbiota in healthy individuals consistently indicated *M. globosa* and *M. restricta* as the predominant species, with a combined detection rate of over 50% (in most of the studies) [7,31,32,34,35,49-51]. Whereas the involvement of the *Malassezia* species in SD and PV has been quite well recognized [35,50,52-58], the clinical role of these fungi in AD and PS is still controversial. The *Malassezia* yeasts are currently considered as contributory factors to the induction and exacerbation of both these conditions. The present study was to determine the composition of *Malassezia* microbiota on the skin of patients with AD and PS, and healthy volunteers from Poland. The choice of the study population was driven by two facts. First, there are much less data on the *Malassezia* microflora in AD and PS, than in other *Malassezia*-related diseases (i.e. PV, and SD). Second, AD and PS are the two most common chronic skin diseases, whose incidence has been on the rise in recent years in Poland. Among the Polish population, the prevalence of AD is around 1.4% in adults, and thrice as much (4.7%) in children aged between 3 to 16 years (but up to 32% in infants and young children, that is aged between 0–6 years) [59,60]. Psoriasis, on the other hand, is estimated to affect up to 1 million people in Poland (*ca.* 2.6% of general population) [61].

The *Malassezia* yeasts were cultured from almost half (48.6%) of the harvested skin samples, with the back being most heavily colonized body site, accounting for *ca.* 46% of the *Malassezia* cultures. The predominant *Malassezia* species in two clinical groups and the healthy control group was *M. sympodialis*. The recovery rate for this species among AD patients, PS patients, and healthy subjects was 100%, 70%, and 76.9%, respectively, and the overall recovery rate for *M. sympodialis* was 82.9%. The finding of such a high prevalence of *M. sympodialis* was rather unexpected, since other *Malassezia* species have usually been much more abundant in all three aforementioned groups, as reported by other authors. In a study of Nakabayashi *et al.*, *M. sympodialis* was only the third most common species in lesional skin of AD Japanese patients (7% of samples), following *M. furfur* (21%), and *M. globosa* (14%) [50]. In a study from Sweden, *M. sympodialis* was absent from lesional sites of AD patients, whereas other *Malassezia* species (i. e. *M. globosa*, *M. obtusa*, *M. restricta*, and *M. slooffiae*) occurred at low rates of 3-11% [62]. Two further studies that used culture-independent, DNA-based methods for the detection of *Malassezia* species, showed *M. globosa* and *M. restricta* as the predominant species in AD. They were detected at frequencies ranging from 87.5% to 100%, while *M. sympodialis* at 40.6% and 58.3% [35,51]. However, in a Canadian study of Gupta *et al.*, it was *M. sympodialis* that predominated in AD patients, with a detection rate of 51.5% [53]. Likewise, *M. sympodialis* was the dominant species among Korean AD patients, yet the isolation rate was low (16.3%) [33]. Among very few reports on the prevalence and species composition of *Malassezia* yeasts in PS patients, two were almost completely negative for the presence of *M. sympodialis*; in a study from Bosnia and Herzegovina, the predominant species in PS patients was *M. globosa* (55%) followed by *M. slooffiae* (17%) and *M. restricta* (10%) [63], while in a study from Iran, *M. globosa*, as the commonest species in PS (47%), was followed by *M. furfur* (39%) and *M. restricta* (11%) [64]. Similar data were obtained from a Japanese, culture-independent study of Takahata *et al.*, who found *M. globosa* and *M. restricta* as the sole two *Malassezia* species in psoriatic scale samples, with similarly high detection frequencies of 98% and 92%, respectively [38]. However, in another study from Japan, as well as in a Canadian, culture-based study, *M. sympodialis* was found the third (50%), after *M. restricta* (91%) and *M. globosa* (68%) or the second (31%), after *M. globosa* (58%) most frequently isolated *Malassezia* species from psoriatic lesions [53,65]. As for the healthy skin, none of the hitherto performed studies have shown the predominance of *M. sympodialis*, as that seen in the present work. This species has usually ranked third in overall abundance among *Malassezia* species colonizing normal human skin, with the detection rate spanned from 10% to *ca.* 40% [7,31,32,35,50]. Two major components of the *Malassezia* biota of healthy individuals, that is *M. globosa* and *M. restricta* were seriously underrepresented in the current study, with an overall isolation rate of 15.4% and 7.7%, respectively. The disparities between the studies, as discussed above, in frequencies of *Malassezia* species isolations from different dermatological affections and body sites may be attributable to several factors, including geographical and ethnic origin, clinical and demographic characteristics and even lifestyle habits of the subjects under the study, but also certain methodological issues, such as the use of different sampling techniques (swabbing, scraping) or culture media (modified Dixon agar, Leeming Notman agar). However, the distribution of *Malassezia* species is probably most influenced by a method used for species identification. Although the traditional identification schemes, based on morphological characteristics and biochemical activities, are in many clinical laboratories the only diagnostic methods available, they suffer from apparent limitations. Phenotypic tests are time-consuming, labour-intensive and often produce variable or inconclusive results, especially for newly described species; the final result relies on subjective interpretation by a laboratory expert. These methods are thus successively being complemented or replaced by DNA-based molecular techniques, of which PCR-RFLP analysis and PCR sequencing have most extensively been used [18,26,29-34,39-41]. Conceptually and technically PCR sequencing is the simplest. It is also the fastest and the most specific identification approach. An important advantage of DNA sequencing over PCR-RFLP is that the latter often involves a lengthy and laborious analysis of complex banding patterns, not always leading to a conclusive result. Moreover, DNA sequencing possesses a much higher discriminatory capacity, allowing intraspecies polymorphisms to be revealed. Some authors have already reported on the rDNA sequence heterogeneity within various *Malassezia* species, proving the existence of several individual genotypes within the species [26,39,40]. The intra-specific genetic diversity was also evidenced in this study. Two types of ITS sequences for *M. sympodialis* and two types of D1/2 sequences for *M. globosa* were demonstrated. Given the ability of DNA sequencing for strain typing and its potential use in phylogenetic and population genetics studies, along with the costs of sequencing rapidly plummeting, the method may soon become an integral part not only of a species identification algorithm but also of a routine epidemiological investigation.

The phenotypic and molecular identification results were discordant in *ca.* 35% of cases (12/35). The reason for this might either be the misidentification or the co-occurrence of different *Malassezia* species in one culture. The latter explanation is even more likely, as in the third of the discrepant cases, molecular methods did not invalidate the presence of a species identified by conventional phenotypic approach but only uncovered another, co-occurring *Malassezia* species. This in turn relates to the fact that the establishment of an axenic culture of a *Malassezia* species, uncontaminated by other *Malassezia* and non-*Malassezia* yeasts is rather challenging. A mixture of *Malassezia* species may not only be present in a clinical sample but even in a seemingly pure single colony on a culture medium. The co-isolation of two *Malassezia* species from the same specimen was recorded in 4 (11.4%) cases evaluated in this study. A higher prevalence of mixed *Malassezia* cultures was reported by other authors. For instance, in a Korean study of Lee *et al.*, 15% of SD patients and 21% of healthy volunteers showed co-colonization of two or more *Malassezia* species [34]. In two European studies, *M. globosa*, the most commonly observed species, was associated in culture with other *Malassezia* species in 18% of PV patients from Greece [52] and 40% of PV patients from Spain [55]. Interestingly, in two cases in this study, *M. sympodialis* was co-cultured with a non-*Malassezia* species, namely *Cryptococcus diffluens* in an AD patient and *Aureobasidium pullulans* in a PS patient. Finding of *C. diffluens* on AD-affected skin is perfectly in line with previous research demonstrating this species to be a frequent colonizer of the skin surface of AD patients [66]. As for *A. pullulans*, it is a ubiquitous dematiaceous fungus that has emerged as an opportunistic human pathogen, especially among immunocompromised patients; it is a frequently isolated skin contaminant but rarely a causative agent of fungemia, systemic infections and abscesses in different viscera [67]. The discordance between phenotypic and molecular identification may also relate to the growth rate of different *Malassezia* species. It means that in a mixed culture, the fast-growing species, such as *M. sympodialis* may conceal the presence of the slow growers, such as *M. globosa*, *M. restrica*, or *M. obtusa*. This is also a possible explanation for the overall high frequency of *M. sympodialis* isolations in this study. Against this possibility is the fact that always a selected single separated colony from a primary culture served as an inoculum for the culture used for species identification tests. The six mixed-species cultures represent the only cases in which a primary culture colony already contained a mixture of distinct yeast species. Nevertheless, it seems that a molecular-based but culture-independent method would serve as a more accurate and reliable approach for the assessment of the diversity of *Malassezia* microbiota [28,35,38,51]. The use of culture-based approach for characterizing *Malassezia* communities from skin samples posed a limitation to the present study. Due to the fastidious nature of *Malassezia* fungi and difficulties in culture arising therefrom, the obtained results may understate the size and complexity (species structure) of the *Malassezia* microbiota.

Culture-based methods essentially select for those species that readily grow under the typical nutritional and physiological conditions supported by commonly used artificial media. These species may not represent the most abundant or influential organisms within a given locality [68].

There is a paucity of reports on drug resistance in *Malassezia* spp., and this mainly stems from the lack of a standardized protocol for *Malassezia* susceptibility testing. The observed variability of the results from laboratory to laboratory precludes any association of *in vitro* and *in vivo* responses of *Malassezia* yeasts to antifungals. In this study, the Neo-Sensitabs tablet diffusion assay was employed to test the susceptibilities of selected *Malassezia* strains to six drugs most widely used in the treatment of *Malassezia* infections, that is the azoles (FLZ, ECZ, ITZ, KTZ, and MNZ) and cyclopiroxolamine (CPO). All the analysed isolates were susceptible to those compounds, albeit the triazoles (FLZ and ITZ) and CPO were found to be more active than the azole derivatives (ECZ, MNZ, and KTZ). Noteworthy, strains of *M. furfur* generally appeared less susceptible than strains of *M. slooffiae* or *M. sympodialis*, indicating that certain *Malassezia* species develop mechanisms of drug tolerance more easily than other species do. Some variations between different *Malassezia* species in the susceptibilities to antifungal agents were also recorded by other authors [69,70]. Although the molecular bases of drug resistance in *Malassezia* fungi are largely unknown, there is an optimism that this will change now with an increasing body of data from the whole genome sequencing projects [71,72]. Recently, Kim *et al.* have demonstrated that genetic alterations in the amino acid sequence of a putative lanosterol 14α-demethylase (CYP51) from *M. globosa* may be responsible for resistance to azoles by blocking substrate access channels of the enzyme [73].

Conclusions

To conclude, this study provides an important insight into the species composition of *Malassezia* microbiota in human skin. The most important findings can be summarized in three points. First, *M. sympodialis* was the predominant species in both normal and pathologic (AD- and PS-affected) skin. Furthermore, AD patients yielded exclusively *M. sympodialis* isolates, whereas isolates of *M. furfur* were observed only in PS patients. Whether this mirrors any predilection of particular *Malassezia* species for certain clinical conditions, and whether the overall dominance of *M. sympodialis* reflects geographical specificity needs to be evaluated on a much larger scale. Second, although the overall concordance between phenotypic and molecular methods was quite high (65%), with the discordant results being rather due to the presence of multiple species in a single culture (co-colonization) than true misidentification, for the identification of *Malassezia* species, molecular typing approach is preferred, as its results are more reliable and straightforward. Third, all *Malassezia* isolates were susceptible to cyclopiroxolamine and azole drugs, with *M. furfur* isolates being somewhat more drug tolerant than other *Malassezia* species.

Abbreviations

AD: Atopic dermatitis; AFLP: Amplified fragment length polymorphism; BSA: Body surface area; CHS2: Chitin synthase; CLSI: Clinical and Laboratory Standards Institute; CPO: Ciclopirox; DGGE: Denaturing gradient gel electrophoresis; ECZ: Econazole; FLZ: Fluconazole; ITS: Internal transcribed spacer; ITZ: Itraconazole; KTZ: Ketoconazole; MDA: Modified Dixon's agar; MEE: Multilocus enzyme electrophoresis; MNZ: Miconazole; NCBI: National Center for Biotechnology Information; PASI: Psoriasis area and severity; PCR-RFLP: PCR-based restriction fragment length polymorphism; PCR-SSCP: PCR-based single strand confirmation polymorphism; PFGE: Pulsed-field gel electrophoresis; PS: Psoriasis; PV: Pityriasis versicolor; RPB1: RNA polymerase subunit 1; SCORAD: Severity scoring of atopic dermatitis; SD: Seborrheic dermatitis.

Competing interests

The authors declare that they have no competing interests.

Authors' contributions

TJ participated in the design of the study, supervised all experimental procedures, and wrote the entire manuscript. ER collected samples, performed drug susceptibility testing, participated in the design of the study and species identification. AZ performed the sequencing analyses. KR did the PCR-RFLP assays. AM and JB revised the manuscript critically for important intellectual content. All authors read and approved the final manuscript.

Acknowledgements

The authors are indebted to Asst. Prof. Aristea Velegraki (Department of Microbiology, Medical School, Aristotle University of Thessaloniki, Thessaloniki, Greece) for her kind revision of the manuscript.

Author details

[1]Department of Applied Microbiology, Institute of Microbiology, Faculty of Biology, University of Warsaw, I. Miecznikowa 1, 02-096 Warsaw, Poland. [2]Department of Mycology, Chair of Microbiology, Collegium Medicum, Jagiellonian University, Cracow, Poland.

References

1. Gao Z, Perez-Perez GI, Chen Y, Blaser MJ: **Quantitation of major human cutaneous bacterial and fungal populations.** *J Clin Microbiol* 2010, **48:**3575–3581.
2. Crespo-Erchiga V, Florencio VD: ***Malassezia* yeasts and pityriasis versicolor.** *Curr Opin Infect Dis* 2006, **19:**139–147.
3. Hay RJ: ***Malassezia*, dandruff and seborrhoeic dermatitis: an overview.** *Br J Dermatol* 2011, **165:**2–8.
4. Amado Y, Patiño-Uzcátegui A, de García MC C, Tabima J, Motta A, Cárdenas M, Bernal A, Restrepo S, Celis A: **Seborrheic dermatitis: predisposing factors and ITS2 secondary structure for *Malassezia* phylogenic analysis.** *Med Mycol* 2013, **51:**868–875.
5. Kanda N, Tani K, Enomoto U, Nakai K, Watanabe S: **The skin fungus-induced Th-1 and Th-2 related cytokine, chemokine and psostaglandin E2 production in peripheral blood mononuclear cells from patients with atopic dermatitis and psoriasis vulgaris.** *Clin Exp Allerg* 2002, **32:**1243–1250.
6. Baroni A, Paoletti I, Ruocco E, Agozzino M, Tufano MA, Donnarumma G: **Possible role of *Malassezia furfur* in psoriasis: modulation of TGF-beta1, integrin, and HSP70 expression in human keratinocytes and in the skin of psoriasis-affected patients.** *J Cut Pathol* 2004, **31:**35–42.
7. Ko JH, Lee YW, Choe YB, Ahn KJ: **Epidemiologic study of *Malassezia* yeasts in patients with *Malassezia* folliculitis by 26S rDNA PCR-RFLP analysis.** *Ann Dermatol* 2011, **23:**177–184.
8. Zhao Y, Li L, Wang JJ, Kang KF, Zhang QQ: **Cutaneous malasseziasis: four case reports of atypical dermatitis and onychomycosis caused by *Malassezia*.** *Int J Dermatol* 2010, **49:**141–145.
9. Bernier V, Weill FX, Hirigoyen V, Elleau C, Feyler A, Labrèze C, Sarlangue J, Chène G, Couprie B, Taïeb A: **Skin colonization by *Malassezia* species in neonates. A prospective study and relationship with neonatal cephalic pustulosis.** *Arch Dermatol* 2002, **138:**215–218.
10. Ginarte M, Fabeiro JM, Toribio J: **Confluent and reticulated papillomatosis (Gougerot-Carteaud) successfully treated with tacalcitol.** *J Dermatolog Treat* 2002, **13:**27–30.
11. Chryssanthou E, Broberger U, Petrini B: ***Malassezia pachydermatis* fungaemia in a neonatal intensive care unit.** *Acta Paediatr* 2001, **90:**323–327.
12. Archer-Dubon C, Icaza-Chivez ME, Orozco-Topete R, Reyes E, Baez-Martinez R, Ponce de León S: **An epidemic outbreak of *Malassezia* folliculitis in three adult patients in an intensive care unit: a previously unrecognized nosocomial infection.** *Int J Dermatol* 1999, **38:**453–456.
13. Guého E, Midgley G, Guillot J: **The genus *Malassezia* with description of four new species.** *Antonie Van Leeuwenhoek* 1996, **69:**337–355.
14. Sugita T, Takashima M, Shinoda T, Suto H, Unno T, Tsuboi R, Ogawa H, Nishikawa A: **New yeast species, *Malassezia dermatis*, isolated from patients with atopic dermatitis.** *J Clin Microbiol* 2002, **40:**1363–1367.
15. Sugita T, Takashima M, Kodama M, Tsuboi R, Nishikawa A: **Description of a new yeast species, *Malassezia japonica*, and its detection in patients with atopic dermatitis and healthy subjects.** *J Clin Microbiol* 2003, **41:**4695–4699.
16. Sugita T, Tajima M, Takashima M, Amaya M, Saito M, Tsuboi R, Nishikawa A: **A new yeast, *Malassezia yamatoensis*, isolated from a patient with seborrheic dermatitis, and its distribution in patients and healthy subjects.** *Microbiol Immunol* 2004, **48:**579–583.
17. Hirai A, Kano R, Makimura K, Duarte ER, Hamdan JS, Lachance MA, Yamaguchi H, Hasegawa A: ***Malassezia nana* sp. nov., a novel lipid-dependent yeast species isolated from animals.** *Int J Syst Evol Microbiol* 2004, **54:**623–627.
18. Cabañes FJ, Theelen B, Castellá G, Boekhout T: **Two new lipid-dependent *Malassezia* species from domestic animals.** *FEMS Yeast Res* 2007, **7:**1064–1076.
19. Cabañes FJ, Vega S, Castellá G: ***Malassezia cuniculi* sp. nov., a novel yeast species isolated from rabbit skin.** *Med Mycol* 2011, **49:**40–48.
20. Casagrande BF, Flückiger S, Linder MT, Johansson C, Scheynius A, Crameri R, Schmid-Grendelmeier P: **Sensitization to the yeast *Malassezia sympodialis* is specific for extrinsic and intrinsic atopic eczema.** *J Invest Dermatol* 2006, **126**(11):2414–2421.
21. Scheynius A, Johansson C, Buentke E, Zargari A, Linder MT: **Atopic eczema/dermatitis syndrome and *Malassezia*.** *Int Arch Allergy Immunol* 2002, **127:**161–169.
22. Guého E, Batra R, Boekhout T: **The genus *Malassezia* Baillon (1889).** In *The Yeasts, a Taxonomic Study.* 5th edition. Edited by Kurtzman CP, Fell JW, Boekhout T. Amsterdam: Elsevier; 2011:1807–1833.
23. Boekhout T, Kamp M, Guého E: **Molecular typing of *Malassezia* species with PFGE and RAPD.** *Med Mycol* 1998, **36:**365–372.
24. Senczek D, Siesenop U, Böhm KH: **Characterization of *Malassezia* species by means of phenotypic characteristics and detection of electrophoretic karyotypes by pulsed-field gel electrophoresis (PFGE).** *Mycoses* 1999, **42:**409–414.
25. Theelen B, Silvestri M, Guého E, van Belkum A, Boekhout T: **Identification and typing of *Malassezia* yeasts using amplified fragment length polymorphism (AFLP), random amplified polymorphic DNA (RAPD) and denaturing gradient gel electrophoresis (DGGE).** *FEMS Yeast Res* 2001, **1:**79–86.
26. Gupta AK, Boekhout T, Theelen B, Summerbell R, Batra R: **Identification and typing of *Malassezia* species by amplified fragment length polymorphism and sequence analyses of the internal transcribed spacer and large-subunit regions of ribosomal DNA.** *J Clin Microbiol* 2004, **42:**4253–4260.
27. Midreuil F, Guillot J, Guého E, Renaud F, Mallié M, Bastide JM: **Genetic diversity in the yeast species *Malassezia pachydermatis* analysed by multilocus enzyme electrophoresis.** *Int J Syst Bacteriol* 1999, **49:**1287–1294.
28. Gaitanis G, Velegraki A, Frangoulis E, Mitroussia A, Tsigonia A, Tzimogianni A, Katsambas A, Legakis NJ: **Identification of *Malassezia* species from patient skin scales by PCR-RFLP.** *Clin Microbiol Infect* 2002, **8:**162–173.
29. Guillot J, Deville M, Berthelemy M, Provost F, Guého E: **A single PCR-restriction endonuclease analysis for rapid identification of *Malassezia* species.** *Lett Appl Microbiol* 2000, **31:**400–403.
30. Mirhendi H, Makimura K, Zomorodian K, Yamada T, Sugita T, Yamaguchi H: **A simple PCR-RFLP method for identification and differentiation of 11 *Malassezia* species.** *J Microbiol Methods* 2005, **61:**281–284.
31. Jang SJ, Lim SH, Ko JH, Oh BH, Kim SM, Song YC, Yim SM, Lee YW, Choe YB, Ahn KJ: **The investigation on the distribution of *Malassezia* yeasts on the normal Korean skin by 26S rDNA PCR-RFLP.** *Ann Dermatol* 2009, **21:**18–26.
32. Oh BH, Song YC, Lee YW, Choe YB, Ahn KJ: **Comparison of nested PCR and RFLP for identification and classification of *Malassezia* yeasts from healthy human skin.** *Ann Dermatol* 2009, **21:**352–357.
33. Yim SM, Kim JY, Ko JH, Lee YW, Choe YB, Ahn KJ: **Molecular analysis of *Malassezia* microflora on the skin of the patients with atopic dermatitis.** *Ann Dermatol* 2010, **22:**41–47.
34. Lee YW, Byun HJ, Kim BJ, Kim DH, Lim YY, Lee JW, Kim MN, Kim D, Chun YJ, Mun SK, Kim CW, Kim SE, Hwang JS: **Distribution of *Malassezia* species on the scalp in Korean seborrheic dermatitis patients.** *Ann Dermatol* 2011, **23:**156–161.
35. Tajima M, Sugita T, Nishikawa A, Tsuboi R: **Molecular analysis of *Malassezia* microflora in seborrheic dermatitis patients: comparison with other diseases and healthy subjects.** *J Invest Dermatol* 2008, **128:**345–351.
36. Morishita N, Sei Y, Sugita T: **Molecular analysis of *Malassezia* microflora from patients with pityriasis versicolor.** *Mycopathologia* 2006, **161:**61–65.
37. Gemmer CM, DeAngelis YM, Theelen B, Boekhout T, Dawson Jr TL Jr: **Fast, noninvasive method for molecular detection and differentiation of Malassezia yeast species on human skin and application of the method to dandruff microbiology.** *J Clin Microbiol* 2002, **40:**3350–3357.
38. Takahata Y, Sugita T, Hiruma M, Muto M: **Quantitative analysis of *Malassezia* in the scale of patients with psoriasis using a real-time polymerase chain reaction assay.** *Br J Dermatol* 2007, **157:**670–673.
39. Makimura K, Tamura Y, Kudo M, Uchida K, Saito H, Yamaguchi H: **Species identification and strain typing of *Malassezia* species stock strains and clinical isolates based on the DNA sequences of nuclear ribosomal internal transcribed spacer 1 regions.** *J Med Microbiol* 2000, **49:**29–35.
40. Sugita T, Kodama M, Saito M, Ito T, Kato Y, Tsuboi R, Nishikawa A: **Sequence diversity of the intergenic spacer region of the rRNA gene of *Malassezia globosa* colonizing the skin of patients with atopic dermatitis and healthy individuals.** *J Clin Microbiol* 2003, **41:**3022–3027.
41. Kano R, Aizawa T, Nakamura Y, Watanabe S, Hasegawa A: **Chitin synthase 2 gene sequence of *Malassezia* species.** *Microbiol Immunol* 1999, **43:**813–815.
42. Hanifin J, Rajka G: **Diagnostic features of atopic dermatitis.** *Acta Derm Venereol* 1980, **60:**44–47.
43. European Task Force on Atopic Dermatitis: **Severity scoring of atopic dermatitis: the SCORAD index.** *Dermatology* 1993, **186:**23–31.
44. Ramsay B, Lawrence CM: **Measurement of involved surface area in patients with psoriasis.** *Br J Dermatol* 1991, **124:**565–570.
45. Fredriksson T, Pettersson U: **Oral treatment of pustulosis palmo-plantaris with a new retinoid, Ro 10-9359.** *Dermatologica* 1979, **158:**60–64.
46. Clinical and Laboratory Standards Institute/National Committee for Clinical Laboratory Standards: *Method for Antifungal Disk Diffusion Susceptibility Testing of Yeasts: Approved Guideline*, Document M44-A. Wayne, PA: Clinical and Laboratory Standards Institute; 2000.

47. Kurtzman CP, Fell JW, Boekhout T, Robert V: **Methods for isolation, phenotypic characterization, and maintenance of yeasts.** In *The Yeasts, a Taxonomic Study.* 5th edition. Edited by Kurtzman CP, Fell JW, Boekhout T. Amsterdam: Elsevier; 2010:87–111.
48. Ashbee HR, Evans EGV: **Immunology of diseases associated with *Malassezia* species.** *Clin Microbiol Rev* 2002, **15**:21–57.
49. Gupta AK, Kohli Y: **Prevalence of *Malassezia* species on various body sites in clinically healthy subjects representing different age groups.** *Med Mycol* 2004, **42**:35–42.
50. Nakabayashi A, Sei Y, Guillot J: **Identification of *Malassezia* species isolated from patients with seborrhoeic dermatitis, atopic dermatitis, pityriasis versicolor and normal subjects.** *Med Mycol* 2000, **38**:337–341.
51. Sugita T, Suto H, Unno T, Tsuboi R, Ogawa H, Shinoda T, Nishikawa A: **Molecular analysis of *Malassezia* microflora on the skin of atopic dermatitis patients and healthy subjects.** *J Clin Microbiol* 2001, **39**:3486–3490.
52. Gaitanis G, Velegraki A, Alexopoulos EC, Chasapi V, Tsigonia A, Katsambas A: **Distribution of *Malassezia* species in pityriasis versicolor and seborrhoeic dermatitis in Greece. Typing of the major pityriasis versicolor isolate *M. globosa*.** *Br J Dermatol* 2006, **154**:854–859.
53. Gupta AK, Kohli Y, Summerbell RC, Faergemann J: **Quantitative culture of *Malassezia* species from different body sites of individuals with or without dermatoses.** *Med Mycol* 2001, **39**:243–251.
54. Affes M, Salah SB, Makni F, Sellami H, Ayadi A: **Molecular identification of *Malassezia* species isolated from dermatitis affections.** *Mycoses* 2009, **52**:251–256.
55. Crespo Erchiga V, Ojeda Martos A, Vera Casaño A, Crespo Erchiga A, Sanchez Fajardo F: ***Malassezia globosa* as the causative agent of pityriasis versicolor.** *Br J Dermatol* 2000, **143**:799–803.
56. Chaudhary R, Singh S, Banerjee T, Tilak R: **Prevalence of different *Malassezia* species in pityriasis versicolor in central India.** *Indian J Dermatol Venereol Leprol* 2010, **76**:159–164.
57. Tarazooie B, Kordbacheh P, Zaini F, Zomorodian K, Saadat F, Zeraati H, Hallaji Z, Rezaie S: **Study of the distribution of *Malassezia* species in patients with pityriasis versicolor and healthy individuals in Tehran, Iran.** *BMC Dermatol* 2004, **4**:5.
58. Ramadán S, Sortino M, Bulacio L, Marozzi ML, López C, Ramos L: **Prevalence of *Malassezia* species in patients with pityriasis versicolor in Rosario, Argentina.** *Rev Iberoam Micol* 2012, **29**:14–19.
59. Kupryś-Lipińska I, Elgalal A, Kuna P: **Epidemiology of atopic dermatitis in general population of the Lodz province's citizens.** *Pneumonol Alergol Pol* 2009, **77**:145–151.
60. Frankowska J, Kamer B, Trznadel-Budźko E, Rotsztejn H: **The estimation of atopic dermatitis in infants and small children in general practitioner practice – own observations.** *Wiad Lek* 2011, **64**:176–180.
61. Neneman A, Adamski Z: **Clinical and epidemiological systemic disorders in psoriasis patients.** *Forum Med Rodz* 2009, **3**:447–453.
62. Sandström Falk MH, Tengvall Linder M, Johansson C, Bartosik J, Bäck O, 's Särnhult T, Wahlgren CF, Scheynius A, Faergemann J: **The prevalence of *Malassezia* yeasts in patients with atopic dermatitis, seborrhoeic dermatitis and healthy controls.** *Acta Derm Venereol* 2005, **85**:17–23.
63. Prohić A: **Identification of *Malassezia* species isolated from scalp skin of patients with psoriasis and healthy subjects.** *Acta Dermatovenerol Croat* 2003, **11**:10–16.
64. Zomorodian K, Mirhendi H, Tarazooie B, Zeraati H, Hallaji Z, Balighi K: **Distribution of *Malassezia* species in patients with psoriasis and healthy individuals in Tehran.** *J Cutan Pathol* 2008, **35**:1027–1031.
65. Amaya M, Tajima M, Okubo Y, Sugita T, Nishikawa A, Tsuboi R: **Molecular analysis of *Malassezia* microflora in the lesional skin of psoriasis patients.** *J Dermatol* 2007, **34**:619–624.
66. Sugita T, Saito M, Ito T, Kato Y, Tsuboi R, Takeuchi S, Nishikawa A: **The basidiomycetous yeasts *Cryptococcus diffluens* and *C. liquefaciens* colonize the skin of patients with atopic dermatitis.** *Microbiol Immunol* 2003, **47**:945–950.
67. Chan GF, Puad MS, Chin CF, Rashid NA: **Emergence of *Aureobasidium pullulans* as human fungal pathogen and molecular assay for future medical diagnosis.** *Folia Microbiol (Praha)* 2011, **56**:459–467.
68. Grice EA, Segre JA: **The skin microbiome.** *Nat Rev Microbiol* 2011, **9**:244–253.
69. Gupta AK, Kohli Y, Li A, Faergemann J, Summerbell RC: ***In vitro* susceptibility of the seven *Malassezia* species to ketoconazole, voriconazole, itraconazole and terbinafine.** *Br J Dermatol* 2000, **142**:758–765.
70. Hammer KA, Carson CF, Riley TV: ***In vitro* activities of ketoconazole, econazole, miconazole and *Melaleuca alternifolia* (tea tree) oil against *Malassezia* species.** *Antimicrob Agents Chemother* 2000, **44**:67–69.
71. Xu J, Saunders CW, Hu P, Grant RA, Boekhout T, Kuramae EE, Kronstad JW, DeAngelis YM, Reeder NL, Johnstone KR, Leland M, Fieno AM, Begley WM, Sun Y, Lacey MP, Chaudhary T, Keough T, Chu L, Sears R, Yuan B, Dawson TL Jr: **Dandruff-associated *Malassezia* genomes reveal convergent and divergent virulence traits shared with plant and human fungal pathogens.** *Proc Natl Acad Sci USA* 2007, **104**:18730–18735.
72. Gioti A, Nystedt B, Li W, Xu J, Andersson A, Averette AF, Münch K, Wang X, Kappauf C, Kingsbury JM, Kraak B, Walker LA, Johansson HJ, Holm T, Lehtiö J, Stajich JE, Mieczkowski P, Kahmann R, Kennell JC, Cardenas ME, Lundeberg J, Saunders CW, Boekhout T, Dawson TL, Munro CA, de Groot PWJ, Butler G, Heitman J, Scheynius A: **Genomic insights into the atopic eczema-associated skin commensal yeast *Malassezia sympodialis*.** *mBio* 2013, **4**:16. 00572–12.
73. Kim D, Lim YR, Ohk SO, Kim BJ, Chun YJ: **Functional expression and characterization of CYP51 from dandruff-causing *Malassezia globosa*.** *FEMS Yeast Res* 2011, **11**:80–87.

14

TGFβ signaling regulates lipogenesis in human sebaceous glands cells

Adrian J McNairn[1,2†], Yanne Doucet[1,3†], Julien Demaude[4], Marion Brusadelli[1], Christopher B Gordon[5], Armando Uribe-Rivera[5], Paul F Lambert[6], Charbel Bouez[4], Lionel Breton[4] and Géraldine Guasch[1*]

Abstract

Background: Sebaceous glands are components of the skin essential for its normal lubrication by the production of sebum. This contributes to skin health and more importantly is crucial for the skin barrier function. A mechanistic understanding of sebaceous gland cells growth and differentiation has lagged behind that for keratinocytes, partly because of a lack of an in vitro model that can be used for experimental manipulation.

Methods: We have developed an in vitro culture model to isolate and grow primary human sebocytes without transformation that display functional characteristics of sebocytes. We used this novel method to probe the effect of Transforming Growth Factor β (TGFβ) signaling on sebocyte differentiation, by examining the expression of genes involved in lipogenesis upon treatment with TGFβ1. We also repressed TGFβ signaling through knockdown of the *TGFβ Receptor II* to address if the effect of TGFβ activation is mediated via canonical Smad signal transduction.

Results: We find that activation of the TGFβ signaling pathway is necessary and sufficient for maintaining sebocytes in an undifferentiated state. The presence of TGFβ ligand triggered decreased expression in genes required for the production of characteristics sebaceous lipids and for sebocyte differentiation such as *FADS2* and *PPARγ*, thereby decreasing lipid accumulation through the TGFβ RII-Smad2 dependent pathway.

Conclusion: TGFβ signaling plays an essential role in sebaceous gland regulation by maintaining sebocytes in an undifferentiated state. This data was generated using a novel method for human sebocyte culture, which is likely to prove generally useful in investigations of sebaceous gland growth and differentiation. These findings open a new paradigm in human skin biology with important implications for skin therapies.

Keywords: Human Sebaceous gland cells, Sebocytes, TGFβ signaling, Cell differentiation, Proliferation, Lipogenesis, Skin appendages

Background

In humans, sebaceous glands associated with hair follicles are distributed throughout all the skin and found in greatest abundance on the face and scalp and are absent from the palms and soles [1]. Sebaceous glands can also form independently from the hair follicle and form specialized glands such as Meibomian glands of the eyelid, ectopic sebaceous gland of the glans penis [2] and Fordyce's spots of the oral epithelium. Sebaceous glands are microscopic glands which secrete an oily substance (sebum) in the hair follicles to lubricate the skin and hair of animals [3]. Their function within the epidermis is to prevent the skin from dehydration and protect the body against infections and physical, chemical and thermal assaults of the environment. The main components of human sebum are triglycerides and fatty acids (57.5%), wax esters (26%), and squalene (12%) [4]. The production of sebum is regulated throughout life, and decreases dramatically with age [5]. This is associated with increased dryness and fragility of the skin. Moreover, several human diseases, such as acne vulgaris, atopic dermatitis, seborrheic dermatitis and primary cicatricial alopecia are thought to be associated with deregulation of the sebaceous glands [4,6,7].

* Correspondence: geraldine.guasch@cchmc.org
†Equal contributors
[1]Division of Developmental Biology, Cincinnati Children's Hospital Medical Center, 3333 Burnet Avenue, Cincinnati, OH 45229, USA
Full list of author information is available at the end of the article

There is a crucial interdependency of sebaceous glands with hair follicles and epidermis as sebocyte dysfunction results in degeneration of hair follicle structures and a defective skin barrier [7,8]. This is illustrated in the *asebia* mutant mouse, which lacks the SCD1 enzyme that desaturates fatty acids. This mutant displays rudimentary sebaceous glands and alteration in the profile of skin surface lipids leading to chronic inflammatory reactions, alopecia and dermal scarring [8].

Successful growth of primary human cells often constitutes a breakthrough in a specific area of human biology with important clinical implications. Tissue stem cells such as those of the blood and the epidermis have already been successfully used in clinics for decades [9,10]. In particular, epidermal cells (keratinocytes) can be cultured in vitro and can be efficiently manipulated to form a three dimensional epidermis [11,12]. Despite these advancements, the successful methods for culturing human primary sebocytes without the use of mouse feeder layers are not established. Selective cultivation of human sebocytes has been attempted in the past using mitomycin-treated 3T3 feeder layers by covering the microdissected sebaceous gland explant with glass slides but primary sebocytes survived only two passages after which they underwent differentiation [13]. Human sebaceous gland cell lines have been established in the past from adult human facial skin and periauricular area [14-17], but their immortalization with Simian virus-40 large T antigen or HPV16/E6E7 genes, which bypass the p53 and retinoblastoma protein mediated restriction point, results in cellular transformation that has limited their use for analyzing their cell cycle and differentiation regulation. Here, we culture human primary sebocytes using a novel method, which can in the future, be incorporated into skin reconstructs and provide a basis for understanding the molecular pathways which regulate human sebaceous gland biology.

A potential candidate for human sebocyte regulation suggested by several lines of evidence is Transforming Growth Factor β (TGFβ) [18,19] but the lack of primary human cultures has impaired an in-depth investigation of the molecular mechanism whereby TGF β signaling controls sebaceous gland differentiation. The TGF β pathway is ubiquitous and involved in the control of growth and differentiation of multiple cell and tissue types. The two major receptors of the TGFβ signaling pathway, TGFβ Receptor I (TGFβ RI) and TGFβ Receptor II (TGFβ RII), are expressed in mouse sebaceous glands [20,21]. In human and mouse epithelial cell lines, TGFβ acts as a potent inhibitor of proliferation mediated at least in part via down-regulation of c-Myc expression [22,23]. Intriguingly, c-Myc overexpression in a mouse model induces an increase in sebaceous gland size due to activation of sebocyte differentiation at the expense of hair differentiation [16,24]. Moreover, disruption of epidermal Smad4, the common mediator of TGFβ signaling, leads to hyperplasia of interfollicular epidermis, hair follicle, and sebaceous glands through c-Myc upregulation [25].

To determine the effect of TGFβ signaling on sebocyte differentiation, we investigated the effect of TGFβ ligands on the primary human sebocytes we established using a novel culture system and skin samples from pediatric donors.

Results

Primary sebocytes established from pediatric donors express markers of sebaceous gland differentiation

To determine the pathways that regulate primary human sebocytes growth and differentiation, we developed a novel culture method by mimicking the microenvironment of the sebaceous glands in vitro. Skin explants from donors ranging from 9 months to 12 years of age were microdissected (Figure 1a-b) and the sebaceous glands were placed between fibronectin-coated glass coverslips to reproduce an in vivo environment (Figure 1c-d). Using this technique, primary sebocyte cultures were derived from eight donors representing four skin tissue types: five scalp, one breast, one chest, and one face sample. While this technique enabled us to continually passage sebocytes beyond 15 passages, all experiments were performed on passage 2 and later passages (3 to 5) without the use of extracellular matrix or supporting irradiated fibroblasts.

To verify that the cell cultures were indeed sebocytes, we examined the expression of known sebocyte markers. Immunofluorescence staining and immunoblot demonstrated that those cells homogeneously express peroxisome proliferator-activated receptor gamma (PPARγ) an adipogenic transcription factor expressed in differentiating sebocytes [26], in vitro (Figure 1d and Figure 2a, Scalp-derived Sebaceous Gland cells SSG3) and in vivo (Additional file 1: Figure S1a-b) but not in human keratinocytes (NIKS) [27]. Real-time PCR confirmed that primary SSG3 expressed a similar level of PPARγ as the immortalized sebocyte line SEB-1 [15] (Figure 2b). However, SEB-1 expresses Keratin 8, a protein associated with skin appendages tumors [28], whereas SSG3 cells do not express Keratin 8 (Figure 2a), akin to sebaceous gland in vivo [29]. Additionally, SSG3 cells express other markers of sebocytes such as Blimp1 and epithelial membrane antigen EMA/Muc1 (Additional file 1: Figure S1c, d and e). In agreement with recent reports [16,30], Blimp1 is expressed in the inner root sheath of the hair follicle and in terminally differentiated cells of the sebaceous glands in human scalp sections from which SSG3 cells were derived (Additional file 1: Figure S1c). All the results shown in scalp-derived sebocytes have been confirmed to be similar in the breast, chest and face derived-sebocytes (Additional file 1: Figure S1g). The only

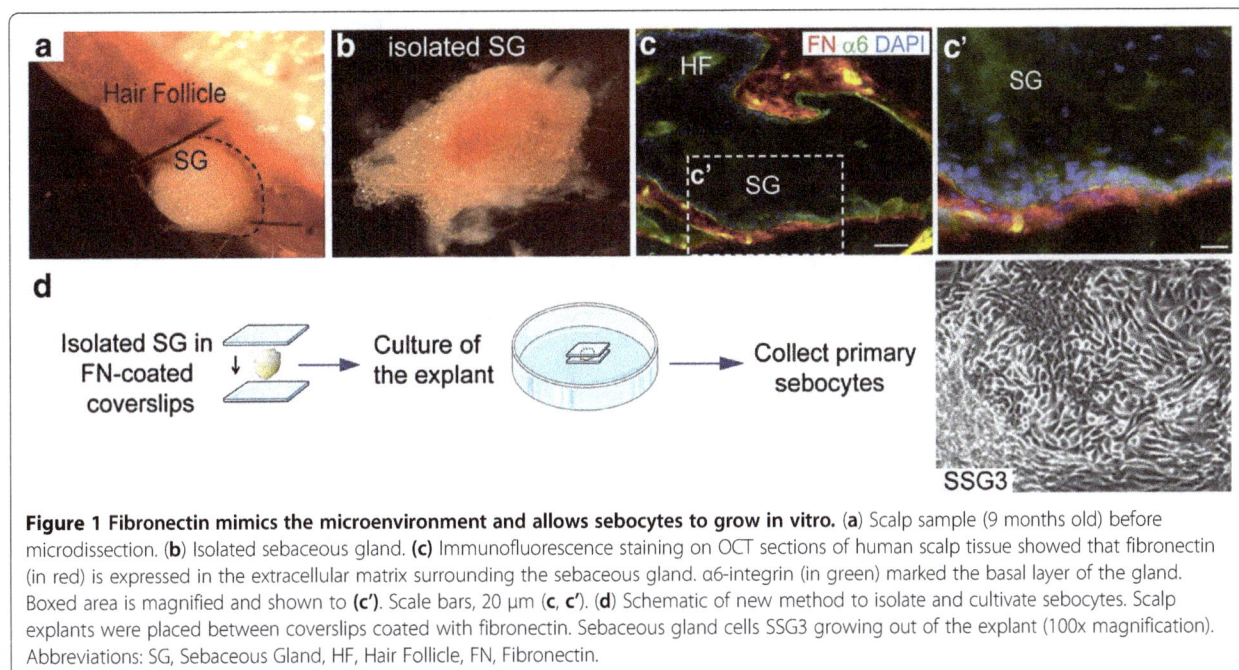

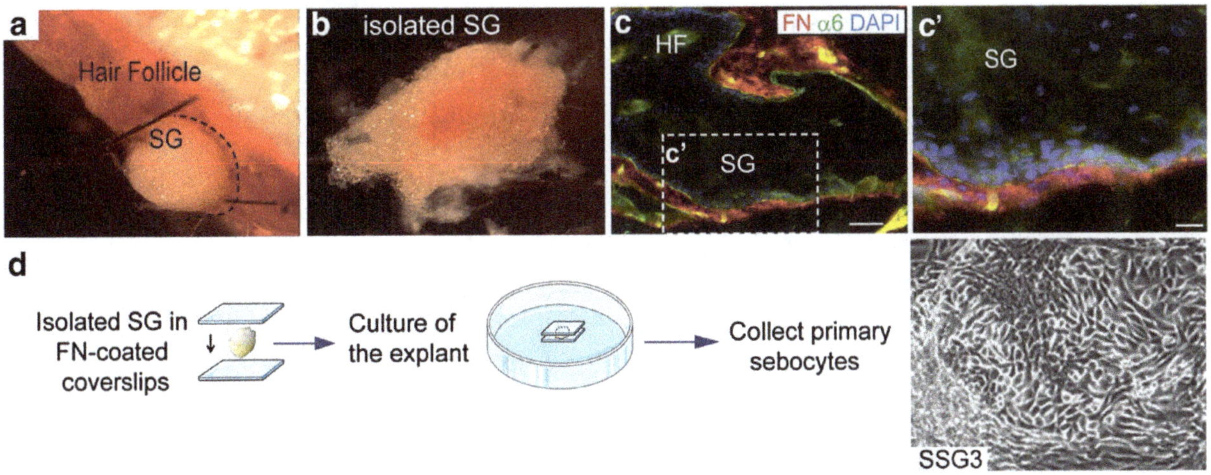

Figure 1 Fibronectin mimics the microenvironment and allows sebocytes to grow in vitro. (**a**) Scalp sample (9 months old) before microdissection. (**b**) Isolated sebaceous gland. **(c)** Immunofluorescence staining on OCT sections of human scalp tissue showed that fibronectin (in red) is expressed in the extracellular matrix surrounding the sebaceous gland. α6-integrin (in green) marked the basal layer of the gland. Boxed area is magnified and shown to **(c')**. Scale bars, 20 μm (**c**, **c'**). (**d**) Schematic of new method to isolate and cultivate sebocytes. Scalp explants were placed between coverslips coated with fibronectin. Sebaceous gland cells SSG3 growing out of the explant (100x magnification). Abbreviations: SG, Sebaceous Gland, HF, Hair Follicle, FN, Fibronectin.

exception is the expression of Keratin 7, a marker of the undifferentiated sebocytes, detected at higher expression in protein lysates of the face-derived sebocytes compared to the scalp, the breast and the chest (Additional file 1: Figure S1f-g). The difference in Keratin 7 expression may depend on the location from which the cells derived (Additional file 1: Figure S1d). To conclude, we have established primary human sebocytes that express typical sebocyte markers and represent a good model for studying sebocyte function.

Primary sebocytes can differentiate in vitro

To confirm that the primary human sebocytes are functional in vitro, we analyzed their ability to differentiate and produce human-specific lipids. The lipophilic dye Nile red can be used to stain terminally differentiating sebocytes [31] (Additional file 2: Figure S2a). Linoleic acid is an essential polyunsaturated fatty acid used for biosynthesis of arachidonic acid and other polyunsaturated fatty acids that can trigger the differentiation of sebocytes in vitro [32]. We therefore analyzed the cellular lipid distribution by Nile red after two days of linoleic acid treatment at physiological levels and show that SSG3 produce lipids in response to linoleic acid (Additional file 2: Figure S2b). Moreover, we detected cytosolic lipid droplets by electron microscopy in untreated cells (Additional file 2: Figure S2c) as well as an increase of lipid droplets with higher electron density after linoleic acid treatment (Additional file 2: Figure S2c"). Humans possess a unique *Δ6 desaturase/FADS2* gene [33] involved in linoleic acid metabolism and sebum production. *FADS2* is detectable mainly in differentiated sebocytes that have reached lipid synthesis capacity, providing a functional marker of activity and differentiation in sebocytes. We have found that *FADS2* is highly expressed in SSG3 cells compared to SEB-1 (Figure 2c). These results demonstrate that the SSG3 cells exhibit gene expression patterns characteristics of cells involved in sebocyte differentiation. Moreover, we found that the differentiation induced by linoleic acid treatment in SSG3 cells is followed by an increase in *PPARγ* at 48 h (Figure 2d) and an increase of *FADS2* after 24 h and 48 h of treatment when cells have reached a high level of cytoplasmic lipid production (Figure 2e).

To further confirm the presence of human specific lipids, gas chromatography of SSG3 cells was performed. We found differences in the composition of fatty acids, in particular, sapienic acid, predominantly found in sebum in vivo [33], and palmitoleic acid. They are synthesized by two desaturases, Δ6/FADS2 and Δ9 respectively [34] (Figure 2f). The desaturation in Δ6 position instead of Δ9 is specific to human sebum [34]. Sapienic acid is detected only in SSG3 cells (2.150%) compared to NIKS (0.795%). In contrast, palmitoleic acid is predominantly found in NIKS (6.959%) compared to SSG3 cells (1.202%) (Figure 2g and h). Next, to determine the functionality of SSG3 cells, we quantified the ratio of Δ6/Δ9 desaturase that is an index of sebocyte maturation and associated metabolic process [35]. We found that this ratio in SSG3 cells is largely superior to the NIKS (178.868 and 11.424 respectively) reflecting the functionality of the scalp-derived sebocytes (Figure 2g). The lipid analysis also revealed that only fatty acids with even-numbered carbon chains, a characteristic of in vivo sebum, are present in SSG3 (Figure 2h). We conclude

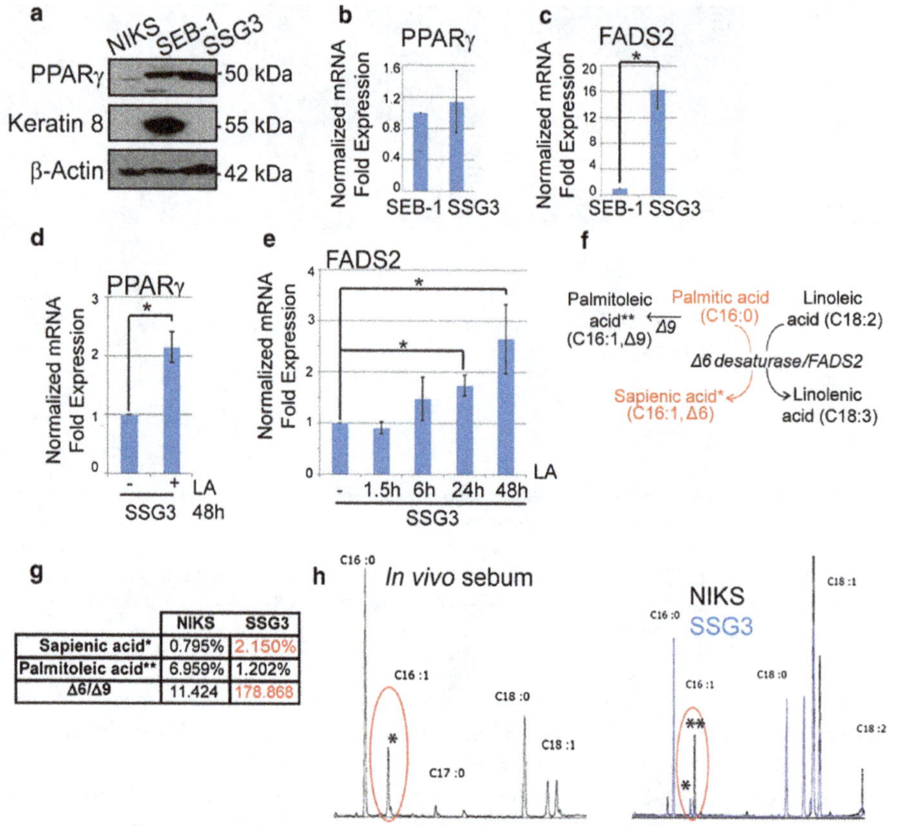

	NIKS	SSG3
Sapienic acid*	0.795%	2.150%
Palmitoleic acid**	6.959%	1.202%
Δ6/Δ9	11.424	178.868

Figure 2 Primary sebocytes isolated from scalp sebaceous glands can differentiate in vitro and produce sebum-characteristic lipids. (**a**) SSG3 expresses PPARγ but not Keratin 8 in contrast to SEB-1. (**b-c**) Real-time PCR shows that *PPARγ* is equally expressed in SEB-1 and SSG3 whereas *FADS2* is more highly expressed in SSG3 cells than SEB-1. RNA from SEB-1 and SSG3 derived from the scalp explant at passage 3 were normalized to *GAPDH* expression. Data shown represent three independent experiments each performed in triplicate (mean +/−SD, n=3). * p-value <0.05 (unpaired two-tailed student's *t* test). (**d**) Cells were cultivated for 48 h with or without 0.1 mM of linoleic acid (LA). Differentiation through LA activation is followed by an increase in *PPARγ* expression in SSG3 cells. * p-value <0.05 paired two-tailed student's *t* test). (**e**) 24 h and 48 h of LA treatment induce a significant increase of *FADS2* expression in SSG3 cells. * p-value <0.05 (paired two-tailed student's *t* test). (**f**) The Δ6 desaturase/FADS2 catalyzes the transformation of palmitic acid into sapienic acid. (**g**) Lipid analysis showing the percentage of Δ9 and Δ6 in the pellet of NIKS and SSG3 and the ratio Δ6/Δ9. (**h**) The sapienic acid (*) can be detected in SSG3 as in vivo sebum, whereas in NIKS, the palmitoleic acid (**) is the abundant lipid detected.

that the primary human sebocyte cultures we have established not only express genes involved in sebum production and lipid synthesis but can also produce sebum-specific lipids. We next investigated the mechanism by which cellular differentiation and lipid production are regulated in primary human sebocytes.

TGFβ signaling is active in sebaceous gland in vivo *and* in vitro

A previous study using whole sebaceous gland explants treated with various cytokines, suggested TGFβ as a potential candidate for human sebocyte regulation [19]. TGFβ ligands bind to a bidimeric receptor complex composed of TGFβ RI and TGFβ RII to phosphorylate and activate receptor-bound Smad (Smad2/3) transcription factors enabling them to translocate into the nucleus and regulate TGFβ-responsive genes [36]. TGFβ RII is essential for the activation of the Smad2 pathway [23,37]. Therefore we analyzed the presence of TGFβ RII and the functionality of the pathway in vivo and in vitro by the presence of phosphorylated Smad2/3 as readout for TGFβ activation. Using immunofluorescence, we first verified that TGFβ RII is expressed throughout the sebaceous gland with the exception of the differentiated, lipid filled sebocytes present in the center of the gland (Figure 3a and 3a'). Further, we determined that the TGFβ pathway is active in the gland in vivo by detecting the expression of nuclear phosphorylated Smad2 in the undifferentiated and maturing sebocytes but not in terminally differentiated sebocytes present in the center of the gland (Figure 3b and 3b'). In vitro, Smad2 is phosphorylated in response to exogenously added recombinant TGFβ1 in SSG3 sebocytes, indicating the TGFβ pathway is intact and active in our in vitro system (Figure 3c).

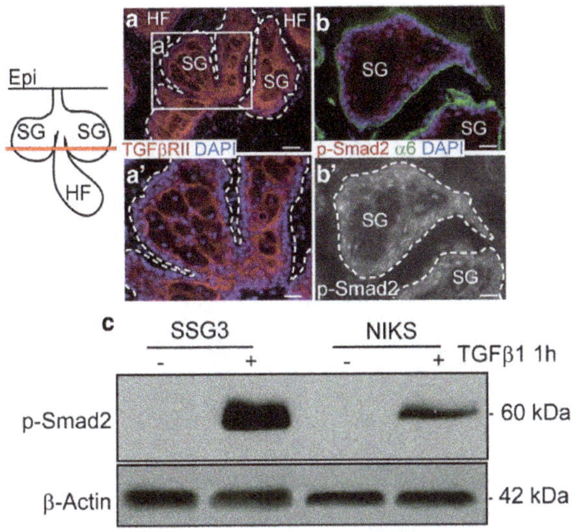

Figure 3 TGFβ signaling is active in sebaceous gland in vivo and in vitro. Sebaceous glands were sectioned in horizontal plane (red line in the diagram). (**a**) OCT sections of human scalp tissue stained with TGFβ RII (red) show expression of the receptor throughout the sebaceous gland with the exception of the differentiated cells in the center. Boxed area is magnified and shown to (**a'**). (**b**) TGFβ pathway is active in vivo as denoted by the expression of nuclear phosphorylated Smad2 (red). α6: α6-integrin stains in green the basal layer of the sebaceous gland. Scale bars, 50 μm (**a**), 20 μm (**a'**, **b**, **b'**). Abbreviations: Epi, Epidermis; HF, Hair Follicle; SG, Sebaceous Gland. (**c**) The indicated sebocyte cultures were treated with 5ng/ml of TGFβ1 ligand for one hour and whole cell extracts were examined by immunoblot to determine the activation of the TGFβ pathway.

Effect of TGFβ signaling on sebocyte differentiation genes

We next probed the effect of TGFβ signaling on their differentiation, by examining the expression of genes involved in lipogenesis upon treatment with TGFβ1. As shown in Figure 4a and b, when cells are stimulated with TGFβ1 for 24 h, the mRNA expression of *FADS2* and *PPARγ* are significantly decreased in SSG3 cells suggesting that TGFβ1 may prevent cell differentiation. Similar results were obtained in primary sebocytes derived from breast and face (Additional file 3: Figure S3), suggesting that the response to TGFβ is indicative of sebocytes in general and not due to the skin tissue type. To test if these effects are dependent on the canonical TGFβ pathway, we used shRNA to knockdown *TGFβ receptor II*, thus effectively inhibiting Smad2 phosphorylation [23]. *TGFβ RII* expression was similarly reduced in SSG3 cells using two independent TGFβ RII shRNA (Figure 4c). Phosphorylated-Smad2 was decreased in shRNA expressing cells compared to controls after TGFβ activation (Figure 4d), as expected. We also detected a decrease of *TGFβ RII* in control cells treated with TGFβ1 for 24 h (Figure 4c) reflecting the possible degradation of the receptor [38]. Moreover, the reduced *TGFβ RII* expression inhibited the ability of SSG3 cells to significantly decrease *FADS2* and *PPARγ* gene expression when cells are treated with TGFβ1 (Figure 4e and f). Our results indicate that the TGFβ pathway can directly control the expression of genes required for the differentiation of sebocytes.

Next we have determined how the inhibition of TGFβ signaling affects the functionality of SSG3 cells at a cellular level by analyzing the presence of cytoplasmic lipids in SSG3 shRNA expressing cells with reduced *TGFβ RII*. *TGFβ RII* depletion is associated with the increase of lipid inclusions positively stained with Nile red, Oil red O, and identified by electron microscopy compared to SSG3 cells expressing a shRNA control (Figure 5b and c and Additional file 4: Figure S4). The lipid droplets labeled with Nile red were analyzed by flow cytometry (Figure 5d). Similar to cells treated with linoleic acid, an increase in fluorescence and granularity (representing the lipid droplets) of the cells was detected in SSG3 *TGFβ RII* shRNA expressing cells compared to the shRNA control.

Additionally, we found that whereas TGFβ1 treatment has no effect on the lipid production in the shRNA cells (Figure 5b), it induces a decrease in lipid inclusion in SSG3 infected with a non-targeting shRNA control (Figure 5a). These results suggest that inhibition of *FADS2* and *PPARγ* at the transcriptional level is mediated via canonical Smad signal transduction. Together, our findings show that activation of the TGFβ signaling pathway down-regulates the expression of genes involved in the production of characteristic sebaceous lipids. We found that *TGFβ RII* gene, which is essential for the activation of the Smad2 pathway, limits lipid production in primary human sebocytes. These findings illustrate the role of TGFβ in maintaining human sebocytes in an undifferentiated state by inhibiting their differentiation and highlight the relevance of this pathway in human sebaceous gland biology.

Discussion

Here we have developed a novel method of culturing human sebocytes without transformation and using a feeder layer-free culture system to examine the role of the TGFβ pathway in the control of differentiation. Primary sebaceous gland cells do not express Keratin 8 in contrast to previously immortalized sebocytes. Keratin 8 is not normally expressed in normal sebaceous gland in vivo [29] and our results indicate that the transformation process in the immortalized line has likely altered the expression of several fundamental cell markers. Moreover, we showed different responsiveness to linoleic acid and TGFβ1 treatment between the primary sebocytes and the immortalized cells (data not shown) suggesting that the cellular properties of those cells substantially differ.

Through our analysis, we have identified that certain markers of sebocytes are differentially expressed depending

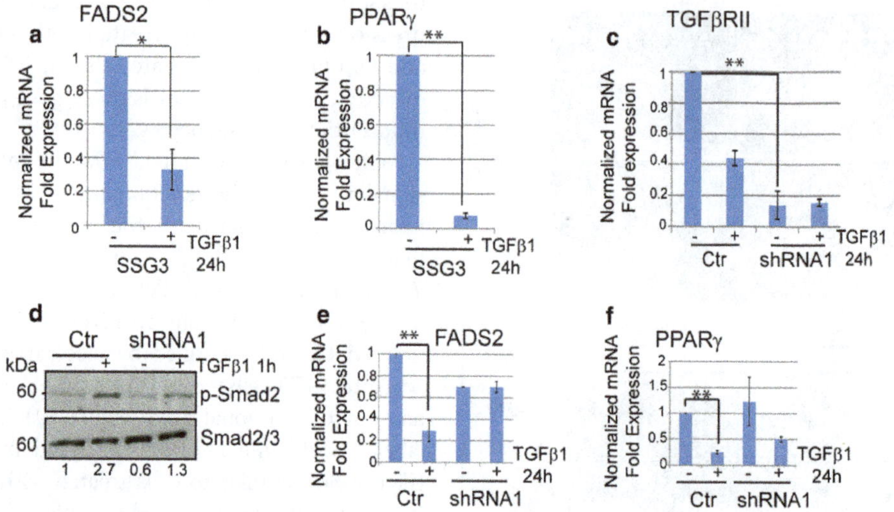

Figure 4 TGFβ signaling triggered decreased expression of lipogenic genes through the TGFβ RII-Smad2 dependent pathway. (**a, b**) SSG3 cells were treated with 5 ng/ml of TGFβ1 for 24 hours and used for qPCR. Data were normalized to *GAPDH* expression and relative expression determined using untreated cells as a reference. *FADS2* and *PPARγ* expression were found to be significantly downregulated in response to TGFβ1 treatment in SSG3 cells. (**c**) *TGFβ RII* expression in SSG3 cells expressing *TGFβ RII* shRNA1 and a control shRNA (Ctr) shows the efficiency of the knockdown. (**d**). Immunoblot confirms the decrease of p-Smad2 activity in shRNA expressing cells stimulated with TGFβ1 5ng/ml for 1 h. Values, noted below the immunoblot, represent the relative density quantified with ImageJ using the ratio p-Smad2/Smad2/3 from each condition. (**e, f**). Decrease of *FADS2* and *PPARγ* at the transcriptional level is mediated via canonical Smad signal transduction. The expression was normalized to control (Ctr) untreated. The significant decrease in *PPARγ* and *FADS2* genes in control SSG3 cells after treatment with TGFβ1, is not detected in *TGFβ RII*-deficient SSG3 cells. * p-value <0.05, ** p-value < 0.001 (paired two-tailed Student's t test).

upon the location on the body (scalp, chest, face), and localization within the sebaceous gland. These results highlight the need for studies covering a range of patient ages to fully comprehend the regulation of the sebaceous glands. However, our work shows that the effect of TGFβ1 activation on sebocyte differentiation is similar in sebocytes derived from three areas (scalp, breast and face) suggesting the specificity of that effect is independent of location. Previous reports have largely focused on cells and glands derived from older adults and post-menopausal women [14-16]. While we have not identified differences in sex, the age of the individual from which the sebaceous gland is derived seems to be of significance. It is known that the sebaceous glands undergo dramatic changes over the course of one's lifespan, with high sebum production occurring in infancy, a reduction during early childhood, followed by a steady increase through puberty into early adulthood. Using pediatric donors we ensured that the skin is not exposed to the hormonal changes that adult or old donor skin goes through. In the future it may be interesting to use our novel method to isolate sebocytes from old donors to examine the effect of age on TGFβ responsiveness in sebocytes.

We have begun to unravel one mechanism of differentiation of human sebaceous glands that culminates in sebum production. Our data suggest that TGFβ signaling maintains sebocytes in an undifferentiated state by decreasing the expression of *FADS2* and *PPARγ* thereby decreasing lipid accumulation through the TGFβ RII-Smad2 dependent pathway. The successful growth of these primary human sebocytes has important clinical application such as the possibility of designing new strategies of culturing engineered skin to enable and maintain the presence of sebaceous glands in skin grafts for burn victims [10,39]. In addition to cell autonomous regulators and signals inducing proliferation and maturation among sebaceous cells, the complex microenvironment surrounding the sebaceous gland might have a profound effect on homeostasis of the tissue. Molecular crosstalk between the dermis and the epithelial cells is crucial for the initiation and maintenance of the hair follicles [40]. It seems most likely that similar mechanisms of communication between sebocytes and the surrounding dermal tissue exist. For instance, in the mouse, TGFβ1 is known to be released by the inner root sheath of the hair follicle, thereby providing a means for a bidirectional interaction between the sebaceous gland and the hair follicle epithelium [20]. Similarly, in the dermis, human fibroblasts secrete TGFβ [41,42] which may then act on keratinocytes and sebocytes. Another component in the microenvironment that could also be part of this crosstalk are the arrector pili muscle cells recently shown to be controlled by bulge stem cells in mouse [43]. Being located in close proximity to the sebaceous gland, arrector pili muscles could help release sebum onto the skin surface [44].

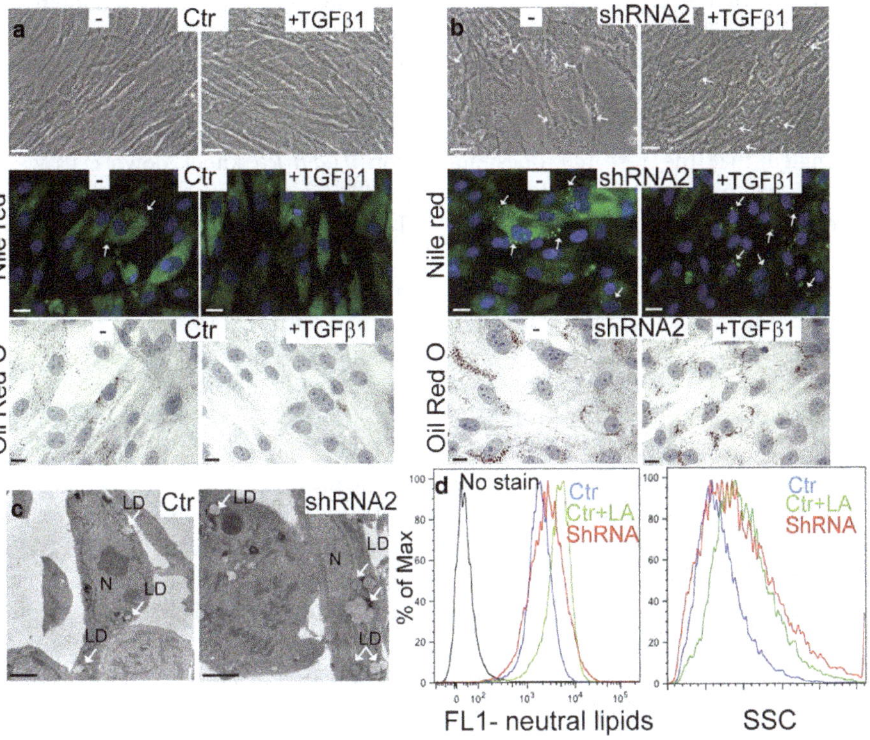

Figure 5 Inhibition of TGFβ signaling induces lipogenesis in primary SSG3 cells. (**a, b**) SSG3 cells stably expressing a shRNA against *TGFβ RII*, show accumulation of lipid droplets on brightfield images (scale bars, 20 μm), by Nile red (scale bars, 20 μm) and Oil red O stainings (scale bars, 10 μm). White arrows show the presence of multiple lipid droplets in the shRNA expressing cells compared to the control (Ctr). 24 h of TGFβ1 (5 ng/ml) treatment decreases the basal level of lipid production in control cells but does not affect cells expressing the *TGFβ RII* shRNA, mainly seen by Oil red O. (**c**) Electron microscopy showing the increase of lipid droplets in SSG3 cells (denoted by white arrows) expressing the shRNA compared to the control. Scale bars, 2 μm. LD, Lipid Droplets. N, Nucleus. (**d**) Flow cytometry of SSG3 cells expressing the shRNA labeled with Nile red. FL-1 measures the neutral lipids and SSC reflects the granularity of the cells. 10,000 cells have been acquired for each condition. As a positive control, SSG3 treated by 0.1 mM linoleic acid (LA) for 24 h show increase of fluorescence and granularity representing the lipid droplets. Note the increase of fluorescence and the increase of granularity in shRNA expressing *TGFβ RII* compared to the cells expressing a shRNA control. We obtained similar result with two different shRNA expressing *TGFβ RII* (Additional file 4: Figure S4).

Impairment of the skin barrier due to the deregulation of sebum production when associated with bacteria colonization and inflammation, can be the cause of serious skin conditions in people. For instance, hyperseborrhea combined with the presence of *Propionibacterium acnes* and inflammation can lead to acne vulgaris [4] and *Staphylococcus aureus* can aggravate atopic dermatitis [6]. Sebocytes can produce antimicrobial peptides such as defensin-1 and -2 upon exposure to *Propionibacterium acnes* or lipopolysaccharides [45,46] to prevent from bacteria colonization [47] and from an upregulation of sebum production [48]. Studies have revealed that TGFβ induces the expression of human β-defensin-2 in endothelial cells [49] and influences inflammatory response [50]. Therefore it will be interesting to further investigate the impact of TGFβ on immune responses in sebaceous gland and its implication in antimicrobial peptides secretion by sebocytes. With the novel isolation strategy we described here, different interactions with the microenvironment can now be investigated.

Conclusions

By describing an innovative way to grow and successfully passage human primary sebocytes, we have overcome a major hurdle in the field of epithelial cell culture. We characterized the role of TGFβ signaling pathway in the inhibition of lipogenesis in these cells by showing that reduced expression of *TGFβ RII* increases lipid production. Our work, can not only improve our understanding of the physiology of the sebaceous gland in normal and pathological conditions [45] but also potentially expand this knowledge to other glands like eccrine and apocrine glands and use these cells to improve the quality of the skin grafts.

Methods

Cell Culture

The sebaceous gland populations were generated from human scalp (SSG3), face, chest and breast from both male and female donors. The skin samples were collected as a surgical waste with information provided regarding the age and sex of the donors with Institutional Review Board (IRB) approval at Cincinnati Children's Hospital Medical Center. Cincinnati Children's Hospital is a Pediatric Hospital that allowed us to collect samples from donors ranging 9 months old to 12 years old. The IRB determined that the research does not meet the regulatory criteria for research involving human subjects as there were no interaction with the donors and no identifiable private information. After treating the skin with dispase overnight at 4°C, intact sebaceous glands were isolated with microsurgical instruments under a dissecting microscope (Figure 1b). To mimic the microenvironment of the sebaceous gland, the explants were sandwiched between glass coverslips coated with human fibronectin (10 μg/ml, Millipore, Billerica, MA) (Figure 1d). The explants were cultivated in sebocyte medium as described [15] (DMEM/Ham's F-12 (3:1), Epidermal Growth Factor (EGF 3 ng/ml, Austral Biologicals, San Ramon, CA), cholera toxin (1.2×10-10M, Sigma, St. Louis, MO), adenine (24 μg/ml, Sigma, St. Louis, MO), insulin (10 ng/ml Sigma), hydrocortisone (45.2 ng/ml, Sigma), FBS (2.5% Hyclone, San Jose, CA), antibiotic/antimycotic (100×, Invitrogen, Grand Island, NY). After 1–2 weeks of growth in culture, cellular outgrowth became apparent from the periphery of the gland lobules. The explants were removed and the isolated cells cultured on the fibronectin-coated coverslips.

Western blotting

Proteins were separated by electrophoresis on 8-10% acrylamide gels, transferred to nitrocellulose membranes and subjected to immunoblotting. Membranes were blocked for one hour with 5% non-fat milk or 5% BSA in PBS containing 0.1% Tween-20. Primary antibodies were used at concentrations described below and HRP-coupled secondary antibodies were used at 1/2,000 in 5% non-fat milk. Immunoblots were developed using standard ECL (Amersham, Pittsburg, PA) and Luminata TM crescendo and classico (Millipore, Billerica, MA). Two-color immunoblot detection was performed using LI-COR Odyssey CL× (Biosciences, Lincoln, NE). Membranes were blocked in Odyssey blocking buffer (Li-Cor) and secondary antibodies conjugated to IRDye 680LT and 800CW were used (1/10,000; Li-Cor). Protein levels were quantified using the Odyssey Infrared Imaging System (Li-Cor).

Retroviral Infection

To ablate *TGFβ RII* in SSG3 cells, we used shRNA vectors from the CCHMC Heart Institute lenti-shRNA library core (shRNA TGFβ RII #197031 and 194992 and a shRNA control). The human library was purchased from Sigma-Aldrich (MISSION shRNA). Lentivirus was produced by the Viral Vector Core at the Translational Core Laboratories, Cincinnati Children's Hospital Research Foundation. Cells were grown to 80% confluency in 6-well plates before being infected with the lentivirus for 48 h. Infected cells were selected with 1 μg/ml puromycin (Sigma, St. Louis, MO) for 48 h. Following selection, *TGFβ RII* knock down cells were grown in regular media for 48 h before being activated with 5 ng/ml TGFβ1 for 24 h.

Histology and Immunofluorescence

Human tissues were frozen unfixed in OCT compound (Tissue-Tek, Sakura, Torrance, CA) for cryosectioning. Immunostainings were performed as previously described [51].

Antibodies

Primary antibodies against the following proteins were used at the dilution indicated: PPARγ (Santa-Cruz Biotechnology Inc., Santa Cruz, CA, H-100 1/250 for immunofluorescence, 1/500 for immunoblot), Blimp1 (Cell Signaling Technology, Beverly, MA, 1/500 for immunofluorescence, 1/1,000 for immunoblot), Fibronectin (Santa-Cruz Biotechnology Inc., Santa Cruz, CA, EP5 1/150), Muc1 (Millipore, Billerica, MA 1/500), cMyc (Cell Signaling Technology, Beverly, MA, 1/800 for immunofluorescence, 1/1,000 for immunoblot), TGFβ RII (Santa-Cruz Biotechnology Inc., Santa Cruz, CA, sc-220 1/1,000), p-Smad2 (Cell Signaling Technology, Beverly, MA, 1/100 for immunofluorescence, 1/1,000 for immunoblot), Smad2/3 (BD Biosciences, San Jose, CA, 1/500), α6 integrin (CD49f, BD Biosciences, San Jose, CA, 1/100), Keratin 8 (this antibody, developed by Dr. Brulet and Dr. Kemler, was obtained from the NICHD Developmental Studies Hybridoma Bank maintained by the University of Iowa, 1/1,000), β-actin (Sigma, St. Louis, MO, 1/2,000), Keratin 7 (Cell Signaling Technology, Beverly, MA, 1/1,000), 4′,6-diamidino-2-phenylindole (DAPI) was utilized as a marker of cell nuclei (Sigma Chemical Co., St. Louis, MO, 1/5,000). Secondary antibodies Alexa Fluor 488 or 555 (Molecular Probes, Grand Island, NY) were used at a dilution of 1/1,000. Fluorescence images were acquired with a fluorescent microscope AxioImager M1 (Zeiss, Oberkochen, Germany) and pictures were taken with an axioCam MRm camera (Zeiss, Oberkochen, Germany).

Real-time PCR

Total RNA was isolated using a Qiagen Rneasy Mini Kit and used to produce cDNA (Maxima first strand cDNA synthesis kit, Fermentas, San Jose, CA). Reverse transcription (RT) reactions were diluted to 10 ng/μl and 1μl of each RT was used for real-time PCR. Real-time PCR was performed using the CFX96 real-time PCR System, CFX Manager Software and the SsoFast EvaGreen

Supermix reagents (Biorad, Hercules, CA). All reactions were run in triplicate and analyzed using the ΔΔCT method with relative expression normalized to GAPDH. Primers used:

GAPDH-F: ACATCGCTCAGACACCATG, GAPDH-R: TGTAGTTGAGGTCAATGAAGGG

PPARγ-F: GAGCCCAAGTTTGAGTTTGC, PPARγ-R: GCAGGTTGTCTTGAATGTCTTC,

FADS2-F: TGTCTACAGAAAACCCAAGTGG, FADS 2-R: TGTGGAAGATGTTAGGCTTGG,

TGFβ RII-F: CTGTGGATGACCTGGCTAAC, TGFβ RII-R: CATTTCCCAGAGCACCAGAG

Lipogenesis assays

For Nile red staining, cells or OCT sections were fixed 10 minutes at room temperature in 4% formaldehyde. After 3 washes in 1XPBS, Nile red staining was performed with 0.1 μg/ml of Nile red (Sigma, St. Louis, MO) in 0.15 M NaCl for 15 minutes at room temperature. For Oil red O staining, cells were fixed 15 minutes in 10% formalin, wash with water for 10 minutes and 60% isopropanol before being stained with Oil red O (0.7% in 60% isopropanol) for 45 minutes. Cells were rinsed with 60% isopropanol and the nuclei stained with haematoxylin. To trigger differentiation of sebocytes in vitro, 0.1 mM linoleic acid (Sigma, St Louis, MO) was added directly to sebocyte media. To prepare cells for extraction of lipids, $2\text{-}3\times10^7$ of cells were pelleted, washed with 1XPBS and lipids were preserved in the dark at −80°C under argon until analysis. The qualitative and quantitative composition of lipids in scalp-derived human sebocytes was determined using an Agilent 5973N Gas chromatograph/Mass spectrometer with a SPE cartridge (solid phase extraction) and was performed by Synelvia S.A.S (Labege, France).

Nile Red analysis by FACS

Cells were cultured in 6-well plates at 80% confluence and infected with the lentivirus expressing the shRNAs as previously described. After puromycin selection for 48 h, cells were washed in 1X PBS and treated with working medium with or without Linoleic acid (0.1 mM) for 24 h. The cells were trypsinized, washed once with 1X PBS and neutral lipids were labeled with the fluorescent dye Nile red (1 μg/ml in PBS). 10,000 cells per sample were analyzed using a FACS Canto I equipped with a blue laser (488 nm excitation).

Electron microscopy

Cells were grown at 80% confluency in sebocyte media and rinsed once with 0.175 M sodium cacodylate buffer. Cells were fixed in 3% glutaraldehyde/0.175 M cacodylate buffer (Electron Microscopy Sciences, Hatfield, PA) for 1 hour at 4°C. Dishes were washed twice with 0.175 M sodium cacodylate buffer. Cells were post fixed in 1% osmium tetroxide/cacodylate buffer for 1 hour at 4°C before being washed three times with 0.175 M sodium cacodylate buffer. After the final wash with 1.5 ml, cells were scraped and centrifuged for 5 min at 10,000 RPM. The cell pellet was then resuspended in 1 ml 1% agarose (Type IX ultra-low gelling tempt, Sigma) overnight at 4°C. The samples were then processed through a graded series of alcohols, infiltrated and embedded in LX-112 resin. After polymerization at 60°C for three days, ultrathin sections (100 nm) were cut using a Reichert-Jung Ultracut E microtome and counterstained in 2% aqueous uranyl acetate and Reynolds lead citrate. Images were taken with a transmission electron microscope (Hitachi H-6750) equipped with a digital camera (AMT 2k×2K tem CCD).

Statistics

Data are expressed as means +/− SD. Comparison between two cell types was performed using unpaired two-tailed student's *t* test. Paired two-tailed student's *t* test was used when we compared the effect of a treatment on the same cell type. $p<0.05$ was considered significant.

Additional files

Additional file 1: Figure S1. Primary human sebocytes derived from scalp, breast, chest and face tissues express typical sebocyte markers. (a) Hematoxylin and Eosin staining of the scalp sample. Scale bar, 50 μm. (b) Immunofluorescence staining showed that PPARγ (red) is expressed in human sebaceous glands from the scalp explant at the periphery stained with α6-integrin (green) and at the center of the gland. Scale bar, 50 μm. Boxed area is magnified and shown to (b'). (c) Blimp1 (red) expression is mostly found in the differentiated cells of the sebaceous gland and in the inner root sheath of the hair follicle. α6-integrin (green) marked the basal layer of the gland. (d) Keratin 7 (red) expression varies depending on the location of the gland (scalp, breast and chest) as shown by immunofluorescence. (e-g) Sebocytes derived from the scalp, breast, chest and face explants expressed sebocytes markers by two-color immunoblot (Blimp1, c-Myc, Muc1, PPARγ and K7). SSG4 represents primary sebocytes derived from a four year old-scalp sample. Scale bars, 50 μm (b), 50 μm (c and d). Abbreviations: SG, Sebaceous Gland; HF, Hair Follicle; α6, α6-integrin; K7, Keratin 7.

Additional file 2: Figure S2. Primary sebocytes can differentiate in vitro. (a) Human scalp sections showing evidence of lipid accumulation (Nile red stain). Scale bar, 50 μm (b) SSG3 cells derived from the scalp explants were treated with 0.1 mM linoleic acid (LA) for 48 h to differentiate the cells and stained with Nile red to detect lipids. Images were taken with the same exposure time in untreated and linoleic acid-treated conditions. Brightfield pictures showed accumulation of cytoplasmic lipid droplets after linoleic acid treatment as denoted by the black arrows. Scale bars, 50 μm (c) Electron microscopy showing cytoplasmic lipid droplets in untreated sebocytes SSG3 derived from the scalp explants. Scale bar, 20 μm. Boxed area is magnified and shown to (c') scale bar, 500 nm. (c") After linoleic acid treatment increased high-electron density lipid droplets are detected in SSG3 cells and magnified in c"'. Scale bars for c" and c"' are 2 μm. Abbreviations: HF, Hair Follicle. SG, Sebaceous Gland. LD, Lipid Droplets. N, Nucleus. Mi, Mitochondria. RER, Rough Endoplasmic Reticulum . SER, Smooth Endoplasmic Reticulum.

Additional file 3: Figure S3. TGFβ signaling triggered decreased expression of lipogenic genes in breast and face-derived sebocytes. RNA was isolated from sebocytes-derived from breast and face untreated or treated with 5 ng/ml of TGFβ1 for 24 h and used for real-time PCR. Two experiments were performed and all qPCR reactions were performed in triplicate. Data were normalized to *GAPDH* expression for each cell population and changes in relative expression were determined using untreated cells as a reference point. (a) *FADS2* and (b) *PPARγ* expression was found to be decreased significantly in response to TGFβ1 treatment as shown in scalp-derived sebocytes (Figure 4a-b) suggesting that the inhibitory effect of TGFβ is not due to the skin tissue type. *p-value<0.05 (paired two-tailed Student's *t* test).

Additional file 4: Figure S4. Inhibition of TGFβ signaling induces lipogenesis in primary SSG3 cells. (a) SSG3 cells, stably expressing a shRNA against *TGFβ RII* (shRNA1), show accumulation of lipid droplets on brightfield image (white arrows) and by Nile red staining (shown in green) compared to cells infected with shRNA control. Scale bars, 20 μm. (b-c), Electron microscopy showing the increase of lipid droplets in SSG3 cells (denoted by white arrows) expressing the shRNA against *TGFβ RII* (shRNA2) compared to the control. Myelin figures, which indicate lipids synthesis, are detected in SSG3 cells expressing the shRNA. Abbreviations: N, nucleus. LD, Lipid Droplets. Scale bars for b and c are 2 μm and 500 nm for c'.

Competing interests
GG has no conflict of interest. JD, CB and LB are employed by L'Oreal and have conflict of interests.

Authors' contributions
AJM, YD, JD, MB, CB, LB and GG contributed to experimental design. AJM, YD and MB performed the experiments. CBG and AUR provided the human samples and advised on tissues preparation. PFL provides the NIKS cells. AJM, YD, JD, MB, LB and GG assisted in data analysis. GG wrote and prepared the manuscript with critical comments from all authors. GG and LB have contributed equally to supervise the project. All authors read and approved the final manuscript.

Acknowledgements
We would like to thank Dr. Diane Thiboutot (Penn State) for providing the SEB-1 cells. Laura Runck (Guasch Lab) for helping with the histology of the sections. Georgianne Ciraolo (CCHMC Pathology Department) for performing the preparation of the samples for the electron microscopy, Xiaoling Zhang and Monica Delay (CCHMC Flow Cytometry Core) for support with the analysis of the Nile Red, and the viral vector core (CCHMC) for producing the lentivirus. Drs. Christopher Wylie and Susanne Wells for critical reading of the manuscript. This work was supported by L'Oreal.

Author details
[1]Division of Developmental Biology, Cincinnati Children's Hospital Medical Center, 3333 Burnet Avenue, Cincinnati, OH 45229, USA. [2]Current Address: Department of Biomedical Sciences, College of Veterinary Medicine, Cornell University, Ithaca, NY 14853, USA. [3]Current Address: Department of Dermatology, Columbia University, College of Physicians and Surgeons, New York, NY 10032, USA. [4]L'OREAL Research & Innovation, 90 rue du General Roguet, 92583, CLICHY, FRANCE. [5]Division of Plastic Surgery, Children's Hospital Medical Center, 3333 Burnet Avenue, Cincinnati, OH 45229, USA. [6]University of Wisconsin School of Medicine and Public Health, Madison, WI, USA.

References
1. Thody AJ, Shuster S: **Control and function of sebaceous glands.** *Physiological reviews* 1989, **69**(2):383–416.
2. Hyman AB, Brownstein MH: **Tyson's "glands."** *Ectopic sebaceous glands and papillomatosis penis. Archives of dermatology* 1969, **99**(1):31–36.
3. Smith KR, Thiboutot DM: **Thematic review series: skin lipids. Sebaceous gland lipids: friend or foe?** *J Lipid Res* 2008, **49**(2):271–281.
4. Picardo M, Ottaviani M, Camera E, Mastrofrancesco A: **Sebaceous gland lipids.** *Dermatoendocrinol* 2009, **1**(2):68–71.
5. Pochi PE, Strauss JS, Downing DT: **Age-related changes in sebaceous gland activity.** *J Invest Dermatol* 1979, **73**(1):108–111.
6. Huang JT, Abrams M, Tlougan B, Rademaker A, Paller AS: **Treatment of Staphylococcus aureus colonization in atopic dermatitis decreases disease severity.** *Pediatrics* 2009, **123**(5):e808–e814.
7. Stenn KS: **Insights from the asebia mouse: a molecular sebaceous gland defect leading to cicatricial alopecia.** *J Cutan Pathol* 2001, **28**(9):445–447.
8. Zheng Y, Eilertsen KJ, Ge L, Zhang L, Sundberg JP, Prouty SM, Stenn KS, Parimoo S: **Scd1 is expressed in sebaceous glands and is disrupted in the asebia mouse.** *Nat Genet* 1999, **23**(3):268–270.
9. Shizuru JA, Negrin RS, Weissman IL: **Hematopoietic stem and progenitor cells: clinical and preclinical regeneration of the hematolymphoid system.** *Annu Rev Med* 2005, **56**:509–538.
10. Ronfard V, Rives JM, Neveux Y, Carsin H, Barrandon Y: **Long-term regeneration of human epidermis on third degree burns transplanted with autologous cultured epithelium grown on a fibrin matrix.** *Transplantation* 2000, **70**(11):1588–1598.
11. Barrandon Y, Green H: **Three clonal types of keratinocyte with different capacities for multiplication.** *Proc Natl Acad Sci U S A* 1987, **84**(8):2302–2306.
12. Barrandon Y: **Crossing boundaries: stem cells, holoclones, and the fundamentals of squamous epithelial renewal.** *Cornea* 2007, **26**(9 Suppl 1):S10–S12.
13. Abdel-Naser MB: **Selective cultivation of normal human sebocytes in vitro; a simple modified technique for a better cell yield.** *Exp Dermatol* 2004, **13**(9):562–566.
14. Zouboulis CC, Seltmann H, Neitzel H, Orfanos CE: **Establishment and characterization of an immortalized human sebaceous gland cell line (SZ95).** *J Invest Dermatol* 1999, **113**(6):1011–1020.
15. Thiboutot D, Jabara S, McAllister JM, Sivarajah A, Gilliland K, Cong Z, Clawson G: **Human skin is a steroidogenic tissue: steroidogenic enzymes and cofactors are expressed in epidermis, normal sebocytes, and an immortalized sebocyte cell line (SEB-1).** *J Invest Dermatol* 2003, **120**(6):905–914.
16. Lo Celso C, Berta MA, Braun KM, Frye M, Lyle S, Zouboulis CC, Watt FM: **Characterization of bipotential epidermal progenitors derived from human sebaceous gland: contrasting roles of c-Myc and beta-catenin.** *Stem Cells* 2008, **26**(5):1241–1252.
17. Xia L, Zouboulis CC, Ju Q: **Culture of human sebocytes in vitro.** *Dermatoendocrinol* 2009, **1**(2):92–95.
18. Furue M, Kato M, Nakamura K, Nashiro K, Kikuchi K, Okochi H, Miyazono K, Tamaki K: **Dysregulated expression of transforming growth factor beta and its type-I and type-II receptors in basal-cell carcinoma.** *Int J Cancer* 1997, **71**(4):505–509.
19. Downie MM, Sanders DA, Kealey T: **Modelling the remission of individual acne lesions in vitro.** *Br J Dermatol* 2002, **147**(5):869–878.
20. Wollina U, Lange D, Funa K, Paus R: **Expression of transforming growth factor beta isoforms and their receptors during hair growth phases in mice.** *Histol Histopathol* 1996, **11**(2):431–436.
21. Paus R, Foitzik K, Welker P, Bulfone-Paus S, Eichmuller S: **Transforming growth factor-beta receptor type I and type II expression during murine hair follicle development and cycling.** *J Invest Dermatol* 1997, **109**(4):518–526.
22. Pietenpol JA, Stein RW, Moran E, Yaciuk P, Schlegel R, Lyons RM, Pittelkow MR, Munger K, Howley PM, Moses HL: **TGF-beta 1 inhibition of c-myc transcription and growth in keratinocytes is abrogated by viral transforming proteins with pRB binding domains.** *Cell* 1990, **61**(5):777–785.
23. Guasch G, Schober M, Pasolli HA, Conn EB, Polak L, Fuchs E: **Loss of TGFbeta signaling destabilizes homeostasis and promotes squamous cell carcinomas in stratified epithelia.** *Cancer Cell* 2007, **12**(4):313–327.
24. Arnold I: **Watt FM: c-Myc activation in transgenic mouse epidermis results in mobilization of stem cells and differentiation of their progeny.** *Curr Biol* 2001, **11**(8):558–568.
25. Yang L, Wang L, Yang X: **Disruption of Smad4 in mouse epidermis leads to depletion of follicle stem cells.** *Mol Biol Cell* 2009, **20**(3):882–890.
26. Rosenfield RL, Deplewski D, Kentsis A, Ciletti N: **Mechanisms of androgen induction of sebocyte differentiation.** *Dermatology* 1998, **196**(1):43–46.
27. Allen-Hoffmann BL, Schlosser SJ, Ivarie CA, Sattler CA, Meisner LF, O'Connor SL: **Normal growth and differentiation in a spontaneously immortalized near-diploid human keratinocyte cell line, NIKS.** *J Invest Dermatol* 2000, **114**(3):444–455.
28. Tsubura A, Okada H, Sasaki M, Dairkee SH, Morii S: **Immunohistochemical demonstration of keratins 8 and 14 in benign tumours of the skin appendage.** *Virchows Archiv A, Pathological anatomy and histopathology* 1991, **418**(6):503–507.

29. Troyanovsky SM, Guelstein VI, Tchipysheva TA, Krutovskikh VA, Bannikov GA: **Patterns of expression of keratin 17 in human epithelia: dependency on cell position.** *J Cell Sci* 1989, **93**(Pt 3):419–426.
30. Magnusdottir E, Kalachikov S, Mizukoshi K, Savitsky D, Ishida-Yamamoto A, Panteleyev AA, Calame K: **Epidermal terminal differentiation depends on B lymphocyte-induced maturation protein-1.** *Proc Natl Acad Sci U S A* 2007, **104**(38):14988–14993.
31. Braun KM, Niemann C, Jensen UB, Sundberg JP, Silva-Vargas V, Watt FM: **Manipulation of stem cell proliferation and lineage commitment: visualisation of label-retaining cells in wholemounts of mouse epidermis.** *Development* 2003, **130**(21):5241–5255.
32. Rosenfield RL, Kentsis A, Deplewski D, Ciletti N: **Rat preputial sebocyte differentiation involves peroxisome proliferator-activated receptors.** *J Invest Dermatol* 1999, **112**(2):226–232.
33. Ge L, Gordon JS, Hsuan C, Stenn K, Prouty SM: **Identification of the delta-6 desaturase of human sebaceous glands: expression and enzyme activity.** *J Invest Dermatol* 2003, **120**(5):707–714.
34. Pappas A, Anthonavage M, Gordon JS: **Metabolic fate and selective utilization of major fatty acids in human sebaceous gland.** *J Invest Dermatol* 2002, **118**(1):164–171.
35. Ottaviani M, Camera E, Picardo M: **Lipid mediators in acne.** *Mediators Inflamm* 2010.
36. Massague J, Gomis RR: **The logic of TGFbeta signaling.** *FEBS Lett* 2006, **580**(12):2811–2820.
37. Wrana JL, Attisano L, Wieser R, Ventura F, Massague J: **Mechanism of activation of the TGF-beta receptor.** *Nature* 1994, **370**(6488):341–347.
38. Mitchell H, Choudhury A, Pagano RE, Leof EB: **Ligand-dependent and -independent transforming growth factor-beta receptor recycling regulated by clathrin-mediated endocytosis and Rab11.** *Mol Biol Cell* 2004, **15**(9):4166–4178.
39. Eisinger M, Li WH, Rossetti DD, Anthonavage M, Seiberg M: **Sebaceous gland regeneration in human skin xenografts.** *J Invest Dermatol* 2010, **130**(8):2131–2133.
40. Rendl M, Lewis L, Fuchs E: **Molecular dissection of mesenchymal-epithelial interactions in the hair follicle.** *PLoS Biol* 2005, **3**(11):e331.
41. Wong T, McGrath JA, Navsaria H: **The role of fibroblasts in tissue engineering and regeneration.** *Br J Dermatol* 2007, **156**(6):1149–1155.
42. Nolte SV, Xu W, Rennekampff HO, Rodemann HP: **Diversity of fibroblasts–a review on implications for skin tissue engineering.** *Cells Tissues Organs* 2008, **187**(3):165–176.
43. Fujiwara H, Ferreira M, Donati G, Marciano DK, Linton JM, Sato Y, Hartner A, Sekiguchi K, Reichardt LF, Watt FM: **The basement membrane of hair follicle stem cells is a muscle cell niche.** *Cell* 2011, **144**(4):577–589.
44. Poblet E, Jimenez F, Ortega F: **The contribution of the arrector pili muscle and sebaceous glands to the follicular unit structure.** *J Am Acad Dermatol* 2004, **51**(2):217–222.
45. Chronnell CM, Ghali LR, Ali RS, Quinn AG, Holland DB, Bull JJ, Cunliffe WJ, McKay IA, Philpott MP, Muller-Rover S: **Human beta defensin-1 and −2 expression in human pilosebaceous units: upregulation in acne vulgaris lesions.** *J Invest Dermatol* 2001, **117**(5):1120–1125.
46. Nagy I, Pivarcsi A, Kis K, Koreck A, Bodai L, McDowell A, Seltmann H, Patrick S, Zouboulis CC, Kemeny L: **Propionibacterium acnes and lipopolysaccharide induce the expression of antimicrobial peptides and proinflammatory cytokines/chemokines in human sebocytes.** *Microbes Infect* 2006, **8**(8):2195–2205.
47. Lee DY, Yamasaki K, Rudsil J, Zouboulis CC, Park GT, Yang JM, Gallo RL: **Sebocytes express functional cathelicidin antimicrobial peptides and can act to kill propionibacterium acnes.** *J Invest Dermatol* 2008, **128**(7):1863–1866.
48. Zouboulis CC: **Propionibacterium acnes and sebaceous lipogenesis: a love-hate relationship?** *J Invest Dermatol* 2009, **129**(9):2093–2096.
49. Kawsar HI, Ghosh SK, Hirsch SA, Koon HB, Weinberg A, Jin G: **Expression of human beta-defensin-2 in intratumoral vascular endothelium and in endothelial cells induced by transforming growth factor beta.** *Peptides* 2010, **31**(2):195–201.
50. Ishinaga H, Jono H, Lim JH, Kweon SM, Xu H, Ha UH, Koga T, Yan C, Feng XH, Chen LF, *et al*: **TGF-beta induces p65 acetylation to enhance bacteria-induced NF-kappaB activation.** *EMBO J* 2007, **26**(4):1150–1162.
51. Runck LA, Kramer M, Ciraolo G, Lewis AG, Guasch G: **Identification of epithelial label-retaining cells at the transition between the anal canal and the rectum in mice.** *Cell Cycle* 2010, **9**(15):3039–3045.

15

A systematic literature review of pediculosis due to head lice in the Pacific Island Countries and Territories: what country specific research on head lice is needed?

Rick Speare[1,2*], Humpress Harrington[3], Deon Canyon[4] and Peter D Massey[5]

Abstract

Background: Lack of guidelines on control of pediculosis in the Solomon Islands led to a search for relevant evidence on head lice in the Pacific Island Countries and Territories (PICTs). The aim of this search was to systematically evaluate evidence in the peer reviewed literature on pediculosis due to head lice (*Pediculus humanus* var *capitis*) in the 22 PICTs from the perspective of its value in informing national guidelines and control strategies.

Methods: PubMed, Web of Science, CINAHL and Scopus were searched using the terms (pediculosis OR head lice) AND each of the 22 PICTs individually. PRISMA methodology was used. Exclusion criteria were: i) not on topic; ii) publications on pediculosis not relevant to the country of the particular search; iii) in grey literature.

Results: Of 24 publications identified, only 5 were included. Four related to treatment and one to epidemiology. None contained information relevant to informing national guidelines.

Conclusions: Current local evidence on head lice in the PICTs is minimal and totally inadequate to guide any recommendations for treatment or control. We recommend that local research is required to generate evidence on: i) epidemiology; ii) knowledge, attitudes and practices of health care providers and community members; iii) efficacy of local commercially available pharmaceutical treatments and local customary treatments; iv) acceptability, accessibility and affordability of available treatment strategies; and iv) appropriate control strategies for families, groups and institutions. We also recommend that operational research be done by local researchers based in the PICTs, supported by experienced head lice researchers, using a two way research capacity building model.

Keywords: Head lice, Pediculosis, *Pediculus humanus* var *capitis*, Pacific Island Countries and Territories, Systematic literature review, Papua New Guinea, Solomon Islands, French Polynesia

Background

When the local community at Atoifi in the Solomon Islands decided to control head lice, they could find no national guidelines. This raised the important question of whether countries and their residents need local evidence to control pediculosis, which is a global problem due to *Pediculus humanus* var *capitis* [1].

Country-specific data is essential for planning communicable disease control programs, even for pediculosis [2]. For more serious diseases the importance of local data is well established. For example, intestinal parasite control activities have to be informed by country, regional and even locally-specific data collected on a regular basis to determine the local epidemiology and extent of parasitic infections with long-term repeated surveillance to inform strategies as the situation changes [3,4]. Quantitative data can be used in modeling to make disease control more cost-effective; e.g., measles vaccination programs [5] and the HIV Spectrum and Estimation and Projection Package programs [6]. In a similar way country-specific

* Correspondence: rickspeare@gmail.com
[1]College of Public Health, Medical and Veterinary Sciences, James Cook University, Townsville 4811, Australia
[2]Tropical Health Solutions, 72 Kokoda St, Idalia, Townsville 4811, Australia
Full list of author information is available at the end of the article

and local data arguably can improve control strategies for pediculosis [2]. The value of local research in informing practice was reinforced by a survey in South Africa carried out by the provincial communicable disease program that showed only children of European and Indian ancestry in a mixed race school had pediculosis [7]. This resulted in targeting of Mpumulanga Province's health departmental control efforts for pediculosis away from the black African students to the other racial groups. From a communicable disease control perspective evidence needed to control pediculosis can be placed in several categories: biology, epidemiology, impact, diagnosis, treatment, societal context and policies.

Head lice have been a topic of research since before the 20th century. Initial studies focussed on biology, epidemiology and techniques to kill lice with the emphasis from the 1940s shifting to research on efficacy of pharmaceutical treatments [8-10]. The emergence of insecticide resistance to organochlorines (DDT and BHC) in the 1970s [11], and then to permethrin in the 1990s [12], expanded the search for alternative insecticidal therapies, and exploration of the mechanisms of action of chemically defined insecticides [13]. Accompanying this was research on control strategies at the community level, particularly in the UK, using physical removal of head lice [14]. In the 21st century research on treatments expanded to include topical silicon-based oils [15] and oral ivermectin [16,17]. Other research included the psychological effect of pediculosis [18] and beliefs and practices of community members from developed and developing countries [19-21].

Various developed countries have published guidelines for management and control of head lice, largely based on the evidence generated by research. A set of international guidelines provided general guidance across many sectors from government to parents [22]. The importance of local data was emphasised for: 1) understanding the pattern of insecticide resistance against the locally marketed products; 2) epidemiological studies in situations where control is ineffective; 3) formulating local recommendations which recognised local cultural factors. The guidelines emphasised the important role of universities and other research institutions in conducting research across the spectrum of pediculosis in their own country.

Although most head lice research is from a developed country perspective, some of the emerging economies, especially in Latin America, Asia and the Middle East, have begun to publish original research. However, head lice research in the developing countries in Africa and Oceania remains rare [2]. The unspoken assumption seems to be that these regions have bigger and more important issues to deal with than pediculosis.

Anecdotal evidence suggests that pediculosis is widespread in the 22 PICTs. However, there appears to be little evidence to support this statement apart from the frequent scene of heads being manually searched and head lice crushed or even eaten (Figure 1).

The biology of head lice (*Pediculus humanus* var *capitis*) is the same globally, but the epidemiology varies with society and cultural behaviour. Feasible treatment options are highly context dependent owing to access to pediculocides, affordability and culturally acceptable behaviour (e.g., head shaving). Insecticide resistance patterns globally are correlated with the use of topical insecticides [23], but these are rarely used in poor societies [20]. Since controlling pediculosis is not a simple task, parents experience difficulty in managing the many aspects of pediculosis control [19,20]. Head lice guidelines that are practical and tailored to fit each groups' special circumstances can assist parents, often through ensuring that health care providers communicate appropriate and relevant advice.

Pediculosis due to head lice is classified as one of the six Epidermal Parasitic Skin Diseases, an informal subcategory of the Neglected Tropical Diseases [24]. In developing countries, pediculosis appears often to be dismissed as being too minor a problem for health departments faced with managing overwhelming health problems with limited resources. However, the majority of parents and guardians in resource poor countries would arguably prefer feasible options to assist them to manage pediculosis [20].

Since we had difficulty locating evidence to inform local head lice guidelines in the Solomon Islands, we decided to do a systematic literature review of pediculosis in the PICTs. The aim of this review was to evaluate evidence in the peer reviewed literature on pediculosis due to head lice in the 22 nations that form the PICTs.

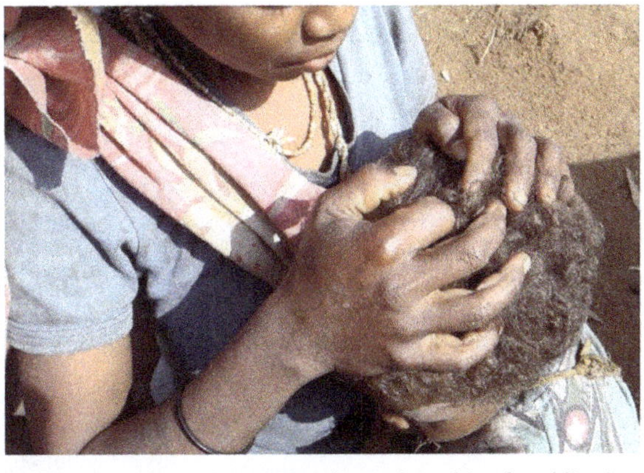

Figure 1 Teenage girl searching for and crushing head lice in a young child (East Kwaio mountains, Malaita Province, Solomon Islands).

Methods

The PRISMA methodology was used to search the peer-reviewed literature [25]. Search terms used were (pediculosis OR head lice) AND the following countries individually: (American Samoa), (Cook Islands), Fiji, (French Polynesia), Guam, Kiribati, (Mariana Islands), (Marshall Islands), Micronesia, Nauru, (New Caledonia), Niue, Palau, (Papua New Guinea), Pitcairn, Samoa, (Solomon Islands), Tokelau, Tonga, Tuvalu, Vanuatu, and Wallis. The following electronic databases were searched between 10-22 August 2013: PubMed, CINAHL, Web of Science, Scopus, and Google Scholar. The reference lists of included papers were subsequently searched for additional papers not found by the database searches.

Inclusion criteria were: the topic of the publication was pediculosis or head lice; the report was about one or more of the 22 PICTs. Exclusion criteria were: i) not on topic; ii) publications on pediculosis not relevant to the country of the particular search even if the publication referred to another PICT since this record was captured under the other PICT; iii) no English title or abstract; iv) in grey literature (i.e., not in a peer reviewed journal or a monograph).

Based on titles irrelevant publications were rejected at country search level. Duplicates from different sources were then collapsed at country level. If content appeared relevant, abstracts were considered, non-relevant articles excluded and reasons for exclusion recorded. Full texts of all remaining publications were obtained and assessed.

The nature of the literature was classified as: i) original research, ii) reviews, iii) program descriptions or iv) commentary/discussion paper using an adapted research identification schema with original research further classified as: (i) descriptive; (ii) measurement study; (iii) operations/intervention research [26].

Results

Five relevant publications were located from an original 28 hits from the database searches (Figure 2). Reasons for rejection of the 19 excluded papers were: i) not on topic = 11; ii) publications on pediculosis not relevant to the country of the particular search = 8.

The five included publications originated from three of the 22 PICTs (French Polynesia, Papua New Guinea (PNG), Solomon Islands) and are summarised in Table 1.

The only clinical trial was an unblinded single arm therapeutic trial of the efficacy of oral ivermectin in treating pediculosis in French Polynesia [27]. A large cross-sectional survey reported in 1985 examined 10,244 people in the Western Province of Solomon Islands for skin conditions [28]. It found that pediculosis was "universally present among both sexes and all ages". However, the prevalence of pediculosis was not determined; no additional details were provided. A genetic study on insecticide susceptibility of head lice used a very small sample of 3 lice from PNG [23]. Although it found that insecticide resistance genes were not present in these lice, it was not designed to assess the extent of resistance or decrease in susceptibility (if any) in PNG. Two other studies from PNG dealt with treatment of pediculosis. One was a case report of fatal poisoning from paraquat (a herbicide) misused to self-treat pediculosis [29]. The other was a brief comment that bark of a tree was used in Morobe Province to treat head lice [30]. No evidence on efficacy was provided.

Discussion

This review found only five publications on pediculosis or head lice from the 22 PICTs. The only epidemiological study was published more than 30 years ago and unfortunately did not quantify the prevalence of pediculosis [28].

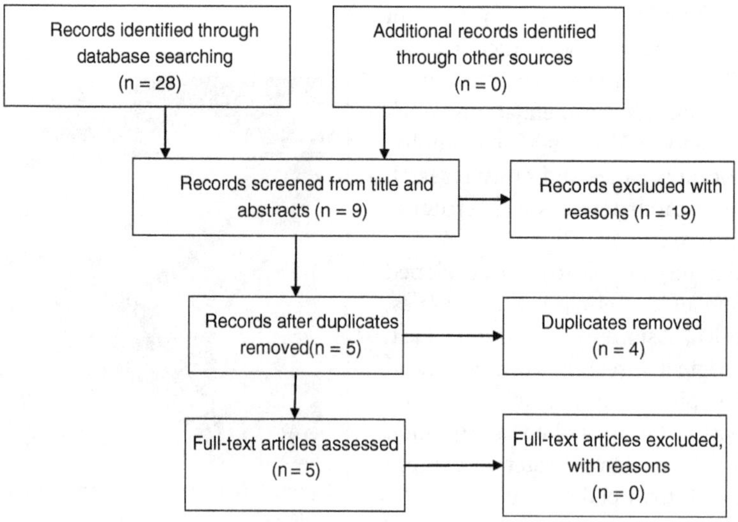

Figure 2 PRISMA flow chart of record retrieval and exclusion.

Table 1 Publications on head lice or pediculosis in Pacific Island Countries or Territories

Author (year) citation number	Content	Type of study	Participants	Country	Classification of study	Comment
Wohlfahrt (1982) [29]	Death with skin ulceration and respiratory failure after self-application of paraquat to head to treat pediculosis	Case report	1 adult male	Papua New Guinea (Western Highlands Province)	Original research; descriptive	No value in informing local guidelines
Eason & Tasman-Jones (1985) [28]	Pediculosis prevalence in Western Province	Cross sectional survey	10,224 total (5,160 < 15 years of age)	Solomon Islands (Western Province)	Original research; measurement	No value in informing local guidelines
Glaziou et al. (1994) [27]	Evaluating the efficacy of oral ivermectin (single oral dose of 0.2 mg/kg) to treat pediculosis	Unblinded single arm therapeutic trial	26 total – 2 males & 24 females aged 5-17 years	French Polynesia	Original research; intervention	Minimal value in informing local guidelines
Thomas (2006) [30]	Ethnomedicine review on use of bark from Galbulimima tree. Mixed with tobacco to treat head lice; no details	Second hand report	No participants	Papua New Guinea (Data collected from Morobe Province)	Commentary	Minimal value in informing local guidelines
Hodgdon et al. (2010) [23]	Genetic study of *kdr* resistance genes in head lice from many countries	Louse genetics	3 lice from 1 person	Papua New Guinea (location not given)	Original research; measurement	No value in informing local guidelines

Of four papers relevant to treatment of pediculosis, only one was a therapeutic trial [27]. This study demonstrated that lice in French Polynesia could be killed by oral ivermectin with at day 14 elimination of adult lice and nymphs in 100% and 43% of subjects respectively. Side effects were minimal, but the study had important limitations. Another paper found no permethrin resistance (*kdr*) genes in three PNG head lice and the other two treatment papers were case reports. All five reviewed publications have minimal or no value for planning head lice control strategies or informing local guidelines.

One possible limitation to this review is that this systematic review did not include non-peer reviewed literature. However, since the goal was to determine what evidence was available to formulate strategies and guidelines, the focus on peer-reviewed sources would be expected to provide the highest level of evidence available.

If we adopt the perspective of a ministry of health in any country in the PICTs and use the categories of research evidence originally proposed, what country specific data are needed? The international guidelines are useful here, but they recommend further research in all aspects of head lice and their control [22]. The only research topic that is prioritised in the international guidelines is resistance to locally available pharmaceutical products.

We do not consider that research on all aspects of pediculosis control is needed in resource poor countries where research funds and skills are in short supply. The following comments highlight important gaps in understanding in areas where we consider that local research will add useful evidence to guide pediculosis control. Although the comments are targeted towards the PICTs, they possibly have value for other developing countries that do little research on pediculosis.

The biology of head lice is well known and the available knowledge can be assumed to be relevant locally. Research on biology is arguably not required at the country level. Epidemiology is location specific and in the absence of any evidence, making assumptions from another countries' data is unreliable. The impact of pediculosis on individuals is not well known globally, but presumably there will be lower levels of anxiety in people in the PICTs than in developed countries. There is less need to research this aspect. Diagnostic techniques are well researched and this knowledge can be adopted locally in the PICTs. However, which techniques are feasible is influenced by local socio-economic factors. For example, the baseline diagnostic technique in the PICTs is visual census, with access to nit combs and conditioner being uncommon. Detection of lice by use of conditioner and nit comb is the most sensitive diagnostic technique; however, affordability of and access to conditioner and nit combs in the PICTs make this diagnostic technique inaccessible to most. Research is needed on what diagnostic techniques are feasible and acceptable in the PICTs.

Treatment of pediculosis in the PICTs is anecdotally reported to be largely by physical capture of lice (Figure 1), with very limited access to and use of pharmaceuticals. For example, in the Solomon Islands topical 1% permethrin is available from the Ministry of Health by prescription only. Cost of treatment relative to income is a critical factor in choice of therapy and must be considered as evidence in formulating government recommendations, particularly for societies with low average incomes like in the PICTs. Local research on access to and affordability of commercially available treatments is required. Assumptions on the efficacy of treatments based on research evidence from other countries will be unreliable; hence, local research is needed. In addition rural populations have local plant based treatments for pediculosis. These are accessible and inexpensive but local research is needed to test efficacy.

Country specific research on feasible management options for pediculosis is needed. The societal context is highly country specific. How people perceive pediculosis and what they want to do about it determines the feasibility of approaches to management and control [20]. Research is essential on this societal context. Research on effectiveness of policies is also needed. Of course the macro-policies of the ministries of health and education and the micro-policies of individual schools and other institutions should be based on relevant country-specific evidence. However, evaluation of policy interventions is essential and this can only be done by country-specific research. Strengthening the capacity of people within resource poor settings to undertake health research is critical to improving health equity and embedding mutuality throughout the research capacity strengthening process is beneficial [31,32].

Conclusion

We conclude that there is minimal current local evidence to guide decisions on head lice control in the Pacific Island Countries and Territories. We recommend that basic evidence be generated on: i) epidemiology; ii) knowledge, attitudes and practices of health care providers and community members; iii) efficacy of local commercially available pharmaceutical treatments and local customary treatments; iv) acceptability, accessibility and affordability of available treatment strategies, including non-pharmaceutical measures; and iv) appropriate control strategies for families, groups and institutions. We also recommend that the required research be done by local researchers based in the PICTs, supported by researchers experienced in head lice research, using a two way research capacity strengthening model [30]. The research should have an operational focus to provide results that will assist health decision makers to develop feasible national guidelines and residents of these nations to have access to relevant knowledge and resources to control head lice.

Competing interests

All authors declare that they have no competing interests.

Authors' contributions

RS designed the review, carried out the literature search, assessed retrieved papers and drafted the manuscript. HH designed the review, and assessed the retrieved papers. DC assessed the retrieved papers. PM assessed the retrieved papers. All authors contributed to the final manuscript and all read and approved the final manuscript.

Acknowledgements

This study received financial support from TDR, the Special Programme for Research and Training in Tropical Diseases, co-sponsored by UNICEF, UNDP, the World Bank and WHO (grant 1-811001688) and Tropical Health Solutions Pty Ltd.

Author details

[1]College of Public Health, Medical and Veterinary Sciences, James Cook University, Townsville 4811, Australia. [2]Tropical Health Solutions, 72 Kokoda St, Idalia, Townsville 4811, Australia. [3]Atoifi College of Nursing, Atoifi, Malaita Province, Solomon Islands. [4]Office of Public Health Studies, University of Hawaii at Manoa, 1960 East-West Rd, Biomed Building #T103, Honolulu, HI 96822, USA. [5]Health Protection, Hunter New England Population Health, Tamworth 2340, Australia.

References

1. Gratz NG: *Human lice their prevalence, control and resistance to insecticides: a review 1985-1997.* Geneva: World Health Organization; 1997.
2. Falagas ME, Matthaiou DK, Rafailidis PI, Panos G, Pappas G: **Worldwide prevalence of head lice.** *Emerg Infect Dis* 2008, **14:**1493–1494. doi:10.3201/eid1409.080368.
3. Shin E, Guk S, Kim H, Lee S, Chair J: **Trends in parasitic disease in the Republic of Korea.** *Trends Parasitol* 2007, **24:**143–150. doi:10.1016/j.pt.2007.12.003.
4. Steinmann P, Utzinger J, Du ZW, Zhou XN: **Multiparasitism a neglected reality on global, regional and local scale.** *Adv Parasitol* 2010, **73:**21–50. doi:10.1016/S0065-308X(10)73002-5.
5. Simons E, Mort M, Dabbagh A, Strebel P, Wolfson L: **Strategic planning for measles control: using data to inform optimal vaccination strategies.** *J Infect Dis* 2011, **204**(Suppl 1):S28–S34. doi:10.1093/infdis/jir095.
6. Stover J, Brown T, Marston M: **Updates to the Spectrum/Estimation and Projection Package (EPP) model to estimate HIV trends for adults and children.** *Sex Transm Infect* 2012, **88**(Suppl 2):i11–i16. doi:10.1136/sextrans-2012-050640.
7. Govere JM, Speare R, Durrheim DN: **The prevalence of pediculosis in rural South African school children.** *S Afr J Sci* 2003, **99:**21–23.
8. Nuttal GHF: **The biology of *Pediculus humanus*.** *Parasitol* 1917, **10:**181–185.
9. Buxton PA: *The louse: an account of the lice which infest man, their medical importance and control.* London: Edward Arnold & Co; 1947.
10. Busvine JR, Burn JL, Gamlin R: **Experiments with DDT and *gamma*-BHC (Gammexane) for use against head lice.** *Med Officer* 1948, **79:**121–127.
11. Maunder JW: **Resistance to organochlorine insecticides in head lice, and trials using alternative compounds.** *Med Officer* 1971, **125:**27–29.
12. Mumcuoglu KY, Hemingway J, Miller J, Ioffe-Uspensky I, Klaus S, Ben-Ishai F, Galun R: **Permethrin resistance in the head louse *Pediculus capitis* from Israel.** *Med Vet Entomol* 1995, **9:**427–432, 447. PMID:8541597.
13. Heukelbach J, Canyon DV, Oliveira FA, Muller R, Speare R: ***In vitro* efficacy of over-the-counter botanical pediculicides against the head louse *Pediculus humanus* var *capitis* based on a stringent standard for mortality assessment.** *Med Vet Entomol* 2008, **22:**264–272. doi:10.1111/j.1365-2915.2008.00738.x.
14. Ibarra J, Fry F, Wickenden C, Jenner M, Franks A: **The impact of well-developed preventative strategies on the eradication of head lice.** *Perspect Public Health* 2009, **129:**165–173. doi:10.1177/1466424008094804.
15. Burgess IF, Brunton ER, Burgess NA: **Single application of 4% dimeticone liquid gel versus two applications of 1% permethrin creme rinse for treatment of head louse infestation: A randomised controlled trial.** *BMC Dermatol* 2013, **13:**5. doi:10.1186/1471-5945-13-5.
16. Currie MJ, Reynolds GJ, Glasgow NJ, Bowden FJ: **A pilot study of the use of oral ivermectin to treat head lice in primary school students in Australia.** *Pediatric Dermatol* 2010, **27:**595–599. doi:10.1111/j.1525-1470.2010.01317.x.
17. Pilger D, Heukelbach J, Khakban A, Oliveira FA, Fengler G, Feldmeier H: **Household-wide ivermectin treatment for head lice in an impoverished community: randomized observer-blinded controlled trial.** *Bull World Health Organ* 2010, **88:**90–96. doi:10.2471/BLT.08.051656.
18. Parison J, Canyon D, Speare R: **Head lice: the feelings people have.** *Int J Dermatol* 2013, **52:**169–171. doi:10.1111/j.1365-4632.2011.05300.x.
19. Parison J, Speare R, Canyon DV: **Uncovering family experiences with head lice: the difficulties of eradication.** *Open Dermatol J* 2008, **2:**9–17.

20. Heukelbach J, Ugbomoiko US: **Knowledge, attitudes and practices regarding head lice infestations in rural Nigeria.** *J Infect Dis Child* 2011, **5:**652–657. doi:10.3855/jidc.1746 PMID:21918306.
21. Rukke BA, Birkemoe T, Soleng A, Lindstedt HH, Ottesen P: **Head lice in Norwegian households: actions taken, costs and knowledge.** *PLoS One* 2012, **7:**e32686. doi:10.1371/journal.pone.0032686.
22. Mumcuoglu KY, Barker SC, Burgess IE, Combescot-Lang C, Dalgleish RC, Larsen KS, Miller J, Roberts RJ, Taylan-Ozkan A: **International guidelines for effective control of head louse infestations.** *J Drugs Dermatol* 2007, **6:**409–414. PMID:17668538.
23. Hodgdon HE, Yoon KS, Previte DJ, Kim HJ, Aboelghar GE, Leed SH, Clarka JM: **Determination of knockdown resistance allele frequencies in global human head louse populations using the serial invasive signal amplification reaction.** *Pest Manag Sci* 2010, **66:**1031–1040. doi:10.1002/ps.1979.
24. Feldmeier H, Heukelbach J: **Epidermal parasitic skin diseases: a neglected category of poverty-associated plagues.** *Bull World Health Organ* 2009, **87:**152–159. doi:10.2471/BLT.07.047308.
25. PRISMA: **[Internet] PRISMA statement.** http://www.prisma-statement.org/.
26. Redman-MacLaren ML, MacLaren DJ, Asugeni R, Fa'anuabae CE, Harrington H, Muse A, Speare R, Clough AR: **"We can move forward": challenging historical inequity in public health research in Solomon Islands.** *Inter J Equity Health* 2010, **9:**25. doi:10.1186/1475-9276-9-25.
27. Glaziou P, Nyguyen LN, Moulia-Pelat JP, Cartel JL, Martin PM: **Efficacy of ivermectin for the treatment of head lice (Pediculosis capitis).** *Trop Med Parasitol* 1994, **45:**253–254. PMID:7899799.
28. Eason RJ, Tasman-Jones T: **Resurgent yaws and other skin diseases in the Western Province of the Solomon Islands.** *P N G Med J* 1985, **28:**247–250. PMID:2940770.
29. Wohlfahrt DJ: **Fatal paraquat poisonings after skin absorption.** *Med J Aust* 1982, **1:**512–513. PMID:7099093.
30. Thomas B: **Galbulimima bark and ethnomedicine in Papua New Guinea.** *P N G Med J* 2006, **49:**57–59. PMID:18396614.
31. Mony PK, Kurpad A, Vaz M: **Capacity building in collaborative research is essential.** *Br Med J* 2005, **331:**843–844. doi:10.1136/bmj.331.7520.843-b.
32. Redman-MacLaren ML, MacLaren DJ, Humpress H, Asugeni R, Timothy-Harrington R, Kekeubata K, Speare R: **Mutual research capacity strengthening: a qualitative study of two-way partnerships in public health research in Solomon Islands.** *Int J Equity Health* 2012, **11:**79. doi:10.1186/1475-9276-11-79.

16

Exposure to indoor tanning in France: a population based study

Tarik Benmarhnia, Christophe Léon and François Beck*

Abstract

Background: Tanning lamp sessions have increased in Europe in recent years. Recent epidemiological studies have confirmed a proven link between melanoma and artificial UV exposure. However, in France, little information is available to determine the exposure of the population. This article presents the results from the 'Baromètre cancer 2010' concerning the proportion of users exposed to artificial UV radiation in France, their characteristics and level of information on the risks associated.

Methods: A two stage random sampling telephone survey assisted by CATI system (household, individual) was performed from 3 April 2010 to 7 August 2010 on a sample of 3,359 people aged 15 to 75 years old.

Results: In 2010, 13.4% of the French population reported to have tanning lamp sessions at least once in their lifetime and 3.5% of the total population reported the use of artificial UV radiation over the last twelve months. Exposure over the last twelve months is most commonly seen among females (5.0%) and young population between 20–25 years old (9.6%). In addition, 3.5% of those under 18 years report having attended UV booths at least once during their lifetime even though they are forbidden to minors. Moreover, more than one the third of users reported more than 10 exposures within a year. The places of exposure cited most often were beauty salons (50%) and tanning centers (46%). Only 49.2% of those surveyed felt that they were well informed on the risks of cancer associated with UV booths. Furthermore, the population was found to have misconceptions about artificial UV radiation. One quarter of the population, believe that artificial UV radiation use before vacation protects the skin from sunburn.

Conclusions: This first study on artificial UV radiation exposure in France has better quantified and characterized the users. It has also defined the state of knowledge and the perception of risk by the general French population. This work will contribute to determine actions of prevention to reduce cancer risk related to artificial UV radiation.

Keywords: Artificial UV radiation, Survey, Random sampling, Exposure, Opinions, Knowledge, Beliefs

Background

The western population's craze for sun since the 1980s has led to the rapid expansion of tanning sessions. The market for artificial UV tanning is not as large in France as in other European countries (Germany, Italy and Scandinavian countries).

This sector seems nonetheless poised to grow significantly in the future. A 2010 census estimated nearly 18,000 listed UV booths nationwide [1].

In 2004, in a telephone survey conducted by the National Institute for Prevention and Health Education (INPES) with a sample of 1002 people aged 15 and over, 55% of French people said they like to be tanned; 19% reported frequent sun exposure, 17% used cosmetics "tanning accelerators" (Monoi, oil, etc..) and 3% made tanning lamp sessions [2].

Skin cancers (basal cell, carcinoma, squamous cell carcinoma and melanoma) are the most common cancers, with nearly 80,000 new cases a year in France. They are also among the types of cancer that have increased the most over the last 50 years. The most severe form called cutaneous melanoma has seen its number of new cases triple between 1980 and 2005 [3]. According to the International Agency for Research on Cancer (IARC), nearly 70% of cutaneous melanoma cases are caused by sun exposure [4]. Recent epidemiological studies have confirmed

* Correspondence: francois.beck@inpes.sante.fr
National Institute for Prevention and Health Education (INPES), 42, Bld de la Libération, St Denis Cedex 93203, France

a proven link between melanoma and artificial UV exposure. An IARC meta-analysis published in 2006 found the risk of melanoma is increased by 75% when the first exposure is before the age of 35 years (RR = 1.75 with CI 95%: 1.35-2.26) [5]. Moreover, two recent systematic reviews and meta-analysis found that sunbed use is associated with a significant increase in risk of melanoma, basal and squamous cell skin cancer [6,7]. They also only found that the risk is higher with use in early life.

Advances in scientific knowledge on the carcinogenic effects of UV rays (UVA and UVB) led the IARC, in July 2009, to include artificial UV radiation in the group of confirmed carcinogens for humans (group 1), just like radiation from the sun [8].

These last years, some studies have reported the frequency of tanning bed use in different contexts [9,10]. They reported the prevalence of tanning bed use, individual characteristics associated with this practice. For example, Börner et al. [9], found positive relationships of appearance and health related beliefs with tanning bed use and some misconceptions in users about the positive effect of artificial UV radiation A systematic literature review reported that users are characterized by a lack of knowledge about health risks of UV, and prompted by the frequent use of sunbeds by friends or family members and the experience of positive emotions and relaxation by indoor tanning [11]. These characteristics are context dependant however [12], and it is important to study specific user profiles in the French context, given the fact that today, limited data are available to accurately describe the frequency of use of UV booths in France and user profiles. Level of knowledge about the risks associated with artificial UV radiation as well as the reasons that bring a certain clientele to use UV booths are poorly documented. For the first time as part of this study, the French population was surveyed on its use of tanning sessions. The first goal was to determine the proportion of French users of artificial UV radiation as well as their characteristics and level of knowledge of the risks associated with artificial UV use. Some local studies have explored beliefs and practices about tanning bed use in France, but never in a population-based study [13,14]. This study provides a first look at the national current situation among 15–75 year olds, which will eventually help us to evaluate changes in exposure of the population as a result of future regulatory, information or risk awareness actions.

Methods

The 'Baromètre Cancer 2010' is a two-stage random sampling survey (household then individual) performed using a *Computer-Assisted Telephone Interviewing* (CATI) system. The survey, assigned to GFK-ISL Institute, was carried out from 3 April to 7 August 2010 [15].

For a survey frame as exhaustive as possible, 'Baromètre Cancer 2010' has integrated, in addition to households with a fixed line (even those ex-directory), households contactable by mobile phone only and those with unbundled ADSL access. Phone numbers were generated randomly in order to be able to interview households corresponding to unlisted phone numbers. The study protocol included a formal request to participate, explaining the objectives of the study that was delivered by mail before (or after for subjects with confidential numbers whose address was unknown) the first telephone call. Eligible households were required to include at least one person in the study age group (15 to 75 years old) and speak French. Within the household, the person surveyed was randomly selected from among the eligible family members using the next-birthday method [16]. Anonymity and respect of privacy were protected by a procedure that deleted the phone numbers.

The data were weighted by the number of eligible individuals and phone lines in a household and were also adjusted for 2008 French population structure (available from the National Institute of Statistics and Economic Studies) according to age, gender, educational level, geographical region, urbanization level and phone equipment. Verbal consent from participants was asked at the survey beginning and the project obtained ethics approval from the French commission on data privacy and public liberties (CNIL - *Commission Nationale Informatique et Liberté*). As with all French telephone surveys, the participation of persons solicited was more difficult than for previous waves: refusal rate was about 40% for both samples (mobile and landline) [17]. For the questionnaire on exposure to artificial UV radiation a total of 3,359 people aged 15 to 75 years old were interviewed. The questionnaire lasted on average 36 minutes.

Statistical analyzes were performed with the software Stata (Version 10SE). The calculation of confidence intervals and comparison tests were performed using the statistic used in surveys by random selection. Chi-square test was used for comparisons of categorical variables and the variables in classes ordered with $p = 0.05$ for maximum significance level. A logistical regression allowed quantifying with precision relations between variables, controlling the effects of the model structure.

Results

Sociodemographic characteristics of people having tanning sessions during their lifetime

In total, 13.4% (n = 517) of the people surveyed reported having used artificial UV radiation during their lifetime. Such use was associated with striking sociodemographic characteristics. Gender appears to be one of the most influential factors, women have already been exposed nearly 3 times more than men (19.4% vs. 7.1%; $p < 0.001$). The differences in practice according to gender were observed for the age groups comprised between 20 and 75 years of age (Figure 1). After 45 years old, women are 4 times exposed than men (17.8% vs. 4.7%; p < 0,001) whereas before 45 years old they are 2 times (20.8% vs. 9.1%; p < 0,001). One alarming observation concerned use in people below the age of 18 years: although the use of UV booths is prohibited for minors, 3.5% of them reported having used one during their lifetime.

UV use is often associated with the social level of individuals. The percentage of people having used UV radiation during their lifetime increased with the income per consumption unit (29.8% for women with an income above 1,800 Euros per consumption unit). Though this was true for women (p < 0.001), the trend was not significant in men.

People without a high school degree used UV radiation less during their lifetime than others (9.9% vs. 18.3% respectively; p < 0.001).

Exposure to artificial UV radiation over the last 12 months

In addition to data on the exposure to sunbed use at least once during a lifetime, it is important to determine current use (over the last 12 months) as well as the frequency of exposure.

Over the last 12 months prior to the survey, 3.5% of the people surveyed reported having used sunbed use (n = 122), which represents slightly more than a quarter of people who have been exposed to UV during their lifetime. Again here, use of this practice is more pronounced in women than in men (5.0% vs. 2.0% respectively; p < 0.001) (Figure 2). In 2010, the practice predominated in the young population of 20–25 year olds with exposure over the last 12 months of 13.7% in women compared to 6.1% in men (p < 0.05). People 25 years old and above were much less concerned. The distribution of recent exposures also followed a gradient according to income.

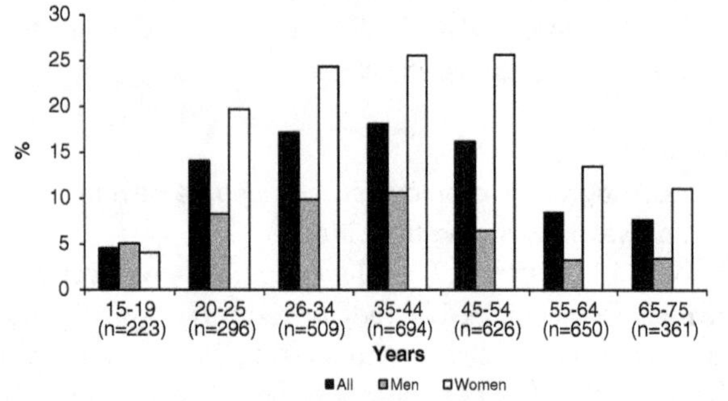

Figure 1 Practice of artificial UV tanning during lifetime among the 15–75 years old group by sex and age.

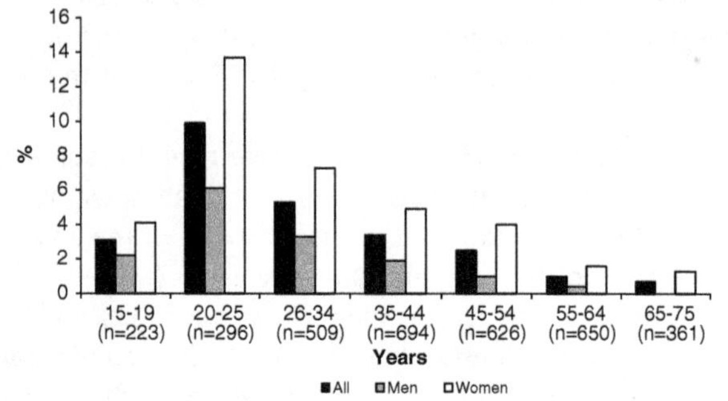

Figure 2 Practice of artificial tanning in the past 12 months among 15–75 years old group by sex and age.

Among people having used sunbed over the last 12 months, we observed large variations in the frequency of use. While 19.4% were only exposed once during the year, 26.4% were exposed more than once a month. Among the 20–25 year olds, 22.2% were exposed once during the year and 26.2% were exposed more than once a month (without significant difference between the age groups).

Over the last 12 months prior to the survey, we observed the same proportion of people that used such equipment between 1 and 3 times (29.3%) and more than 10 times (32.6%). This suggests two types of behaviour that are quite distinct. The first corresponds to occasional use (fewer than 3 times a year) and the second represents regular use (more than 10 times a year).

Places of exposure to artificial UV

One of the characteristics of sunbed use is the diversity of locations that offer this service (tanning centers, beauty salons, gyms, pools, etc.). For this reason, the (no exclusive) question regarding the places of exposure was asked to users in order to evaluate their habits (Table 1). Tanning centers and beauty salons were preferred by people having used sunbed over the last 12 months (46% and 50% of those surveyed reported having gone to these locations, respectively).Among people aged under 18 years old (n = 3), all of them used sunbed in tanning centers.

Table 1 Locations of exposure to artificial UV radiation (several possible responses)

Places of exposure	*Proportion of users (n = 122)*
Beauty salons	50%
Tanning centres	46%
Pools or spas	4.5%
Doctor's office	3.5%
Gyms	2.6%
Home	1.5%

Knowledge and popular misconceptions relative to cancer risks associated with UV booths

This study shows that 49.2% of the people surveyed felt that they were well informed on the risks of cancer associated with UV booths (52.7% of women vs. 45.4% of men; p < 0.001).

The people who have used sunbed over the last 12 months believe that they are better informed on the risks of cancer than people who haven't had tanning sessions (61.7% vs. 47.7%; p < 0.05).

In total, 89.2% of the people surveyed believed that exposure to sunbed is a possible cause of cancer. The people having used sunbed during their lifetime were slightly less, in proportion, than the others to take into account the risks of cancer (85.9% vs. 89.7%; p < 0.05).

Statement: "Using UV before going on vacations helps prepare the skin to protect it from sunburns". 24.1% agreed with this statement, without any significant difference by gender and age. On the other hand, marked differences were observed between the group of people having used UV radiation and the group of people having never used sunbed. 42.9% of the first group agreed with this statement, compared with 21.2% in the second group (p < 0.001). Finally, there was no significant difference between sunbed regular users (more than 10 times) (48.9% agreed with this statement) compared with 61.0% among sunbed occasional users (fewer than 3 times a year).

Determining factors of artificial UV exposure

The determining factors of UV exposure over the last 12 months were analyzed according to the level of information and popular misconceptions relative to the risks of cancer associated with artificial sunbed use, while controlling the structure effects related to sex, age and household income (Table 2). Analysis of the determining factors of exposure identified certain types of users. First of all, we found a clear difference between men and women (OR = 2.8 [1.7; 4.4], where women are much larger consumers of tanning equipment. Exposure to sunbed use is less important if age increase (OR = 0.95 [0.94; 0.96]). Furthermore, a clear social gradient was observed on the measured data. This practice seems associated with income, people with income greater than or equal to 1800 Euros by consummation unit and more are more concerned (OR = 2.3 [1.3; 4.1]). People feeling well informed (OR = 2.0 [1.3; 3.3]) and believing that sunbed use prepares the skin and avoids sunburn (OR = 4.3 [2.7; 6.7]) and do not know that UV is not a possible cause of cancer (OR = 1.7 [0.9; 3.1]) seem to favor their use.

Table 2 Logistic regression for the use of UV in the past 12 months (n = 3321)

Explicative variables	n observed	% weighted	OR	CI 95%
Sex		***		
man (ref.) (n = 1472)	30	2.0	- 1 -	
woman (n = 1887)	92	5.0	2,8	[1.7; 7.4]
Age (continous)				
(n = 3359)	122		0.95	[0.94; 0.96]
Household Income				
less than 1 100 Euros (ref.) (n = 921)	31	2.8	- 1 -	
1100 to 1800 Euros (n = 1156)	40	3.4	1.4	[0.8; 2.4]
1800 Euros and more (n = 1006)	41	4.5	2.3	[1.3; 4.1]
missing (n = 276)	10	3.8	1.1	[0.4; 2.9]
Information about the risks of cancer associated with UV		***		
poorly informed (ref.) (n = 1642)	42	2.6	- 1 -	
well informed (n = 1686)	80	4.6	2	[1.3; 3.3]
UV exposition is a possible cause of cancer		***		
yes (ref.) (n = 2966)	96	3.3	- 1 -	
no (n = 356)	25	5.6	1.7	[0.9; 3.1]
Using UV before going on vacations helps prepare the skin to protect it from sunburns		***		
don't agree (réf.) (n = 2501)	51	2.1	- 1 -	
agree (n = 820)	71	8.2	4.3	[2.7; 6.7]

*** : p < 0.001 ; ** : p < 0.01 ; * p < 0.05; results obtained by Chi^2 test Pearson for the column % (percentage from bivariate analysis).
Hosmer-Lemeshow goodness-of-fit test:
F-adjusted test statistic = 1159.2532.
p-value = 0,000000.

Discussion

This study presents, for the first time, data on both artificial UV radiation exposure in the French population and on the perception of the risk for cancer, as well as tanning bed use determinants. Young women, between the ages to 20 and 25 years, are a group characterized by a frequent use as 13.7% of them was exposed over the last 12 months. Nearly one out of three users exposed over the last 12 months went to UV booths more than 10 times a year.

A number of limitations of this study should be noted. First, we had a refusal rate of 40%. This rate, which is current in recent French general population surveys, could be differential regarding to some sunbed use characteristics, and in this case could influence our results. However, we expect this bias is limited because the person surveyed was randomly selected and we can assume that this refusal response was randomly distributed in the population. Second, this study characterizes only the beliefs and practices about tanning bed use, but we did not include data on physical exposure to artificial UV (UV intensity combined with exposure time). In fact, the artificial UV tanning sector has been expanding for several years in many European countries. Although it is less developed in France, this market has shown signs of significant growth over the last ten years (increase in the number of devices available and increase in the number of specialized centers) [17]. Professionals in this sector are leading a very active communication campaign to attract new and increasingly younger clients, based on non-scientifically proven information. Many popular misconceptions are spread among the population such as "exposure to artificial UV radiation helps to prepare the skin for the sun and prevent sunburns" or the role of artificial UV in fighting vitamin D deficiencies. Any reference to a beneficial effect for health is prohibited by law ('Article 12 du décret n°97-617 du 30 mai 1997'). Yet, such information is commonly spread via internet and in many articles addressed to the general public. Moreover, European standard for cosmetic sunbeds, EN 60 335-2-27, states that information regarding risks of sunbed use shall be part of the users instruction [18]. These results suggest public health policies efforts in this way.

This study identified two highly distinct types of use. The first concerns people who use tanning beds occasionally. The second concerns people using such equipment frequently, often several times per month. Public health interventions will need to take into consideration the existence of both categories of users. In addition, we should highlight the existence of artificial UV use in a population below the age of 18 years, though this practice is forbidden as reported in a recent French study [19].

Regulatory control should thus be reinforced in order to put an end to the previously mentioned popular misconceptions by increasing awareness among the general population and users and informing them of the risks associated with this practice. The most important risks are health-related, such as, skin cancer, cataracts, the weakening of immune defenses and, in some cases, phototoxicity and photoallergy [4,17,20].

The aesthetic consequences of UVA exposure, such as photo-induced accelerated skin aging after 10-20 years, might also constitute a possible lever to reduce use of tanning booths. Prevention efforts could be implemented in association with recommendations for sun exposure, notably via health professionals (general physicians, dermatologists, pharmacists physiotherapists, nurses).

Moreover, other studies of this type should be conducted in the future to measure changes in prevalence, beliefs, knowledge and other tanning bed use determinants. Incorporating findings related to tanning dependency, peer group affiliation, media influences and other constructs will also improve our understanding and ability to develop efficacious interventions to reduce engagement in this health risk behavior.

A systematic review of intervention efforts to reduce indoor tanning was conducted and the authors [21] concluded that there was very limited research on indoor tanning interventions. Further studies should produce evidence based knowledge about the reduction to sunbed use exposure.

Conclusions

This study gives an overview of the current situation regarding practices, knowledge and perception of artificial UV associated risks among the general French population and proposes some possible options for prevention of cancer risks associated with artificial UV radiation. These population exposure results will serve to study the importance of artificial UV radiation in the progression of melanoma incidence in France and in Europe. It could also be interesting to investigate the age of first use as the 2006 IARC meta-analysis showed that exposure before the age of 35 led to a higher increase in the risk of melanoma and that the risk level also increased with longer periods of exposure [4].

Therefore, exposure to artificial UV radiation is truly a public health menace and challenge put before authorities [22]. Hence, it seems relevant to provide targeted information to users concerning the risks associated sunbed use and the risks of the sun and tanning booths in particular. Furthermore, European and national regulations controlling the artificial tanning sector should be enhanced.

Abreviations

UV: Ultra violet; INPES: Institut National de Prévention et d'Education à la Santé; IARC: International Agency for Research on Cancer; RR: Relative risk;

CATI: Computer-Assisted Telephone Interviewing; ADSL: Asymmetric digital subscriber line; INSEE: Institut National de la Statistique et des Etudes Economiques.

Competing interest

The authors declare they have no competing financial interests.

Authors' contributions

All authors contributed to the development of the study aims. CL realized statistical analyses and reviewed the final manuscript. FB supervised the study and acted as guarantor. TB wrote the first and final versions of the manuscript. All authors read and approved the final manuscript.

Acknowledgements

This study was supported financially by INPES funds in the context of the 'Baromètre Cancer 2010' realization. Some results have been previously published in French in the French journal "Bulletin Epidemiologique Hebdomadaire" We are grateful to Isabelle Tordjman and Julie Gaillot, from the Cancer National Institute (InCA) for their help in the first version of this manuscript.

References

1. Direction générale de la concurrence, de la consommation et de la répression des fraudes (DGCCRF): *Note d'information DGCCRF n° 2010–195 du 25 octobre 2010: recensement des appareils de bronzage UV sur le territoire national.* DGCCRF: Paris; 2010 [In French].
2. Bottéro J, Léon C, Fournier C: *Connaissances, attitudes et comportements vis-à-vis des risques liés à l'exposition aux ultraviolets, France, 2004. Bulletin Epidémiologique Hebdomadaire, 18 décembre 2007,* Volume 50. 2007:420–422. www.invs.sante.fr/beh/2007/50/beh_50_2007.pdf. [In french].
3. Belot A, Grosclaude P, Bossard N, Jougla E, Benhamou E, Delafosse P, Guizard AV, Molinié F, Danzon A, *et al*: **Cancer incidence and mortality in France over the period 1980–2005.** *Rev Epidemiol Santé Publique* 2008, **56**(3):159–75.
4. International agency for research on cancer (IARC): *Attribuable causes of cancer in France in the year 2000.* Lyon: IARC; 2007:177.
5. International agency for research on cancer (IARC): *Exposure to artificial UV radiation and skin cancer.* Lyon: IARC; 2006:76.
6. Boniol M, Autier P, Boyle P, Gandini S: **Cutaneous melanoma attributable to sunbed use: systematic review and meta-analysis.** *Br Med J* 2012, **345**:e4757.
7. Wehner MR, Shive ML, Chren MM, Han J, Qureshi AA, Linos E: **Indoor tanning and non-melanoma skin cancer: systematic review and meta-analysis.** *Br Med J* 2012, **345**:e5909.
8. El GF, Baan R, Straif K, Grosse Y, Secretan B, Bouvard V, *et al*: **A review of human carcinogens-part D: radiation.** *The Lancet Oncology* 2009, **10**(8):751–752.
9. Börner FU, Schütz H, Wiedemann P: **A population-based survey on tanning bed use in Germany.** *BMC Dermatol* 2009, **9**(1):6.
10. Heckman CJ, Manne SL, Kloss JD, Bass SB, Collins B, Lessin SR: **Beliefs and Intentions for Skin Protection and UV Exposure in Young Adults.** *Am J Heal Behav* 2011, **35**(6):699–711.
11. Schneider S, Zimmermann S, Diehl K, Breitbart EW, Greinert R: **Sunbed use in German adults: risk awareness does not correlate with behaviour.** *Acta dermato-venereologica* 2009, **89**(5):470–475.
12. Gordon LG, Hirst NG, Green AC, Neale RE: **Tanning behaviors and determinants of solarium use among indoor office workers in Queensland, Australia.** *J Heal Psychol* 2012, **17**(6):856–865.
13. Ezzedine K, Malvy D, Mauger E, Nageotte O, Galan P, Hercberg S, Guinot C: **Artificial and natural ultraviolet radiation exposure: beliefs and behaviour of 7200 French adults.** *J Eur Acad Dermatol Venereol* 2008, **22**(2):186–194.
14. Isvy A, Beauchet A, Saiag P, Mahé E: **Medical students and sun prevention: knowledge and behaviours in France.** *J Eur Acad Dermatol Venereol* 2012, **27**(2):e247–51.
15. Beck F, Gautier A: ***Baromètre cancer 2010****, INPES.* St Denis: coll. Baromètres santé; 2011:275 [In french].
16. Salmon CT, Nichols JS: **The next-birthday method of respondent selection.** *Public Opinion Quarterly* 1983, **47**(2):270–276.
17. Institut national du cancer (INCa): *Installation de bronzage UV: état des lieux des connaissances sur les risques de cancer et recommandation.* Boulogne Billancourt: INCa; 2010:62 [In French].
18. European Committee for Electrotechnical Standardisation, Household and similar electrical appliances – Safety: *Part 2–27: Particular requirements for appliances for skin exposure to ultraviolet and infrared radiation, EN 60335-2-27.* Brussels: CENELEC; 2010.
19. Tella E, Beauchet A, Vouldoukis I, Séi JF, Beaulieu P, Sigal ML, Mahé E: **French teenagers and artificial tanning.** *J Eur Acad Dermatol Venereol* 2012, : [Epub ahead of print].
20. Agence française de sécurité sanitaire environnementale (AFSSE), Institut de veille sanitaire (INVS), Agence française de sécurité sanitaire des produits de santé (AFSSAPS): *Rayonnements ultraviolets - État des connaissances sur l'exposition et les risques sanitaires.* Saint Maurice: INVS; 2005:168 [In french].
21. Turrisi R, Hillhouse J, Mallett K, Stapleton J, Robinson J: **A Systematic Review of Intervention Efforts to Reduce Indoor Tanning.** In *Shedding light on artificial tanning.* Edited by Heckman C, Manne S. New York: Springer; 2012:135–146.
22. De Maleissye MF, Fay-Chatelard F, Beauchet A, Saiag P, Mahé E: **Compliance with indoor tanning advertising regulations in France.** *Br J Dermatol* 2011, **64**:880–2.

17

Effect of etanercept therapy on psoriasis symptoms in patients from Latin America, Central Europe, and Asia: a subset analysis of the PRISTINE trial

L. Kemeny[1*], M. Amaya[2], P. Cetkovska[3], N. Rajatanavin[4], W-R. Lee[5], A. Szumski[6], L. Marshall[6], E. Y. Mahgoub[6] and E. Aldinç[7]

Abstract

Background: Psoriasis prevalence and characteristics in Asia, Central Europe, and Latin America have not been thoroughly investigated and there are no large trials for biologic treatments for patients from these regions. The goal of this analysis was to report clinical response to anti-tumor necrosis factor-alpha treatment in these patients.

Methods: Patients from Argentina, Czech Republic, Hungary, Mexico, Taiwan, and Thailand ($N = 171$) were included in this subset analysis of the PRISTINE trial. Patients with stable moderate-to-severe plaque psoriasis were blinded and randomized to receive etanercept 50 mg once weekly (QW) or biweekly (BIW) for 12 weeks, followed by 12 weeks of open-label QW treatment with etanercept 50 mg through week 24 (QW/QW vs. BIW/QW). Concomitant methotrexate (≤20 mg/week) and mild topical corticosteroids or other agents were permitted at the physician's discretion, in accordance with therapeutic practice.

Results: As early as week 8, 26.7 % in the etanercept QW group and 44.0 % in the BIW group achieved Psoriasis Area and Severity Index (PASI) 75. At weeks 12 and 24, respectively, PASI 75 increased to 39.5 % and 62.8 % in the QW/QW group and 66.7 % and 83.3 % in the BIW/QW group. PASI 75 was significantly different between treatment groups from week 8 through the end of study ($p < 0.05$). The Kaplan-Meier estimate of the proportions achieving PASI 75 in QW/QW and BIW/QW groups, respectively, was 27.4 % and 45.8 % through week 8; 41.9 % and 68.7 % through week 12; and 72.5 % and 95.2 % through week 24.

Conclusions: Treatment with etanercept 50 mg provided rapid relief of psoriasis symptoms in patients from Asia, Central Europe, and Latin America. A more rapid response was observed in patients who received BIW treatment for the first 12 weeks which was sustained after reducing to QW dosing for the subsequent 12 weeks. Response rates were similar to those observed in the overall PRISTINE population.

Keywords: Etanercept, Psoriasis treatment, Asia, Central Europe, Latin America

* Correspondence: Kemeny.lajos@med.u-szeged.hu
[1]Department of Dermatology and Allergology, University of Szeged, Szeged, Hungary
Full list of author information is available at the end of the article

Background

Psoriasis is a chronic inflammatory skin condition characterized by exacerbations and remissions and estimated to affect approximately 125 million people (2–3 %) worldwide [1]. In the United States, where such data are available, the prevalence of psoriasis varies among ethnicity, with 0.47 % of Chinese [2], 1.3 % of African Americans and 1.6 % of Hispanic affected compared with 3.6 % of Caucasians [1]. As such, it is possible that patients from different parts of the world may respond differently to treatment.

The goal of treatment in psoriasis is to alleviate symptoms as rapidly as possible and maintain the response over time. Current treatment guidelines in both the United States and Europe support the combination of topical and systemic therapies, including biologic agents, in order to achieve these goals [3–6]. Although the effectiveness of biologic agents is well-established through clinical trials in the United States and Europe [5–7], these agents have not been studied extensively in many parts of the world.

The PRISTINE trial was a multinational, randomized, double-blind study in patients with moderate-to-severe plaque psoriasis in which investigators evaluated the efficacy and safety of two dosing regimens of etanercept [8]. This trial included patients from Argentina, Czech Republic, Hungary, Mexico, Taiwan, and Thailand. The objective of the subset analysis reported here was to evaluate the efficacy of etanercept therapy in patients from countries in Asia, Central Europe, and Latin America.

Methods

Study details

The details of the PRISTINE trial have been previously published [8]. Briefly, patients ≥18 years of age with stable moderate-to-severe plaque psoriasis were randomized to receive 50 mg etanercept subcutaneously either once weekly (QW) or twice weekly (BIW) for 12 weeks, after which all patients received open-label, 50 mg etanercept subcutaneously QW for an additional 12 weeks, i.e. QW/QW or QW/BIW dosing groups (Fig. 1). Concomitant methotrexate was allowed (≤20 mg/week) if doses were stable from at least 28 days prior to baseline through the end of study. Only mild topical corticosteroids were permitted on scalp, axillae and groin for first 12 weeks; topical medications (corticosteroids of all potencies, vitamin D analogues and combination products) were allowed as needed, at physician's discretion, during the second 12 weeks, consistent with therapeutic practice. Of the 273 patients enrolled in the PRISTINE trial, 171 patients were eligible for this subset analysis.

The study protocol was reviewed and approved by an independent Ethics Committee prior to initiation. The study was conducted in compliance with the ethical principles of the Declaration of Helsinki and the International Conference on Harmonization Good Clinical Practice Guidelines. The PRISTINE trial is registered on ClinicalTrials.gov, identifier NCT00663052.

Study endpoints

Primary efficacy was measured as the proportion of patients achieving 50 %, 75 %, or 90 % improvement in

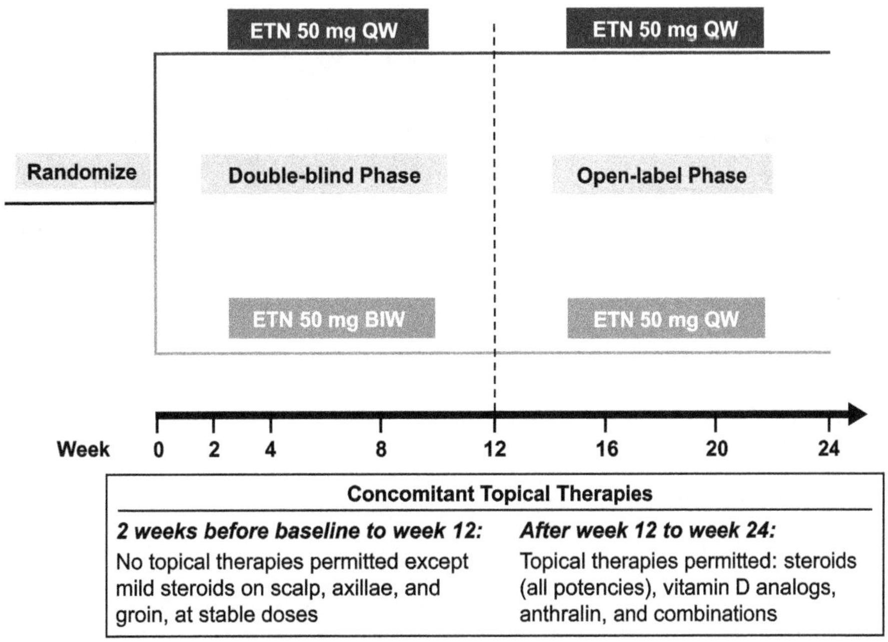

Fig. 1 PRISTINE study design. BIW: twice weekly; QW: once weekly

Psoriasais Area and Severity Index (PASI), PASI 50, PASI 75, and PASI 90, respectively, at weeks 8, 12, and 24. Other efficacy endpoints included the percentage of patients who achieved a status of "clear" or "almost clear" on the Physician's Global Assessment (PGA) of psoriasis, time to achieving PGA first "clear" or "almost clear" status, and percentage reduction in affected body surface area (BSA). Health-related quality of life (HRQoL) measures included Dermatology Life Quality Index (DLQI) [9], EuroQoL-5 Dimension (EQ-5D™) [10, 11], Work Productivity and Activity Impairment scale (WPAI) [12] and Functional Activity in Chronic Therapy (FACIT) [13].

Statistical analyses

For continuous efficacy parameters, treatment groups were compared in 1-way analysis of variance for baseline parameters or in analysis of covariance models of week 12/24 change from baseline parameters with treatment group as a factor and baseline measurement as a covariate. For dichotomous or categorical parameters, Fisher's exact test was used. The last observation was carried forward for patients for whom data were not available at any time point.

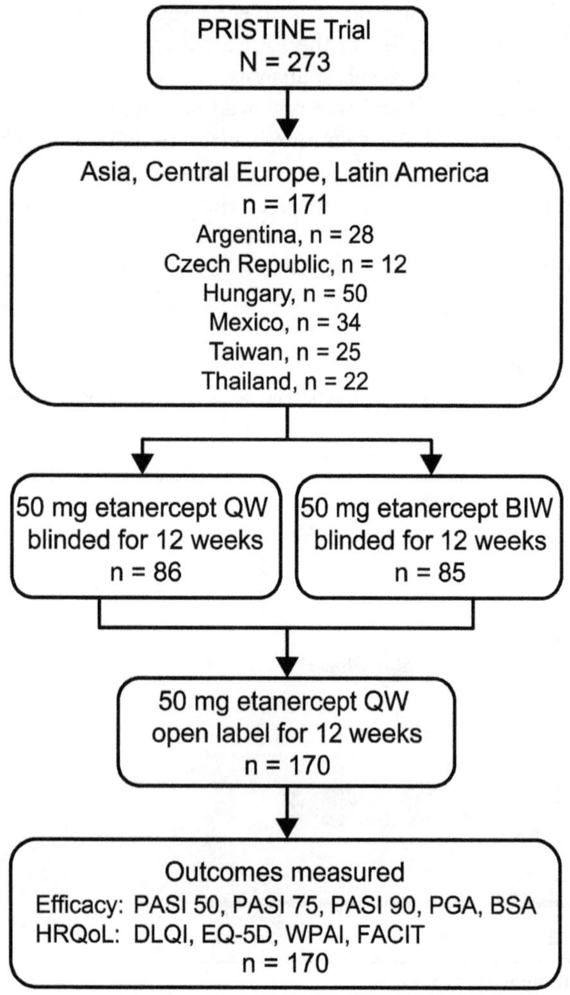

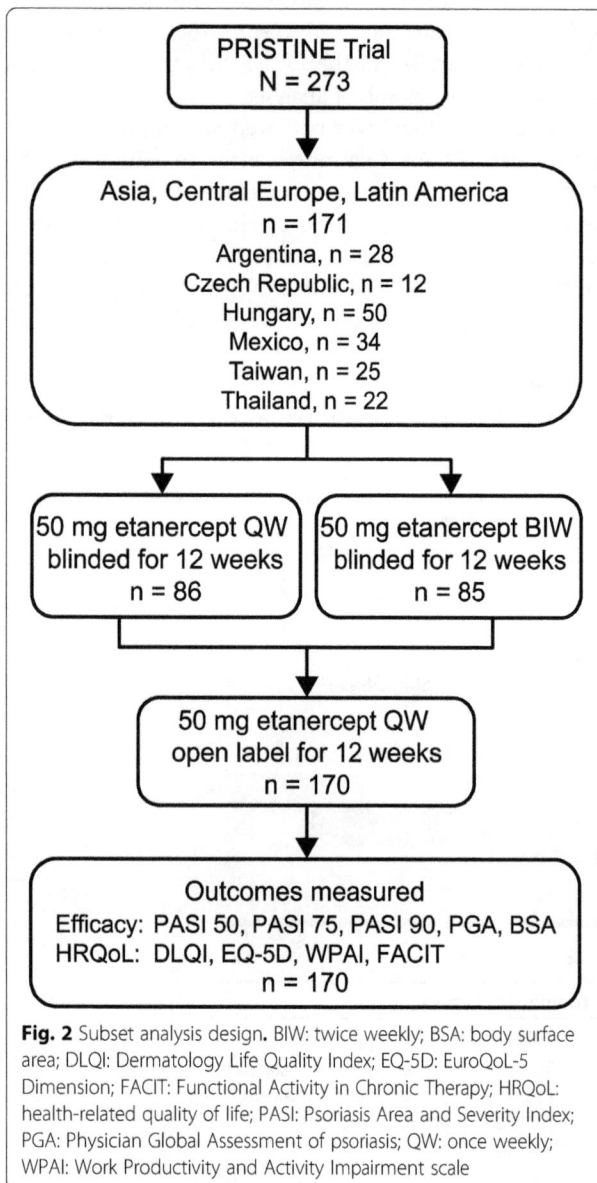

Fig. 2 Subset analysis design. BIW: twice weekly; BSA: body surface area; DLQI: Dermatology Life Quality Index; EQ-5D: EuroQoL-5 Dimension; FACIT: Functional Activity in Chronic Therapy; HRQoL: health-related quality of life; PASI: Psoriasis Area and Severity Index; PGA: Physician Global Assessment of psoriasis; QW: once weekly; WPAI: Work Productivity and Activity Impairment scale

Table 1 Baseline characteristics of all randomized patients from Asia, Central Europe, and Latin America ($n = 171^a$)

Characteristic	QW/QW ($n = 86$)	BIW/QW ($n = 85$)	p value
Age, years	45.8 (13.0)	44.8 (12.0)	0.581
Male gender, n (%)	64 (74.4)	63 (74.1)	1.000
Race, n (%)			0.898
White	44 (51.2)	46 (54.1)	
Asian	25 (29.1)	22 (25.9)	
Other	17 (19.8)	17 (20.0)	
Body weight, kg	87.3 (19.3)	84.5 (17.1)	0.311
Body mass index, kg/m^2			
Male	28.9 (5.1)	28.2 (4.4)	0.438
Female	32.8 (8.4)	30.4 (6.7)	0.295
Waist to hip ratio			
Male	1.0 (0.1)	1.0 (0.1)	0.289
Female	0.9 (0.1)	0.9 (0.1)	0.501
Current smokers, n (%)	29 (33.7)	25 (29.4)	0.622
Psoriasis disease duration, years	17.0 (10.8)	15.8 (7.8)	0.440
PASI total score	22.2 (9.7)	22.4 (9.4)	0.905
PGA score	3.4 (0.8)	3.4 (0.7)	0.955
Affected body surface area, %	38.0 (22.6)	36.9 (19.6)	0.743
History of psoriatic arthritis, n (%)	32 (37.2)	32 (37.7)	1.000
Duration of psoriatic arthritis, years	7.5 (7.1)	7.7 (5.6)	0.903
Secondary diagnosis of diabetes, n (%)	9 (10.5)	12 (14.1)	0.494
Secondary diagnosis of hypertension, n (%)	37 (43.0)	37 (43.5)	1.000
DLQI score	14.8 (8.4)	14.8 (7.2)	0.967
EQ-5D score	0.6 (0.3)	0.6 (0.3)	0.856
WPAI: % activity impairment due to problem	39.3 (31.2)	42.6 (30.5)	0.487
WPAI: % impairment while working due to problem	23.2 (25.0)	25.8 (24.8)	0.603
WPAI: % overall work impairment due to problem	27.1 (26.0)	27.1 (24.8)	0.999
WPAI: % work time missed due to problem	8.3 (20.7)	4.8 (19.5)	0.378
FACIT score	35.9 (11.4)	37.3 (9.4)	0.368

[a]Data are given as mean (SD) unless otherwise specified
BIW twice weekly, *DLQI* Dermatology Life Quality Index, *EQ-5D* EuroQOL 5 Dimension, *FACIT* Functional Activity in Chronic Therapy, *PASI* Psoriasis Area and Severity Index, *PGA* Physician Global Assessment of psoriasis, *QW* once weekly, *WPAI* Work Productivity and Activity Impairment scale

Results

Patients

Of the 273 patients enrolled in the PRISTINE trial, all 171 patients from Asia (Taiwan, $n = 25$; Thailand, $n = 22$), Central Europe (Czech Republic, $n = 12$; Hungary, $n = 50$), and Latin America (Argentina, $n = 28$; Mexico, $n = 34$) were included in the analysis. Since the number of patients from each region was small, they were pooled together for this subset analysis (Fig. 2).

The baseline demographics were similar between the etanercept 50 mg QW/QW and BIW/QW treatment groups (Table 1). In addition, the history of psoriasis, the extent of the disease, the presence and duration of psoriatic arthritis, and baseline HRQoL measures were also similar between the two groups of patients (Table 1). The baseline characteristics of the patients in this subset were comparable to those from the overall PRISTINE population (Table 2).

Table 2 Baseline characteristics of patients from Asia, Central Europe, and Latin America compared with total PRISTINE population[a]

Characteristic	Patients from Asia, Central Europe, and Latin America ($n = 171$)	Full PRISTINE population ($n = 273$)
Age, years	45.3 (12.5)	43.9 (12.7)
Male gender, n (%)	127 (74.3)	190 (69.6)
Ethnicity, n (%)		
White	90 (52.6)	174 (63.7)
Asian	47 (27.5)	64 (23.4)
Other	34 (19.9)	35 (12.8)
Body weight, kg	85.9 (18.3)	85.1 (18.6)
Body mass index, kg/m^2		
Male	28.5 (4.8)	28.3 (4.6)
Female	31.6 (7.6)	29.6 (7.5)
Waist to hip ratio		
Male	1.0 (0.1)	1.0 (0.1)
Female	0.9 (0.1)	0.9 (0.1)
Prior smokers, n (%)	57 (33.7)	109 (40.2)
Psoriasis disease duration, years	16.4 (9.4)	17.3 (10.6)
PASI total score	22.3 (9.6)	21.2 (9.4)
PGA score	3.4 (0.8)	3.4 (0.8)
Affected body surface area, %	37.4 (21.1)	33.0 (20.2)
History of psoriatic arthritis, n (%)	64 (37.4)	84 (30.8)
Duration of psoriatic arthritis, years	7.6 (6.3)	8.2 (8.0)
Secondary diagnosis of diabetes, n (%)	21 (12.3)	26 (9.5)
Secondary diagnosis of hypertension, n (%)	74 (43.3)	97 (35.5)

[a]Data are given as mean (standard deviation) unless otherwise specified
PASI Psoriasis Area and Severity Index, *PGA* Physician Global Assessment of psoriasis

Efficacy analyses

There were more patients achieving PASI 50, PASI 75, and PASI 90 in the group that received etanercept 50 mg BIW than in the group that received etanercept 50 mg QW over the time course of the study (Fig. 3). Statistically significant difference between the two treatment groups was evident as early as week 4 in PASI 50. Statistically significant difference in PASI 75 was observed by week 8 and in PASI 90 by week 12 (Fig. 3). After 12 weeks of treatment, i.e. at the end of the

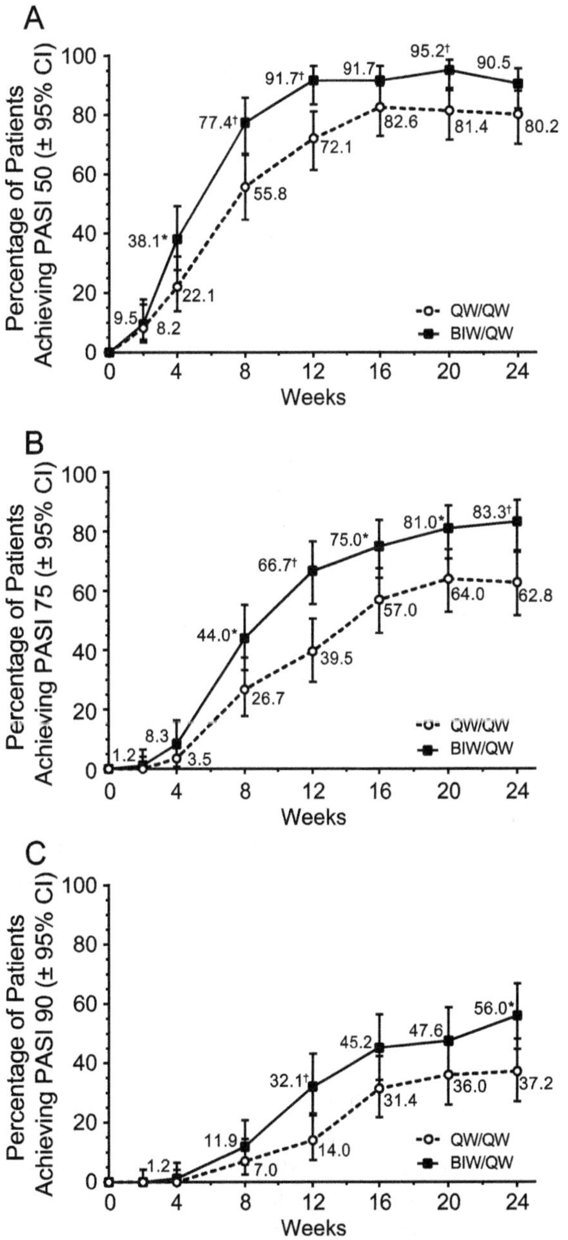

Fig. 3 Percentage of PASI 50 **a**, 75 **b**, and 90 **c** responders by treatment group (LOCF data). *$p < 0.05$; †$p < 0.01$. BIW: twice weekly; LOCF: last observation carried forward; PASI: Psoriasis Area and Severity Index; QW: once weekly

Table 3 Kaplan-Meier rate estimates: proportions of patients achieving first PASI 50, 75, and 90, by treatment group

PASI Response	% of Patients (95 % CI)					
	Week 0–8		Week 0–12		Week 0–24	
	QW/QW $n = 86$	BIW/QW $n = 84$	QW/QW $n = 86$	BIW/QW $n = 84$	QW/QW $n = 86$	BIW/QW $n = 84$
PASI 50	59.5\ (49.3, 70.0)	79.5 (70.3, 87.4)	75.5 (65.8, 84.1)	92.8 (85.9, 97.0)	90.5 (82.8, 95.6)	98.8 (94.2, 99.9)
PASI 75	27.4 (19.1, 38.3)	45.8 (35.8, 57.1)	41.9 (32.2, 53.2)	68.7 (58.6, 78.3)	72.5 (62.5, 81.6)	95.2 (89.1, 98.4)
PASI 90	7.2 (3.3, 15.2)	13.3 (7.6, 22.7)	15.6 (9.4, 25.3)	32.5 (23.6, 43.7)	47.7 (37.5, 59.1)	61.5 (51.2, 71.8)

BIW twice weekly, *CI* confidence interval, *PASI* Psoriasis Area and Severity Index, *QW* once weekly

blinded phase of the study, 72 %, 40 % and 14 % of patients in the QW/QW group and 92 %, 67 % and 32 % in the BIW/QW group achieved PASI 50, PASI 75 and PASI 90, respectively. Kaplan-Meier estimates of the proportions of patients achieving first PASI 50, PASI 75 and PASI 90 responses by weeks 8, 12 and 24 also indicate a strong beneficial response in both treatment groups (Table 3). Improvements from baseline were also observed in PGA and BSA scores ($p < 0.0001$) at weeks 12 and 24 in both treatment groups (Fig. 4). By week 12, 36 % and 56 % of patients in the QW/QW and BIW/QW groups, respectively, exhibited a PGA status of clear or almost clear (Table 4). By week 24, the number of patients with clear or almost clear status increased to 57 % and 71 % in the QW/QW and BIW/QW groups, respectively. For the achievement of first PGA of clear/almost clear response, there was a statistically significant difference between the time-to-event curves for the QW/QW and BIW/QW treatment arms ($p = 0.0112$) and a significantly higher median time-to-response for the QW/QW group (113 days; 95 % confidence interval [CI]: 85–141) compared with the BIW/QW group (85 days; 95 % CI: 59–86). The efficacy parameters are summarized in Table 4.

HRQoL analyses

Statistically significant ($p < 0.001$) improvements from baseline in all measures of HRQoL were observed in both treatment groups by week 12 and were maintained to week 24 (Table 5). In addition, the difference in the observed improvement in DLQI and EQ-5D scores at week 12 between the two treatment groups was statistically significant ($p < 0.05$).

Safety analyses

Individual safety analysis by country or region was not performed since the trial was designed to randomize all enrolled patients and not stratified by geographic location. The complete safety data for the PRISTINE trial have been reported before [8]. Briefly, etanercept was well tolerated. The most commonly reported (≥5 % of patients) treatment-emergent adverse events were nasopharyngitis, headache, elevated blood insulin, diarrhea, injection-site erythema, pharyngitis, arthralgia, fatigue and injection-site reaction. Seven patients of 273 (2.6 %) reported serious adverse events and nine patients discontinued treatment due to an adverse event. There was no incidence of tuberculosis, opportunistic infections, or deaths reported.

Discussion

Guidelines for the treatment of psoriasis have been well established in the United States and Western Europe [3–6] and, more recently, in the Czech Republic [14] and Mexico [15]. These same treatment paradigms have

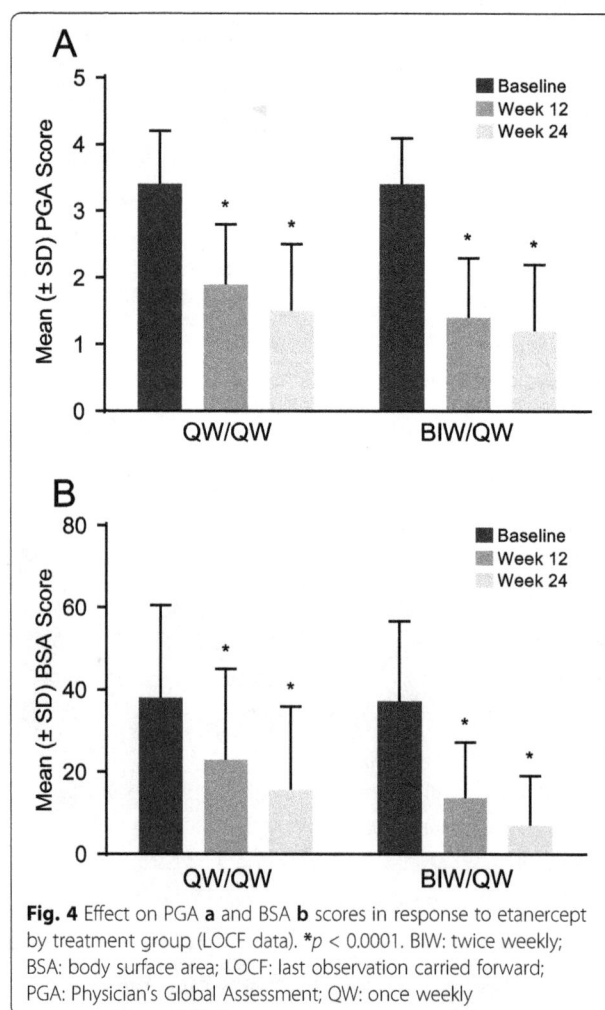

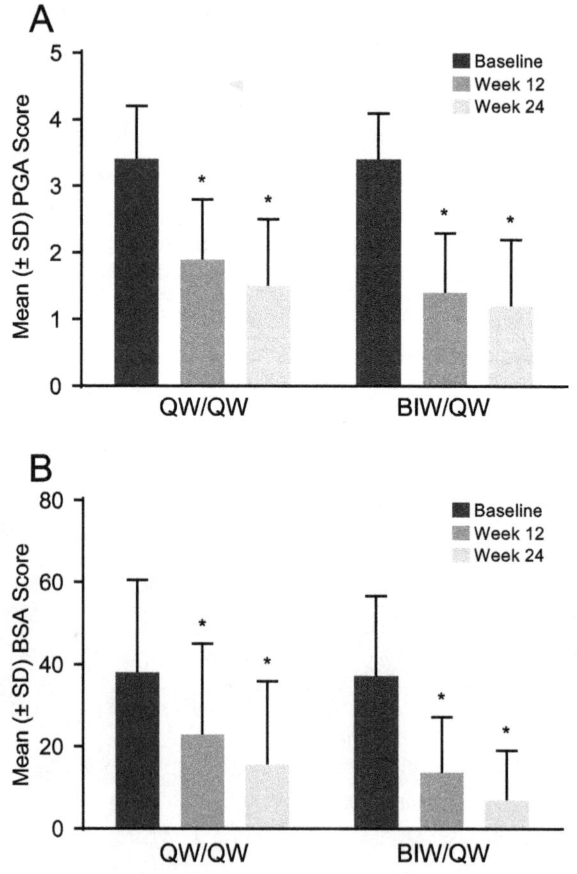

Fig. 4 Effect on PGA **a** and BSA **b** scores in response to etanercept by treatment group (LOCF data). *$p < 0.0001$. BIW: twice weekly; BSA: body surface area; LOCF: last observation carried forward; PGA: Physician's Global Assessment; QW: once weekly

Table 4 Summary of improvements in efficacy measures in response to etanercept by treatment group

Response/Parameter	Week 12		Week 24	
	QW/QW $n = 86$	BIW/QW $n = 84$	QW/QW $n = 86$	BIW/QW $n = 84$
PASI 50, % of patients (95 % CI)	72.1 (61.4, 81.2)	91.7* (83.6, 96.6)	80.2 (70.2, 88.0)	90.5 (82.1, 95.8)
PASI 75, % of patients (95 % CI)	39.5 (29.2, 50.7)	66.7* (55.5, 76.6)	62.8 (51.7, 73.0)	83.3* (73.6, 90.6)
PASI 90, % of patients (95 % CI)	14.0 (7.4, 23.1)	32.1* (22.4, 43.2)	37.2 (27.0, 48.3)	56.0* (44.7, 66.8)
Adjusted mean change from baseline in total PGA score, mean (SEM)	−1.5† (0.1)	−2.0*† (0.1)	−1.9† (0.1)	−2.2*† (0.1)
PGA clear/almost clear, % of patients (95 % CI)	36.0† (26.0, 47.1)	56.0*† (44.7, 66.8)	57.0† (45.8, 67.6)	71.4† (60.5, 80.8)
Adjusted mean % change in affected body surface area, mean (SEM)	−14.6† (1.7)	−23.2*† (1.7)	−21.7† (1.5)	29.6*† (1.5)

Missing data were imputed using the last observation carried forward method
*$p < 0.05$ between treatment groups at the same time point. †$p < 0.01$ from baseline within treatment group
BIW twice weekly, *PASI* Psoriasis Area and Severity Index, *PGA* Physician's Global Assessment, *QW* once weekly, *SEM* standard error of the mean

been used in other parts of the world with the expectation that there would be similar responses. However, there have been few, if any, formal evaluations of responses to any specific treatment in patients from other parts of the world. The fact that the prevalence of psoriasis in Hispanic, African Americans, and other ethnic groups is less than half of that observed in Caucasians (1.4 %–1.6 % vs. 3.6 %, respectively) [1] suggests that it may be important to at least review and re-evaluate the responses of patients from other ethnic backgrounds and countries.

In this post-hoc, subset analysis, we examine the responses of patients from six countries (Argentina, Czech Republic, Hungary, Mexico, Taiwan, and Thailand) in three regions of the world (Asia, Central Europe, and Latin America) in which there are no current guidelines for the treatment of psoriasis other than in the Czech Republic [14] and Mexico [15]. Of the 273 patients originally enrolled in the PRISTINE trial, 171 patients were from these three regions. However, since the number of patients from each of the six countries was small, they were pooled for descriptive statistical analyses.

The percentages of patients achieving PASI 50, PASI 75 or PASI 90 in response to etanercept treatment were numerically greater in this subset than the corresponding percentages in the overall PRISTINE population [8] at both the 12- and 24-week time points. Similarly, the percentage of patients achieving a PGA status of clear or almost clear in response to etanercept treatment was also numerically greater in this subset than in the overall PRISTINE study population. Even though some outcomes appear to have slightly better responses numerically for this subpopulation compared with the overall study population [8], the underlying cause for these differences is unclear. This could be related to shorter psoriatic arthritis disease duration; slightly higher disease severity, e.g. BSA and PASI, at baseline for this subpopulation, allowing for greater improvement; slightly higher body mass index and smaller waist-to-hip ratio among the females in this subpopulation; slightly fewer Caucasians; slightly higher number of patients with secondary diagnosis of psoriatic arthritis, diabetes or hypertension; or random chance. Since the study was designed to randomize all enrolled patients without stratification by their geographic location, the patients from these six countries were not homogenously distributed between the two treatment groups. Thus, any analysis comparing the responses of the subpopulation from these six

Table 5 Summary of improvements in HRQoL measures in response to etanercept by treatment group

Adjusted mean change from baseline	Week 12		Week 24	
	QW/QW $n = 86$	BIW/QW $n = 84$	QW/QW $n = 86$	BIW/QW $n = 84$
DLQI, mean (SEM)	−8.4† (0.5)	−10.8† (0.5)	−9.5† (0.6)	−11.0† (0.6)
EQ-5D, mean (SEM)	0.2 (0.0)	0.3* (0.0)	0.2* (0.0)	0.3* (0.0)
WPAI: % activity impairment due to problem, mean (SEM)	−19.1† (2.3)	−25.1† (2.3)	−22.1† (2.2)	−27.3† (2.3)
WPAI: % impairment while working due to problem, mean (SEM)	−7.5 (2.5)†	−16.3 (2.6)*†	−11.8 (2.0)†	−18.8 (2.0)*†
WPAI: % overall work impairment due to problem, mean (SEM)	−7.8 (3.3)†	−15.1 (3.2)†	−13.5 (2.8)†	−16.3 (2.8)†
WPAI: % work time missed due to problem, mean (SEM)	−3.4 (2.6)†	0.4 (2.5)†	−6.1 (2.3)†	0.6 (2.3)*†
Total FACIT, mean (SEM)	3.2† (0.7)	4.5† (0.7)	4.5† (0.8)	4.3† (0.8)

Missing data were imputed using the last observation carried forward method
*$p < 0.05$ between treatment groups at the same time point. †$p < 0.01$ from baseline within treatment group
BIW twice weekly, *DLQI* Dermatology Life Quality Index, *EQ-5D* EuroQoL 5 Dimension, *FACIT* Functional Activity in Chronic Therapy, *HRQoL* health-related quality of life, *QW* once weekly, *SEM* standard error of the mean, *WPAI* Work Productivity and Activity Impairment scale

countries with those from the rest of the enrolled patients could introduce bias in the results which could be random or due to regional differences, e.g., accepted standard of care.

The Kaplan-Meier estimates for time to first response also demonstrate the rapidity with which patients in this subset experienced the benefits of etanercept treatment. As might be expected, the response time was shorter for those receiving etanercept BIW (median time 85 days, 95 % CI: 59–86 days) compared with those receiving etanercept QW during the first 12 weeks of the study (median time 113 days, 95 % CI: 85–141 days). This difference was statistically significant based on non-overlapping 95 % CIs suggesting faster and greater benefit to patients from the BIW dosing regimen than QW dosing regimen.

Analysis of HRQoL measures demonstrated statistically significant ($p < 0.01$) improvement of scores from baseline in response to etanercept treatment for all parameters in both treatment groups at both 12 weeks and 24 weeks. Furthermore, the differences in the improvements observed for DLQI and EQ-5D scores at week 12 between the BIW and QW treatment groups were statistically significant ($p < 0.05$). These data parallel the data observed for the efficacy analyses for this subset of patients.

Conclusion

The subset analysis reported here demonstrates that patients with moderate-to-severe plaque psoriasis from six countries in Asia, Central Europe and Latin America respond to etanercept treatment in a manner similar to that observed in patients from the United States and Western Europe. In all analyses, compared with QW treatment, BIW treatment appears to be more beneficial with more rapid and greater response. The results for this Asian, Central European and Latin American subpopulation of the PRISTINE trial, as well as the overall study population, showed etanercept was well tolerated by patients at both the BIW and QW dosages and there were no differences in safety parameters between the two treatment groups [8]. In conclusion, this analysis suggests that the guidelines for the treatment of psoriasis in the United States and Europe can be applied to populations from other parts of the world as well.

Abbreviations

BIW: Twice weekly; BSA: Body surface area; CI: Confidence interval; DLQI: Dermatology life quality index; EQ-5D: EuroQoL-5 dimension; FACIT: Functional activity in chronic therapy; HRQoL: Health-related quality of life; PASI: Psoriasis area and severity index; PGA: Physician global assessment of psoriasis; QW: Once weekly; WPAI: Work productivity and activity impairment.

Competing interests

L. Kemeny, M. Amaya, P. Cetkovska, N. Rajatanavin, and W-R. Lee report no competing interests.
L. Marshall, E. Y. Mahgoub, and E. Aldinç are all employees of Pfizer, which sponsored the original trial and this subpopulation analysis.
A. Szumski is an employee of Inventiv Health Inc who is a paid contract worker to Pfizer in the development of this manuscript.
This study was sponsored by Pfizer.

Authors' contributions

LK, MA, PC, NR, and W-RL were all active investigators on the PRISTINE trial, recruited and treated patients in their respective countries, participated in the design and interpretation of this subset analysis, helped draft the manuscript, and approved the final manuscript. LM, EYM, and EA participated in the design and interpretation of this subset analysis, helped draft the manuscript, and approved the final manuscript. AS carried out the statistical analysis, participated in the interpretation of this subset analysis, helped draft the manuscript, and approved the final manuscript.

Acknowledgements

Medical writing support was provided by Mukund Nori, PhD, MBA, CMPP, of Engage Scientific Solutions and was funded by Pfizer, New York, NY, USA.

Author details

[1]Department of Dermatology and Allergology, University of Szeged, Szeged, Hungary. [2]Hospital San Lucas, Monterrey, Nuevo Leon, Mexico. [3]Department of Dermatovenereology, Charles University Hospital, Pilsen, Czech Republic. [4]Division of Dermatology, Ramathibodi Hospital, Mahidol University, Bangkok, Thailand. [5]Department of Dermatology, Shuang Ho Hospital, Taipei, Taiwan. [6]Global Innovative Pharma, Pfizer, Collegeville, PA, USA. [7]Global Innovative Pharma, Pfizer, New York, NY, USA.

References

1. Rachakonda TD, Schupp CW, Armstrong AW. Psoriasis prevalence among adults in the United States. J Am Acad Dermatol. 2014;70(3):512–6.
2. Ding X, Wang T, Shen Y, Wang X, Zhou C, Tian S, et al. Prevalence of psoriasis in China: a population-based study in six cities. Eur J Dermatol. 2012;22(5):663–7.
3. Nast A, Boehncke W-H, Mrowietz U, Ockenfels H-M, Philipp S, Reich K, et al. S3 – Guidelines on the treatment of psoriasis vulgaris (English version). Update. J German Soc Dermatol. 2012;10:S1–s95.
4. Menter A, Korman NJ, Elmets CA, Feldman SR, Gelfand JM, Gordon KB, et al. Guidelines of care for the management of psoriasis and psoriatic arthritis: Section 5. Guidelines of care for the treatment of psoriasis with phototherapy and photochemotherapy. J Am Acad Dermatol. 2010;62(1):114–35.
5. Smith CH, Anstey AV, Barker JNWN, Burden AD, Chalmers RJG, Chandler DA, et al. British Association of Dermatologists' guidelines for biologic interventions for psoriasis 2009. Br J Dermatol. 2009;161(5):987–1019.
6. Menter A, Gottlieb A, Feldman SR, Van Voorhees AS, Leonardi CL, Gordon KB, et al. Guidelines of care for the management of psoriasis and psoriatic arthritis: Section 1. Overview of psoriasis and guidelines of care for the treatment of psoriasis with biologics. J Am Acad Dermatol. 2008;58(5):826–50.
7. Menter A. The status of biologic therapies in the treatment of moderate to severe psoriasis. Cutis. 2009;84(4 Suppl):14–24.
8. Strohal R, Puig L, Chouela E, Tsai TF, Melin J, Freundlich B, et al. The efficacy and safety of etanercept when used with as-needed adjunctive topical therapy in a randomised, double-blind study in subjects with moderate-to-severe psoriasis (the PRISTINE trial). J Dermatolog Treat. 2013;24(3):169–78.
9. Badia X, Mascaro JM, Lozano R. Measuring health-related quality of life in patients with mild to moderate eczema and psoriasis: clinical validity, reliability and sensitivity to change of the DLQI. The Cavide Research Group. Br J Dermatol. 1999;141(4):698–702.
10. EuroQol–a new facility for the measurement of health-related quality of life. The EuroQol Group. Health Policy. 1990; 16(3):199–208.
11. Rabin R, de Charro F. EQ-5D: a measure of health status from the EuroQol Group. Ann Med. 2001;33(5):337–43.
12. Reilly MC, Zbrozek AS, Dukes EM. The validity and reproducibility of a work productivity and activity impairment instrument. Pharmacoeconomics. 1993;4(5):353–65.

13. Webster K, Cella D, Yost K. The Functional Assessment of Chronic Illness Therapy (FACIT) Measurement System: properties, applications, and interpretation. Health Qual Life Outcomes. 2003;1:79.
14. Cetkovská P, Kojanová M. Czech recommendations for biological therapy of severe plaque psoriasis. Čes-slov Derm. 2012;87(1):1–76.
15. Amaya-Guerra M, Barba F, Blancas González F, Gómez Flores M, Gómez Trigo A, González Soto R, et al. Consenso Mexicano para el Manejo de Terapia Biológica en Psoriasis. Rev Cent Dermatol Pascua. 2004;13(3):172–84.

18

Evaluation of therapeutic potential of VB-001, a leave-on formulation, for the treatment of moderate adherent dandruff

Anamika Bhattacharyya[1], Nilu Jain[1], Sudhanand Prasad[1], Shilpi Jain[1], Vishal Yadav[1], Shamik Ghosh[1*] and Shiladitya Sengupta[2*]

Abstract

Background: Dandruff is a common scalp condition characterized by excessive scaling and itch. Aberrant colonization of the scalp by commensal *Malassezia* spp. is a major contributor in the multifactorial etiology of dandruff. Literature based understanding of *Malassezia* linked pathophysiology of dandruff allowed us to comprehend a strategy to potentiate the efficacy of a known antifungal agent used in dandruff therapy. The aim of this study was to determine the efficacy and skin safety of VB-001 antidandruff leave-on formulation in comparison with marketed antidandruff ZPTO shampoo in patients with moderate adherent dandruff of the scalp.

Methods: Healthy males or females aged ≥ 15 years and ≤ 65 with a clinical diagnosis of moderate adherent dandruff of the scalp were recruited for the study to monitor the effects of topical VB-001 versus those of marketed antidandruff ZPTO shampoo.

Results: 168 subjects were randomized to the treatment (VB-001, $n = 84$) and control (ZPTO shampoo, $n = 84$) groups. The efficacy of each product was evaluated by comparing proportion of subjects who have shown reduction in flaking by ASFS (adherent scalp flaking score) and pruritus by IGA (investigator global assessment) score. VB-001 imparted consistently better reduction in ASFS and enabled early reduction of pruritus in comparison to marketed ZPTO shampoo.

Conclusion: VB-001, a leave-on formulation with ingredients chosen to selectively disturb the *Malassezia* niche on dandruff scalp by denying extra nutritional benefits to the microbe, provides unique advantages over existing best in class ZPTO shampoo therapy. It has the potential to emerge as an attractive novel treatment for moderate adherent dandruff.

Keywords: Scalp, Dandruff, Malassezia, Anti-fungals

Background

Dandruff is a common scalp disorder characterized by flaking, often pruritic skin and affecting more than half of the human population [1]. The onset and development of dandruff is determined by multiple factors including abnormal colonization of skin by *Malassezia* spp. [2], sebum production [3] and individual predisposition [4, 5]. Sebaceous lipids on the skin surface support colonization and growth of *Malassezia* by fulfilling the latter's obligate need for fatty acids as the microbe lacks fatty acid synthase genes [6]. To compensate, *Malassezia* secretes multiple lipases [6] to metabolize triglycerides in sebum and release free fatty acids for its use. Apart from acting as food for growth of *Malassezia*, these free fatty acids are thought to act as skin irritants and induce inflammatory responses typical of dandruff [3]. In susceptible individuals, the effect is amplified as the fungus not only resides on the skin surface, but reaches deeper due to inherent epidermal barrier defects of the individual.

* Correspondence: shamik.ghosh@vyome.in; shiladit@mit.edu
[1]Vyome Biosciences Pvt. Ltd, Plot# 465, F.I.E., Patparganj Industrial Area, Delhi 110092, India
[2]Medicine & HST, Brigham and Women's Hospital, Harvard Medical School, Room 317, 65 Landsdowne Street, Cambridge, MA 02139, USA

Understandably, a common approach for the treatment of dandruff and its symptoms is to use anti-fungal agents in topical formulations to eradicate *Malassezia* from the scalp [7]. Few of the most commonly used and effective anti-fungal agents for dandruff are zinc pyrithione (ZPTO), selenium sulfide, ciclopirox and ketoconazole in wash-off formulations [8]. Despite high in vitro potency of these antifungal agents against *Malassezia* species, currently available wash-off antidandruff formulations are often limited in efficacy due to short contact time and thus fail to completely eliminate the fungus from skin. Interestingly, certain previous studies [9, 10] as well as our own in vitro screening assays (data not shown) have shown susceptibility of *Malassezia* spp. to certain medium chain fatty acids. In the light of this information, inclusion of medium chain fatty acids (or their derivatives) in topical formulations can be considered for treating *Malassezia*-induced skin infections.

The scope to formulate a more efficacious anti-dandruff product (compared to existing ones) devoid of growth promoting fatty acids (that act as food for the microbe) but including inhibitory fatty acids for *Malassezia* spp. was explored. The idea was to attempt changing the microenvironment of the dandruff-causing fungus on scalp through molecular replacement of sebaceous nutrients with a detrimental medium chain fatty acid derivative thus allowing overall higher anti-dandruff efficacy in the presence of a known antifungal agent. Thus, a leave-on antidandruff product VB-001 was formulated combining piroctone olamine and a derivative of a medium chain fatty acid, the combination showing enhanced in vitro fungal killing compared to a formulation containing piroctone olamine alone (data not shown).

The aim of this study was to evaluate the efficacy of VB-001 against a marketed reference antidandruff ZPTO shampoo (1%) in patients with moderate adherent dandruff. VB-001 demonstrated better clinical efficacy compared to the marketed wash-off antidandruff formulation containing 1% ZPTO.

Methods

Objectives

The general objective of this study was to determine the efficacy and in-use skin safety of VB-001 antidandruff leave-on formulation in comparison with marketed antidandruff ZPTO shampoo in patients with moderate adherent dandruff of the scalp. The specific objectives were to determine if outcomes in patients treated with VB-001 differed significantly from those in patients treated with antidandruff shampoo in terms of: (i) Mean adherent scalp flaking score (ASFS) after 2 weeks of daily application of VB-001 for a minimum period of 8 h per day (overnight) compared to a rinse-off antidandruff shampoo used on alternate days. (ii) Score of pruritus (Investigators' Global Assessment-IGA) 2 weeks after daily application of VB-001 for a minimum period of 8 h per day (overnight) compared to a marketed antidandruff shampoo used on alternate days (iii) Change in hair fall, subject satisfaction including hair sensorial evaluation measured by scalp related quality of life index on days 0, 5, 9 and 14. (iv) High resolution photographic monitoring of worst affected area on days 0, 5, 9 and 14 (v) In-use skin safety and tolerability in patients exposed to VB-001 at day 5, 9 and 14 (vi) The incidence of adverse events.

Patients and study design

This study was a randomized, parallel group, active controlled trial. Protocol approval was obtained from an independent ethics committee established following the guidelines of Helsinki Declaration (1975) before the initiation of the clinical trial (details on Clinical Trial Registry India: CTRI/2013/01/003283). Informed consent from adults and informed assent from children aged ≥ 15 years were likewise secured prior to treatment.

Healthy males or females aged ≥ 15 years and ≤ 65 with a clinical diagnosis of moderate adherent dandruff of the scalp were recruited for the study to monitor the effects of topical antidandruff leave-on formulation VB-001 versus those of marketed antidandruff ZPTO shampoo on moderate adherent dandruff of the scalp at various dermatology clinics in Mumbai and Nashik, India.

Both newly diagnosed and OPD follow-up patients of moderate adherent dandruff of the scalp were screened for enrollment following stated inclusion criteria. Before the initiation of the study, participating doctors and other evaluators were made completely aligned on the scoring matrix to reduce interpretational variability. Six zones on each patient scalp were pre-defined for assessment (right frontal, left frontal, right parietal/temporal, left parietal/temporal, right occipital, left occipital). Comb was used to part the hair in each area to give a clear view of the patient scalp. Each section of the scalp was assessed for the presence of dandruff flakes that were adhering to the scalp skin using a 0 to 5 scale (0 means no flakes and 5 means intense flaking) as described in Table 1. Loose flakes in the hair were not considered in the grading. The final or total ASFS was determined by adding the grades for all six zones on the scalp. Thus, based on the stated grading system, patients with a minimum total ASFS of 6 and not exceeding 14; baseline scaling score of at least 3 and not more than 4 of adherent flaking in at least one zone of the scalp (6 zones- two frontal, two parietal plus temporal and two occipital) were diagnosed with moderate adherent dandruff of the scalp and considered eligible for inclusion. IGA for pruritus score of at least 1 was set as another inclusion criterion. Inclusion screening ensured that the patients had not used an antidandruff agent in the 14 days preceding the trial and they were willing to refrain from

Table 1 ASFS grading scale applicable to the study

Grade	Standard Established
0	No scales
1	Thin scales
2	Diffused thin scales
3	Thick heaped-up scales but not forming plaques
4	Diffused thick heaped-up scales but not forming plaques
5	Very thick heaped-up scales forming plaques

use of all other topical medications that would affect the results of the trial, including medicated shampoos/oils or antibiotics, during the treatment and observation periods (from day 0 to day 14).

Exclusion criteria precluded the participation of: patients who had a history or presence of Parkinson's disease, HIV, infections or disorders of the central nervous system, history of overt bacterial, viral or fungal infections of the head/neck, a history or presence of compromising dermatosis elsewhere on the skin; patients with actinically damaged skin; patients with any skin condition that would interfere with the diagnosis or assessment of adherent dandruff; e.g., psoriasis, acne, atopic dermatitis; patients with clinically significant systemic disease (e.g., immunological deficiencies, AIDS, current malignancies, uncontrolled diabetes mellitus); patients who had used within 1 month prior to baseline any treatment that would affect the results of the trial, including 1) systemic antifungal, 2) systemic steroids 3) systemic antibiotics 4) systemic anti-inflammatory agents or 5) cytostatic or immune-modulating drugs (e.g. cyclosporine, tacrolimus, pimecrolimus) 6) topical steroids 7) topical retinoids 8) topical anti-inflammatory agents 9) topical antibiotics or 10) topical treatment of adherent dandruff (e.g., coal tar preparations, antidandruff shampoos/oils/gels/creams/conditioners 11) antihistamines; and patients with any other major medical problem that the investigator deemed likely to increase the risk for adverse events associated with the intervention and pregnant or lactating women by history.

Materials

VB-001 antidandruff leave-on formulation was developed at Vyome Biosciences Pvt. Ltd by including an ester derivative of a medium chain fatty acid (considered as a GRAS excipient) to a mixture of piroctone olamine (POL) dissolved in absolute alcohol, followed by the addition of a well-accepted topical formulation base to obtain a clear, transparent formulation, free from undissolved solid material. The comparator antidandruff ZPTO shampoo was obtained from marketed batch of a reputed brand. VB-001 was packaged into uniform transparent plastic bottles with a small opening and antidandruff shampoo was repacked in white plastic bottles with a small opening. There were clear differences between VB-001 and antidandruff shampoo in appearance and viscosity.

To harmonize the study and for patient compliance, two more non-antidandruff products from reputed brands were included in both the study arms; a non-antidandruff shampoo for VB-001 arm and a non-antidandruff conditioner for antidandruff shampoo arm. Both non antidandruff products were repacked in similar white plastic bottles as the ones used for antidandruff shampoo. Although the study was an open label, repacking was done just to avoid cognitive bias.

Randomization, treatment allocation and blinding

The patients were recruited in the ratio of 1:1 between the arms. A randomization sheet was generated manually based on ASFS. Patients were allocated to one of the two groups to receive either test product (VB-001) or the comparator product (ZPTO shampoo). The final group wise distribution of the patients recruited at the three centers is depicted in Fig. 1a. The codes were not disclosed to the investigator until the end of study.

Study Intervention

Each subject was given one bottle (250 ml) of VB-001 or marketed antidandruff shampoo at each visit. For the VB-001 group, the patients were instructed to apply 10 ml of investigational product daily with massage onto the scalp and leave overnight (at least for 8 h leave-on). These patients were further instructed to wash their head on the next day of investigational product application with marketed non-antidandruff shampoo given to them. The patients assigned to the marketed antidandruff shampoo group were instructed to apply sufficient quantity with gentle massage onto scalp, lather and rinse off thoroughly with water on alternate days. These patients were further instructed to gently massage the given non-antidandruff conditioner onto the shampoo cleaned wet hair and rinse off thoroughly with water. Patients in both groups were advised not to apply any other product with antidandruff effect during the study period. All subjects followed their respective procedures for 2 weeks.

Clinical assessment

Subjects were evaluated at baseline and on day 5, 9 and 14 by the principle investigator. The primary end points of the study were the assessment of clinical efficacy of the investigational product and marketed antidandruff shampoo in terms of demonstrated improvement in dandruff score and pruritus in both groups. Secondary end points included efficacy and safety of investigational product from baseline in terms of changes in hair sensorial, hair fall and the incidence of adverse events during the study in both groups. The study end points were

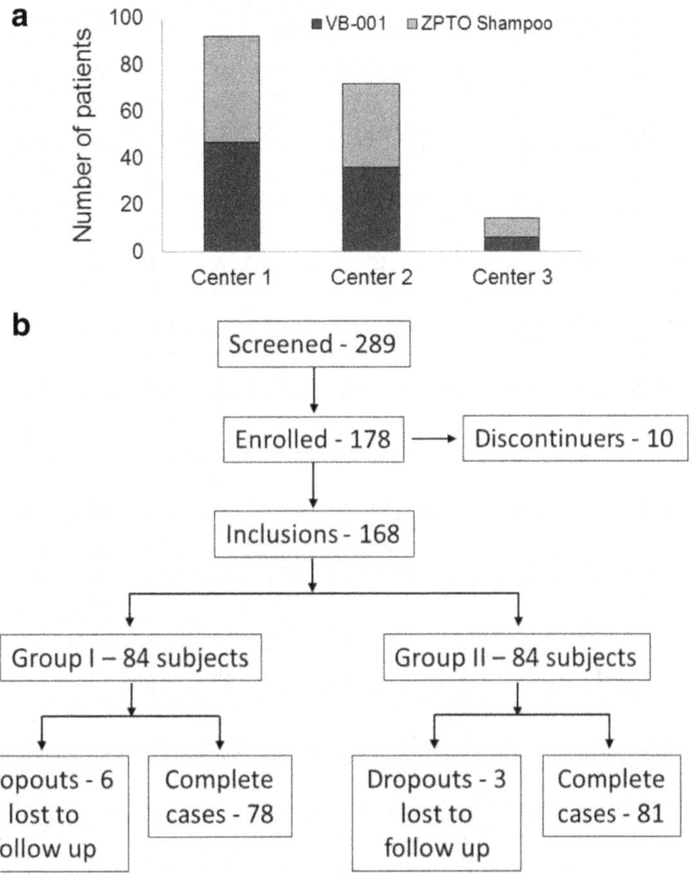

Fig. 1 Study population. **a** Graphical representation of the patient randomization at the three centers where the trial was conducted. **b** Trial profile showing subject population. Groups I and II represent VB-001 and ZPTO antidandruff shampoo groups respectively

recorded and digital photographs of affected areas of the scalp were obtained at every visit in both groups.

The clinical severity of dandruff was measured using mean ASFS on scalp using a scale (0: No score- 5: Very thick heaped up scales forming plaques). The scores on 6 zones (right frontal, left frontal, right parietal/temporal, left parietal/temporal, right occipital, left occipital) of scalp were individually measured and total score recorded at baseline. Any further improvement was measured at day 5, 9 and 14. Clinical efficacy of pruritus was measured using IGA for pruritus and subjects with IGA for pruritus score of at least 1 were considered at baseline. Further improvement was measured at 5, 9 and 14 days.

A scalp related quality of life questionnaire was circulated among subjects in order to capture their perception on change in hair fall, overall satisfaction and hair sensorial on day 0, 5, 9 and 14. The Digital Viewer III 2.0 M digital magnascope is a simple microscope and was used to obtain magnified images of hair and scalp. High resolution photographic monitoring of worst affected area was performed on days 0, 5, 9 and 14 using the digital magnascope. The in-use skin safety and tolerability in subjects exposed to VB-001 as adverse events or skin intolerances were reported during the study period. The efficacy and safety assessments used in this study were standard, i.e., widely used and generally recognized as reliable, accurate, and relevant (able to discriminate between effective and ineffective agents).

Stopping guidelines

No stopping guidelines were envisaged for this study.

Eligible subjects, who for whatever reason, did not report to the clinic to receive the first application of test product and comparator product after having been selected for the study were referred to as discontinuers in the report. A volunteer who was withdrawn from the study, for whatever reason, was classified as a drop out, and identified as such in the relevant Case Report Form (CRF).

Sample size

The sample size was calculated accepting a power of 80%, with an alpha of 0.05, using the formula for computing the difference between two proportions the aim was to recruit 84 subjects per arm to allow for a 10% drop out rate.

Data processing and analysis

Data from the study were subjected to both per protocol (PP) analysis and intention to treat (ITT) analysis and results were found to be comparable. Further interpretation of data was drawn based on PP analysis wherein all ASFS and pruritus scores for each patient on each visit was normalized to their individual baseline (day 0) score and the normalized data sets were further analyzed for differences. Tests of significance for difference between the two groups were performed using Student's *t*-test while analyzing the normalized ASFS and pruritus data. Analysis of the data from the quality of life questionnaire were performed using ANOVA Kruskal Wallis test. Further, the data for monitoring hair fall and hair softness was analyzed using Chi square test as they represented categorical variables.

Results

Study population

Of the 289 individuals who were screened, 178 met the entry criteria and were eligible subjects but 10 subjects, for whatever reason, did not report to the clinic to receive the first application of test product or comparator product after having been selected for the study were referred to as discontinuers in the report and 168 subjects were randomized to the treatment (VB-001, $n = 84$) and control (marketed antidandruff shampoo, $n = 84$) groups (Fig. 1b). Of these, 9 were lost to follow-up and were considered drop outs. A PP analysis was performed in which 159 subjects were included. No statistical difference was observed in the baseline demographics of the study population as summarized in Table 2.

Table 2 Demographic characteristic of the study population ($n = 168$) at baseline

Parameters		VB-001 Group	ZPTO Shampoo Group	p value (Between groups)
No. of cases		84	84	
Age (Yrs)	Mean	26.20	25.31	-
	SD	09.37	07.37	
	Range	15–58 yrs	15–46 yrs	
Gender (%)	Male	10 (11.9)	14 (16.7)	-
	Female	74 (88.1)	70 (83.3)	
Mean total ASFS (Mean ± SD)		11.09 ± 1.55	10.86 ± 1.53	0.3479 (NS)
Mean score for pruritus (Mean ± SD)		1.19 ± 0.40	1.17 ± 0.38	0.7471 (NS)
Mean scalp related quality of life index score-II (Mean ± SD)		12.05 ± 3.18	11.67 ± 3.13	0.4489 (NS)

NS non significant by ANOVA Kruskal Wallis test

Clinical effects

VB-001 imparted consistently better reduction in ASFS

Mean total ASFS decreased from baseline in both VB-001 and marketed antidandruff ZPTO shampoo groups (Fig. 2a). However, the percentage reductions from baseline in the VB-001 group were significantly higher at all measurement time-points. The post-treatment reduction in the mean ASFS value from baseline in the VB-001 group was 76%, which was significantly higher ($P < 0.001$) than that observed in the marketed antidandruff ZPTO shampoo group (68%) as depicted in Fig. 2a. High-resolution photographic monitoring of worst affected scalp area revealed a dramatic reduction in adherent flaking over time following treatment in both groups (Fig. 2b).

In addition, when the efficacy of each product was assessed by comparing the proportion of subjects who achieved reduction in ASFS (score < 5) it was found that 47% of the patients (37 out of 78) in VB-001 group and 34% (28 out of 81) in marketed antidandruff ZPTO shampoo group showed an ASFS of less than 5 on day 9. In VB-001 group 90% subjects and 79% in marketed

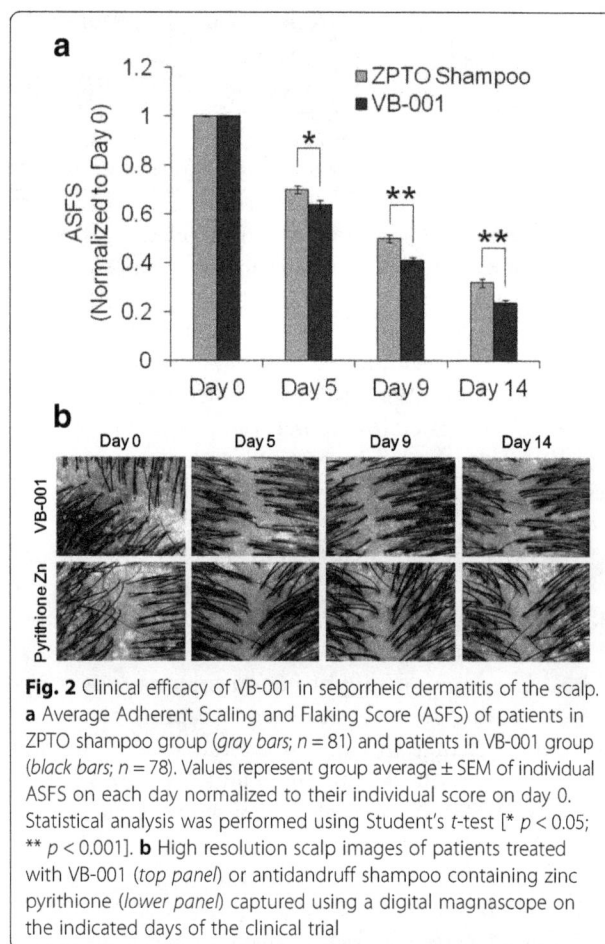

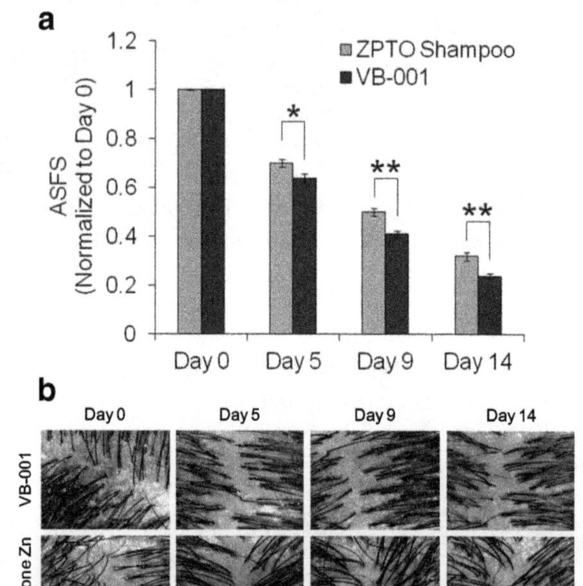

Fig. 2 Clinical efficacy of VB-001 in seborrheic dermatitis of the scalp. **a** Average Adherent Scaling and Flaking Score (ASFS) of patients in ZPTO shampoo group (*gray bars*; $n = 81$) and patients in VB-001 group (*black bars*; $n = 78$). Values represent group average ± SEM of individual ASFS on each day normalized to their individual score on day 0. Statistical analysis was performed using Student's *t*-test [* $p < 0.05$; ** $p < 0.001$]. **b** High resolution scalp images of patients treated with VB-001 (*top panel*) or antidandruff shampoo containing zinc pyrithione (*lower panel*) captured using a digital magnascope on the indicated days of the clinical trial

antidandruff ZPTO shampoo group showed a good response (ASFS < 5) at day 14 (Fig. 3 and Table 3).

VB-001 treatment enabled an early reduction in pruritus

Pruritus symptom was analyzed by score of pruritus- Investigator global assessment (IGA). Mean score for pruritus (normalized to baseline) decreased from baseline to day 14 in both groups (Fig. 4). The percentage reductions from baseline in the VB-001 group were significantly higher at day 5 and day 9 time-points. Mean score for pruritus showed a significant fall of 35% among VB-001 group and 18% in ZPTO shampoo group from baseline after 5 days of treatment which was significantly more for VB-001 group than the shampoo group ($P < 0.01$). Similarly, after 9 days of treatment, mean score for pruritus showed a significant fall from baseline in both the groups i.e. 75% among VB-001 group and 61% in ZPTO shampoo group which was significantly more ($P < 0.05$) in VB-001 group than ZPTO shampoo group (Fig. 4). However, at the end of day 14, mean score for pruritus showed a significant fall of 89.1% and 87.2% from baseline among VB-001 group and ZPTO shampoo group respectively. There was no significant difference between VB-001 group and ZPTO shampoo group at day 14.

In addition, the efficacy of each product was assessed by comparing the proportion of subjects who achieved reduction in itching (score = 0) which was remarkable at day 5 and day 9 in the VB001 group. 26.9% of the subjects in VB-001 showed complete cure in pruritus on day 5 compared to only 9.9% in the ZPTO shampoo group (Fig. 5 and Table 3). Similarly, on day 9, a greater percentage of subjects (67.9%) in the VB-001 group showed complete cure in pruritus compared to the 53.1% in ZPTO shampoo group. On day 14 both VB-001 group (87.2% subjects)

Table 3 Proportion of subjects showing reduction in flaking and itching in both groups

Day	VB-001 (%)	ZPTO shampoo (%)
	ASFS < 5	
Day 5	7	6
Day 9	47	34
Day 14	90	79
	Pruritus IGA Score = 0	
Day 5	27	10
Day 9	68	53
Day 14	87	85

and marketed antidandruff shampoo group (85.2% subjects) showed an excellent response (Fig. 5).

VB-001 improved patient experience during antidandruff therapy

To establish subject satisfaction in both groups the sensorial effects and hair fall change was measured by Scalp Related Quality Of Life Index. The result for the mean total score of scalp related quality of life index showed that there was a significant improvement in mean total score of Scalp Related Quality of Life Index in both groups as compared to baseline at all time points (day 5, day 9 and day 14). At day 5 and day 9, the results were comparable between both groups. After 14 days of treatment, however, mean scalp related quality of life index score-II showed a significant increase of 51.6% and 45.1% from baseline in VB-001 group and ZPTO shampoo group, respectively (Table 4). The rise was significantly more in VB-001 group than ZPTO shampoo group. Additionally, 14 days post treatment, 41% of

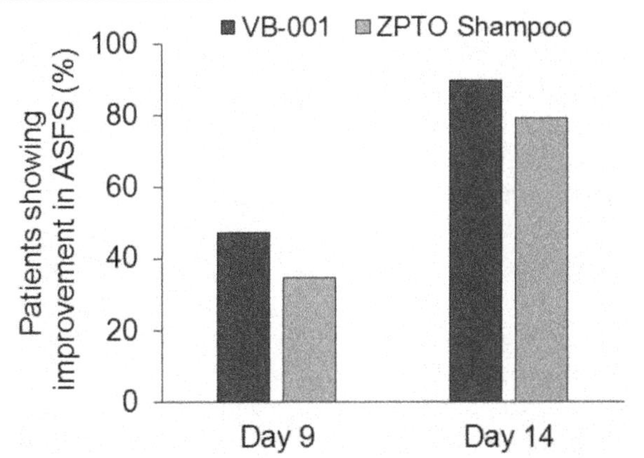

Fig. 3 Comparison of patients showing improvement in scalp flaking during the course of the study. Bar graphs show percentage of patients reaching an ASFS of less than 5 at the indicated days of the trial in VB-001 group versus ZPTO shampoo group

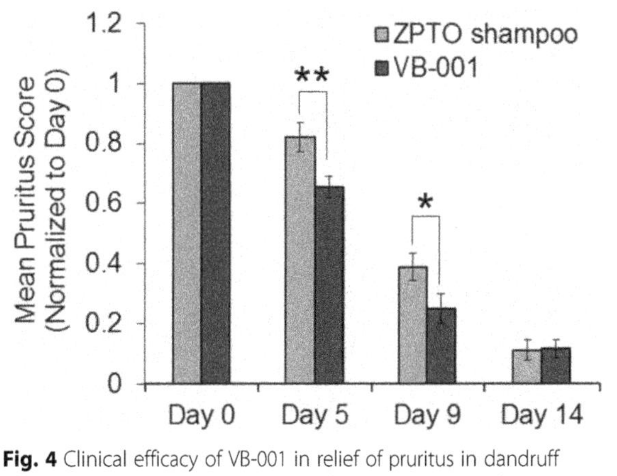

Fig. 4 Clinical efficacy of VB-001 in relief of pruritus in dandruff afflicted scalp. Mean pruritus score of patients in ZPTO shampoo group (*gray bars*) and patients in VB-001 group (*black bars*). Values represent group average ± SEM of individual pruritus score on each day normalized to their individual score on day 0. Statistical analysis was performed using Student's *t*-test [* $p < 0.05$; ** $p < 0.01$]

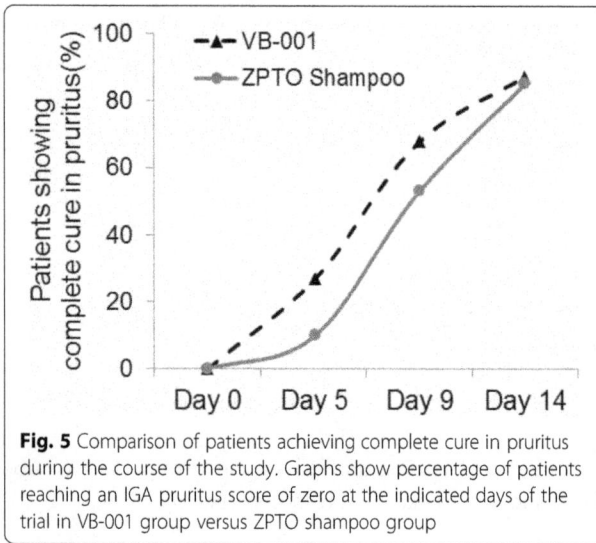

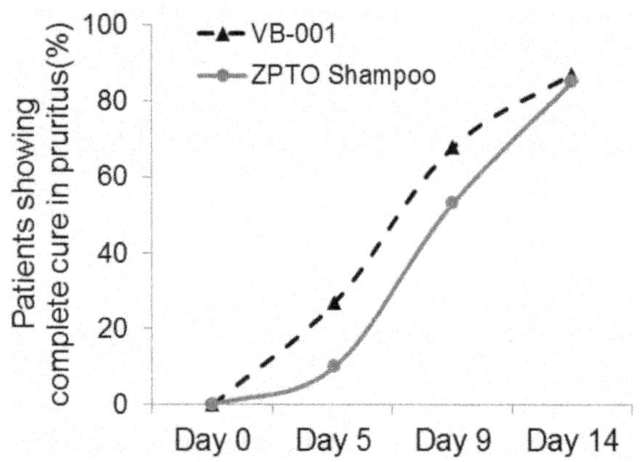

Fig. 5 Comparison of patients achieving complete cure in pruritus during the course of the study. Graphs show percentage of patients reaching an IGA pruritus score of zero at the indicated days of the trial in VB-001 group versus ZPTO shampoo group

subjects in VB-001 group reported a visible reduction in hair fall which was significantly more than the 18.5% subjects in the antidandruff shampoo group. Finally, 83.3% of subjects in VB-001 group reported softness of hair which was significantly more than the 67.9% subjects in the ZPTO shampoo arm (Table 4).

Safety

There were no adverse events or skin intolerances reported during the study period. Both product regimens were well tolerated by the subjects.

Discussion

The accepted scientific consensus is that *Malassezia* is the causative agent for dandruff and thus for multiple decades the preferred modes of treatment have included the use of anti-fungal agents [7, 8], many of which show good efficacy. However, the current understanding is that dandruff occurs in susceptible individuals who have decreased scalp lipid levels and inherent defects in stratum corneum (SC) permeability barrier [4, 5]. Such defects in skin allow pathogenic colonization by the otherwise commensal *Malassezia* spp. which exacerbates the damage in an already impaired SC barrier to present features of dandruff. Recovery of skin from dandruff-associated symptoms by use of topical anti-fungal agents is primarily due to removal of *Malassezia* and the resultant secondary effects from clearing of the microbe [7]. However, recurrence of dandruff is common in individuals treated solely with an anti-fungal agent possibly due to (apart from other reasons) persistent SC defects that are not addressed by the anti-fungal treatment.

Table 4 Treatment success in both groups

Efficacy Parameter	VB-001 (*N* = 78)	ZPTO shampoo (*N* = 81)	*P* value
Mean ASFS (normalized) difference (Baseline-Day 14)	75.6%	67.9%	0.0005[a]
Mean pruritus score (normalized) difference (Baseline-Day 9)	75%	61%	0.03[a]
Mean scalp related quality of life index score difference (Baseline-Day 14)	51.6%	45.1%	0.03[b]
Visible hair fall reduction at day 14 (% of subjects)	41%	18.5%	<0.05[c]
Softness at day 14 (% of subjects)	83.3%	67.9%	<0.05[c]

[a]Significant by *t*-test; [b]Significant by ANOVA Kruskal Wallis; [c]Significant by Chi square test

Multiple evidences, as reviewed by many [7, 8], suggest that the use of synthetic anti-fungal agents efficiently works against the microbe but commonly used vehicle formulation(s) alter the lipid balance in the affected SC and subsequent trans-epidermal water loss (TEWL) issue remains unaddressed [4]. Harsh treatment from surfactants in traditional shampoo formulations further disturbs the free lipid levels on an already damaged SC [11, 12]. Such deteriorated scalp condition also instigates hyper-proliferation of keratinocytes, changes the maturation pattern of corneocytes and subsequently leads to the manifestation of inflammation [13]. Additionally, many currently available anti-dandruff treatment options show limited efficacy due to factors like short contact time (wash-off formulations), rising fungal resistance to various anti-fungals, formulation challenges etc. Hence there is clear scope to improve anti-dandruff treatment options using formulations that target the pathogen as well as the host predisposition.

VB-001 is a well-researched topical formulation designed by keeping in mind the recent literature about *Malassezia* genetics/physiology [6] and the evolving understanding about the benefits of a leave-on product in the treatment of dandruff. The clinical study results presented herein indicate that although both treatments showed beneficial effects on ASFS, pruritus and scalp related quality of life index score, VB-001 was significantly better in improving all outcomes compared to a leading ZPTO anti-dandruff shampoo formulation. The most apparent outcome was the early onset of relief of symptoms in the VB-001-treated group compared to the ZPTO shampoo-treated group. The effect of VB-001 started as early as day 5 for relief of pruritus symptoms. The faster onset of action is possibly attributable to the longer contact time of the antifungal agent in VB-001 (leave-on formulation). An early onset of the relief of symptoms is much coveted by patients and often dictates compliance to a certain therapeutic regimen. Such data encourages further development of similar formulations to achieve overall better efficacy & patient satisfaction. On the contrary, shampoo formulations are known to have a very short resident time on the scalp and additionally require a rinsing step that makes achievement of effective concentrations of actives a challenging task.

Additionally, VB-001 includes a potent anti-*Malassezia* medium chain fatty acid derivative as a GRAS (generally regarded as safe) excipient and demonstrated enhanced in vitro fungal killing activity when compared to a similar formulation containing the active (piroctone olamine) alone (data not shown). The overall extra efficacy of VB-001 reported in this study may be ascribed, in part, to the presence of this excipient. Finally, VB-001 is unique in its composition by being devoid of long chain fatty acids (LCFAs) or their derivatives. This feature ensures that the formulation does not provide any nutritional benefits to *Malassezia* residing on the scalp as LCFAs are known to promote growth of this yeast [9]. Hence modification of the scalp microenvironment through molecular replacement of sebaceous fatty acids with the anti-*Malassezia* fatty acid derivative may enable efficient clearance of the fungus and thus translate into the observed therapeutic benefits.

With respect to host parameters, although there are reports which suggest that the new generation of ZPTO shampoo takes care of many of the barrier defect issues [14, 15] but it seems to be an indirect effect following elimination of the causal pathogen from the scalp. On the other hand, a leave-on formulation with proper balance of all or some of the three main classes of moisturizing agents (occlusives, humectants and emollients) would leave a layer on the scalp which would help slow down the movement of water in and out of the scalp [12, 13] and enhance the patient experience. Oil based formulations have been earlier reported to impart properties of occlusives, coat the SC and retard TEWL [16]. Recent reports of skin cleansing agents also suggest that the addition of saturated fatty acids like palmitic or stearic acid can replenish the lost lipid from the scalp and rejuvenate skin health [17]. But the addition of LCFAs to antidandruff formulations may inadvertently provide nutritional advantages to the pathogen that the treatment is intended to control. VB-001, on the other hand, is devoid of any long chain fatty acid and yet it performed better than the marketed ZPTO shampoo formulation in all scalp related quality of life parameters evaluated in the study. Therefore, VB-001, a non-greasy, oil-based leave-on formulation with carefully chosen ingredients may provide unique advantages over the existing best in class therapy by not only depriving *Malasezzia* from its coveted nutrients but also addressing the pre-existing issue of loss in skin hydration.

Although randomization of the trial was done manually, both the treatment groups were more or less matched in terms of baseline demographics. However, there were big differences in the rate of recruitment of male and female patients in the study. In order to minimize any discrepancy in the outcome, the ratio of male to female was maintained in a similar range for both groups (Table 2).

The open label feature of the study was a limitation of the trial. However, the study design involved the testing of VB-001 against a comparator product (best in class), wherein the comparator was used as per published protocol that produces maximal efficacy. Additionally, this was not only a formulation versus formulation study but also a regimen versus regimen study. It was assumed that the marketed comparator had optimized their frequency of use in the wash-off format to achieve desirable results. The goal was to test whether the new leave-on product is as good as or better than the existing wash-off shampoo product. This makes the study design rigorous despite the open label.

Conclusion

VB-001 is, thus, a novel, clinically proven effective and safe formulation, and has the potential to emerge as an attractive novel treatment for moderate adherent dandruff.

Abbreviations

ASFS: Adherent scalp flaking score; CTRI: Clinical trials registry -India; GRAS: Generally regarded as safe; IGA: Investigators' global assessment; ITT: Intention to treat; LCFA: Long chain fatty acid; OPD: Out-patient department; PP: Per protocol; SC: stratum corneum; TEWL: Trans-epidermal water loss; ZPTO: Zinc pyrithione

Acknowledgements

The authors are grateful to Dr. Abhijit Bapat for extending his expert opinion in designing the clinical trial.

Funding

The study was funded by Vyome Biosciences Pvt. Ltd. Employees and Vyome Founder-Director are responsible for the initial design, approval of study plan and final analysis of the data for publications. Final study design, patient recruitment, data collection and statistical analysis have been performed by the clinical research organization.

Authors' contributions

SS and SG are responsible for conceptualizing the trial design. AB and SG are responsible for data analysis, data interpretation and drafting the article. NJ and SP are responsible for planning and developing VB-001 formulation. VY is responsible for ensuring that all the design components perceived at the conception of the study were being properly followed by the Clinic. SJ and SS are responsible for critical revision of the article and enriching its intellectual content. All authors read and approved the final manuscript.

Competing interests

AB, SJ, VY, and SG are employees of Vyome Biosciences Pvt. Ltd. SS is the founder, director and holds equity in Vyome Biosciences Pvt. Ltd. NJ and SP are former employees of Vyome Biosciences Pvt. Ltd.

References

1. Piérard-Franchimont C, Xhauflaire-Uhoda E, Piérard GE. Revisiting dandruff. Int J Cosmet Sci. 2006;28(5):311–8.
2. McGinley KJ, Leyden JJ, Marples RR, Kligman AM. Quantitative microbiology of the scalp in non-dandruff, dandruff, and seborrheic dermatitis. J Invest Dermatol. 1975;64(6):401–5.
3. Ro BI, Dawson TL. The role of sebaceous gland activity and scalp microfloral metabolism in the etiology of seborrheic dermatitis and dandruff. J Investig Dermatol Symp Proc. 2005;10(3):194–7.
4. Harding CR, Moore AE, Rogers JS, Meldrum H, Scott AE, McGlone FP. Dandruff: a condition characterized by decreased levels of intercellular lipids in scalp stratum corneum and impaired barrier function. Arch Dermatol Res. 2002;294(5):221–30.
5. DeAngelis YM, Gemmer CM, Kaczvinsky JR, Kenneally DC, Schwartz JR, Dawson Jr TL. Three etiologic facets of dandruff and seborrheic dermatitis: Malassezia fungi, sebaceous lipids, and individual sensitivity. J Investig Dermatol Symp Proc. 2005;10(3):295–7.
6. Xu J, Saunders CW, Hu P, Grant RA, Boekhout T, Kuramae EE, et al. Dandruff-associated Malassezia genomes reveal convergent and divergent virulence traits shared with plant and human fungal pathogens. Proc Natl Acad Sci U S A. 2007;104(47):18730–5.
7. Shuster S. The aetiology of dandruff and the mode of action of therapeutic agents. Br J Dermatol. 1984;111(2):235–42.
8. Ranganathan S, Mukhopadhyay T. Dandruff: the most commercially exploited skin disease. Indian J Dermatol. 2010;55(2):130–4.
9. Papavassilis C, Mach KK, Mayser PA. Medium-chain triglycerides inhibit growth of Malassezia: implications for prevention of systemic infection. Crit Care Med. 1999;27(9):1781–6.
10. Mayser P. Medium chain fatty acid ethyl esters - activation of antimicrobial effects by Malassezia enzymes. Mycoses. 2015;58(4):215–9.
11. Misra M, Ananthapadmanabhan KP, Hoyberg K, Gursky RP, Prowell S, Aronson M. Correlation between surfactant-induced ultrastructural changes in epidermis and transepidermal water loss. J Soc Cosmet Chem. 1997;48(5):219–34.
12. Del Rosso JQ, Levin J. The clinical relevance of maintaining the functional integrity of the stratum corneum in both healthy and disease-affected skin. J Clin Aesthet Dermatol. 2011;4(9):22–42.
13. Turner GA, Hoptroff M, Harding CR. Stratum corneum dysfunction in dandruff. Int J Cosmet Sci. 2012;34(4):298–306.
14. Warner RR, Schwartz JR, Boissy Y, Dawson Jr TL. Dandruff has an altered stratum corneum ultrastructure that is improved with zinc pyrithione shampoo. J Am Acad Dermatol. 2001;45(6):897–903.
15. Billhimer W, Erb J, Bacon R. Shampooing with pyrithione zinc reduces trans-epidermal water loss in scalp of dandruff-involved patients. J Am Acad Dermatol. 2006;54 Suppl 3:AB131.
16. Schliemann-Willers S, Wigger-Alberti W, Kleesz P, Grieshaber R, Elsner P. Natural vegetable fats in the prevention of irritant contact dermatitis. Contact Dermatitis. 2002;46(1):6–12.
17. Mukherjee S, Edmunds M, Lei X, Ottaviani MF, Ananthapadmanabhan KP, Turro NJ. Stearic acid delivery to corneum from a mild and moisturizing cleanser. J Cosmet Dermatol. 2010;9(3):202–10.

19

Estimation of individual cumulative ultraviolet exposure using a geographically-adjusted, openly-accessible tool

Gefei A. Zhu[1†], Inbar Raber[1†], Sukolsak Sakshuwong[2], Shufeng Li[1], Angela S. Li[1], Caroline Tan[1] and Anne Lynn S. Chang[1*]

Abstract

Background: Estimates of an individual's cumulative ultraviolet (UV) radiation exposure can be useful since ultraviolet radiation exposure increases skin cancer risk, but a comprehensive tool that is practical for use in the clinic does not currently exist.

The objective of this study is to develop a geographically-adjusted tool to systematically estimate an individual's self-reported cumulative UV radiation exposure, investigate the association of these estimates with skin cancer diagnosis, and assess test reliability.

Methods: A 12-item online questionnaire from validated survey items for UV exposure and skin cancer was administered to online volunteers across the United States and results cross-referenced with UV radiation indices. Cumulative UV exposure scores (CUES) were calculated and correlated with personal history of skin cancer in a case–control design. Reliability was assessed in a separate convenience sample.

Results: 1,118 responses were included in the overall sample; the mean age of respondents was 46 (standard deviation 15, range 18 – 81) and 150 (13 %) reported a history of skin cancer. In bivariate analysis of 1:2 age-matched cases ($n = 149$) and controls ($n = 298$), skin cancer cases were associated with (1) greater CUES prior to first skin cancer diagnosis than controls without skin cancer history (242,074 vs. 205,379, $p = 0.003$) and (2) less engagement in UV protective behaviors ($p < 0.01$). In a multivariate analysis of age-matched data, individuals with CUES in the lowest quartile were less likely to develop skin cancer compared to those in the highest quartile. In reliability testing among 19 volunteers, the 2-week intra-class correlation coefficient for CUES was 0.94.

Conclusions: CUES is a useable and comprehensive tool to better estimate lifetime ultraviolet exposure, so that individuals with higher levels of exposure may be identified for counseling on photo-protective measures.

Keywords: Clinical research, Survey, Case–control, Sun exposure, Skin cancer, Ultraviolet radiation

Background

Ultraviolet (UV) radiation exposure increases risk for cutaneous cancers and photo-aging, [1–7] however, systematic estimation of whether an individual has higher-than-average sun exposure is difficult in the clinical setting. UV radiation is an environmental carcinogen, much like cigarette smoke is an environmental carcinogen whose exposure can be estimated using lifetime cumulative "pack-years" in the clinical setting [8]. The objective of this study was to create a tool that systematically estimates cumulative UV exposures, and accounts for geographic locale.

Calculating an individual's lifetime UV radiation exposure can be challenging [9] in the clinical setting, as it requires information on (1) the frequency and duration of UV exposures which can vary over a person's lifetime, and (2) the residential history, since UV index varies by

* Correspondence: alschang@stanford.edu
†Equal contributors
[1]Department of Dermatology, Stanford University School of Medicine, 450 Broadway St., Redwood City, CA 94063, USA
Full list of author information is available at the end of the article

geographic location. In the research setting, data on (1) has been gathered through face-to-face [3, 5, 6, 10–15] or telephone interviews, [16, 17] which can take 45 min just to collect sun exposure-related variables, [13] and is too time-consuming for a fast paced dermatology clinic. Individual diary formats and dosimetry are suitable for collecting data for short periods of time, but not feasible for recording lifetime exposures [18–21] over decades. Finally, though shorter instruments exist, such as the Sun Exposure Behavior Inventory, [22] these questionnaires do not collect an complete residential and exposure history to allow for assessment of lifetime ultraviolet exposure.

With regard to data collection and analysis, an accurate, clinically-useful tool should rapidly parse residential histories, including the durations of residence, and link them to UV indices, as all these factors can vary significantly across a lifetime [20, 22, 23]. Individuals living in the United States frequently change their geographic region of residence over their lifetimes, with over one-third of the population residing in a state different than the one they were born in [24, 25]. Therefore, accounting for regional differences in UV index when estimating an individual's lifetime UV radiation exposure is critical. Indeed, the average annual UV index varies widely within the United States, from 1.9 in Anchorage, Alaska, to 3.3 in Seattle, Washington to 9.3 in Honolulu, Hawaii and must be accounted for when assessing cumulative exposure (Additional file 1: Table S1).

In this three-part study, we developed an internet-based, self-administered questionnaire for (1) estimating cumulative UV exposure (which we term the cumulative UV exposure score or CUES) and (2) assessed for associations with sun protective behaviors and skin cancer to establish a connection with clinically relevant endpoints, and (3) since sun protective behaviors are known to change after skin cancer diagnosis, [19, 26–28] we retrospectively assessed the CUES before and after first skin cancer diagnosis to examine whether CUES could detect a significant difference, as would be expected from data in the medical literature.

Methods

Recruitment of participants

Following approval by the Stanford University Institutional Review Board (Protocol #29695), volunteers for this case–control study were recruited online between March and November 2014 to ensure geographic diversity in residence and travel throughout the United States. Volunteers were contacted using ResearchMatch, a national health volunteer registry created by several academic institutions and supported by the United States National Institutes of Health as part of the Clinical Translational Science Award (CTSA) program. ResearchMatch curates a database of volunteers who have consented to be contacted by researchers about health-related studies for which they may be eligible.

Individuals aged 18 years or older who have not resided outside of the United States for more than one year in their lifetime were eligible for the study. Those residing outside the United States for greater than one year were excluded, as UV index data from countries outside the United States were not always directly comparable due to differences in measurement methodology. All eligible subjects within the 50 states were sent an email with an invitation to complete the study questionnaire. The random selection feature was utilized in the recruitment process.

ResearchMatch did not allow us to confirm whether recruitment emails were received, opened, or read by recipients, precluding calculation of a traditional response rate. In addition, we were unable to access the demographics of individuals who did not participate in the study to probe for potential bias of responders versus non-responders. Subjects were not compensated for their participation in this study.

Study cases were defined as those with a personal history of skin cancer diagnosed after age 18, and controls were defined as those without a personal history of skin cancer. Because initial testing indicated that CUES is strongly correlated with age, cases and controls were matched on age. Specifically, age at first skin cancer diagnosis among cases was matched with age at time of survey administration among controls. For each case, two age-matched controls were randomly selected from the study cohort using standard propensity score matching.

To test the reliability of the questionnaire responses, a convenience sample of 19 individuals who were 18 years and older from the Stanford academic community, and separate from ResearchMatch participants, was asked to complete the questionnaire twice with an intervening two-week period between administrations, with results compared between the two time points. The sample size of 19 and the two-week time separation were determined after literature review of other questionnaire reliability studies. Since there are no published reports of *minimum* time interval and sample size requirements specifically related to ultraviolet radiation exposure surveys, we utilized test-retest time interval and sample size reported in similar types of studies consisting of self-reported data outside of dermatology. The two-week time interval between test and retest for reliability studies is a generally accepted time frame referenced in multiple clinical studies [29–32]. For sample size determination for test-retest reliability studies, a well-designed study by Hobart and colleagues [33] have reported similar intra-class correlation coefficients across a sample size of 20 versus 120 in a study of self-reported patient symptoms.

Questionnaire development and administration

Following a PubMed search and review of validated sun-exposure and skin cancer questionnaire items, a survey was created consisting of 17 total items. Out of the 17 questions, the first eleven items were used to ascertain clinically relevant phenomena such as history of skin cancer or sun protective behaviors for the purposes of this study.

In actual non-study use, we envision that only items under the heading "Estimated outdoor exposure time" and "Estimated location data" would need to be answered to calculate CUES (although the first eleven items could be clinically useful for the health care provider, they are not needed to calculate CUES). Skip patterns were automatically implemented and the actual number of questions answered could be as few as 10, depending on the responses entered. The questionnaire was administered using a dynamic website interface (see screenshots included in the Additional file 2 and live online demo at http://gefeizhu.github.io/cues-study/). Demographic information collected from respondents was limited to age and self-reported Fitzpatrick skin type, based on questions on propensity for tanning and burning [34, 35]. Next, respondents were asked about whether there was a personal or family history of skin cancer, and if so, what type of cancer (possible choices were "basal cell carcinoma," "squamous cell carcinoma," "melanoma," "other," or "don't know"). Respondents with a personal history of skin cancer were asked about age and type of skin cancer at first diagnosis. All respondents answered questions on lifetime frequency of (1) tanning bed use (possible choices were "0," "1 – 5," "6 – 10," "11 – 100, "and "greater than 100"), (2) blistering sunburns (possible choices were "0," "1 – 5," "6 – 10," and "greater than 10"), (3) use of sunscreen, (4) use of long-sleeved shirts, (5) use of a hat, and (6) shade-seeking behaviors (possible choices for items 3 – 6 were "never," "rarely," sometimes," "often," and "always"); some of these items were adapted from previously validated instruments [16, 22] and modified for use in our questionnaire. For individuals with a personal history of skin cancer, the 6 items mentioned above appeared twice to capture behaviors both before and after the date of diagnosis of their first skin cancer. To minimize recall bias, identical before and after question pairs related to sun protective behaviors and skin blistering were separated by four questions not related to the question pairs.

Respondents were asked about duration of sun exposure during peak sunlight hours (10 am – 4 pm) during weekdays and weekends, expressed in hours per day. To facilitate recall, exposure duration data were collected for discrete age ranges (0 – 13, 13 – 20, 20 – 40, 40 – 65, 65 – 80, and 80+) that roughly correspond with life milestones.[10, 31, 36] To account for geographic differences in UV exposure across the lifetime, respondents were queried on location of residence and the ages during which they lived in each location. The questionnaire was programmed to require a full and complete lifetime residential history before respondents were allowed to submit the responses.

The final item of the online survey tool solicited subjective feedback from respondents in narrative form.

Integration of data validation tools into our online questionnaire allowed for real-time delivery of feedback to respondents, minimized unanalyzable and missing data (99.8 % of all responses were included for analysis, see Results section) and ensured proper implementation of inclusion and exclusion criteria.

Calculation of Cumulative UV Exposure Score (CUES)

CUES was calculated from data taken in the sections of the questionnaire entitled "Estimated outdoor exposure time" and "Estimated location data". The most recent data available from the National Oceanic and Atmospheric Administration (2009–2012) at the time of questionnaire development was used to calculate average annual UV indices for 58 anchor cities across the United States (Additional file 1: Table S1). During this period, the lowest UV index was 1.9 (Anchorage, AK) and the highest UV index was 10.3 (San Juan, PR). The UV index is a standardized, linear measure of erythemally-weighted irradiance which can theoretically fall between 0 (at night) and 43 [37] but annual UV indices in the United States generally fall between 1 and 11, with each unit equal to 0.025 W/m^2 [38]. CUES was calculated according to CUES = Σ (Hours of Exposure × UV Index). CUES, which has formal units of $W*h/m^2$, is directly proportional to standard radiant exposure units (J/m^2). As the CUES is an estimate only, and not data from dosimetry, we omit the actual units in the report of the CUES. Rather the CUES can be viewed as a relative measure, akin to the pack-year.

The participant's lifetime was divided into one-year intervals, each of which was assigned a duration of exposure and a location of exposure based on questionnaire responses. Next, the location of exposure (in "City, State" format) was resolved into longitude and latitude coordinates using the publically-available Google Maps application program interface (API) and the closest anchor city was determined using the Haversine formula for great-circle distances. For each one-year interval, the hours of exposure was multiplied by the UV index for the nearest anchor city to obtain an annual UV dose estimate. This method was repeated for each one-year interval and the annual doses were summed to obtain a CUES. To minimize human error during this process, data acquisition, validation and CUES calculation was completely automated using an open source JavaScript program developed by the authors. We have provided the ~1,700 lines of code used to collect questionnaire data and calculate CUES as an open access resource at https://github.com/gefeizhu/cues-study so that future UV indices can be substituted, should they change significantly.

Association of CUES with clinically relevant endpoints

We compared the CUES of individuals with skin cancer history prior to their first skin cancer diagnosis with the CUES of individuals without skin cancer history, in age-matched fashion. This enabled us to assess whether CUES could detect differences in lifetime ultraviolet exposures between those with and without skin cancer, recapitulating a well-known association in the medical literature [5, 6, 39].

Second, since sun protective behaviors and UV exposures have been reported in the literature to change after skin cancer diagnosis, [28, 40, 41] we assessed the ability of our instrument to detect differences in CUES among cases before and after first skin cancer diagnosis, as well as changes in tanning and sun protective behaviors before and after first skin cancer diagnosis.

Statistical analysis

Student's t-tests or chi-square tests were used in bivariate analyses on most continuous and categorical variables, respectively, for comparisons between individuals with a personal history of skin cancer and those without. Because age and CUES were not normally distributed, Wilcoxon's rank-sum tests were used as nonparametric alternatives to t-tests in these comparisons. Individuals could report one or more types of family history of skin cancer, and therefore two-sample Student's t-tests were used to compare these variables.

Each case was matched with 2 controls on age using standard propensity score matching. One case was excluded because the respondent had a first diagnosis of skin cancer before age 18. To estimate the odds of developing skin cancer, conditional logistic regression was applied in univariate and multivariate analyses. Interactions and multi-collinearity were assessed in determining the final multivariate model. Wilcoxon's signed-rank test was used to compare CUES and Bowker's test was used to compare sun protective behaviors, tanning bed use, and lifetime history of blistering sunburns before and after diagnosis of skin cancer among cases.

Test-retest reliability was assessed by calculating an intraclass correlation coefficient (ICC) for the CUES score and weighted kappa coefficients for categorical survey items. In general, kappa scores of 0.75 or greater reflect excellent agreement, scores of 0.40 to 0.75 reflect fair-to-good agreement, and scores below 0.4 reflect poor agreement [42]. The raw and standardized Cronbach's alpha for the questionnaire items was 0.59.

In light of the Cronbach's alpha score, factor analysis was performed on use of hat, use of long-sleeved clothing, shade-seeking behavior, use of sunscreen, Fitzpatrick skin type, lifetime history of blistering sunburns, and use of tanning beds to assess dimensionality. After applying eigenvalue selection criteria, one factor was retained, comprising: use of hat, use of long-sleeved clothing, shade-seeking behavior, use of sunscreen, Fitzpatrick skin type, lifetime number of blistering sunburns, and use of tanning beds.

All statistical analyses were conducted using SAS (Version 9.4, SAS Institute, Inc., Cary, North Carolina).

Results

ResearchMatch sent emails to 60,480 individuals for this study. 1,120 (1.9 %) completed the study questionnaire, of which 1,118 (99.8 %) were completely filled out and met inclusion criteria by age and residential history.

This group was analyzed for the study and individuals residing in 47 states (see Additional file 3: Figure S1 for distribution of states). Both of the excluded questionnaires reported location(s) of residence outside of the United States for ≥1 year. A standard response rate could not be calculated from the online format, as there was no way to ascertain that the email had been read by the potential respondents in their inboxes.

The mean age of all study participants was 46 years (range 18 – 81), and 150 (13 %) individuals reported a personal history of skin cancer. Approximately 70 % of individuals participating in this study self-reported Fitzpatrick skin type 2–3, with 20 % self-reporting Fitzpatrick skin type 4–6. Other demographic information is presented in Table 1. The annual UV indices in the reported locales of study participants in the United States ranged from 1.88 to 10.29. (Additional file 1: Table S1).

In bivariate analyses, individuals with a personal history of skin cancer were significantly older than those without a personal history of skin cancer (mean age 61.6 vs. 45.4, $p < 0.0001$), were more likely to have a family history of skin cancer (55 % vs. 30 %, $p < 0.0001$), and more likely to have Fitzpatrick skin types I or II (59 % vs. 43 %, $p = 0.001$).

To further characterize the relationship between development of skin cancer and clinical and UV exposure-related behavioral variables, factor analysis was performed on the questionnaire items. One factor was identified, with standardized scoring coefficients presented in

Table 1 Characteristics for all participants by personal history of skin cancer, $N = 1,118$

Parameter	Negative personal history of skin cancer (*n* = 968)	Positive personal history of skin cancer (*n* = 150)	*p*
Age, mean (SD), in years	45.4 (14.6)	61.6 (11.6)	<0.0001
Family history of skin cancer, n (%)	286 (30)	82 (55)	<0.0001
Type of family history of skin cancer, n (%)[c]			
Basal cell carcinoma	123 (43)	66 (80)	<0.0001
Squamous cell carcinoma	58 (20)	31 (38)	0.0012
Melanoma	73 (26)	19 (23)	0.6528
Other	1 (0.4)	1 (1.2)	0.3464
Don't know	80 (28)	7 (8)	0.0002
Skin type (Fitzpatrick), n (%)			0.001
1	71 (7)	9 (6)	
2	350 (36)	80 (53)	
3	315 (33)	35 (23)	
4 + 5 + 6	232 (24)	26 (17)	
Tanning bed use by number of visits,[a] n (%)			0.1017
0	537 (55)	100 (67)	
1–5	157 (16)	18 (12)	
6–10	85 (9)	11 (7)	
11–100	152 (16)	19 (13)	
>100	37 (4)	2 (1)	
Lifetime number of blistering sunburns, n (%)			<0.0001
0	165 (17)	14 (9)	
1–5	524 (54)	72 (48)	
6–10	162 (17)	25 (17)	
>10	117 (12)	39 (26)	
Age at first skin cancer diagnosis, mean (SD), in years	NA	51.4 (13.8)	NA
Type of first skin cancer diagnosis, n (%)			
Basal cell carcinoma	NA	93 (62)	NA
Squamous cell carcinoma		20 (13)	
Melanoma		17 (11)	
Other		7 (5)	
Don't know		13 (9)	
Factor score, median (range)[d]	0.2 (−2.0 – 2.2)	−0.2 (−2.3 – 1.4)	<0.0001
Lifetime total hours of exposure, median (range)	37,128 (2,496 – 156,520)	55,172 (14,976 – 157,248)	<0.0001
CUES[b], median (range)	180,708 (11,288 – 778,332)	241,873 (44,858 – 898,344)	<0.0001

[a]Total number of tanning bed visits per lifetime (negative personal history of skin cancer) or total number of tanning bed visits up until first skin cancer diagnosis (positive personal history of skin cancer)
[b]Total CUES (negative personal history of skin cancer) or CUES prior to first skin cancer diagnosis (positive personal history of skin cancer)
[c]Individuals could report a family history of more than one type of cancer, therefore chi-squared testing was not possible
[d]A single factor was identified during factor analysis, which incorporated Fitzpatrick skin type, use of tanning bed, lifetime number of blistering sunburns, use of hat, use of long-sleeved clothing, shade-seeking behavior, and use of sunscreen

Additional file 4: Table S2. Median factor scores of individuals with a personal history of skin cancer were significantly lower than those without (median −0.2 vs. 0.2, $p < 0.0001$), suggesting an inverse relationship between factor scores and skin cancer risk (Table 1).

Association of CUES with personal history of skin cancer

The median CUES of individuals with a personal history of skin cancer was significantly higher than those without personal history of skin cancer (241,873 vs. 180,708, $p = 0.0001$), as was the total hours of exposure (55,172 vs. 37,128, $p < 0.0001$). The CUES distributions of individuals with and without a personal history of skin cancer overlapped significantly, as expected for a disease process with a multifactorial etiology (Table 1).

To assess if CUES is associated with development of skin cancer, a case–control format was utilized. In this part of the study, 149 cases (individuals with a personal history of skin cancer) were matched to 298 controls (individuals with no personal history of skin cancer), with exclusion of only one individual who reported a history of skin cancer prior to age 18 years. CUES at time of first skin cancer diagnosis (for those with a personal history of skin cancer) and total CUES (for those without) were divided into quartiles and used as the predictor of interest. In age-matched case–control analyses, individuals in the lowest quartile of CUES were less likely to report a positive history of skin cancer compared to those in the highest quartile (OR 0.4, 95 % CI 0.2 – 0.7). Cases had significantly greater CUES prior to first skin cancer diagnosis compared to total CUES of controls in matched analyses (242,074 vs. 205,379, $p = 0.003$) (Table 2).

A multivariate model using conditional logistic regression showed that CUES was an independent risk factor for development of skin cancer, while controlling for family history of skin cancer and the factor score, which included Fitzpatrick skin type and several ultraviolet exposure-related variables (Additional file 4: Table S2). Individuals with CUES in the 1st quartile (adjusted odds ratio [AOR] 0.5, 95 % CI 0.2 – 0.97) were less likely to develop skin cancer compared to those in the highest quartile independent of covariates (Table 2).

Association of sun protective behaviors with personal history of skin cancer

In univariate analyses, cases were more likely to report "rarely" using hats (OR 1.9, 95 % CI 1.1 – 3.2) compared to controls. Cases were *less* likely to report "often" seeking shade (OR 0.3, 95 % CI 0.2 – 0.6), "often" (OR 0.3, 95 % CI 0.1 – 0.6) or "always" (OR 0.2, 95 % CI 0.1 – 0.6) using long-sleeved clothing, and "often" (OR 0.3, 95 % CI 0.2 – 0.8) or "always" (OR 0.03, 95 % CI 0.003 – 0.23) using sunscreen. Positive history of tanning bed use was not significantly different between cases and controls (Table 2).

In multivariate analysis using conditional logic regression, Fitzpatrick skin type and many UV exposure-related variables were collapsed into a single factor score. Cases reported a significantly lower factor score compared to controls (AOR 0.5, 95 % CI 0.4 – 0.7), consistent with the UV exposure-related risk factors included in the calculation of this factor (Table 2 and Additional file 4: Table S2).

After a skin cancer diagnosis, individuals with a personal history of skin cancer reported significantly increased engagement in sun-protective behaviors, including tanning bed avoidance ($p = 0.0005$), use of sunscreen ($p < 0.0001$), use of long-sleeved clothing ($p < 0.0001$), use of hat ($p < 0.0001$), shade seeking behavior ($p < 0.0001$), and reduced number of blistering sunburns ($p < 0.0001$). Additionally, there was a concordant decrease in the median annual CUES calculated after skin cancer diagnosis compared to before (4,970 vs. 3,087, $p < 0.0001$) (Table 3).

To promote the ease of use of the CUES score, a summary of scores (rounded to the nearest thousand units) relative to study participants is provided in Table 4, so that individuals can see whether their scores are above the median of study participants across the United States.

Reliability of CUES

To assess the reliability of CUES, a convenience sample of 19 individuals was recruited outside of ResearchMatch from the Stanford academic community and asked to fill out identical questionnaires before and after a 2 week period to assess the reliability of survey items. The weighted kappa/ICC for CUES was 0.94, (95 % CI, 0.86 – 0.98) indicating excellent reliability. Weighted kappa scores for other questionnaire items ranged from 0.43 (95 % CI 0.23 – 1.00) for shade seeking behavior to 1.00 (95 % CI 1.00 – 1.00) for family history of skin cancer (Table 5). While the weighted kappa for CUES is good, the small sample size from the Stanford academic community could limit its generalizability to the national survey population.

Feedback from respondents indicated the questionnaire and its online implementation was easy to understand, logical, and brief. All the respondents took less than 10 min to complete the survey.

Discussion

We report an open-source questionnaire-based method of calculating cumulative UV radiation exposure that can be used to identify individuals with higher lifetime UV radiation exposures (e.g. >240,000 units, the median CUES of those with a history of skin cancer) and accounts for the variety of geographic differences across the United States. Increased CUES was associated with a positive personal history of skin cancer in the overall sample ($n = 1{,}118$) (Table 1) as well as the age-matched case–control subset analysis ($n = 447$) in univariate and multivariate analyses (Table 2). We also report a decrease in annual CUES and a concordant increase in sun protective habits following skin cancer diagnosis,(Table 3), thereby demonstrating the ability of CUES to detect

Table 2 Sun-Protective behaviors and CUES among skin cancer cases and age-matched controls, $N = 447$

Parameter	Controls ($n = 298$)	Cases ($n = 149$)	Unadjusted Odds Ratio (95 % confidence interval)[a]	Adjusted Odds Ratio (95 % confidence interval)[b,c]
Fitzpatrick Skin Type, n (%)				
1	25 (8)	8 (5)	Ref	Incorporated into factor score[e]
2	112 (38)	80 (54)	2.26 (0.97 – 5.26)	
3	102 (34)	35 (23)	1.10 (0.46 – 2.63)	
4 + 5 + 6	59 (20)	26 (17)	1.40 (0.58 – 3.41)	
Use of tanning bed, n (%)				
0	177 (59)	99 (66)	Ref	Incorporated into factor score[e]
1–5	42 (14)	18 (12)	0.76 (0.41 – 1.42)	
6–10	29 (10)	11 (7)	0.66 (0.30 – 1.42)	
11–100	43 (14)	19 (13)	0.77 (0.42 – 1.42)	
>100	7 (2)	2 (1)	0.54 (0.11 – 2.59)	
Lifetime number of blistering sunburns, n (%)				
0	41 (14)	14 (9)	Ref	Incorporated into factor score[e]
1 -5	156 (52)	72 (48)	1.3 (0.7 – 2.6)	
- 10	58 (19)	24 (16)	1.2 (0.5 – 2.6)	
>10	43 (14)	39 (26)	2.6 (1.2 – 5.5)	
Use of hat, n (%)				
Never	78 (26)	32 (21)	Ref	Incorporated into factor score[e]
Rarely	77 (26)	63 (42)	1.89 (1.11 – 3.23)	
Sometimes	80 (27)	25 (17)	0.74 (0.39 – 1.41)	
Often	45 (15)	23 (15)	1.20 (0.62 – 2.32)	
Always	18 (6)	6 (4)	0.79 (0.28 – 2.21)	
Use of long-sleeved clothing, n (%)				
Never	13 (4)	19 (13)	Ref	Incorporated into factor score[e]
Rarely	34 (11)	31 (21)	0.70 (0.29 – 1.66)	
Sometimes	58 (19)	39 (26)	0.56 (0.25 – 1.26)	
Often	112 (38)	37 (25)	0.29 (0.14 – 0.63)	
Always	81 (27)	23 (15)	0.24 (0.11 – 0.55)	
Shade seeking, n (%)				
Never	25 (8)	25 (17)	Ref	Incorporated into factor score[e]
Rarely	68 (23)	50 (34)	0.80 (0.42 – 1.54)	
Sometimes	120 (40)	52 (35)	0.50 (0.27 – 0.93)	
Often	79 (27)	21 (14)	0.31 (0.16 – 0.63)	
Always	6 (2)	1 (1)	0.18 (0.02 – 1.76)	
Use of sunscreen, n (%)				
Never	16 (5)	13 (9)	Ref	Incorporated into factor score[e]
Rarely	55 (18)	44 (30)	1.01 (0.44 – 2.34)	
Sometimes	84 (28)	62 (41)	0.90 (0.41 – 1.97)	
Often	97 (33)	29 (19)	0.34 (0.15 – 0.82)	
Always	46 (15)	1 (1)	0.03 (0.003 – 0.23)	
Factor score, median (range)[e]	0.2 (−2.0 – 2.2)	−0.2 (−2.3 – 1.4)	0.56 (0.43 – 0.72)	0.54 (0.41 –0.71)

Table 2 Sun-Protective behaviors and CUES among skin cancer cases and age-matched controls, $N = 447$ *(Continued)*

Family history of skin cancer, n (%)	92 (31)	81 (54)	2.63 (1.73 – 3.99)	3.06 (1.92 – 4.88)
CUES[d], median (range)	205,379 (28,439 – 764,540)***	242,074 (44,858 – 898,344)***		
CUES[d], quartilized, n (%)				
4th Quartile	112 (25)	112 (25)	Ref	Ref
1st Quartile	111 (25)	111 (25)	0.36 (0.19 – 0.69)	0.48 (0.24 – 0.97)
2nd Quartile	112 (25)	112 (25)	0.62 (0.34 – 1.12)	0.76 (0.38 – 1.49)
3rd Quartile	112 (25)	112 (25)	0.63 (0.37 – 1.10)	0.75 (0.41 – 1.37)
Lifetime total hours of exposure, median (range)	43,342 (6,630 – 156,520)	55,328 (14,976 – 157,248)		

[a]Univariate logistic regression
[b]Multivariate logistic regression
[c]Adjusted for quartilized CUES, family history of skin cancer, and a single factor comprising Fitzpatrick skin type, use of tanning bed, lifetime number of blistering sunburns, use of hat, use of long-sleeved clothing, shade-seeking, and use of sunscreen
[d]Total CUES (controls) or CUES prior to first skin cancer diagnosis (cases)
***$p = 0.003$ by Wilcoxon rank-sum test
[e]A single factor was identified during factor analysis, which incorporated Fitzpatrick skin type, use of tanning bed, lifetime number of blistering sunburns, use of hat, use of long-sleeved clothing, shade-seeking, and use of sunscreen

changes in sun exposure after skin cancer diagnoses that is well known from previous studies [19, 26–28].

Current methods in the clinic to estimate an individual's UV exposure are often uni-dimensional (such as "how many blistering sunburns have you had in your lifetime?") or subjective (such as "do you spend a lot of time outdoors?"), and CUES enables systematic estimation that can be performed in the clinic waiting room such as with a patient's own smartphone or tablet by logging onto the publically available website. CUES can then be incorporated as part of the discussion with dermatologists on whether more aggressive sun-protective measures may be beneficial. Of course, skin cancer risk is multifactorial, and includes factors other than cumulative UV exposure such as patient's co-morbid medical conditions, family history, or Fitzpatrick skin type. Moreover, CUES does not contribute information about the intermittency of exposure events, which has been positively correlated with an increased risk of developing melanoma [43]. This tool does not replace clinical judgment to assess individual risk for skin cancer.

Nevertheless, a potential use of the CUES may be to motivate at-risk patients to reduce ongoing UV exposure through immediate, personalized feedback in clinic or through other means of conveying such information (e.g. secure email or messaging systems). The ability of immediate feedback to alter sun protective behaviors has been shown, for instance through a mobile phone application that delivered real-time, location-based UV index data and encouraged sun protection [44]. Whether receipt of a CUES upon completion of the survey tool improves sun protective behaviors is the subject of a forthcoming study.

Several important simplifying assumptions were made in designing this study. First, since average annual UV indices were used, we did not account for important diurnal, seasonal or yearly differences in the UV index. Second, we were not able to adjust our CUES using traditional means, such as applying corrections for body posture (the UV index is typically measured using dosimeters installed on a horizontal surface). Finally, we assumed that self-reported frequencies of exposure (expressed in hours per week) were constant for epochs spanning several years. Though future refinements may enable these assumptions to be diminished or eliminated, a statistically-significant difference in CUES was detectable between those with more or less sun-protective behaviors and with skin cancer diagnosis, even with the aforementioned assumptions.

CUES is not intended to substitute for precise measurements of UV exposure through dosimetry. While dosimetry is the gold standard method of estimating UV exposure in short-term research studies, it is not currently realistic for individuals to carry a dosimeter over many decades. Dosimetry is also problematic due to possible heterogeneity in the location the device is worn between studies and the potential lack of adherence in wearing the device. We do not claim that CUES is a physical measure of actual UV exposure by the survey respondents but is rather an estimate based on self-reported data. In lieu of testing the content validity of our measure, we elected to validate CUES by reporting its ability to detect a well-established association between UV exposure and sun protective behaviors and skin cancer.

Moreover, since CUES is not a precise measure of actual UV dosage, we avoided reporting the formal units

Table 3 Sun-Protective behaviors and CUES before and after skin cancer diagnosis among cases, $N = 149$

Parameter	Before skin cancer	After skin cancer	Percentage of absolute agreement	*P*
Annual CUES, median (range) units*	4,970 (1,057 – 16,042)	3,087 (0 – 13,353)		
Use of tanning bed, n (%)				
0	100 (67)	136 (91)	64 %	0.0005
1–5	17 (11)	0 (0)		
6–10	11 (7)	5 (3)		
11–100	18 (12)	6 (4)		
>100	2 (1)	1 (1)		
Use of sunscreen, n (%)				
Never	13 (9)	2 (1)	29 %	<0.0001
Rarely	44 (30)	9 (6)		
Sometimes	62 (42)	39 (26)		
Often	29 (19)	69 (46)		
Always	2 (1)	31 (21)		
Use of long-sleeved clothing, n (%)				
Never	19 (13)	7 (5)	41 %	<0.0001
Rarely	31 (21)	11 (7)		
Sometimes	39 (26)	28 (19)		
Often	37 (25)	45 (30)		
Always	24 (16)	59 (40)		
Use of hat, n (%)				
Never	32 (21)	10 (7)	29 %	<0.0001
Rarely	64 (43)	15 (10)		
Sometimes	25 (17)	37 (25)		
Often	23 (15)	55 (37)		
Always	6 (4)	33 (22)		
Shade seeking, n (%)				
Never	25 (17)	10 (7)	35 %	<0.0001
Rarely	50 (34)	16 (11)		
Sometimes	52 (35)	43 (29)		
Often	22 (15)	64 (43)		
Always	1 (1)	17 (11)		
Lifetime number of blistering sunburns, n (%)				
0	14 (9)	127 (85)	12 %	<0.0001
1 – 5	72 (48)	19 (13)		
6 – 10	25 (17)	1 (1)		
>10	39 (26)	3 (2)		

P-value determined by Bowker's test

of the CUES. Our intention is for CUES to be used to identify patients at risk for skin cancer in a similar way as "pack-years" is used to stratify lung cancer risk in smokers. While CUES does not reflect a physical measurement of UV dose received by an individual, CUES can be easily incorporated into epidemiological studies in which lifetime UV exposure is a covariate or independent variable of interest. We envision that the CUES will primarily be of interest to clinicians, as it relies on self-reported data ascertainable in clinic waiting rooms. Of course, the CUES is a crude measurement when compared to studies employing dosimetry, diaries, or interviews, which allow for precise quantitation of UV exposure in physical units. However, such methodological rigor does not add to clinical utility, just as knowing the precise number of cigarettes smoked does not

Table 4 How your CUES compares to individuals in the study

Your CUES[a]	How Your CUES compares to Individuals in the study
<205,000 units	Below median score for those without history of skin cancer
205,001–242,000 units	Above median score for those without history of skin cancer and below the median score for those with skin cancer
>242,001 units	Above median score for those with skin cancer

[a]The CUES reported in this table have been rounded to the nearest thousand

substantially alter to the management of a smoker who is known to have a high pack-year history.

There are several important limitations in this study. First, we were unable to detect increased odds of developing skin cancer among individuals reporting tanning bed use, either in the entire sample (Table 1) or in case–control analyses (Table 2). We stratified tanning bed use by age, such as aged ≤54 or >54 years, the median age in our study, but this did not yield different results (data not shown). The strong relationship between tanning bed use and UV-dependent skin cancers, particularly melanoma, is well established in the literature [45]. Our inability to recapitulate these findings in this study is likely a combination of (1) low sample size, given that only 9 individuals reported using tanning beds >100 times in their lifetimes, (2) heterogeneity in the dose and spectral characteristics of tanning bed UV radiation, [46] and (3) our inability to specify the age(s) at which our respondents used tanning beds, as tanning during adolescence and young adulthood is more strongly associated with subsequent skin cancers [45, 47].

A second limitation is potential selection bias, in that only 1.9 % of individuals contacted by ResearchMatch completed the questionnaire. It is possible that there were important undetected differences between responders and nonresponders, however, the ResearchMatch platform did not allow for this type of assessment.

A third and most important limitation is the possibility of recall bias, which is inherent in the retrospective and self-reported nature of this study. This was carefully considered in the design of the study, and measures were taken to minimize this bias, namely (A) separating pairs of identical questions asking about sun protective behaviors and tanning bed use before and after diagnosis of skin cancer among those with a positive history and (B) constraining exposure duration responses to fixed age epochs (0 – 13, 13 – 20, 20 – 40, 40 – 65, 65 – 80, and 80+) rather than having the epochs fall before and after first skin cancer diagnosis. This study would not be feasible to conduct in prospective fashion due to the need to follow large numbers of individuals nationally over many decades with dosimetry data or serial questionnaire administrations. It is not possible to prospectively "blind" patients to their own diagnosis of skin cancer, and therefore it would be impossible to remove this potential recall bias. The retrospective format of CUES is consistent with how it would be used in the clinical setting, that is, as a tool that could be used before or after eliciting the past medical history, itself a retrospective but necessary part of everyday clinical care that is also prone to recall bias.

In fact, multiple clinical measures in fields outside of dermatology in common use rely on patient self-report, such as the New York Heart Association (NYHA) functional classification in cardiology or the Eastern Cooperative Oncology Group (ECOG) performance status score used in oncology. These measures, like the CUES, are subject to recall bias but are used ubiquitously in their respective clinical contexts due to their utility. Nevertheless, we envision that recall bias could be explored in future studies, for example by comparing self-reported data with

Table 5 Test-retest reliability, $N = 19$

Survey Item	Weighted kappa/ICC	95 % Confidence intervals	Percentage of absolute agreement
CUES	0.94[a]	0.86–0.98	NA
Fitzpatrick skin type	0.90	0.79–1.00	72 %
Family history of skin cancer	1.00	1.00–1.00	100 %
Use of sunscreen	0.84	0.71–0.98	72 %
Use of long-sleeved clothing	0.73	0.55–0.91	72 %
Use of hat	0.96	0.88–1.00	94 %
Shade seeking	0.43	0.23–1.00	83 %
History of blistering sunburns	0.87	0.70–1.00	83 %
Residential history	0.99	0.99–1.00	94 %

[a]Intraclass correlation coefficient (ICC)

observer-reported data such as those provided by family members or caregivers, though such data also carry the risk of bias.

Conclusions

Finally, we make the CUES calculation tool freely available online in two ways. First, the source code is available for modification, for instance, should UV indices change in the future or if customization is needed for specific populations. Second, the CUES calculator can be accessed at the link reported in the Methods section for individual calculation, the result of which can be provided to a dermatologist or other health care provider by the patient in their discussion of photo-protective measures or skin cancer risk.

Additional files

Additional file 1: Table S1. Calculated Annual Average UV Indices for 58 Anchor Cities in the United States. UV indices in this study ranged from 1.88 to 10.29.

Additional file 2: Supplemental Materials. (PDF 954 kb)

Additional file 3: Figure S1. The Pacific Northwest includes WA, OR and CA. Atlantic Northeast includes MA, NY, DE, RI, Washington DC, ME, CT and NH. Atlantic South includes FL, AL, LA, SC, NC, GA, VA. Central U.S. includes all other states besides those previously mentioned.

Additional file 4: Table S2. Scoring Coefficients Used in Factor Analysis.

Abbreviations

AOR: Adjusted odds ratio; API: Application program interface; CTSA: Clinical Translational Science Award; CUES: Cumulative ultraviolet exposure score; h: Hour; J: Joule; m: Meter; SD: Standard deviation; UV: Ultraviolet; W: Watt.

Competing interests

The authors declare that they have no competing interests.

Authors' contributions

GAZ and IR participated in the design of the study and performed the statistical analysis. SS developed the software tool. GAZ, IR, ASL, and CT participated in data collection. ALSC conceived of the study and provided supervision of the study; she participated in its design, coordination, drafting of the manuscript and provided critical comments. All authors read and approved the final manuscript.

Author details

[1]Department of Dermatology, Stanford University School of Medicine, 450 Broadway St., Redwood City, CA 94063, USA. [2]Department of Computer Science, 353 Serra Mall, Stanford, CA 94305, USA.

References

1. Armstrong BK, Kricker A. The epidemiology of UV induced skin cancer. J Photochem Photobiol B Biol. 2001;63(1–3):8–18.
2. Flament F, Bazin R, Laquieze S, Rubert V, Simonpietri E, Piot B. Effect of the sun on visible clinical signs of aging in Caucasian skin. Clin Cosmet Investig Dermatol. 2013;6:221–32.
3. Kricker A, Armstrong BK, English DR, Heenan PJ. A dose-response curve for sun exposure and basal cell carcinoma. Int J Cancer. 1995; 60(4):482–8.
4. Moan J, Grigalavicius M, Baturaite Z, Dahlback A, Juzeniene A. The relationship between UV exposure and incidence of skin cancer. Photodermatol Photoimmunol Photomed. 2015;31(1):26–35.
5. Rosso S, Zanetti R, Martinez C, Tormo MJ, Schraub S, Sancho-Garnier H, et al. The multicentre south European study 'Helios'. II: Different sun exposure patterns in the aetiology of basal cell and squamous cell carcinomas of the skin. Br J Cancer. 1996;73(11):1447–54.
6. Vitasa BC, Taylor HR, Strickland PT, Rosenthal FS, West S, Abbey H, et al. Association of nonmelanoma skin cancer and actinic keratosis with cumulative solar ultraviolet exposure in Maryland watermen. Cancer. 1990; 65(12):2811–7.
7. Xiang F, Lucas R, Hales S, Neale R. Incidence of nonmelanoma skin cancer in relation to ambient UV radiation in white populations, 1978–2012: empirical relationships. JAMA Dermatol. 2014;150(10):1063–71.
8. International Agency for Research on Cancer (IARC). Agents Classified by the IARC Monographs, Volumes 1–112. In.; 4/7/2015.
9. Worswick SD, Cockburn M, Peng D. Measurement of ultraviolet exposure in epidemiological studies of skin and skin cancers. Photochem Photobiol. 2008;84(6):1462–72.
10. English DR, Armstrong BK, Kricker A. Reproducibility of reported measurements of sun exposure in a case-control study. Cancer Epidemiol Biomarkers Prev. 1998;7(10):857–63.
11. English DR, Armstrong BK, Kricker A, Winter MG, Heenan PJ, Randell PL. Case-control study of sun exposure and squamous cell carcinoma of the skin. Int J Cancer. 1998;77(3):347–53.
12. Fears TR, Bird CC, Guerry D, Sagebiel RW, Gail MH, Elder DE, et al. Average midrange ultraviolet radiation flux and time outdoors predict melanoma risk. Cancer Res. 2002;62(14):3992–6.
13. Karagas MR, Zens MS, Nelson HH, Mabuchi K, Perry AE, Stukel TA, et al. Measures of cumulative exposure from a standardized sun exposure history questionnaire: a comparison with histologic assessment of solar skin damage. Am J Epidemiol. 2007;165(6):719–26.
14. Kricker A, Armstrong BK, English DR, Heenan PJ. Does intermittent sun exposure cause basal cell carcinoma? a case-control study in Western Australia. Int J Cancer. 1995;60(4):489–94.
15. Tatalovich Z, Wilson JP, Mack T, Yan Y, Cockburn M. The objective assessment of lifetime cumulative ultraviolet exposure for determining melanoma risk. J Photochem Photobiol B Biol. 2006;85(3):198–204.
16. Kricker A, Vajdic CM, Armstrong BK. Reliability and validity of a telephone questionnaire for estimating lifetime personal sun exposure in epidemiologic studies. Cancer Epidemiol Biomarkers Prev. 2005;14(10): 2427–32.
17. Thomas NE, Kricker A, From L, Busam K, Millikan RC, Ritchey ME, et al. Associations of cumulative sun exposure and phenotypic characteristics with histologic solar elastosis. Cancer Epidemiol Biomarkers Prev. 2010; 19(11):2932–41.
18. Glanz K, Gies P, O'Riordan DL, Elliott T, Nehl E, McCarty F, et al. Validity of self-reported solar UVR exposure compared with objectively measured UVR exposure. Cancer Epidemiol Biomarkers Prev. 2010;19(12):3005–12.
19. Idorn LW, Datta P, Heydenreich J, Philipsen PA, Wulf HC. A 3-year follow-up of sun behavior in patients with cutaneous malignant melanoma. JAMA Dermatol. 2014;150(2):163–8.
20. Kimlin MG, Lucas RM, Harrison SL, van der Mei I, Armstrong BK, Whiteman DC, et al. The contributions of solar ultraviolet radiation exposure and other determinants to serum 25-hydroxyvitamin D concentrations in Australian adults: the AusD Study. Am J Epidemiol. 2014;179(7):864–74.
21. Thieden E, Collins SM, Philipsen PA, Murphy GM, Wulf HC. Ultraviolet exposure patterns of Irish and Danish gardeners during work and leisure. Br J Dermatol. 2005;153(4):795–801.
22. Jennings L, Karia PS, Jambusaria-Pahlajani A, Whalen FM, Schmults CD. The Sun Exposure and Behaviour Inventory (SEBI): validation of an instrument to assess sun exposure and sun protective practices. J Eur Acad Dermatol Venereol. 2013;27(6):706–15.
23. Grasso AA, Blanco S, Fantini G, Torelli F, Grasso M. Relationship between sun exposure and kidney cancer: preliminary experience with the evaluation of recreational UV exposure. Urologia. 2014;81(2):115–9.
24. United States Census Bureau. Domestic Migration Across Regions, Divisions, and States: 1995 to 2000. Washington, D.C.; 2003.

25. United States Census Bureau. Lifetime Mobility in the United States: 2010. Washington, D.C.; 2011.
26. Freiman A, Yu J, Loutfi A, Wang B. Impact of melanoma diagnosis on sun-awareness and protection: efficacy of education campaigns in a high-risk population. J Cutan Med Surg. 2004;8(5):303–9.
27. Idorn LW, Datta P, Heydenreich J, Philipsen PA, Wulf HC. Sun behaviour after cutaneous malignant melanoma: a study based on ultraviolet radiation measurements and sun diary data. Br J Dermatol. 2013;168(2):367–73.
28. Soto E, Lee H, Saladi RN, Gerson Y, Manginani S, Lam K, et al. Behavioral factors of patients before and after diagnosis with melanoma: a cohort study - are sun-protection measures being implemented? Melanoma Res. 2010;20(2):147–52.
29. Marx RG, Menezes A, Horovitz L, Jones EC, Warren RF. A comparison of two time intervals for test-retest reliability of health status instruments. J Clin Epidemiol. 2003;56(8):730–5.
30. Paiva CE, Barroso EM, Carneseca EC, de Padua SC, Dos Santos FT, Mendoza Lopez RV, et al. A critical analysis of test-retest reliability in instrument validation studies of cancer patients under palliative care: a systematic review. BMC Med Res Methodol. 2014;14:8.
31. Russell M, Marshall JR, Trevisan M, Freudenheim JL, Chan AW, Markovic N, et al. Test-retest reliability of the cognitive lifetime drinking history. Am J Epidemiol. 1997;146(11):975–81.
32. Streiner DL, Norman GR. Health Measurement Scales: A Practical Guide to Their Development and Use. Oxford University Press; 1995.
33. Hobart JC, Cano SJ, Warner TT, Thompson AJ. What sample sizes for reliability and validity studies in neurology? J Neurol. 2012;259(12):2681–94.
34. Fitzpatrick TB. The Validity and Practicality of Sun-Reactive Skin Types I Through VI. Arch Dermatol. 1988;124(6):869.
35. He SY, McCulloch CE, Boscardin WJ, Chren MM, Linos E, Arron ST. Self-reported pigmentary phenotypes and race are significant but incomplete predictors of Fitzpatrick skin phototype in an ethnically diverse population. J Am Acad Dermatol. 2014;71(4):731–7.
36. Kricker AA A, Armstrong BK, Jones ME, Burton RC. Health, Solar UV Radiation and Environmental Change. Lyon, France: World Health Organization; 1993.
37. Cabrol NA, Feister U, Häder D-P, Piazena H, Grin EA, Klein A. Record solar UV irradiance in the tropical Andes. Frontiers in Environmental Science. 2014;2:19.
38. World Health Organization (WHO). Global Solar UV Index: A Practical Guide. Geneva 2002.
39. Rosso S, Zanetti R, Pippione M, Sancho-Garnier H. Parallel risk assessment of melanoma and basal cell carcinoma: skin characteristics and sun exposure. Melanoma Res. 1998;8(6):573–83.
40. Rhee JS, Davis-Malesevich M, Logan BR, Neuburg M, Burzynski M, Nattinger AB. Behavior modification and risk perception in patients with nonmelanoma skin cancer. WMJ. 2008;107(2):62–8.
41. Rhee JS, Matthews BA, Neuburg M, Smith TL, Burzynski M, Nattinger AB. Quality of life and sun-protective behavior in patients with skin cancer. Arch Otolaryngol Head Neck Surg. 2004;130(2):141–6.
42. Fleiss JL. Statistical methods for rates and proportions. 2nd ed. New York: Wiley; 1981.
43. Elwood JM, Jopson J. Melanoma and sun exposure: an overview of published studies. Int J Cancer. 1997;73(2):198–203.
44. Buller DB, Berwick M, Lantz K, Buller MK, Shane J, Kane I, et al. Smartphone mobile application delivering personalized, real-time sun protection advice: A randomized clinical trial. JAMA Dermatology. 2015;151(5):497–504.
45. International Agency for Research on Cancer Working Group on artificial ultraviolet I, skin c. The association of use of sunbeds with cutaneous malignant melanoma and other skin cancers: A systematic review. Int J Cancer. 2007;120(5):1116–22.
46. Lazovich D, Vogel RI, Berwick M, Weinstock MA, Anderson KE, Warshaw EM. Indoor tanning and risk of melanoma: a case-control study in a highly exposed population. Cancer Epidemiol Biomarkers Prev. 2010;19(6):1557–68.
47. Zhang M, Qureshi AA, Geller AC, Frazier L, Hunter DJ, Han J. Use of tanning beds and incidence of skin cancer. J Clin Oncol. 2012;30(14):1588–93.

Patch testing in Iranian children with allergic contact dermatitis

Hossein Mortazavi[1,2], Amirhooshang Ehsani[1,2], Seyed Sajed Sajjadi[2], Nessa Aghazadeh[1,2,3*] and Ebrahim Arian[4]

Abstract

Background: Allergic contact dermatitis is a common disorder in adults and children alike and appears to be on the increase. The purpose of this study was to determine the sensitization trends in Iranian children with contact dermatitis.

Methods: The result of 109 patch tests performed using the 24 allergens of the European Standard Series in patients below 18 years old from September 2007 to March 2009 were recorded and analyzed. The tests were evaluated at 48 and 72 h after performing.

Results: The study population consisted of 72 (66.1 %) females and 37 (33.9 %) males. Hands were the most commonly affected anatomic site. In the final evaluation of the tests on day three, 51 (46.8 %) individuals showed a positive reaction to at least one allergen. Females were significantly more likely to show a positive response to at least one allergen (p-value = 0.031, odds ratio: 2.46). The most common allergens were nickel sulfate, cobalt, methylisothiazolinone, and colophony with 21 (19.3 %), 11 (10.1 %), 7 (6.4 %), and 6 (5.5 %) positive reactions, respectively. Contact allergy to nickel sulfate was more common in females than males (23.6 % vs. 10.8 %). There was no statistically significant relationship between personal or family history of atopy and a positive reaction to patch testing. The clinical and practical relevance were assessed for nickel and cobalt with a clinical current relevance in 11 (52.3 %) and 4 (36.4 %), respectively.

Conclusions: Nickel sulfate, cobalt, methylisothiazolinone, and colophony are the most common allergens responsible for induction of allergic contact dermatitis in Iranian children and adolescents. Females tended to show more positive reactions to allergens.

Keywords: Allergic contact dermatitis, Patch testing, Children, Adolescent, Contact allergens

Background

Allergic contact dermatitis (ACD) is an inflammatory skin disease caused by a T-cell-mediated delayed-type hypersensitivity reaction [1]. In ACD, the hapten is initially introduced to the epidermal langerhans cells. These cells migrate to the regional lymph nodes and the allergen is subsequently processed by the T-lymphocytes. Upon re-exposure of the allergen, CD8+ T-cells response is mediated by the CD4+ T-cell subset [2].

ACD affects up to 20 % of the pediatric population [3]. According to previous studies, 14.5 to 70.7 % of children with a clinical diagnosis of contact dermatitis have positive reactions to one of the applied allergens for patch testing [4, 5]. Based on a recent review of five patch test studies in children, the most commonly reported allergens in children are neomycin, balsam of Peru, fragrance mix, lanolin, cocamidopropylbetaine, formaldehyde, corticosteroids, methylchlorisothiazolinone/methylisothiazolinone, propylene glycol, and benzalkonium chloride [6]. Properly performed and interpreted patch testing is the gold standard for identification and documentation of allergic sensitization and its inducing agents in children and adults [7, 8]. Although patch testing in children is not approved by the FDA, it has proven to be a safe procedure both in adults and children [9]. There are no rules and limitations for patch testing in children in Iran. Therefore, we often use it on similar approved indication for adults.

The purpose of this study was to determine the causes of allergic contact dermatitis and identify the pattern of

* Correspondence: nessa.a@gmail.com; n-aghazadeh@sina.tums.ac.ir
[1]Autoimmune Bullous Diseases Research Center, Razi Dermatology Hospital, Tehran University of Medical Sciences, Tehran, Iran
[2]Razi Dermtology Hospital, Tehran University of Medical Sciences, Tehran, Iran
Full list of author information is available at the end of the article

allergen responsiveness in Iranian children and adolescents affected by ACD.

Methods

The study was approved by Tehran University of Medical Scienced board of ethics. Registered data of 109 patch tests performed in individuals younger than 18 years old diagnosed clinically and/or histopathologically with allergic contact dermatitis and referred by dermatologists for patch testing were collected and analyzed. We used the ESS (European Standard Series Hermal, Reinbek, Germany) at similar allergen concentrations as for adults. The allergens were applied on the healthy skin of the patients' backs and left for 48 h. Readings were performed at 48 h, 72 h and after patch testing (on day 2 and day 3). Reactions were classified and documented according to the criteria of the International Contact Dermatitis Research Group (ICDRG) as follows: (0 = negative), (+/− = doubtful), (+ = erythema), (++ = papule vesicle formation), and (+++ = bulla formation or ulceration) [7].

Statistical analysis

Data management and descriptive statistical analysis were performed using the SPSS 16 statistical program. Chi-square and Fisher's exact tests were used and a *P-value* less than 0.05 was considered a statistically significant difference.

Results

The study population consisted of 37 (33.9 %) males and 72 (66.1 %) females. The mean age was 14.4 with a standard deviation of 3.4 years (range: 5–18 years). A positive personal history of atopy was recorded in 48 patients (44.0 %). Forty one (37.6 %) had a positive family history of atopy. Anatomic sites of involvement in order of frequency are shown in Table 1. Hands were the most common site of involvement (Additional files 1 and 2).

Table 1 Anatomic sites of involvement in order of frequency

Anatomic sites of involvement	Frequency
Hand	84 (77.1 %)
Face	30 (27.5 %)
Calf	23 (21.1 %)
Foot	17 (15.6 %)
Back	9 (8.2 %)
Forearm	9 (8.2 %)
Abdomen	8 (8.7 %)
Knee	7 (7.6 %)
Thorax	7 (7.6 %)
Arm	6 (6.5 %)
Body	6 (6.5 %)

Results of patch test reading on day 2 and re-evaluation on day 3 (72 h) with regard to one or more reaction to allergens or negative or doubtful results in male and female patients are shown in Table 2.

Females were significantly more likely to show a positive response to at least one allergen (*p*-value = 0.031, odds ratio: 2.46, 95 %, and confidence interval (CI): 1.07–5.64). We found no significant difference in the frequency of positive patch test responses among patients with and without personal or family history of atopy (Table 3).

The overall results of patch test reading on day 2 and re-evaluation on day 3 based on gender are shown in Table 4. The ten most common inciting allergen in our series were nickel sulfate (21,19.3 %), cobalt chloride (11,10.1 %), methylisothiazolinone (7,6.4 %), colophony (6,5.5 %), potassium dichromate (5,4.6 %), paraben mix (4,3.7 %), 4-tert-butylphenon (4,3.7 %), fragrance mix (4,3.7 %), thiuram mix (3,2.8 %), mercapto mix (3,2.8 %), 4-phenylendiamine base (2,1.8 %), and formaldehyde (2,1.8 %) (Additional file 2).

Positive allergic reaction to nickel was more common in females than in males, however, without statistical significance (23.6 % vs. 10.8 %, *p*-value = 0.130) (Table 4).

We could only assess the clinical and practical relevance in the two most important allergens (nickel and cobalt), and we observed clinical current relevance in 11 (52.3 %) and 4 (36.4 %) for nickel and cobalt, respectively.

Results of patch test reading according to age groups are shown in Table 5.

For most allergens (except cobalt chloride, methylisothiazolinone, paraben mix, and fragrance mix), the percentages of positive response in the older age group (11–18 years) were higher than children below 10 years.

The most common allergen in the younger age group were cobalt chloride (4, 18.2 %), nickel sulfate (3, 13.6 %), methylisothiazolinone (2, 9.1 %), and paraben mix (2, 9.1 %) while in the older group they were as follows: nickel sulfate, cobalt chloride, methylisothiazolinone, colophony, potassium dichromate.

Discussion

In this study we have identified the inciting allergen according to patch tests in 109 children with ACD. Contact dermatitis in children has been studied less extensively than adults in the existing literature [10, 11].

In the current study, overall 48.6 % of patients had one or more positive patch test results. The positive response rate to patch test allergens ranges from 15 to 62.3 % in different studies [5, 12, 13].

Nickel was the most common allergen in our study, a common finding with most previous reports [10, 14, 15]. Although some authors have reported the rate of false-positive and irritant reactions to nickel is higher among

Table 2 The overall positive, doubtful and negative responses to patch test allergens among male and female patients

Gender	Positive	Percent	Negative	Percent	Doubtful	Percent
Male ($N = 37$)	12	32.4	12	32.4	13	35.2
Female ($N = 72$)	39	54.2	25	34.7	8	11.1
Total ($N = 109$)	51	46.8	37	33.9	21	19.3

children [16], other studies suggest that this high rate might be due to use of adult concentration of allergen for patch testing [17], and the recent series do not confirm this [6]. We could not demonstrate clinical relevance in about half of the cases in our study. In our series nickel sulfate, cobalt chloride, methylisothiazolinone, colophony, potassium dichromate, paraben mix, 4-tert-butylphenon, fragrance mix, thiuram mix, mercapto mix, phenylendiamine base, and formaldehyde were the most common allergens in decreasing order of frequency.

The most commonly reported allergens in a study in Singapore were Nickel (40 %), Thimerosal (15 %), Colophony (9 %), Lanolin (8 %), Cobalt (8 %), Fragrance mix (5 %), and Neomycin (4 %) [18]. While in another study in Turkey, the most commonly documented inciting allergens were Nickel sulfate (46 %), Cobalt chloride (9.5 %), p-Phenylenediamine (9.5 %), Neomycin sulfate 20 % (7 %), Formaldehyde 1 % (4.6 %), Fragrance mix 8 % (3.9 %), CL-methylisothiazolinone 0.01 % (3.1 %), Mercapto mix 2 % (3.1 %), Quaternium 15 % (2.3 %), Benzocaine 5 % (2.3 %), and Potassium dichromate 0.5 % (1.5 %) [19]. In a recent review of five pediatric patch test studies to, the top ten allergens were neomycin, balsam of Peru, fragrance mix, lanolin, cocamidopropylbetaine, formaldehyde, corticosteroids, methylchlorisothiazolinone/methylisothiazolinone, propylene glycol, and benzalkonium chloride [6]. The observed differences in the frequency of the allergens responsible for induction of ACD between the present study and other studies may be explained by a variety of reasons. First and foremost, the prevalence of sensitivity to an individual allergen depends not only on the intrinsic allergenicity of the compound but also on the level of allergen exposure to the population, which may vary from country to country [20–23]. Another important issue is that investigators often employ a variety of test panels and allergen concentrations in different studies, therefore rendering comparisons difficult [23]. There are disagreements as to whether there is seasonal and temporal variation in reactivity to allergens [24]. Moreover, reactivity to some allergens may be influenced by ethnic factors [25].

Gender differences in rates of reactions to a variety of contact allergens have been previously reported [2, 5]. In our study females were significantly more likely to have positive tests. This finding is consistent with previously published studies [5, 12, 15]. Nevertheless, in one study no difference between sex and reactivity to the applied allergens was observed [26].

In the current study, nickel sensitivity was also found to be more frequent in females; however, without statistical significance (Table 4). Ear piercing has been considered as the most common cause of nickel sensitization and the reason for its higher rate in females, with the risk of nickel allergy rising with the number of piercings [12]. Piercing is a common tradition in Iran and is usually performed in girls early in life often followed by long term wearing of golden earing to keep the hole open. Low-carat gold may contain nickel [19] In contrast to studies reporting more potassium dichromate reactivity in adult males, we found no male predominance for this allergen [27, 28].

As previously reported, co-reactivity between cobalt and nickel allergy was observed in our study [2, 18]. We found that in 45.5 % of patients with positive cobalt responses nickel reactivity was also present, while 23.8 % of patients with positive patch tests to nickel also had positive reaction to cobalt. In agreement with our results, Rystedt reported that nickel sensitivity predisposed the patients to cobalt sensitivity [29].

Our results showed that older children tend to show more positive reactions to allergens. This finding is in concordance with a pervious study that showed the rate of patch test positivity was higher in older age groups [12]. Moreover, it should be taken into account that

Table 3 Comparison of reactions to allergens (at least one positive or negative reaction) in patients with or without personal or family history of atopy

		Total	Reaction to allergens		p-value
			Positive (one or more reactions)	Negative	
personal history of atopy	+	48	26 (54.2 %)	22 (45.8 %)	0.171
	-	61	25 (41.0 %)	36 (59.0 %)	
family history of atopy	+	41	23 (56.1 %)	18 (43.9 %)	0.130
	-	68	28 (41.2 %)	40 (58.8 %)	

Table 4 Positive response to allergens of the European standard series in Iranian children with allergic contact dermatitis

Substance	Concentration (%)	Total (*N* = 109)	Percent	Male (*N* = 37)	Percent	Female (*N* = 72)	Percent	*P-Value*	Relevance
Nickel sulfate	5	21	19.3	4	10.8	17	23.6	0.130	11 (52.3 %)
Cobalt chloride	1	11	10.1	5	13.5	6	8.3	0.504	4 (36.4 %)
Methylisothiazolinone	0.05	7	6.4	1	2.7	6	8.3	0.419	NA
Colophony	20	6	5.5	1	2.7	5	6.9	0.662	NA
Potassium dichromate	0.5	5	4.6	3	8.1	2	2.8	0.334	NA
Paraben mix	16	4	3.7	2	5.4	2	2.8	0.603	NA
4-tert-butylphenol formaldehyde resin	1	4	3.7	0	0.0	4	5.6	0.297	NA
Fragrance mix	8	4	3.7	1	2.7	3	4.2	1.000	NA
Thiuram mix	1	3	2.8	1	2.7	2	2.8	1.000	NA
Mercapto mix	1	3	2.8	0	0.0	3	4.2	0.550	NA
4-Phenylenediamine base	1	2	1.8	0	0.0	2	2.8	0.547	NA
Formaldehyde	1	2	1.8	1	2.7	1	1.4	1.000	NA
N-isopropyl-N-phenyl-4-phenylenediamine	0.1	2	1.8	1	2.7	1	1.4	1.000	NA
Wool Alcohol	30	2	1.8	0	0.0	2	2.8	0.547	NA
Sesquiterpene lactone mix	0.1	2	1.8	2	5.4	0	0.0	0.113	NA
Benzocaine	5	2	1.8	0	0.0	2	2.8	0.547	NA
Cliquinol	5	1	0.9	1	2.7	0	0.0	0.339	NA
Balsam of peru	25	1	0.9	0	0.0	1	1.4	1.000	NA
Epoxy resin	1	1	0.9	0	0.0	1	1.4	1.000	NA
Quaterium-15	1	1	0.9	0	0.0	1	1.4	1.000	NA
Mercaptobenzothiazole	2	1	0.9	1	2.7	0	0.0	0.339	NA
Neomycin sulphate	20	1	0.9	0	0.0	1	1.4	1.000	NA
Hydroxyl-methyl-penthyl-cyclo-carboxaldehyde	5	1	0.9	1	2.7	0	0.0	0.339	NA
Primin	0.01	0	0.0	0	0.0	0	0.0	NA	NA

contact dermatitis increases with age and is more common in older individuals [30]. However, according to some researchers an age-dependent decrease in delayed type hypersensitivity may occur with age [30].

In the present study 44.0 % of patients had a personal history of atopy. The relationship between atopy and ACD remains controversial [31, 32]. Although it has been assumed that atopy could be a predisposing factor for the development of ACD, and more reactivity to specific allergens have been reported in atopic patient [33–35]; we found no significant association between personal or family history of atopy and patch test results. In concordance with our findings, some studies indicate that there is a similar prevalence of ACD in individuals with and without atopic diathesis [31, 36]. Hands were the most frequent sites of ACD in our study. Metal preservative and rubber are the most common causes for ACD of this region [11]. Also, in our study metal was the most common causative allergens of ACD.

In the present study, the face was the second most frequent ACD anatomic site. In some studies, the face was the most common site of ACD in children and adolescents [11].

Positive clinical relevance of the positive reactions was considered if the patient described a current or past cutaneous exposure to a product known to contain the allergen to which the patient reacted [7]. For some allergens in the pediatric patient group evaluation of relevance was not possible due to unknown history of exposure.

Methylisothiazolinone is a common preservative found in many cosmetic and toiletry products marketed to both children and adults. It is increasingly known to cause ACD, especially in perioral and perineal regions due to facial or baby wipes [37]. Colophony is a cause of ACD to adhesives and tapes. However, the clinical relevance of a positive patch-test reaction to colophony is often difficult to evaluate [38].

Our study is limited by small sample size, also we were unable to evaluate the relevance for positive patch test for all antigens. Studies with greater sample size and with adequate antigen relevance determination is recommended in Iranian children with ACD.

Table 5 The positive patch test responses according to the inciting allergen and age group (0–10, 11–8 years)

Substance	0–10 (*N* = 22)	Percent	11–18 (*N* = 87)	Percent	*P-Value*
Nickel sulfate	3	13.6	18	20.7	0.55
Cobalt chloride	4	18.2	7	8.0	0.22
Methylisothiazolinone	2	9.1	5	5.7	0.62
Colophony	1	4.5	5	5.7	1.0
Potassium dichromate	0	0.0	5	5.7	0.58
Paraben mix	2	9.1	2	2.3	0.17
4-tert-butylphenon	0	0.0	4	4.6	0.58
Fragrance mix	1	4.5	3	3.4	1.0
Thiuram mix	0	0.0	3	3.4	1.0
Mercapto mix	0	0.0	3	3.4	1.0
Phenylendiamine base	0	0.0	2	2.3	1.0
Formaldehyde	0	0.0	2	2.3	1.0
N-isopropyl-N-phenyl-4-phenylenediamine	0	0.0	2	2.3	1.0
Wool Alcohol	0	0.0	2	2.3	1.0
Sesquiterpene lactone mix	0	0.0	2	2.3	1.0
Benzocaine	0	0.0	2	2.3	1.0
Cliquinol	0	0.0	1	1.1	1.0
Balsam of peru	0	0.0	1	1.1	1.0
Epoxy resin	0	0.0	1	1.1	1.0
Quaterium-18	0	0.0	1	1.1	1.0
Mercaptobenzothiazole	0	0.0	1	1.1	1.0
Neomycin sulphate	0	0.0	1	1.1	1.0
Hydroxyl-methyl-penthyl-cyclo-carboxaldehyde	0	0.0	1	1.1	1.0
Primin	0	0.0	0	0.0	NA

Conclusion

Our results indicate that nickel sulfate, cobalt, methylisothiazolinone, and colophony are the most common allergens responsible for induction of allergic contact dermatitis in Iranian children and adolescents. Females tend to show more positive reactions to allergens. These findings are crucial in the treatment, long term management, and proper education of children with allergic contact dermatitis.

Abbreviation

ACD, allergic contact dermatitis

Acknowledgements

None.

Funding

None.

Authors' contributions

HM participated in the design, analysis and interpretation of data. SSS collected the data and did the statistical analysis. NA interpreted the data and drafted the manuscript. AH critically revised the manuscript and helped in the coordination and data analysis. All authors have read and approved the final manuscript.

Competing interests

The authors declare that they have no competing interests.

Author details

[1]Autoimmune Bullous Diseases Research Center, Razi Dermatology Hospital, Tehran University of Medical Sciences, Tehran, Iran. [2]Razi Dermtology Hospital, Tehran University of Medical Sciences, Tehran, Iran. [3]Children's Medical Hospital, Tehran University of Medical Sciences, Tehran, Iran. [4]Sharif University of Technology, Tehran, Iran.

References

1. Rich RR, Fleisher TA, Shearer WT, Schroeder Jr HW, Frew AJ, Weyand CM. Clinical Immunology, Principles and Practice. 4th ed. China: Elsevier Health Sciences; 2013.
2. Rietschel RL, Fowler JF, Fisher AA. Fisher's contact dermatitis. 6th ed. Hamilton: BC Decker Inc.; 2008.
3. Militello G, Jacob SE, Crawford GH. Allergic contact dermatitis in children. Curr Opin Pediatr. 2006;18(4):385–90.
4. Zug KA, McGinley-Smith D, Warshaw EM, Taylor JS, Rietschel RL, Maibach HI, Belsito DV, Fowler JF, Storrs FJ, DeLeo VA. Contact allergy in children referred for patch testing: North American Contact Dermatitis Group data, 2001–2004. Arch Dermatol. 2008;144(10):1329–36.
5. Mortz CG, Andersen KE. Allergic contact dermatitis in children and adolescents. Contact Dermatitis. 1999;41(3):121–30.
6. Hill H, Goldenberg A, Golkar L, Beck K, Williams J, Jacob SE. Pre-Emptive Avoidance Strategy (P.E.A.S.) - addressing allergic contact dermatitis in pediatric populations. Expert Rev Clin Immunol. 2016;12(5):551–61.
7. Lachapelle J-M, Maibach HI. Patch Testing and Prick Testing: A Practical Guide Official Publication of the ICDRG, third edn. Heidelberg: Springer-Verlag Berlin Heidelberg; 2012.
8. Goldenberg A, Silverberg N, Silverberg JI, Treat J, Jacob SE. Pediatric allergic contact dermatitis: lessons for better care. J Allergy Clin Immunol Pract. 2015;3(5):661–7.
9. Johansen JD, Aalto-Korte K, Agner T, Andersen KE, Bircher A, Bruze M, Cannavó A, Giménez-Arnau A, Gonçalo M, Goossens A. European Society of Contact Dermatitis guideline for diagnostic patch testing–recommendations on best practice. Contact Dermatitis. 2015;73(4):195–221.
10. Simonsen AB, Deleuran M, Johansen JD, Sommerlund M. Contact allergy and allergic contact dermatitis in children–a review of current data. Contact Dermatitis. 2011;65(5):254–65.
11. Brod BA, Treat JR, Rothe MJ, Jacob SE. Allergic contact dermatitis: Kids are not just little people. Clin Dermatol. 2015;33(6):605–12.
12. Clayton T, Wilkinson S, Rawcliffe C, Pollock B, Clark S. Allergic contact dermatitis in children: should pattern of dermatitis determine referral? A retrospective study of 500 children tested between 1995 and 2004 in one UK centre. Br J Dermatol. 2006;154(1):114–7.
13. Zug KA, Pham AK, Belsito DV, DeKoven JG, DeLeo VA, Fowler Jr JF, Fransway AF, Maibach HI, Marks Jr JG, Mathias CT. Patch testing in children from 2005 to 2012: results from the North American contact dermatitis group. Dermatitis. 2014;25(6):345–55.
14. Tuchman M, Silverberg JI, Jacob SE, Silverberg N. Nickel contact dermatitis in children. Clin Dermatol. 2015;33(3):320–6.
15. Sharma VK, Asati DP. Pediatric contact dermatitis. Indian J Dermatol Venereol Leprol. 2010;76(5):514.
16. Shah M, Lewis FM, Gawkrodger DJ. Patch testing in children and adolescents: five years' experience and follow-up. J Am Acad Dermatol. 1997;37(6):964–8.
17. Roul S, Ducombs G, Taieb A. Usefulness of the European standard series for patch testing in children. A 3-year single-centre study of 337 patients. Contact Dermatitis. 1999;40(5):232–5.

18. Goon ATJ, Goh CL. Patch testing of Singapore children and adolescents: our experience over 18 years. Pediatr Dermatol. 2006;23(2):117–20.
19. Onder M, Adisen E. Patch test results in a Turkish paediatric population. Contact Dermatitis. 2008;58(1):63–5.
20. Schnuch A, Geier J, Uter W. National rates and regional differences in sensitization to allergens of the standard series. Population-adjusted frequencies of sensitization (PAFS) in 40,000 patients from a multicenter study (IVDK). Occup Health Ind Med. 1998;2(38):83.
21. Uter W, Hegewald J, Aberer W, Ayala F, Bircher A, Brasch J, Coenraads PJ, Schuttelaar ML, Elsner P, Fartasch M. The European standard series in 9 European countries, 2002/2003–first results of the European Surveillance System on Contact Allergies. Contact Dermatitis. 2005;53(3):136–45.
22. Weston WL, Weston JA. Allergic contact dermatitis in children. Am J Dis Child. 1984;138(10):932–6.
23. Thompson TR, Belsito DV. Regional variation in prevalence and etiology of allergic contact dermatitis. Dermatitis. 2002;13(4):177–82.
24. Kränke B, Aberer W. Seasonal influence on patch test results in central Europe. Contact Dermatitis. 1996;34(3):215–31.
25. DeLeo VA, Taylor SC, Belsito DV, Fowler JF, Fransway AF, Maibach HI, Marks JG, Mathias CT, Nethercott JR, Pratt MD. The effect of race and ethnicity on patch test results. J Am Acad Dermatol. 2002;46(2):S107–12.
26. Seidenari S, Giusti F, Pepe P, Mantovani L. Contact Sensitization in 1094 Children Undergoing Patch Testing over a 7-Year Period. Pediatr Dermatol. 2005;22(1):1–5.
27. Freireich-Astman M, David M, Trattner A. Standard patch test results in patients with contact dermatitis in Israel: age and sex differences. Contact Dermatitis. 2007;56(2):103–7.
28. Greig JE, Carson CF, Stuckey MS, Riley TV. Prevalence of delayed hypersensitivity to the European standard series in a self-selected population. Australas J Dermatol. 2000;41(2):86–9.
29. Rystedt I, Fischer T. Relationship between nickel and cobalt sensitization in hard metal workers. Contact Dermatitis. 1983;9(3):195–200.
30. Kwangsukstith C, Maibach HI. Effect of age and sex on the induction and elicitation of allergic contact dermatitis. Contact Dermatitis. 1995;33(5):289–98.
31. Akhavan A, Cohen SR. The relationship between atopic dermatitis and contact dermatitis. Clin Dermatol. 2003;21(2):158–62.
32. Vender R. The utility of patch testing children with atopic dermatitis. Skin Therapy Lett. 2002;7(6):4–6.
33. Malajian D, Belsito DV. Cutaneous delayed-type hypersensitivity in patients with atopic dermatitis. J Am Acad Dermatol. 2013;69(2):232–7.
34. Shaughnessy CN, Malajian D, Belsito DV. Cutaneous delayed-type hypersensitivity in patients with atopic dermatitis: reactivity to topical preservatives. J Am Acad Dermatol. 2014;70(1):102–7.
35. Shaughnessy CN, Malajian D, Belsito DV. Cutaneous delayed-type hypersensitivity in patients with atopic dermatitis: Reactivity to surfactants. J Am Acad Dermatol. 2014;70(4):704–8.
36. Landeck L, Schalock P, Baden L, González E. Contact sensitization pattern in 172 atopic subjects. Int J Dermatol. 2011;50(7):806–10.
37. Schlichte MJ, Katta R. Methylisothiazolinone: an emergent allergen in common pediatric skin care products. Dermatol Res Pract. 2014;2014:132564.
38. Färm G. Contact allergy to colophony. Clinical and experimental studies with emphasis on clinical relevance. Acta Derm Venereol Suppl. 1997;201:1–42.

21

Expression profiling and bioinformatic analyses suggest new target genes and pathways for human hair follicle related microRNAs

Lara M. Hochfeld[1,2], Thomas Anhalt[1,2], Céline S. Reinbold[3], Marisol Herrera-Rivero[1,2], Nadine Fricker[1,2], Markus M. Nöthen[1,2] and Stefanie Heilmann-Heimbach[1,2*]

Abstract

Background: Human hair follicle (HF) cycling is characterised by the tight orchestration and regulation of signalling cascades. Research shows that micro(mi)RNAs are potent regulators of these pathways. However, knowledge of the expression of miRNAs and their target genes and pathways in the human HF is limited. The objective of this study was to improve understanding of the role of miRNAs and their regulatory interactions in the human HF.

Methods: Expression levels of ten candidate miRNAs with reported functions in hair biology were assessed in HFs from 25 healthy male donors. MiRNA expression levels were correlated with mRNA-expression levels from the same samples. Identified target genes were tested for enrichment in biological pathways and accumulation in protein-protein interaction (PPI) networks.

Results: Expression in the human HF was confirmed for seven of the ten candidate miRNAs, and numerous target genes for miR-24, miR-31, and miR-106a were identified. While the latter include several genes with known functions in hair biology (e.g., *ITGB1, SOX9*), the majority have not been previously implicated (e.g., *PHF1*). Target genes were enriched in pathways of interest to hair biology, such as integrin and GnRH signalling, and the respective gene products showed accumulation in PPIs.

Conclusions: Further investigation of miRNA expression in the human HF, and the identification of novel miRNA target genes and pathways via the systematic integration of miRNA and mRNA expression data, may facilitate the delineation of tissue-specific regulatory interactions, and improve our understanding of both normal hair growth and the pathobiology of hair loss disorders.

Keywords: miRNA, mRNA, Gene regulation, Human hair biology, Correlation analysis

Background

The human hair follicle (HF) passes through cycles of active growth (anagen); regression (catagen); and rest (telogen). Each of these stages is tightly regulated, and is characterised by distinct changes in gene expression, cell proliferation, and differentiation [1, 2].

Micro(mi)RNAs are short (~20-25 nucleotides), non-coding RNAs, which influence gene expression by binding to target messenger(m)RNAs via a complementary seed region, which elicits mRNA degradation or transcriptional inhibition. In recent years, accumulating research data have indicated the importance of miRNAs as potent regulators of numerous developmental and pathobiological processes [3]. Several miRNAs have been implicated in hair biology, e.g., in the control of hair pigmentation, HF cycling, and keratinocyte differentiation [4–6]. For instance, miR-137 is reported to be responsible for coat colour determination in mice [5], while the

* Correspondence: sheilman@uni-bonn.de
[1]Institute of Human Genetics, University of Bonn, Sigmund-Freud-Str. 25, 53127 Bonn, Germany
[2]Department of Genomics, Life and Brain Center, University of Bonn, Sigmund-Freud-Str. 25, 53127 Bonn, Germany
Full list of author information is available at the end of the article

inhibition of miR-31 in murine skin has been shown to result in accelerated anagen progression and abnormal hair shaft morphology [4]. A further study reported, a differential expression for four miRNAs (miR-106a, miR-410, miR-221, miR-125b) in dermal papilla cells (DPCs) from the balding and non-balding scalp areas of eight patients with male pattern baldness (MPB) [7]. However, the majority of available data on the role of miRNAs in hair biology have been obtained from mouse or cell culture experiments, and knowledge of the genes and pathways that are targeted by these miRNAs in the human HF is limited. Such knowledge is essential in terms of understanding the relevance of miRNAs to human hair (patho-) biology.

The aims of the present study were to: 1) perform a systematic investigation of the expression of ten candidate miRNAs (miR-22, miR-24, miR-31, miR-106a, miR-125b, miR-137, miR-205, miR-214, miR-221, miR-410) in human HF samples; 2) correlate these data with corresponding HF mRNA expression levels; and 3) test the identified target genes for enrichment in pathways and protein networks in order to delineate regulatory interactions in the human HF.

Methods

Sample collection and nucleic acid extraction

HF samples were collected from the frontal- and the occipital scalp areas of 25 volunteer healthy male donors of European descent (mean age 24.2 years ± 1.6). RNA and miRNA were extracted from HF tissue using the miRNeasy Mini Kit and the RNeasy® MinElute® Cleanup Kit (Qiagen, Hilden, Germany). The quantity and quality of the extracted RNAs and miRNAs were tested on an ND-1000 spectrophotometer (Peqlab Biotechnologie, Erlangen, Germany) and a BioAnalyzer 2100 (Agilent Technologies, Waldbronn, Germany), respectively. Samples with an RNA concentration of ≥20 ng/μl, an RNA integrity number (RIN) of ≥8 and a miRNA concentration of ≥25 ng/μl were included in the microarray analysis.

miRNA profiling

MiRNA profiling of n = 50 samples (25 frontal, 25 occipital) was performed on the Affymetrix® GeneChip® miRNA 4.0 (Affymetrix, Santa Clara, CA) using a total of 250 ng of HF miRNA. Poly(A) tailing and biotinylation were performed with the Affymetrix® GeneChip® Hybridization, Wash, and Stain Kit, in accordance with the manufacturer's instructions. After scanning, miRNA raw expression values were background subtracted, quantile normalised and log_2-transformed using robust multi-array analysis (RMA) and detection above background (DABG) in the Affymetrix® Expression Console™ (Affymetrix Santa Clara, CA). A total of 48 samples from 24 individuals fulfilled all quality control criteria. Candidate miRNAs were considered to be expressed if they were defined as 'present' in ≥80% of all samples.

mRNA profiling

Whole transcriptome profiling of the corresponding HF RNA samples was performed using the TotalPrep™-96 RNA Amplification Kit and Illumina HT-12v4 Bead Arrays (Illumina Inc., San Diego, CA). Background subtracted expression intensities and detection *P*-values were exported from the Illumina GenomeStudio software. These were then quantile normalised and log_2-transformed using the R package 'limma'. Only probes with all of the following four characteristics were taken into account: (i) a detection *P*-value of <0.05 (indicating significant expression above background) in at least 80% of the samples; (ii) a good or perfect probe quality; (iii) an annotated Entrez gene identifier, as reported in the Bioconductor package illuminaHumanv4.db [8]; and (iv) no single nucleotide polymorphism within the probe sequence (dbSNP Build 142). After filtering, a total of 10,029 expression probes, corresponding to 8,210 gene symbols, remained for the correlation analysis.

Selection of candidate miRNAs

Candidate miRNAs were selected based on the results of a comprehensive PubMed literature search for the role of miRNAs in HF biology. A total of ten candidate miRNAs (miR-22, miR-24, miR-31, miR-106a, miR-125b, miR-137, miR-205, miR-214, miR-221, and miR-410) were selected for investigation in the human HF (PMIDs: 26020521, 20522784, 21362569, 21967250, 22847819, 23974039, 24232098, and 25422376). These miRNAs were represented by 21 expression probes on the Affymetrix miRNA4.0 array (Table 1).

Target gene identification

To identify targets genes, mean miRNA and mRNA expression levels were calculated from the frontal and occipital sample of each of the final 24 participants. The expression levels of 10,029 mRNA probes and seven expressed candidate miRNAs which were represented by 14 mature miRNA forms were correlated using the Pearson correlation analysis method [9]. The respective correlation coefficients (*r*) were computed and the resulting *P*-values were then corrected for multiple testing using Benjamini-Hochberg correction (P_{adj}). All mRNAs with a significant correlation (P_{adj} <0.01) to a candidate miRNA were assumed to be target genes. To exclude correlations driven by differential expression between frontal and occipital samples, the correlation trend was confirmed via single-tissue analysis (Additional file 1: Table S1, Additional file 2: Figure S1).

Table 1 Overview of selected candidate miRNAs: Previously reported role(s) in hair biology and expression status of the analysed miRNAs in the human hair follicle (HF)

Candidate miRNA	Reported role in hair biology	Reference	Mature form on miRNA array	HF Expression	# of uniquely correlated genes
miR-31	Inhibits anagen development by regulating gene expression programmes and alters hair shaft formation in mice	Mardaryev AN et al., 2010	hsa-miR-31-5p	✓	99
			hsa-miR-31-3p	✓	-
miR-24	Overexpression is associated with reduced proliferation and premature HF-keratinocyte differentiation in mice	Amelio I et al., 2013	hsa-miR-24-3p	✓	103
			hsa-miR-24-1-5p	✓	-
			hsa-miR-24-2-5p	✓	5
miR-106a	Upregulated in balding human DPC in comparison to nonbalding DPCs	Goodarzi HR et al., 2012	hsa-miR-106a-5p	✓	53
			hsa-miR-106a-3p	✗	-
miR-22	Overexpression in mice is associated with hair loss due to anagen-to-catagen transition and knockout in mice is associated with delayed catagen entry and accelerated telogen-to-anagen transition	Yuan S et al., 2015	hsa-miR-22-5p	✓	-
			hsa-miR-22-3p	✓	
miR-125b	Represses HF stem cell differentiation in mice; significantly upregulated in balding human DPCs in comparison to nonbalding DPCs	Zhang L et al., 2011; Goodarzi HR et al., 2012	hsa-miR-125b-5p	✓	–
			hsa-miR-125b-1-3p	✗	
			hsa-miR-125b-2-3p	✓	
miR-137	Involved in murine HF pigmentation (melanogenesis)	Dong C et al., 2012	hsa-miR-137	✗	–
miR-205	Essential for development of HF stem cell proliferation during murine embryonic skin development	Wang D et al., 2013	hsa-miR-205-5p	✓	–
			hsa-miR-205-3p	✓	
miR-214	Controls Wnt pathway and β-catenin expression in murine embryonic HF development	Ahmed MI et al., 2014	hsa-miR-214-5p	✗	–
			hsa-miR-214-3p	✗	
miR-221	Upregulated in balding human DPCs in comparison to nonbalding DPCs	Goodarzi HR et al., 2012	hsa-miR-221-5p	✓	–
			hsa-miR-221-3p	✓	1
miR-410	Upregulated in balding human DPC in comparison to nonbalding DPCs	Goodarzi HR et al., 2012	hsa-miR-410-5p	✗	–
			hsa-miR-410-3p	✗	

HF hair follicle, *DPCs* dermal papilla cells, # number

Pathway enrichment of, and protein-protein interactions (PPIs) between, miRNA target genes

For all significantly correlated target genes, testing for pathway enrichment was performed using the Ingenuity Pathway Analysis software (IPA, Qiagen, Hilden, Germany, accessed 31 March 2016); and the Protein ANalysis THrough Evolutionary Relationship database (PANTHER, version 11.1, http://pantherdb.org/, accessed 2nd December 2016) [10]. Only pathways with ≥3 annotated genes and a *P*-value based on right tailed Fisher's exact test <0.05 (IPA) were taken into account.

PPIs were investigated using the Search Tool for the Retrieval of Interacting Genes/Proteins (STRING, version 10, http://string-db.org, accessed 2nd December 2016) [11].

miRNA target prediction

The miRWalk2.0 (http://zmf.umm.uni-heidelberg.de/apps/zmf/mirwalk2, accessed 11 March 2016) [12]; and the TargetScan7.0 (http://targetscan.org, accessed 2nd December 2016) [13] algorithms were used to search for predicted and validated target genes of the expressed candidate miRNAs. Only genes that were predicted by the miRWalk algorithm and three additional implemented databases, or that were predicted to target a conserved site in TargetScan, were taken into account.

Results

Seven of the ten candidate miRNAs were expressed in both the frontal an occipital HF samples. The strongest mean $\log_2$ expression ($\log_2$_value) was found for miR-205 ($\log_2$_value = 3.73 ± 0.01), and miR-24 ($\log_2$_value = 3.69 ± 0.03). Using the present criteria, no expression was observed for miR-137 ($\log_2$_value = -1.77 ± 1.72); miR-214 ($\log_2$_value = 1.50 ± 0.56); or miR-410 ($\log_2$_value = -1.08 ± 0.61) (data not shown).

To investigate the function of these seven miRNAs, and to identify their target genes in the human HF, a correlation analysis of intrasample mean miRNA and mean mRNA expression was performed. Significant correlation between miRNA and mRNA expression was observed for miR-24, miR-31, miR-106a, and miR-221. For miR-24 (i.e., miR-24-3p, miR-24-2-5p), a significant correlation was found with 106 genes: $n = 74$, negatively correlated (neg. cor.); and $n = 32$, positively correlated (pos. cor.). The two most significantly correlated genes were *COL5A2* (Collagen, Type V, Alpha 2; $r = -0.92$, $P_{adj} = 1.70 \times 10^{-5}$); and *SERPING1* (Serpin Family G Member 1; $r = -0.86$, $P_{adj} = 8.77 \times 10^{-4}$). For miR-31, a total of 99 genes (53 neg. cor. and 46 pos. cor.) were identified. Here, the two most significantly correlated genes were *FAM178A* (SMC5-SMC6 complex localisation factor 2; $r = -0.90$, $P_{adj} = 1.51 \times 10^{-4}$); and *PLAA* (Phospholipase A2-Activating Protein; $r = 0.89$, $P_{adj} = 1.82 \times 10^{-4}$). MiR-106a expression was correlated with a total of 53 genes (29 neg. cor. and 24 pos. cor.). Here, the two most significantly correlated genes were *UST* (Uronyl-2-Sulfotransferase; $r = -0.86$, $P_{adj} = 8.77 \times 10^{-4}$); and *COL5A2* ($r = -0.85$, $P_{adj} = 8.77 \times 10^{-4}$) (Additional file 1: Table S1). For miR-221, correlation was found with a single gene - *RPRD2* (Regulation Of Nuclear Pre-MRNA Domain Containing 2; $r = -077$. $P_{adj} = 7.59 \times 10^{-3}$). A total of 40 genes were targets of more than one miRNA. The largest overlap was found between target genes of miR-31 and miR-106a ($n = 29$). Ten genes (*FZD7, JUN, MEIS2, TAX1BP3, RBM17, SFRP1, TP63, ZCCHC11, COL17A1, SMARCA4*) were significantly correlated with miR-24, miR-31, and miR-106a (Fig. 1, Additional file 1: Table S1).

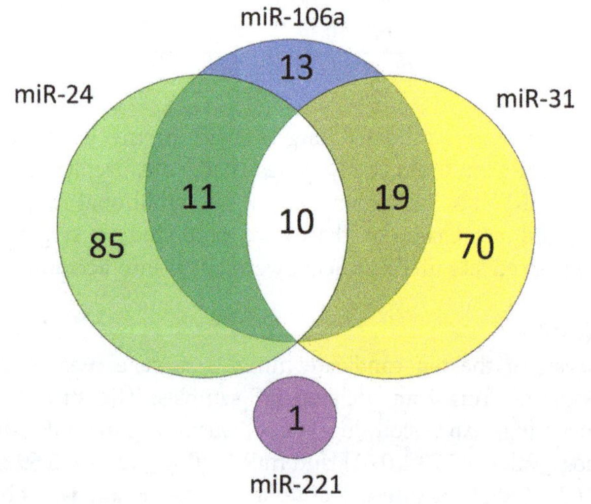

Fig. 1 Overview of all target genes with a significant correlation to miR-24, miR-31, and miR-106a. The largest overlap in target genes was detected for miR-31 and miR-106a (n = 29). MiR-31, miR-24 (i.e., miR-24-3p, miR-24-2-5p), and miR-106a shared the following ten target genes: *FZD7, JUN, MEIS2, TAX1BP3, RBM17, SFRP1, TP63, SMARCA4, COL17A1,* and *ZCCHC11*. The same ten target genes were shared between miR-31 and miR-24. MiR-24 and miR-106a shared a total of 21 target genes. No overlap was found for miR-221 and the three remaining miRNAs

In the investigation of a potential enrichment of miRNA target genes in biological pathways, IPA revealed the strongest enrichment of the respective target genes in 'Hepatic Fibrosis/Hepatic Stellate Cell Activation' (miR-24), and 'JAK/STAT Signalling' (miR-31 and miR-106a). In the PANTHER analysis, 'Integrin Signalling' was the top pathway for the target genes of miR-24, miR-31 and miR-106a. An overview of all identified pathways is provided in Additional file 1: Table S2.

In the miRWalk2.0 [12] and TargetScan7.0 [13] analyses, 40%, 62%, and 42% respectively of the identified target genes for miR-24, miR-31 and miR-106a were not predicted by either tool. The single target gene of miR-221 was predicted by miRWalk only (Additional file 1: Table S3).

The STRING [11] database query revealed numerous interactions between the miRNA-specific-, shared- and all target genes of all four miRNAs. In all PPI-networks, an interaction was observed between JUN and FZD7 via SFRP1 (Fig. 2, Additional file 2: Figure S2).

Discussion

The present study involved comprehensive analysis in the human HF of ten miRNAs previously implicated in hair biology [7, 14]. Expression profiling confirmed the expression of seven of the ten candidate miRNAs, suggesting that these miRNAs may indeed play a role in human hair biology. For miR-24, miR-31, and miR-106a several target genes and pathways of interest were identified (Table 1).

The highest number of target genes was identified for miR-24. Previous research has identified miR-24 as an anti-proliferative miRNA, which promotes keratinocyte differentiation via the modulation of actin filaments [15], and plays a role in hair morphogenesis [6]. For miR-24 (i.e., miR-24-3p, miR-24-2-5p), correlation analysis revealed a total of 106 unique target genes. These include the miRWalk2.0 predicted target *ITGB1,* which encodes the integrin β-1 subunit and has been subject to extensive investigation with respect to skin and hair homeostasis (reviewed in Rippa *et al.*, 2013 [16]). The present pathway analysis also revealed an enrichment of miR-24 target genes in 'Integrin Signalling'. These results suggest that integrin signalling is an essential pathway for keratinocyte differentiation in the human HF, and that this is controlled by miR-24. Furthermore, significant correlations with miR-24 expression were observed for six collagen genes. In descending order of significance, these were: *COL5A2, COL17A1, COL4A6, COL4A5, COL18A1* and *COL4A1.* The respective gene products also form a dense PPI-network (Fig. 2). Previous functional studies have demonstrated hair coat thinning and abnormal HF morphogenesis in mice that overexpress miR-24 in basal keratinocytes. These mice display shorter, misangled, and wavy HFs [6]. A similar hair phenotype is seen in

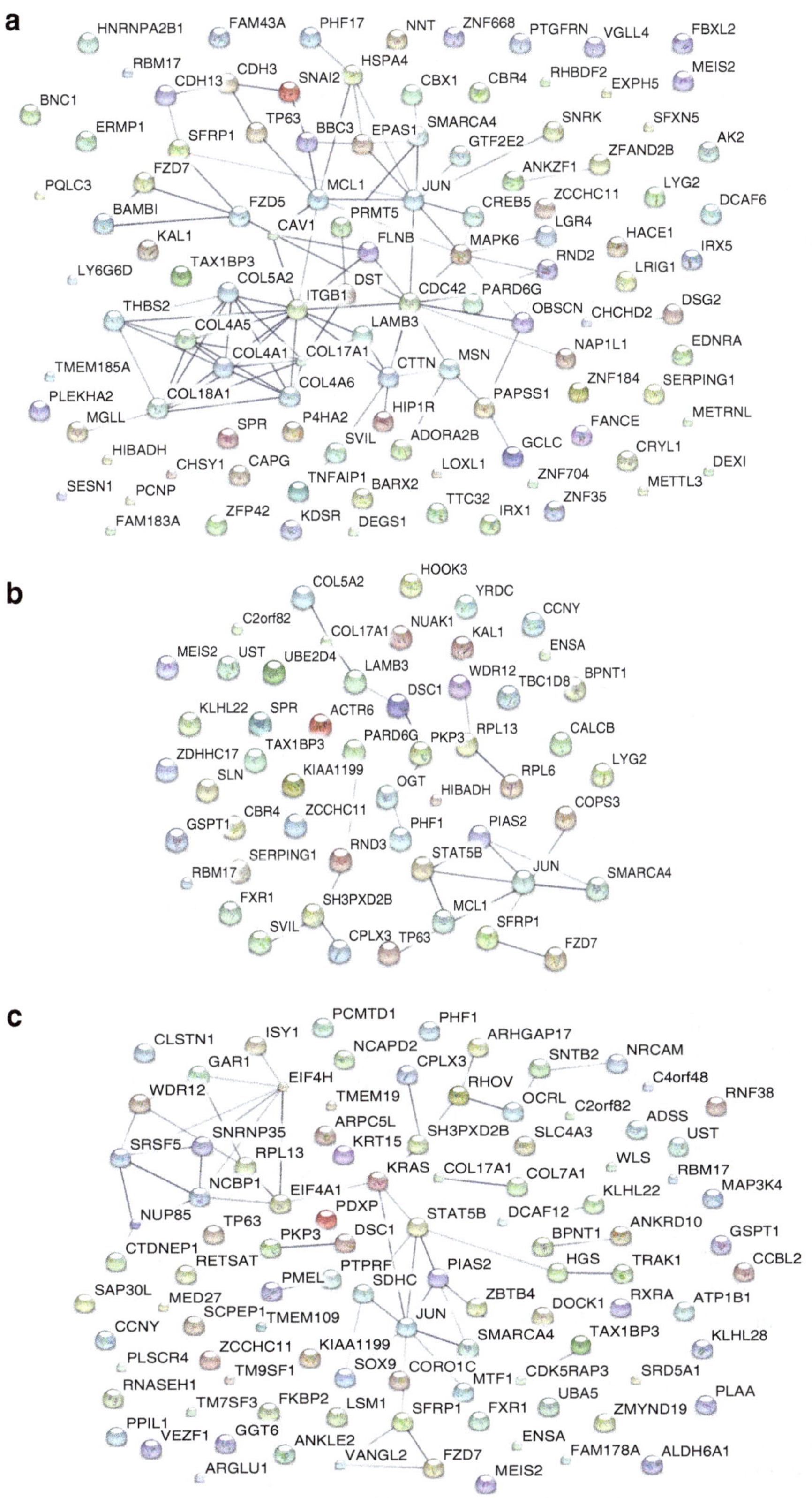

Fig. 2 STRING protein-protein interaction (PPI) query. PPIs of significantly correlated target genes **a** miR-24; **b** miR-106a; and **c** miR-31. Connecting lines represent confidence interactions according to the STRING database. The genes *JUN*, *SFRP1*, and *FZD7* were targets of all three miRNAs and show a consistent PPI in combination with other miRNA-specific target proteins

patients with the chromosome 2q32 deletion syndrome, whose clinical features include thin, sparse, woolly, and slowly growing scalp hair [17, 18]. Interestingly, the affected 2q32 chromosomal region includes *COL5A2*. Another collagen gene, *Col17a1*, is reported to be essential for HF stem cell maintenance [19] and age-associated HF miniaturisation and thinning, as mediated by COL17A1 proteolysis [20]. Moreover, *COL17A1* deficiency is associated with junctional epidermolysis bullosa, a severe skin disease characterised by hair loss [21]. Taken together, these data suggest that miR-24 is an important regulator of hair morphogenesis and maintenance, which achieves its effect via the control of integrin and collagen signalling. The present study also detected an enrichment of miR-24 target genes in the hormone signalling cascades 'Gonadotropin Releasing Hormone (GnRH) Receptor Pathway', and 'Androgen Signalling'. Whereas androgen signalling is essential for hair biology and has been shown to regulate hair growth and cycling at different body sites [22], GnRH signalling antagonises androgen receptor signalling at androgen-sensitive body sites in women, and GnRH antagonists are an effective treatment for hirsutism [23, 24]. Research is warranted to determine whether these hormone pathways also play a role in keratinocyte differentiation.

Research has shown that miR-31 is responsible for both anagen inhibition and normal hair shaft formation [4]. The present analyses identified a total of 99 target genes that may act downstream of miR-31 in these processes. These include Retinoid X Receptor Alpha (*RXRA*), a nuclear receptor which is highly expressed in skin and in HF outer root sheath (ORS) keratinocytes [25, 26]. In mice, ablation of *Rxra* in the skin leads to HF degeneration and subsequent hair loss [27], while conditional knockout in epidermal and ORS keratinocytes results in altered anagen initiation [28]. These findings underline the role of *RXRA* in HF maintenance and hair cycle control. Interestingly, target genes of miR-31 were enriched in *PPAR* and *RAR/RXRA* signalling, thus supporting the hypothesis that *RXRA*-mediated signalling is important for the control of anagen initiation. Moreover, miR-31 target genes were enriched in PDGF (Platelet-Derived Growth Factor), adipogenesis, and JAK/STAT signalling, which have been implicated previously in the control of the HF cycle [29–33]. Studies in murine HFs have demonstrated that several PDGF isoforms induce and maintain murine anagen HFs [31]. Furthermore, PDGF signalling may contribute to the essential role of immature adipocytes in anagen induction [34]. A recent study identified JAK/STAT signalling as a promising therapeutic target for the treatment of hair loss disorders. Here, topical application of JAK/STAT inhibitors to the shaved back skin of mice led to rapid anagen induction [33]. Collectively, the identified target genes and pathways indicate that miR-31 is a potent cross-species inhibitor of the anagen phase. However, functional studies are required to confirm the interaction between miR-31 and these pathways, and to elucidate their role in anagen control in the human HF.

The third miRNA to show significant mRNA correlations in the present analyses, miR-106a, is reported to be upregulated in the balding, as compared to the non-balding, DPCs of males with MPB, which suggests that it may be implicated in MPB pathobiology [7]. Although none of the 53 identified target genes of miR-106a have yet been associated with MPB, two building blocks of the desmosome - Plakophilin 3 (*PKP3*) and Desmocollin 1 (*DSC1*), are reported to play a role in HF morphogenesis [35]. *Pkp3* deficient mice develop an abnormal hair coat and secondary alopecia [36]. Although *Dsc1* deficient mice show normal HF cycling and structures until the age of four weeks, they develop alopecia and HF degeneration in later life [37]. Moreover, one of the pathways identified in the present study was 'WNT Signalling', which is of key importance in terms of HF development and cycling [38–41]. Interestingly, genetic evidence is available for the involvement of WNT signalling in MPB development. Heilmann et al. reported that a single nucleotide polymorphism (rs7349332) located intronically in *WNT10A* was associated with MPB risk ($P \leq 5 \times 10^{-8}$) and resulted in reduced *WNT10A* expression in HFs of risk allele carriers [42]. The present analyses therefore provide strong support for the hypothesis that miR-106a contributes to MPB development via WNT signalling and that the regulation of cell-cell adhesion may be an important factor in MPB.

Intriguingly, ten of the identified target genes were shared between miR-31, miR-24, and miR-106a, suggesting that they may be critical points in the signalling cascades that control HF biology. The overlapping target genes *FZD7*, *SFRP1*, and *TAX1BP3* are involved in WNT/β-catenin signalling, which is an important biological pathway for HF development and maintenance [43–46]. The WNT receptor *FZD7* mediates canonical and non-canonical signalling [47, 48], while *SFRP1* and *TAX1BP3* are reported as WNT antagonists. The respective proteins exert their effects via direct interaction with WNT or FZD proteins [49] and binding to β-catenin [50], respectively. Another interesting shared target gene is *TP63*, since one characteristic of *p63* knockout mice is the absence of HFs [51]. *SMARCA4* is a component of the chromatin remodelling complex, and knock-out experiments in murine bulge cells showed that it is required for hair regeneration and anagen progression [52]. The role of *COL17A1* in hair biology was discussed earlier. The four remaining overlapping target genes have not yet been associated with HF biology. The gene *RBM17* is reported to be involved in mRNA splicing [53], *JUN* belongs to the AP-1 transcription factor family, and is involved in many fundamental cell processes including proliferation, differentiation, and apoptosis and plays an essential role in skin development and the differentiation of epidermal keratinocytes [54–59]. *MEIS2* encodes a TALE homeobox protein, which is a highly conserved transcription factor, and *ZCCHC11* is a zinc finger containing RNA uridyltransferase. Taken together, these results underline the importance of WNT signalling in hair biology and suggest that miRNAs are critical regulators of WNT and TP63 signalling in the human HF.

In addition to these ten shared genes, a total of 30 genes were targeted by two miRNAs. These therefore represent further promising candidate genes, which may impact key functions in healthy hair biology and the pathobiology of hair loss disorders.

According to the STRING database, numerous interactions exist between the identified target genes of each candidate miRNA, and among the 40 shared miRNA target genes. This indicates that these miRNAs are (in)directly involved in various regulatory networks. Notably, all of these networks contain an indirect interaction between *JUN* and *FZD7* via *SFRP1*, suggesting that these genes may play a pivotal role in the miRNA mediated control of HF cycling, keratinocyte differentiation and MPB development (Fig. 2, Additional file 2: Figure S2).

The present analyses failed to confirm the expression of miR-137, miR-214 and miR-410 in the human HF. While miR-137 has been described in the determination of murine coat colour [5], no data are available concerning the expression pattern of miR-137 in the human HF or skin. Research has shown that miR-214 controls WNT/β-catenin signalling in murine embryonic HF development [60]. Further studies are required to determine whether miR-137 is involved in the determination of human hair colour and whether miR-214 plays a role in human HF embryogenesis. MiR-410 expression was found almost exclusively in the DPCs of balding vellus HFs [7]. As the present analyses were restricted to non-balding HFs with sparse DPCs, the failure to detect miR-410 expression in the present samples may point to a very specific role for miR-410 during MPB pathogenesis. Moreover, no significant correlation was found with mRNA expression for miR-22, miR-125b, or miR-205. This may be attributable to limited power of our sample (n = 24) to detect smaller regulatory effects.

Conclusions

In conclusion, the present systematic investigation of the expression of ten miRNAs previously implicated in hair biology and the identification of their target genes, pathways, and regulatory networks provides novel insights into the biological mechanisms that control human HF cycling, HF keratinocyte differentiation, and MPB pathogenesis. Further analyses in larger samples and detailed functional follow up investigations, such as the precise miRNA localisation in the human HF and their expression profile during different hair cycle stages, are now warranted to confirm these findings and to identify additional target genes and regulatory interactions. Increased sample sizes will also allow genome-wide investigations and thus the identification of additional hair-relevant miRNAs, as well as their target genes and regulated pathways. This research will facilitate understanding of human hair (patho-) biology.

Abbreviations

DPC: Dermal papilla cell; HF: Hair follicle; IPA: Ingenuity pathway analysis; miRNA/miR: MicroRNA; MPB: Male pattern baldness; PANTHER: Protein analysis through evolutionary relationship; PPI: Protein-protein interaction; STRING: Search tool for the retrieval of interacting genes/proteins

Acknowledgments

The authors thank the study participants for their cooperation. We thank Christine Schmael for her revision of the manuscript. MMN is a member of the Deutsche Forschungsgemeinschaft (DFG) Excellence Cluster ImmunoSensation.

Funding

The study was supported by the BONFOR programme of the Medical Faculty of the University of Bonn.

Authors' contributions

TA, LMH collected the samples. NF, MHR, CSB, LMH, SHH designed and performed the experiments. LMH, SHH and MMN prepared the manuscript. All authors read and approved the final manuscript.

Competing interests

The author(s) declare that they have no competing interests.

Author details

[1]Institute of Human Genetics, University of Bonn, Sigmund-Freud-Str. 25, 53127 Bonn, Germany. [2]Department of Genomics, Life and Brain Center, University of Bonn, Sigmund-Freud-Str. 25, 53127 Bonn, Germany. [3]Human Genomics Research Group, Department of Biomedicine, University of Basel, Hebelstrasse 20, 4031 Basel, Switzerland.

References

1. Millar SE. Molecular mechanisms regulating hair follicle development. J Invest Dermatol. 2002;118:216–25.
2. Schneider MR, Schmidt-Ullrich R, Paus R. The hair follicle as a dynamic miniorgan. Curr Biol. 2009;19:R132–42.
3. Huntzinger E, Izaurralde E. Gene silencing by microRNAs: contributions of translational repression and mRNA decay. Nat Rev Genet. 2011;12:99–110.
4. Mardaryev AN, Ahmed MI, Vlahov NV, et al. Micro-RNA-31 controls hair cycle-associated changes in gene expression programs of the skin and hair follicle. FASEB J. 2010;24:3869–81.
5. Dong C, Wang H, Xue L, et al. Coat color determination by miR-137 mediated down-regulation of microphthalmia-associated transcription factor in a mouse model. RNA. 2012;18:1679–86.

6. Amelio I, Lena a M, Bonanno E, et al. miR-24 affects hair follicle morphogenesis targeting Tcf-3. Cell Death Dis. 2013;4:e922.
7. Goodarzi HR, Abbasi A, Saffari M, et al. Differential expression analysis of balding and nonbalding dermal papilla microRNAs in male pattern baldness with a microRNA amplification profiling method. Br J Dermatol. 2012;166:1010–6.
8. Barbosa-Morais NL, Dunning MJ, Samarajiwa SA, et al. A re-annotation pipeline for Illumina BeadArrays: improving the interpretation of gene expression data. Nucleic Acids Res. 2010;38:e17.
9. Pearson K. Determination of the coefficient of correlation. Science. 1909;30:23–5.
10. Mi H, Muruganujan A, Thomas PD. PANTHER in 2013: modeling the evolution of gene function, and other gene attributes, in the context of phylogenetic trees. Nucleic Acids Res. 2013;41:D377–86.
11. Szklarczyk D, Jensen LJ. Protein-protein interaction databases. Methods Mol Biol. 2015;1278:39–56.
12. Dweep H, Gretz N. miRWalk2.0: a comprehensive atlas of microRNA-target interactions. Nat Methods. 2015;12:697.
13. Agarwal V, Bell GW, Nam J-W, Bartel DP. Predicting effective microRNA target sites in mammalian mRNAs. Elife 2015; 4. doi:10.7554/eLife.05005
14. Andl T, Botchkareva NV. MicroRNAs (miRNAs) in the control of HF development and cycling: The next frontiers in hair research. Exp Dermatol. 2015;24:821–6.
15. Amelio I, Lena AM, Viticchiè G, et al. miR-24 triggers epidermal differentiation by controlling actin adhesion and cell migration. J Cell Biol. 2012;199:347–63.
16. Rippa AL, Vorotelyak EA, Vasiliev AV, Terskikh VV. The role of integrins in the development and homeostasis of the epidermis and skin appendages. Acta Naturae. 2013;5:22–33.
17. Van Buggenhout G, Van Ravenswaaij-Arts C, Mc Maas N, et al. The del(2)(q32.2q33) deletion syndrome defined by clinical and molecular characterization of four patients. Eur J Med Genet. 2005;48:276–89.
18. Rifai L, Port-Lis M, Tabet A-C, et al. Ectodermal dysplasia-like syndrome with mental retardation due to contiguous gene deletion: further clinical and molecular delineation of del(2q32) syndrome. Am J Med Genet A. 2010; 152A:111–7.
19. Tanimura S, Tadokoro Y, Inomata K, et al. Hair follicle stem cells provide a functional niche for melanocyte stem cells. Cell Stem Cell. 2011;8:177–87.
20. Matsumura H, Mohri Y, Binh NT, et al. Hair follicle aging is driven by transepidermal elimination of stem cells via COL17A1 proteolysis. Science. 2016;80(351):aad4395.
21. Darling TN, Bauer JW, Hintner H, Yancey KB. Generalized atrophic benign epidermolysis bullosa. Adv Dermatol. 1997;13:87–120.
22. Inui S, Itami S. Androgen actions on the human hair follicle: perspectives. Exp Dermatol. 2013;22:168–71.
23. Hohl A, Ronsoni MF, de Oliveira M. Hirsutism: diagnosis and treatment. Arq Bras Endocrinol Metabol. 2014;58:97–107.
24. Andreyko JL, Monroe SE, Jaffe RB. Treatment of hirsutism with a gonadotropin-releasing hormone agonist (nafarelin). J Clin Endocrinol Metab. 1986;63:854–9.
25. Fisher GJ, Talwar HS, Xiao JH, et al. Immunological identification and functional quantitation of retinoic acid and retinoid X receptor proteins in human skin. J Biol Chem. 1994;269:20629–35.
26. Reichrath J, Münssinger T, Kerber A, et al. In situ detection of retinoid-X receptor expression in normal and psoriatic human skin. Br J Dermatol. 1995;133:168–75.
27. Ghyselinck NB, Chapellier B, Calléja C, et al. Genetic dissection of retinoic acid function in epidermis physiology. Ann Dermatologie vénéréologie. 2002;129:793–9.
28. Li M, Chiba H, Warot X, et al. RXR-alpha ablation in skin keratinocytes results in alopecia and epidermal alterations. Development. 2001;128:675–88.
29. Karlsson L, Bondjers C, Betsholtz C. Roles for PDGF-A and sonic hedgehog in development of mesenchymal components of the hair follicle. Development. 1999;126:2611–21.
30. Kamp H, Geilen CC, Sommer C, Blume-Peytavi U. Regulation of PDGF and PDGF receptor in cultured dermal papilla cells and follicular keratinocytes of the human hair follicle. Exp Dermatol. 2003;12:662–72.
31. Tomita Y, Akiyama M, Shimizu H. PDGF isoforms induce and maintain anagen phase of murine hair follicles. J Dermatol Sci. 2006;43:105–15.
32. Schmidt B, Horsley V. Unravelling hair follicle-adipocyte communication. Exp Dermatol. 2012;21:827–30.
33. Harel S, Higgins CA, Cerise JE, et al. Pharmacologic inhibition of JAK-STAT signaling promotes hair growth. Sci Adv. 2015;1:1–13.
34. Festa E, Fretz J, Berry R, et al. Adipocyte lineage cells contribute to the skin stem cell niche to drive hair cycling. Cell. 2011;146:761–71.
35. Nekrasova O, Green KJ. Desmosome assembly and dynamics. Trends Cell Biol. 2013;23:537–46.
36. Sklyarova T, Bonné S, D'Hooge P, et al. Plakophilin-3-deficient mice develop hair coat abnormalities and are prone to cutaneous inflammation. J Invest Dermatol. 2008;128:1375–85.
37. Chidgey M, Brakebusch C, Gustafsson E, et al. Mice lacking desmocollin 1 show epidermal fragility accompanied by barrier defects and abnormal differentiation. J Cell Biol. 2001;155:821–32.
38. Millar SE, Willert K, Salinas PC, et al. WNT Signaling in the Control of Hair Growth and Structure. Dev Biol. 1999;207:133–49.
39. Reddy S, Andl T, Bagasra A, et al. Characterization of Wnt gene expression in developing and postnatal hair follicles and identification of Wnt5a as a target of Sonic hedgehog in hair follicle morphogenesis. Mech Dev. 2001;107:69–82.
40. Andl T, Reddy ST, Gaddapara T, Millar SE. WNT Signals Are Required for the Initiation of Hair Follicle Development. Dev Cell. 2002;2:643–53.
41. Shimizu H, Morgan BA. Wnt Signaling through the β-Catenin Pathway Is Sufficient to Maintain, but Not Restore, Anagen-Phase Characteristics of Dermal Papilla Cells. J Invest Dermatol. 2004;122:239–45.
42. Heilmann S, Kiefer AK, Fricker N, et al. Androgenetic alopecia: identification of four genetic risk loci and evidence for the contribution of WNT signaling to its etiology. J Invest Dermatol. 2013;133:1489–96.
43. Huelsken J, Vogel R, Erdmann B, et al. β-Catenin Controls Hair Follicle Morphogenesis and Stem Cell Differentiation in the Skin. Cell. 2001;105:533–45.
44. Chen D, Jarrell A, Guo C, et al. Dermal β-catenin activity in response to epidermal Wnt ligands is required for fibroblast proliferation and hair follicle initiation. Development. 2012;139:1522–33.
45. Choi YS, Zhang Y, Xu M, et al. Distinct functions for Wnt/β-catenin in hair follicle stem cell proliferation and survival and interfollicular epidermal homeostasis. Cell Stem Cell. 2013;13:720–33.
46. Tsai S-Y, Sennett R, Rezza A, et al. Wnt/β-catenin signaling in dermal condensates is required for hair follicle formation. Dev Biol. 2014;385:179–88.
47. Bhanot P, Brink M, Samos CH, et al. A new member of the frizzled family from Drosophila functions as a Wingless receptor. Nature. 1996;382:225–30.
48. Ueno K, Hirata H, Hinoda Y, Dahiya R. Frizzled homolog proteins, microRNAs and Wnt signaling in cancer. Int J cancer. 2013;132:1731–40.
49. Kawano Y. Secreted antagonists of the Wnt signalling pathway. J Cell Sci. 2003;116:2627–34.
50. Kanamori M, Sandy P, Marzinotto S, et al. The PDZ protein tax-interacting protein-1 inhibits beta-catenin transcriptional activity and growth of colorectal cancer cells. J Biol Chem. 2003;278:38758–64.
51. Mills AA, Zheng B, Wang XJ, et al. p63 is a p53 homologue required for limb and epidermal morphogenesis. Nature. 1999;398:708–13.
52. Xiong Y, Li W, Shang C, et al. Brg1 governs a positive feedback circuit in the hair follicle for tissue regeneration and repair. Dev Cell. 2013;25:169–81.
53. Lallena MJ, Chalmers KJ, Llamazares S, et al. Splicing regulation at the second catalytic step by Sex-lethal involves 3' splice site recognition by SPF45. Cell. 2002;109:285–96.
54. Jochum W, Passegué E, Wagner EF. AP-1 in mouse development and tumorigenesis. Oncogene. 2001;20:2401–12.
55. Rossi A, Jang SI, Ceci R, et al. Effect of AP1 transcription factors on the regulation of transcription in normal human epidermal keratinocytes. J Invest Dermatol. 1998;110:34–40.
56. Angel P, Szabowski A, Schorpp-Kistner M. Function and regulation of AP-1 subunits in skin physiology and pathology. Oncogene. 2001;20:2413–23.
57. Mehic D, Bakiri L, Ghannadan M, et al. Fos and jun proteins are specifically expressed during differentiation of human keratinocytes. J Invest Dermatol. 2005;124:212–20.

58. Zenz R, Wagner EF. Jun signalling in the epidermis: From developmental defects to psoriasis and skin tumors. Int J Biochem Cell Biol. 2006;38:1043–9.
59. Han B, Rorke EA, Adhikary G, et al. Suppression of AP1 transcription factor function in keratinocyte suppresses differentiation. PLoS One. 2012;7:e36941.
60. Ahmed MI, Alam M, Emelianov VU, et al. MicroRNA-214 controls skin and hair follicle development by modulating the activity of the Wnt pathway. J Cell Biol. 2014;207:549–67.

Role models in a preventive program for hand eczema among healthcare workers: a qualitative exploration of their main tasks and associated barriers and facilitators

Anne M Bruinewoud[1], Esther WC van der Meer[1], Joost WJ van der Gulden[2], Johannes R Anema[1,3,4] and Cécile RL Boot[1,3*]

Abstract

Background: Role models often play a role when implementing guidelines in healthcare. However, little is known about how role models perform their respective roles, or about which factors may hamper or enhance their functioning. The aim of the present study was therefore to investigate how role models perform there role as a part of a multifaceted implementation strategy on the prevention of hand eczema, and to identify barriers and facilitators for the performing of their role.

Methods: The role models were selected to become a role model and received a role model training. All role models worked at a hospital. In total, 19 role models, were interviewed. A topic list was used focussing on how the role models performed their role and what they experienced to be facilitators and barriers for their role. After coding the interviews, the codes were divided into themes.

Results: This study shows that the main tasks perceived by the role models were to raise awareness, to transfer information, to interact with colleagues about hand eczema, to provide material, and to perform coordinating tasks. Barriers and facilitators were whether the role suited the participant, affinity with the topic, and risk perception.

Conclusions: Most role models performed only the tasks they learned during their training. They mentioned a wide range of barriers and facilitators for the performing of their role. To enhance the functioning of the role models, a suggestion would be to select role models by taking into account prior coaching experience.

Keywords: Role models, Healthcare workers, Hand eczema, Implementation, Facilitators, Barriers

Background

When implementing guidelines in hospitals, multifaceted implementation strategies have shown to be more effective than single strategies [1]. As recent studies have showed that participatory programmes have been tested successfully in healthcare employees [2, 3], role models often play an important role in interventions. In 2010, Ploeg et al. [4] found that role models can influence the use of guidelines by dissemination of information, by being persuasive practice leaders and by tailoring the guideline implementation strategies to an organizational context. Although the experiences of role models in interventions on occupational skin diseases have been studied in wet work settings [5], it is still unknown which factors may hamper and/or enhance the role model's function in a healthcare setting. To improve interventions that aim to increase adherence to guidelines among hospital staff, deeper insight into these factors is crucial.

Role models are often part of interventions that aim to manage changes in behaviour or to implement guidelines

* Correspondence: crl.boot@vumc.nl
[1]Department of Public and Occupational Health, EMGO Institute for Health and Care Research, VU University Medical Center, Van der Boechorststraat 7, 1081 BT Amsterdam, The Netherlands
[3]Body@Work, Research Center Physical Activity, Work and Health, TNO-VU University Medical Center, Amsterdam, The Netherlands
Full list of author information is available at the end of the article

in healthcare [6, 7]. Role models are seen as one of the most important factors for the successful implementation of recommendations that aim to change workers' behaviour [8] as they influence the subjective norm [9]. According to the Theory of Planned Behaviour [10], the subjective norm is one of three intermediate variables that form the intention to perform desired behaviour [11].

Changing the behaviour of workers within a healthcare setting is difficult, as is demonstrated by the low compliance to guidelines in hospitals [12]. Erasmus et al. [13] concluded that within the field of hand hygiene, a lack of positive role models among hospital staff during daily practice may hinder compliance to the proposed recommendations. This was explained by the finding that participants copy the behaviour of their superiors. Based on the research of Erasmus et al. [13] we hypothesized that the use of role models can positively contribute to the prevention of occupational hand eczema among healthcare workers.

Healthcare workers like nurses are at increased risk for developing hand eczema [14, 15] as occupational exposure to irritants like water greatly increases the likeliness for developing this skin disease [16]. Prevention is necessary, because recent research showed that the prevalence of hand eczema in healthcare workers is double the prevalance in other populations [17] and that the skin disease is one of the most prevalent work-related diseases in Europe [18].

To reduce hand eczema among healthcare workers, a multifaceted implementation strategy was developed in which healthcare workers were trained as role models as a part of this strategy. Previously, role models were often chosen based on their position in the organisation or department [8, 19]. In the present study role models were allocated alternatively, based on their representativeness, their influence on colleagues, and their motivation.

The aim of this study was to *qualitatively* explore what 'placed' role models considered to be their main tasks, and to gain insight into facilitators and barriers that could have influenced their role as a role model.

Methods

Design and participants

The participants of this study participated in the intervention group of the Hands4U study who received a multifaceted implementation strategy. The Hands4U study is a two-armed clustered randomized controlled trial. The goal of this study was to evaluatie the (cost-) effectiveness of the multifaceted implementation strategy and to investigate barriers and facilitators that arise in the use of this strategy. In total, 1649 Dutch healthcare workers participated in the trial of which 876 participated in the intervention group. More details on the Hands4U study have been published elsewhere [20]. Within the multifaceted implementation strategy used in this study, evidence-based recommendations were given about preventive measures for hand eczema [21]. The strategy contained five parts: 1) education; 2) participatory working groups who identified problems with adherence to the recommendations, found solutions for these problems, and implemented these solutions within their department; 3) role models who helped and encouraged their colleagues to increase adherence to the recommendations; 4) reminders (posters); and 5) a leaflet containing the recommendations.

All role models were members of the participatory working groups who followed an hour and a half educational session about hand eczema. The training consisted of a lecture by an occupational nurse and a role play. Topics were: dealing with resistance from colleagues, motivational interviewing, and principles of the stages of change model. Role models were trained on how to promote and enhance the implementation of recommendations for the prevention of hand eczema within their department, and on how to be a role model for their colleagues.

A total number of 70 role models participated in the Hands4U study, working at 23 departments. For the interview recruitment of the role models for the present study, convenience sampling was used. Role models were invited in two ways: 1) by asking them to participate during the last working group meeting, and 2) by sending them an e-mail with the request to participate. Variety in participants was desired, and was based on the following characteristics: the hospital and the department where the participants worked, gender, having patient contact or not, and having an executive function or not. In total, 19 role models from 14 different departments were interviewed. At the time the interviews took place, all participants have been performing their role for a period longer than six months.

Data collection and ethical considerations

The interviews were conducted from December 2011 to January 2013 by EWCM. Before the interview, participants received an informative letter stating that the interview would take approximately 45 minutes. A semi-structured interview guide was used. The interviews were recorded and transcribed into Word-files. The interview covered two topics: 1) barriers and facilitators for the implementation of recommendations for hand eczema, and 2) experiences as a role model, and barriers and facilitators related to this role. The present study focused solely on the second topic. During the interviews, the participants were asked to explain what they considered to be tasks as a role model within their department, and what they perceived to be barriers and facilitators in performing their role as a role model. At the end of the interview, participants were asked whether all important topics were covered and if they wanted to add something to the conversation.

The Medical Ethics Committee of the VU University Medical Center approved this study. Most interviews took place within the participant's department, in a private conference room. Due to the nature of the study, the ethics committee decided that no informed consent was needed.

Data analysis

All interviews were read and quotes about the role model's tasks, facilitators and barriers were identified by AMB, based on the method used in the study of Hooftman et al. [22]. As it is highly important to analyze the data systematically in qualitative research, the analyses were conducted by AMB in close colaboration with the second researcher (ECWM). AMB was not directly involved in the interviewing. The constant comparison method was used for the analyses, in which each item was compared with the rest of the data in order to establish analytical categories [23]. Facilitators were defined as factors that participants perceived as making it easier to perform their role as a role model. The barriers were factors that participants perceived as making it more difficult to perform their role as a role model within their department. First, five interview transcripts were randomly selected and read by AMB. Then, the interview transcripts were open-coded by AMB to identify relevant themes. To ensure that all the themes were identified, the interview transcripts were read and reread several times. Similar themes were clustered into categories and inter-subjective agreement was tested by a second researcher (EWCM) based on the first five interviews, as well as in one other interview that was randomly selected. When there was disagreement, the quote was discussed and afterwards a decision was made about the inclusion or exclusion of the quote. During consensus meetings, the third researcher (CRLB) solved disagreements on the coding and gave advice. The remaining interviews were read and efforts were made to detect quotes of the identified themes and, if applicable, to identify new themes. After analyzing the remaining interviews, we updated the themes and quotes were transcribed into codes categorized by main tasks, facilitators and barriers. Related segments and subthemes were subcategorized by AMB and seperately checked by EWCM and CRLB. Next, all codes were categorized into themes by three researchers (AMB, EWCM and CRLB). All quotes were translated from Dutch into English. There was no software package used to code the data other than Microsoft Word.

Results

Of the 19 role models: 15 were women and four were men. Twelve of the participants worked in a department where there was patient contact (i.e. chirurgical units, intensive care units, dentistry), three worked in a kitchen, two worked in a laboratory, and two worked at the hospital's pharmacy. The participants worked at different cities throughout the Netherlands: 13 in Groningen, and the remaining six worked in Nijmegen, Amsterdam, or Stadskanaal. Six participants had an executive function. Characteristics and quotes of the participants are shown in Table 1. In the following text quote numbers from Table 1 are given in square brackets.

Main tasks of the role models

There were five specific aspects that participants mentioned as their main tasks as a role model:1) to raise awareness and maintain mindfulness in regard to hand eczema; 2) to present information and modeling; 3) to have interaction with colleagues about hand eczema; 4) to provide relevant material; and 5) to perform coordinating tasks for the Hands4U project as a whole.

To raise awareness and maintain mindfulness on hand eczema

There were several ways in which role models tried to raise awareness for the topic of 'hand eczema': by periodically repeating relevant information to colleagues within their department, by directing attention to the theme, by informing new colleagues, and by showing enthusiasm and commitment to the topic. In many cases, the role models agreed with their manager about repeating the information on hand eczema regularly during meetings in order to keep focus on the topic [Table 1, Quote 1]. Furthermore, one participant stated that the enthusiasm of the role models was a determining factor for the implementation of all recomendations.

To present information and modeling

There were three main ways in which the role models provided information. First, transfer of knowledge was seen as a major task. Participants informed their colleagues about the benefits of using moisturizer and disinfectant and how to prevent hand eczema. In addition, participants noticed that it was important that their tone was not demanding because that did not fit with their personality or their role at the department [Table 1, Quote 2]. To be a good example for their colleagues was found to be another task of the role models, as they believed this was needed to convince their colleagues [Table 1, Quote 3]. Letting colleagues know that they have been assigned as a role model was named as a third way of information provision, for instance via a whiteboard announcement in the coffee room, by e-mail, and/or in team meetings.

Table 1 Characteristics and quotes of participants

Quote	Participant number, gender Department (with/no patient contact) Function (executive /not executive)	
1	6, Female With patient contact Executive function	*'When you see something fading away, you notice that with many things, you will have to repeat it.'*
2	1, Male No patient contact Not executive function	*'I am not the kind of person that says: "You have to do this or you have to do that" and that's not the kind of person I want to be. And obviously, I do not have that role at the department... So not top down or in a compulsory way, but more like: "Did you know that hand eczema is often not visible, you might have it without knowing it?"'*
3	13, Female With patient contact Not executive function	*'If you are trying to convince people of the importance, but you do not practice what you preach, they will never listen to you. So I think that's the most important. That they see you do the things you say you do.'*
4	5, Female With patient contact Executive function	*'If I see something, I address people of course. And I say: "He guys, here's the moisturizer, let's use it."'*
5	18, Female No patient contact Executive function	*'Yes, and people ask: "Has the cotton under gloves already been ordered? What is the order status?" Because, of course, you told them that it was going to happen, they know it.'*
6	8, Female No patient contact Executive function	*'Well, that role [the role of the role model] was performed more frequently by W. and P. and I performed the more coordinating tasks.'*
7	1, Male No patient contact Not executive function	*'Personally, I would have liked to know more about hand eczema and maybe the consequences of hand eczema and things like that. Then I would have been able to tell more about it, than I could after the first meeting.'*
8	10, Female With patient contact Not executive function	*'Yes, and also personally I think it is important, because you still want to continue work for many years, so you do not want to have that kind of illness.'*
9	1, Male No patient contact Not executive function	*'What made it easier was that I followed other courses previously, for instance ergonomy training, and first aid, and then you already know what is to be expected from you as a coach.'*
10	18, Female No patient contact Executive function	*'That's because I am in a position where it is perhaps easier for me to address people than for an analyst in the laboratory. That might be the case.'*
11	18, Female No patient contact Executive function	*'J. just arrived, she had just finished her studies and she has just started to work here, and she was also in the working group... I think she was trying to find her own way. She does not have the experience yet to address people or to arrange these kind of things.'*
12	2, Female No patient contact Not executive function	*'We all learned from it. So that's positive as well. If you are going to do something and you think: "Yes, I already know that", then you will not benefit from it. Yes, we all found it quite interesting and fun. Yes, that's an advantage as well.'*
13	14, Female With patient contact Not executive function	*'Well, the manager was also a member of the working group. That makes a difference when you wish to arrange things. Yes, that made it easier.'*
14	15, Male With patient contact Executive function	*'When one of them is suddenly entitled as 'coach', the other one says: 'Why you?' It is like a henhouse here.'*

Table 1 Characteristics and quotes of participants *(Continued)*

15	17, Female With patient contact Not executive function	*'We work at very different locations, we do not have coffee breaks together, so it was difficult how I could announce this to everyone.'*
16	10, Female With patient contact Not executive function	*'When you are working here, it is pretty busy. So it is not always easy to keep it in sight* and that makes it a bit difficult.'
17	9, Female With patient contact Not executive function	*'But then of course, at a certain moment it is up to them to do something about it. You cannot force them, of course, that's not always possible. That's sometimes difficult.'*
18	10, Female With patient contact Not executive function	*'We could have used that one colleague as an example, because it was very clearly visible and then you notice that people think: "Well, that's not something I want, so I will do of course my best to avoid it."*
19	16, Female No patient contact Not executive function	*'"No, I don't have hand eczema," she said. So you can talk and talk, that didn't help a thing. Or let me put it this way: it did not help here. So I consider that effect as very minimal.'*
20	7, Female With patient contact Not executive function	*'It was sometimes really nice to be with the two of us, because when one of us was silent, the other one could come up with other nice arguments.'*
21	10, Female With patient contact Not executive function	*'So that way you can show people examples by using for instance a leaflet... That makes it of course easier to say something or to show people that it can have a result.'*
22	14, Female With patient contact Not executive function	*'Because it is a small and compact department, it has been easy to reach everybody.'*
23	12, Female With patient contact Not executive function	*'Because it is not a major issue, I think, it has been given a relatively high priority, relative to the problem perception, and that can be difficult.'*

Interaction with colleagues about hand eczema

The first aspect mentioned by participants was starting conversations with colleagues within the theme of 'hand eczema'. This was often done when 'unhealthy hand behaviour' like not using moisturizer was noticed by the role model [Table 1, Quote 4]. A second aspect was answering questions from colleagues about hand eczema and the preventive measures associated with it. A participant explained [Table 1, Quote 5]: *'Yes, and people ask: "Has the cotton under gloves already been ordered? What is the order status?" Because, of course, you told them that it was going to happen, they know it'.*

Providing material

Ensuring the availability of essential products for the prevention of hand eczema was considered to be very important by the role models. Providing material like moisturizers and gloves was therefore seen as one of their main tasks.

Coordinating tasks

Being a coordinator for the whole Hands4U project was the last task the role models mentioned. However, this task was mainly mentioned by participants in management positions [Table 1, Quote 6]. It seems that when there were several role models within a department, including a manager, there was a difference in the tasks that they performed.

Facilitators and barriers

Several facilitators and barriers for performing their role were mentioned by the role models (Table 2). These factors were divided into *internal factors* (personal factors) and *external factors* (department factors or factors originating from colleagues or work situations). Some factors that were mentioned as a facilitator were also mentioned as a barrier in opposite direction (e.g. social support by colleagues was considered a facilitator, whereas lack of social support was mentioned as a barrier).

Table 2 Facilitators and barriers

Theme's		Barriers	Facilitators
Internal	Knowledge about hand eczema	X	X
	Affinity with the topic	X	X
	Whether the role suited	X	X
	Attitude towards the role		X
External	Support or resistance colleagues	X	X
	Contact role model and colleagues	X	X
	Risk perception	X	X
	Amount of role models	X	X
	Availability of material		X
	Education		X
	Role suited the department		X
	Priority of hand eczema	X	
	Low risk at department	X	
	Little response of colleagues	X	
	Communication role models	X	

Internal factors

Knowledge about hand eczema

Sufficient knowledge ensured that the role model felt more confident in his/her role and that he/she could come up with good arguments to motivate colleagues to alter their behaviour. Participants who indicated that they had sufficient knowledge about the prevention of hand eczema, reported that they had a higher self-efficacy in sharing this knowledge with their colleagues. When the role model lacked knowledge about (the prevention of) hand eczema, this was experienced as a barrier. One participant explained [Table 1, Quote 7]: *'Personally, I would have liked to know more about hand eczema and maybe the consequences of hand eczema and things like that. Then I would have been able to tell more about it, than I could after the first meeting.'*

Affinity with the topic 'hand eczema'

Acknowledging the need for the prevention of hand eczema as this might be a barrier to continue working was seen as an internal facilitator [Table 1, Quote 8]. On the other hand, a lack of affinity with the topic of 'hand eczema' was considered to be a barrier for performing tasks as a role model. Some participants mentioned that they found it hard to give priority to and stay enthusiastic about a subject that they would not mark as highly important outside of the research project.

Whether the role suited the participant

An internal facilitator was whether the role suited the participant. The participants felt the role suited them when 1) they had experienced the consequences of hand eczema, 2) they had strong communication skills, 3) the role fit with their other tasks, and 4) they had previous experience in a coaching-role. A comment of one of the participants was [Table 1, Quote 9]: *'What made it easier was that I followed other courses previously, for instance ergonomy training, and first aid, and then you already know what is to be expected from you as a coach.'* In addition, participants with experience as a coach reported to feel more confidence in guiding their colleagues in performing desired behaviour. This facilitator was also reported by a participant in an executive position [Table 1, Quote 10]: *'That's because I am in a position where it is perhaps easier for me to address people than for an analyst in the laboratory. That might be the case.'* In cases where the role did not fit the participant, this was experienced as a barrier. Several reasons were mentioned by the participants for why the role did not suit them: 1) the role model did not want to control other people, 2) the role model found it difficult to correct people, and 3) the role model had no experience in a coaching role. Of these factors, the lack of experience in a coaching role was mentioned most often. The manager illustrated why the role of role model was difficult for a young employee [Table 1, Quote 11]: *'J. just arrived, she had just finished her studies and she has just started to work here, and she was also in the working group... I think she was trying to find her own way. She does not have the experience yet to address people or to arrange these kind of things.'* Another participant mentioned that it was difficult performing in the role of a coach when they lacked supervisory experience.

Attitude towards the role

This factor was only mentioned as a facilitator. Role models reported that their attitude positively influenced their role when they 1) were motivated to perform in their role 2) had fun in being a role model [Table 1, Quote 12] and 3) took their tasks seriously.

External factors

Support or resistance from colleagues and supervisors

Colleagues and supervisors could influence the functioning of the role models. On the one hand they could be supportive, which the role models experienced as facilitating, for instance when they wanted to arrange something for the project [Table 1, Quote 13]: *'Well, the manager was also a member of the working group. That makes a difference when you wish to arrange things. Yes, that made it easier.'* On the other hand, a negative attitude towards the role model by department employees was mentioned as a barrier for performing their role. A manager explained that when one worker at his department was suddenly titled as a 'coach', this was not always accepted by his colleagues because they did not understand why they were not chosen [Table 1, Quote 14].

Contact between the role model and his/her colleagues and peers

To be able to perform their tasks, the role models indicated that having contact with their colleagues was of great importance. It was seen as a facilitator when the behaviour of their colleagues was well visible, as this gave them the possibility to address them when they performed unhealthy behaviour in relation to the prevention of hand eczema. On the other hand, not having contact with colleagues was deemed to be a barrier [Table 1, Quote 15]. Another participant explained that because of work pressure and lack of time it was not always possible to keep an eye on the behaviour of colleagues, something that was experienced as a barrier [Table 1, Quote 16]. When colleagues did not pick up or continue the encouraged healthy behaviour, this was experienced as a barrier to role models [Table 1, Quote 17]. When there were two or more role models within a department, and there was insufficient communication between them, this was experienced as a barrier for performing the role.

Risk perception

An external facilitator was the risk perception within the department of the role model. In departments where there was a colleague suffering from hand eczema, the problem was recognized by colleagues. One participant noticed how hand eczema among her colleague increased the awareness at the department [Table 1, Quote 18]; *'We could have used that one colleague as an example, because it was very clearly visible and then you notice that people think: "Well, that's not something I want, so I will do of course my best to avoid it."'* Many role models mentioned that a low risk perception on hand eczema at the department was a barrier for performing their role. Several participants mentioned that their colleagues experienced no risk because they were not familiar with the problem [Table 1, Quote 19].

Number of role models

Two or more role models within a department, was described as a facilitator because they could support each other. A participant explained [Table 1, Quote 20]: *'It was sometimes really nice to be with the two of us, because when one of us was silent, the other one could come up with other nice arguments.'* Taking charge of too many colleagues as a role model was experienced as a barrier.

Availability of material

The availability of study related material like flyers and leaflets about hand eczema, was experienced as a facilitator for performing the role. A participant explained that the role models used flyers to make their colleagues aware of the impact of hand eczema [Table 1, Quote 21].

Education

One participant explained that the educational session within his department contributed to the fact that his colleagues took his tasks more seriously afterwards.

When the role suited the department

Participants mentioned that it was a facilitator when the role suited the department where they worked. This was the case when employees were attainable in case of a small department for example, when there was a culture of speaking up and/or a dynamic atmosphere and when the workers of the department were used to paying attention to new projects [Table 1, Quote 22].

Priority of hand eczema

Several role models explained that the prevention of hand eczema was not relevant for the department because it was not a major issue at that moment [Table 1, Quote 23]. Other priorities within the department, were also viewed as a barrier.

Low risk for hand eczema at the department

Another barrier for performing the role was having a low risk for developing hand eczema at work. At departments where people did not have to complete 'dirty' tasks or where they did not work with patients, employees had to clean their hands less compared to other departments. Therefore, role models did not always have the opportunity to give a good example for their colleagues.

Discussion

The implementation strategy used in this study included role models who were intended to stimulate their colleagues to adhere to recommendations aiming to reduce hand eczema, and to pay attention to their colleagues' risk behaviour. This study aimed to qualitatively explore what the role models perceived to be their main role and tasks, and to identify possible factors that hampered or facilitated their role.

Main tasks of the role models

Creating awareness about 'hand eczema', the transferring of knowledge, and serving as a good example were perceived as important role model tasks. This is partly consistent with Ploeg et al. [4], who reported that dissemination of information by education and mentoring was one of the ways in which role models could influence the diffusion of best practice guidelines. In addition, coordinating the study happened to be one of the main tasks for participants in an executive function. It was not a goal of our study to investigate differences in tasks perceived by employees in a non supervisory position versus a supervisory one, but our findings suggest that differences may exist: role models in an executive function also felt responsible for coordinating tasks within the study, while participants without supervisory tasks often stuck with the tasks they received from role model training. However, it is also possible that managers who performed the role of role model would have taken care of coordinating tasks anyway, as it is often part of their job.

Previous research states that healthcare workers often do not think of themselves as role models and that they underestimate the impact of their behaviour on the behaviour of those they interact with [19]. We found that our participants considered giving a good example one of their main tasks. This finding suggests that a compact education session had an impact on the participants and that they were aware of the fact that their own behaviour might positively influence the behaviour of their colleagues. Remarkably, more participants with no executive function mentioned this task than role models with supervisory tasks. Previous research shows that role models, especially those in an executive function, should be aware of the influence of their behaviour on others, because medical students, for example, mentioned that they copy the behaviour of their superiors [13].

Barriers and facilitators

The internal themes showed that the manner in which role models were selected, has room for improvement. Our participants were selected by their supervisor, based on their expected influence on colleagues and their motivation. Several participants mentioned that they experienced it as a barrier that they had to stay enthusiastic about a topic, that they would not mark as 'highly important' by themselves. Others mentioned that the role did not fit them, because they did not feel comfortable correcting the behaviour of their colleagues. Thus, it seems to be difficult for managers to assess whether someone is actually motivated and capable to perform a particular role. We suggest, for future interventions, that a 'job application' is written up prior to the study, in which interested participants can apply for the role of role model.

Two major facilitating factors for the role models were when the role fit in with other tasks, and when the role model had previous experience in a coaching role. These results suggest that it might be easier to act as a role model when someone is familiar with coaching-tasks, which is often the case when someone has supervisory tasks in their daily work. Furthermore, a manager explained that there was resistance among the employees when someone was suddenly entitled to be a coach. In previous studies where only the more senior health care workers acted as a role model [8, 19, 24] these findings were not reported. Also in our study, no managers reported the barrier of not being able to guide their colleagues to alter their behaviour. Therefore, in future role modeling interventions it might be better to choose workers with experience in coaching-tasks or with an executive function to act as a role model. When role models lack experience with coaching-tasks, a more comprehensive training about coaching needs to be incorporated.

An important external factor was the amount of support the role models received from their supervisor and/or their peers. When the role model felt supported by their colleagues or supervisor, this was experienced as a facilitator. A lack of social support and resistance towards the role model among colleagues was mentioned as a barrier. While the topic of 'dealing with resistance' is briefly discussed during role model training, we advise to pay more attention to resistance during the study. In addition, most barriers were experienced from the moment a role model had actually started to perform his/her role. Therefore it seems appropriate to plan meetings for the role models in which problems like lack of social support can be discussed with the other role models. We hypothesize that these peermeetings during the intervention might have the potential to increase their role confidence.

A low risk perception at the department was perceived as a barrier. Although we did not investigate whether the risk perception of the healthcare workers was correct, other studies indicate that there are many misperceptions among hospital staff regarding hand eczema prevention measures [25]. Colleagues of the role models in our study might have underestimated the risk of developing hand eczema. Educating role models and their colleagues about the occupational risk factors for developing hand eczema and the possibilities for prevention is therefore important. This was confirmed by our finding that several role models stated that they lacked sufficient knowledge about (the prevention of) hand eczema. Although an educational session was part of our implementation strategy, increasing the number of sessions in which the principles of prevention and the consequences of hand eczema are emphasized and refreshed once in a while should be considered. Furthermore, training the role models on peer-to-peer coaching could possibly contribute to a better performance.

Strengths and limitations

Although the experiences of role models have been studied in wet work settings [5], this is the first study in a healthcare setting that examined facilitators and barriers experienced by the role models themselves. The explorative qualitative design provides more insight into the experiences of role models than a quantitative study could do. Thereby, important indepth information was obtained about how role models experienced their role and what they perceived to be barriers and facilitators which can be used for future implementation studies. Another strength is that our study population was heterogeneous: our data reflected perspectives from role models in different functions, positions and gender.

A limitation of our study is that participants might have been more enthusiastic about their role and the Hands4U study than role models who did not answer the request to participate in the interviews. The fact that we do not have data of the total group of role models may have biased our results. Furthermore, bias due to social desirability may have occurred because all interviews were conducted by the principal researcher of the Hands4U study. Participants were familiar with the researcher and her role. As a result, participants might not have mentioned all external barriers (like lack of support from Hands4U). Nevertheless, there was an open atmosphere during all interviews and participants were given the opportunity to add topics at the end. Bias may have occurred because not all interviews were double read and marked. Therefore, some quotes about tasks, barriers and/or facilitators might have been missed. However, as an inter-subjective agreement was tested on six interviews and quickly achieved, we assume that in the other interviews no quotes were missed.

Conclusion

There were several factors that hampered and/or enhanced role models to perform their tasks. Important theme's were: whether the role suited the participant, affinity with the topic of 'hand eczema' and support versus resistance from colleagues. Future interventions should take into account that role models should have experience with coaching-tasks or as a supervisor. As we consider the one hour and a half educational session as rather limited, a more comprehensive educational session could possibly contribute to a better performance of the role models. Furthermore, role models should have affinity with the study topic and be motivated to perform their role. During the intervention phase, role models can be better supported by 'dealing with resistance' training or by increasing their knowledge on the study topic.

Conflict of interest

No conflict of interest has been declared by the authors. This study is conducted within the Hands4U study, which was granted by the Netherlands Organisation for Health Research and Development (ZONMW).

Authors contributions

All authors contributed to the writing of this paper. All authors read and approved the final manuscript. AMB is the principle researcher. EWCM collected the data. Together with EWCM and CRLB, AMB was responsible for the coding of the interviews and the categorization in themes. EWCM, JWJ, JRA, and CRLB supervised the study.

Acknowledgements

We would like to thank the role models who participated in this study.

Author details

[1]Department of Public and Occupational Health, EMGO Institute for Health and Care Research, VU University Medical Center, Van der Boechorststraat 7, 1081 BT Amsterdam, The Netherlands. [2]Department of Primary and Community Care, Centre for Family Medicine, Geriatric Care and Public Health, Radboud University Nijmegen Medical Centre, PO Box 91016500 HB Nijmegen, The Netherlands. [3]Body@Work, Research Center Physical Activity, Work and Health, TNO-VU University Medical Center, Amsterdam, The Netherlands. [4]Research Center for Insurance Medicine AMC-UWV-VU University Medical Center, Amsterdam, The Netherlands.

References

1. Boaz A, Baeza J, Fraser A. Effective implementation of research into practice: an overview of systematic reviews of the health literature. BMC Res Notes. 2013;4(212):1–8.
2. Held E, Mygind K, Wolff C, Gyntelberg F, Agner T. Prevention of work related skin problems: an intervention study in wet work employees. Occup Environ Med. 2002;59:556–61.
3. Evanoff BA, Bohr PC, Wolf LD. Effects of a participatory ergonomics team among hospital orderlies. Am J Ind Med. 1999;35:358–65.
4. Ploeg J, Skelly J, Rowan M, Edwards N, Davies B, Grinspun D, et al. The role of nursing best practice champions in diffusing practice guidelines: a Mixed methods study. Worldviews Evid Based Nurs. 2010;7(4):238–51.
5. Mygind K, Borg V, Flyvholm M-A, Sell L, Frydendall JK. A study of the implementation process of an intervention to prevent work-related skin problems in wet-work occupations. Int Arch Occup Environ Health. 2006;79:66–74.
6. Huis A, Holleman G, van Achterberg T, Grol R, Schoonhoven L, Hulscher M. Explaining the effects of two different strategies for promoting hand hygiene in hospital nurses: a process evaluation alongside a cluster randomised controlled trial. Implement Sci. 2013;8:41.
7. Salmela S, Eriksson K, Fagerström L. Leading change: a three-dimensional model of nurse leaders' main tasks and roles during a change process. J Adv Nurs. 2011;68(2):423–33.
8. Lankford MG, Zembower TR, Trick WE, Hacek DM, Noskin GA, Peterson LR. Influence of role models and hospital design on hand hygiene of health care workers. Emerg Infect Dis. 2003;9(2):217–23.
9. Karimi S, Biemans HJA, Lans T, Chizari M, Mulder M, Naderi Mahdei K. Understanding role models and gender influences on entrepreneurial intentions among college students. Procedia - Social and Behavioral Sciences. 2013;93:204–14.
10. Ajzen I. Attitudes, personality and behavior. Open University Press: Chicago, IL, USA; 1988.
11. O'Boyle CA, Henly SJ, Larson E. Understanding adherence to hand hygiene recommendations: The theory of planned behavior. Am J Infect Control. 2001;29:352–60.
12. Grol R. Implementation of evidence and guidelines in clinical practice: a new field of research? Int J Qual Health Care. 2000;12(6):455–6.
13. Erasmus V, Brouwer W, van Beeck EF, Oenema A, Daha TJ, Richardus JH, et al. A qualitative exploration of reasons for poor hand hygiene among hospital workers: lack of positive role models and of convincing evidence that hand hygiene prevents cross-infection. Infect Control Hosp Epidemiol. 2009;30:415–9.
14. Flyvholm MA, Bach B, Rose M, Jepsen KF. Self-reported hand eczema in a hospital population. Contact Dermatitis. 2007;57:110–5.
15. Nicholson PJ, Llewellyn D, English JS. Evidence-based guidelines for the prevention, identification and management of occupational contact dermatitis and urticaria. Contact Dermatitis. 2010;63:177–86.
16. Thyssen JP, Johansen JD, Linneberg A, Menné T. The epidemiology of hand eczema in the general population - prevalence and main findings. Contact Dermatitis. 2010;62:75–87.
17. Ibler KS, Jemec GB, Flyvholm MA, Diepgen TL, Jensen A, Agner T. Hand eczema: prevalence and risk factors of hand eczema in a population of 2274 healthcare workers. Contact Dermatitis. 2012;67(4):200–7. doi:10.1111/j.1600-0536.2012.02105.x.

18. Skoet R, Olsen J, Mathiesen B, Iversen L, Johansen JD, Agner T. A survey of occupational hand eczema in Denmark. Contact Dermatitis. 2004;51:159–66.
19. Schneider J, Moromisato D, Zemetra B, Rizzi-Wagner L, Rivero N, Mason W, et al. Hand hygiene adherence is influenced by the behavior of role models. Pediatr Crit Care Med. 2009;10(3):360–3.
20. van der Meer EWC, Boot CRL, Jungbauer FHW, van der Klink JJ, Rustemeyer T, Coenraads PJ et al. Hands4U: A multifaceted strategy to implement guideline-based recommendations to prevent hand eczema in health care workers: design of a randomised controlled trial and (cost) effectiveness evaluation. *BMC Public Health* 2011; 11(669) doi: 10.1186/1471-2458-11-669
21. Jungbauer FHW, Piebenga WP, ten Berge EE, Hoogland RW, Posma AL, Randolfi MFC, et al. NVAB-richtlijn: Preventie Contacteczeem [NVAB-guideline: Prevention of Contact Dermatitis]. Utrecht: Kwaliteitsbureau NVAB; 2006.
22. Hooftman WE, Westerman MJ, van der Beek AJ, Bongers PM, van Mechelen M. What makes men and women with musculoskeletal complaints decide they are too sick to work? Scand J Work Environ Health. 2008;34(2):107–12.
23. Glaser BG, Strauss AL. The discovery of grounded theory: strategies for qualitative research. Chicago: Aldine Publishing Company; 1967.
24. Snow M, White RL, Alder SC, Stanford JB. Mentor's hand hygiene practices influence student's hand hygiene rates. Am J Infect Control. 2006;34(1):18–24.
25. Stutz N, Becker D, Jappe U, John SM, Ladwig A, Spornraft-Ragaller P, et al. Nurses' perceptions of the benefits and adverse effects of hand disinfection: alcohol-based hand rubs vs. hygienic handwashing: a multicentre questionnaire study with additional patch testing by the German Contact Dermatitis Research Group. Br J Dermatol. 2008;160:565–72.

SIRT1 activation mediates heat-induced survival of UVB damaged Keratinocytes

Leslie Calapre[1], Elin S. Gray[1], Sandrine Kurdykowski[2], Anthony David[2], Pascal Descargues[2] and Mel Ziman[1,3*]

Abstract

Background: Exposure to heat stress after UVB irradiation induces a reduction of apoptosis, resulting in survival of DNA damaged human keratinocytes. This heat-mediated evasion of apoptosis appears to be mediated by activation of SIRT1 and inactivation of p53 signalling. In this study, we assessed the role of SIRT1 in the inactivation of p53 signalling and impairment of DNA damage response in UVB *plus* heat exposed keratinocytes.

Results: Activation of SIRT1 after multiple UVB *plus* heat exposures resulted in increased p53 deacetylation at K382, which is known to affect its binding to specific target genes. Accordingly, we noted decreased apoptosis and down regulation of the p53 targeted pro-apoptotic gene *BAX* and the DNA repair genes *ERCC1* and *XPC* after UVB *plus* heat treatments. In addition, UVB *plus* heat induced increased expression of the cell survival gene *Survivin* and the proliferation marker Ki67. Notably, keratinocytes exposed to UVB *plus* heat in the presence of the SIRT1 inhibitor, Ex-527, showed a similar phenotype to those exposed to UV alone; i.e. an increase in p53 acetylation, increased apoptosis and low levels of *Survivin*.

Conclusion: This study demonstrate that heat-induced SIRT1 activation mediates survival of DNA damaged keratinocytes through deacetylation of p53 after exposure to UVB *plus* heat

Keywords: Heat stress, UVB, Keratinocytes, Apoptosis, p53, SIRT1, p53 deacetylation

Background

The incidence of skin cancers, particularly of keratinocyte-derived cancers, basal cell carcinoma (BCC) and squamous cell carcinoma (SCC), has increased in the last few decades [1, 2]. Chronic exposure to UV radiation, predominantly UVB, is the most common cause of these cutaneous malignancies [3, 4]. Studies have shown moreover, that high temperature can increase the rate of tumour formation in mice and potentiate the carcinogenic effects of UV [5, 6] and thus, heat stress may also be a risk factor in skin carcinogenesis. Given this evidence, the paucity of studies on the consequences of repeated exposure to both high temperatures and UVB on epidermal cell biology requires addressing [7].

A few studies have shown that exposure to heat stress prior to UVB irradiation protected human and murine keratinocytes against DNA damage [8–10]. The heat-mediated reduction of DNA damage in the form of photoproduct formation, particularly cyclobutane pyrimidine dimers (CPDs), was suggested to be a consequence of increased expression and pre-activation of heat shock proteins (HSPs), thought to diminish the lethality of UV radiation on keratinocytes [9, 11–13]. However, previous studies in our laboratory showed UVB and UVB *plus* heat exposures induce the same level of CPD formation. Conversely, UVB *plus* heat treated samples had a significantly reduced number of apoptotic keratinocytes when compared to cells treated with UVB alone [14].

The reduction in apoptosis and thus the survival of DNA damaged keratinocytes in UVB *plus* heat treated samples was thought to be associated with the presence of phosphorylated Sirtuin 1 (SIRT1) and inactivation of p53 signalling [14]. Since SIRT1 induces deacetylation of the p53 protein [15–17], we hypothesised that SIRT1 activation by heat stress affects the ability of p53 to regulate downstream gene targets. Thus, UVB *plus* heat

* Correspondence: m.ziman@ecu.edu.au
[1]School of Medical Science, Edith Cowan University, 270 Joondalup Drive, Joondalup, Perth, WA 6027, Australia
[3]School of Pathology and Laboratory Medicine, University of Western Australia, Crawley, WA, Australia
Full list of author information is available at the end of the article

treated keratinocytes are unable to mediate an adequate cellular stress response to UVB mediated DNA damage.

SIRT1 is an NAD-dependent histone deacetylase that is known to be increased by heat stress [18, 19], but inhibited by UVB [20]. Its activity is vital for the maintenance of chromosomal integrity and control of various cellular processes including cell metabolism and cellular stress response [21, 22]. The deacetylase activity of SIRT1 regulates several stress-induced transcription factors including p53 [15, 23] and HSF1 [18, 19, 24].

Of particular interest to our study is the ability of SIRT1 to deacetylate the lysine 382 residue of the p53 protein [24–26]. SIRT1-mediated deacetylation of p53 reduces its DNA binding capability, leading to deregulation of expression of p53 dependent genes and impairment of the tumour suppressor functions of the protein [15, 27]. Such functions include the regulation of cell proliferation, DNA damage repair, cell cycle arrest, and apoptosis [28–30]. It appears then that heat-mediated activation of SIRT1 may affect the efficiency of repair of UVB–induced DNA damage and inhibit apoptosis. Survival of DNA damaged cells, that otherwise would have undergone apoptosis, results in the accumulation of UVB-induced mutation in dividing cells [31].

In this study, we aimed to determine whether activation of SIRT1 is the main biomolecular mechanism driving the heat-mediated survival of DNA damaged cells in UVB *plus* heat treated keratinocytes. In particular, we investigated the effects of SIRT1 activation on the on-set of the p53-mediated cellular stress response, approximately 4 h after UV irradiation in normal skin [32, 33], and the efficiency of this system to mediate repair and/or apoptosis in UVB *plus* heat treated keratinocytes harbouring DNA damage. We used ex vivo skins and in vitro primary keratinocytes to assess this, as well as whether UVB *plus* heat leads to the increased presence of unrepaired CPDs, and survival and proliferation of keratinocytes despite DNA damage. Finally, we assessed whether blocking SIRT1 activity abrogates the evasion of apoptosis and cell survival observed after UVB *plus* heat exposures.

Methods

Ex vivo skin model

Thirty-two NativeSkin® (Genoskin, France) ex vivo skin models, taken from non-sun exposed skin of healthy donors, are punch biopsies of normal human skin embedded in a matrix and fixed in a cell culture insert. Informed consent was obtained from donors, and commercialisation and experimental use of the skin biopsies were approved by the Comitė de Protection des Personnes (CPP, France) and the ECU Human Research Ethics Committee.

NHEK

Primary adult human epidermal keratinocytes (NHEK-c, Promocell) were cultured in vitro using Keratinocyte Growth Medium 2 (Promocell, Germany) supplemented with bovine pituitary extract (0.004 ml/ml), recombinant human epidermal growth factor (0.125 ng/ml), recombinant human insulin (5 μg/ml), hydrocortisone (0.33 μg/ml), epinephrine (0.39 μg/ml), human transferrin holo (10 μg/ml), $CaCl_2$ (0.06 mM) and penicillin/streptomycin (Sigma-Aldrich, Australia).

UVB radiation and heat exposure

Skins and primary keratinocytes were exposed to heat stress and UVB *plus* heat according to previous protocols [14]. Samples were then analysed for DNA damage, apoptosis and gene expression at 4 h after the last exposure. UVB and/or heat treated samples were also evaluated for apoptosis and expression of Ki67 2 days post-exposures. For SIRT1 inhibition experiments, 1 μM of Ex-527 was added to the cell culture medium of NHEKs prior to exposures. Each experiment was performed in triplicate and each set of experiments included untreated cells which underwent similar handling.

Immunocytochemistry and Immunohistochemistry

Primary keratinocytes were seeded in a 12-well plate at 100,000 cells/well in LabTek Chambered -Microscopic slides (Thermofisher, Australia) and exposed to UV and/or heat stress. For immunocytochemistry, cells were fixed with 4% paraformaldehyde, washed twice with TBS. Skin tissues were processed and stained according to previous protocols [14]. Primary NHEK and skin sections were incubated with antibodies to either thymine dimer (CPD) (mouse monoclonal, 1:500 dilution; Kamiya Biomedical, USA), p53 antibody (rabbit monoclonal 1:50 dilution; Abcam, USA), p53 acetyl K382 (rabbit monoclonal 1:200, Abcam USA), SIRT1, SIRT1-p, Casp-3 (cleaved), Survivin or anti-pan Cytokeratin and ki67 (rabbit polyclonal, 1:50 dilution; Abcam, USA). The mouse monoclonal antibody to pan-cytokeratin (1:50; Abcam, USA) was used to label keratinocytes. The secondary antibodies anti-mouse Alexa Fluor 488 (for keratin and CPD) and anti-rabbit Alexa Fluor 550 (for caspase 3, p53 and ki67) were used for detection. Three sections were analysed per exposure replicate and five images of randomly selected fields-of-view were captured from each section. To determine percentages of keratinocytes positive for each individual antibody, positive cells were quantified within 5 images randomly chosen per section.

Western blot

Cytosolic and nuclear proteins were isolated from untreated and treated primary keratinocytes using AllPrep

RNA/Protein Kit (Qiagen, Australia) according to manufacturer's instructions. A total of 20 μg protein was loaded onto Mini-PROTEAN TGX Stain-Free Precast Gels (Bio-Rad, USA) and then transferred onto Midi Trans-Blot 0.2 μm nitrocellulose membrane (Bio-Rad). The membrane was probed with rabbit monoclonal p53 antibody or p53 acetyl K382 and detected using Clarity Western ECL Blotting Substrate detection kit (Bio-Rad) as per the manufacturer's instructions. The blot was visualised using the ChemiDoc Touch system (Bio-Rad) and protein levels were assessed and quantified relative to standards using ImageLab software (Bio-Rad).

Apoptosis

In the ex vivo skin models, apoptosis was quantified via the percentage of CPD keratinocytes with active caspase 3 (casp-3), a marker of apoptosis [34]. The level of apoptosis for exposed NHEKs was determined using Annexin V-FITC Apoptosis Detection Kit I (BD Pharmingen, USA) and cells were stained as per the manufacturer's instructions. Samples were analysed using the Gallios™ flow cytometer (Beckman-Coulter). For each sample, 10,000 events were acquired. Annexin V^+PI^-cells represented early apoptotic populations and Annexin V^+PI^+ cells represented either late apoptotic or secondary necrotic populations.

Ex vivo gene expression analysis

RNA was isolated from skin tissues and cells using an AllPrep RNA/DNA Mini Kit (Qiagen). The quality of the RNA extracted from samples was analysed using an Agilent RNA 6000 Bioanalyser Kit. Differential expression of *BAX*, *Survivin* (*BIRC5*), *ERCC1* and *XPC* genes in the UV and/or heat exposed samples were verified by quantitative real-time PCR (qRT-PCR) using the ViiA 7 Real-Time PCR System (Applied Biosystems, USA).

Quantitative RT-PCR was performed based on the manufacturer's instructions using TaqMan probes (Life Technologies, Australia) for *BAX*, Survivin (*BIRC5*), *ERCC1* and *XPC* genes. Human 18S (Taqman, Life Technologies) was used as the endogenous reference gene. Relative quantification of the expression levels of each transcript in each sample were calculated using the Delta-Delta CT method relative to untreated controls.

Statistical analyses

Two-way ANOVA was used to analyse differences across treatment groups, while parametric unpaired t-tests were used to detect differences between specific treatment groups in all experimental categories, with *p*-values <0.05 considered significant.

Results

UVB *plus* heat induced SIRT1 phosphorylation and decreased apoptosis of DNA damaged keratinocytes

We first determined whether activation of SIRT1 is apparent after UVB *plus* heat exposure. Ex vivo skin models and normal primary human epidermal keratinocytes (NHEK) in vitro were exposed to UVB and/or heat once a day for 4 consecutive days. Cells that harboured DNA damage signatures (CPD^+) and activated SIRT1 (SIRT1-p $^+$) were quantified after the last exposure in samples treated with UVB and/or heat relative to untreated controls (Fig. 1a and Additional file 1: Figure S1a).

The percentage of keratinocytes containing CPDs was high in both UVB irradiated (84 ± 7%) and UVB *plus* heat (79 ± 3%) treated skin models (Table 1), and in NHEKs exposed to UVB (91 ± 8%) or UVB *plus* heat (87 ± 3%). UVB *plus* heat treated keratinocytes were observed to contain both SIRT1-p and CPD positive staining in skin models (50 ± 3%) and in vitro NHEKs (55 ± 3%). Notably, neither of the models had SIRT1-p staining in cells irradiated with UVB alone (Fig. 1a, Additional files 1 and 2: Figure S1a and Table S1). SIRT1 activation, however, was also apparent in samples treated with heat alone, clearly linking SIRT1 activation to heat exposure.

UVB *plus* heat treated samples also exhibited a significantly decreased percentage of DNA damaged keratinocytes that were apoptotic (Casp-3/CPD positive cells) compared to those irradiated with UVB alone in ex vivo skin (15 ± 4% vs 37 ± 3%, $p = 0.004$) and in NHEKs (7 ± 4% vs 25 ± 3%, $p = 0.0003$) (Fig. 1b and Table 1). Altogether, these results suggest that SIRT1 phosphorylation is activated in response to repeated UVB *plus* heat exposures and this is associated with evasion of apoptosis within CPD damaged-keratinocytes.

UVB *plus* heat induced deacetylation of p53

The p53 protein is a key regulator of cellular response to stress. The p53 regulation of DNA damage response and cell cycle arrest is coordinated via acetylation and phosphorylation [23, 35]. It has previously been shown that SIRT1 induces deacetylation of p53 [36]. Thus, we determined the percentage of cells expressing total p53 and acetylated p53 (p53-ace382) after repeated UVB and UVB *plus* heat exposure.

There were no significant differences in the percentage of CPD positive cells expressing p53 between UVB and UVB *plus* heat treated keratinocytes ex vivo or in vitro (Fig. 1c, Additional file 1: Figure S1b and Table 1). However, a significantly lower percentage of CPD positive keratinocytes had acetylated p53 in UVB *plus* heat treated samples compared to those irradiated with UVB alone in ex vivo models (40 ± 2% vs 79 ± 6%, $p = 0.002$) and in NHEKs (28 ± 7% vs 75 ± 4%, $p = 0.001$) (Fig. 1d and Additional file 1: Figure S1c). Notably, there was an

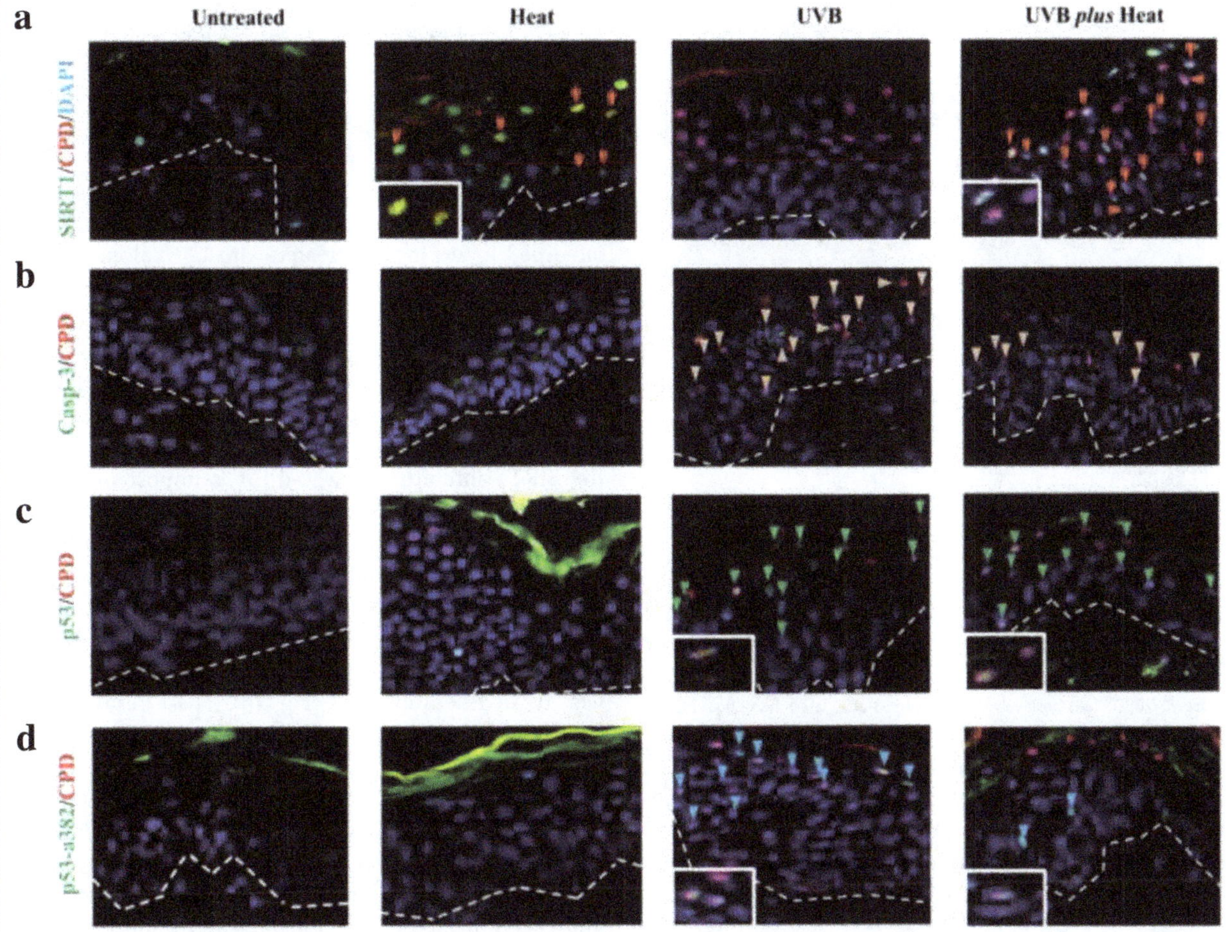

Fig. 1 Exposure to repeated UVB plus heat significantly decreased acetylated p53 levels in keratinocytes. Representative immunohistochemical staining of ex vivo skin either untreated, or exposed to heat, UVB or UVB plus heat, for nuclear DNA (DAPI, *blue*), CPD (*red*) and (**a**) phosphorylated SIRT1 (SIRT1-p), (**b**) caspase (casp-3), (**c**) total p53 or (**d**) acetylated p53 (p53-a382). Inset images are an enlarged view of cells positive for CPD and SIRT1 (*red arrows*), CPD and Casp-3 (*orange arrows*), CPD and p53 (*green arrows*) or CPD and p53-a382 (*blue arrows*). Broken lines denote the epidermal/dermal border. All images are at 400X magnification

inverse relationship between the percentage of CPD positive cells expressing SIRT1-p and those with acetylated p53 in the UVB and UVB *plus* heat treated samples. More importantly, our results demonstrated that repeated exposure of keratinocytes to UVB *plus* heat did not prevent the expression of p53 in these cells, but appeared to affect the acetylation status of the p53 protein.

UVB *plus* heat induces deregulation of p53 downstream target genes

SIRT1-mediated deacetylation of the p53 protein is known to reduce its DNA binding capability, leading to deregulation of expression of p53 dependent genes [15, 37]. We therefore, measured the expression levels of downstream target genes of p53 that may be affected by deacetylation. We first looked at gene expression levels of *BAX*, a regulator of cell apoptosis and *Survivin* (*BIRC5*), a regulator of cell survival, as we previously observed these genes to be affected by UVB *plus* heat treatment of keratinocytes at 48 h after exposure [14]. We found that UVB irradiation caused significant upregulation of *BAX*, but not of *Survivin*, in the ex vivo skins models (Fig. 2a) and in NHEKs (Fig. 2b). By contrast, UVB *plus* heat exposure induced downregulation of *BAX* and significant upregulation of *Survivin* in both the skin and NHEKs.

We then examined the gene expression of *XPC* and *ERCC1*, which are p53-regulated nucleotide excision repair (NER) genes. *XPC* and *ERCC1* are commonly upregulated in UVB irradiated cells and are necessary for the repair of UVB-induced CPD damage [38]. UVB irradiated keratinocytes in ex vivo skin models and in vitro showed significant upregulation of *ERCC1* (3- and 4-fold) and *XPC* (9- and 4-fold) in skin and NHEKs respectively. Notably, this upregulation was not apparent in UVB *plus* heat exposed NHEKs (Fig. 2b), and in fact,

Table 1 Effect of UVB and/or heat exposure in keratinocytes of the ex vivo skin models or NHEK in vitro

Percentage Mean ± S.D.	Untreated	Heat	UVB	UVB *plus* Heat
Skin				
DNA Damaged Cells (%)	0 ± 0	5 ± 3	84 ± 7	79 ± 3
Apoptotic Cells (%)	0 ± 0	14 ± 1	37 ± 3	15 ± 4***
SIRT1-p⁺/CPD⁺ (%)	0 ± 0	32 ± 2	0 ± 0	50 ± 3
Apoptotic Cells (%)	0 ± 0	14 ± 1	37 ± 3	15 ± 4***
p53⁺/CPD⁺ (%)	0 ± 0	0 ± 0	76 ± 3	69 ± 3
p53-ace382⁺/CPD⁺ (%)	0 ± 0	0 ± 0	79 ± 6	40 ± 2**
NHEK				
DNA Damaged Cells (%)	0 ± 0	2 ± 1	91 ± 8	87 ± 3
Apoptotic Cells (%)	2 ± 1	3 ± 1	25 ± 3	7 ± 4
SIRT1-p⁺/CPD⁺ (%)	1 ± 1	34 ± 5	0 ± 0	55 ± 3**
p53⁺/CPD⁺ (%)	0 ± 0	0 ± 0	84 ± 3	79 ± 2
p53-ace382⁺/CPD⁺ (%)	0 ± 0	0 ± 0	75 ± 4	28 ± 7**

Statistically significant differences relative to UVB: ** = *p*-value ≤0.001 or *** = *p*-value ≤0.0001
SIRT1-p⁺/CPD⁺ cells positively stained for SIRT1-p and CPD
p53⁺/CPD⁺ cells positively stained for p53 and CPD
P53-ace382⁺/CPD⁺ cells positively stained for p53-acetylated (lys382) and CPD

ERCC1 and *XPC* were significantly downregulated in UVB *plus* heat treated skin models (Fig. 2a). These results confirm that exposure to UVB *plus* heat stress appears to compromise the p53-mediated DNA repair mechanisms within keratinocytes.

UVB *plus* heat increased ki67 expression in DNA damaged keratinocytes

Next we quantified the percentage of cells that were positive for ki67, a protein commonly used as a marker of proliferation [39–42]. To ensure that cells were provided sufficient time for repair and mitosis and that the effects on repair and proliferation were persistent, quantification of proliferative (ki67-positive) keratinocytes was conducted 2 days after the last exposure. UVB *plus* heat treatment caused a significant increase in the percentage of keratinocytes that were positive for ki67 relative to UVB treated samples in ex vivo skins (36 ± 8% vs 16 ± 10%, $p = 0.0427$) and in vitro (59 ± 3% vs 19 ± 2%, $p = 0.003$) (Fig. 2c-d, Additional file 3: Figure S2). These results show that heat, presumably as a result of the impaired p53-mediated cellular stress response, leads to increased survival and proliferation of keratinocytes.

SIRT1 inhibition reduces UVB *plus* heat-induced inactivation of p53 signalling

To determine whether inhibition of SIRT1 will reverse the pro-survival effects of heat exposure on UVB damaged keratinocytes, we treated NHEKs with Ex-527, a known inhibitor of SIRT1. Previous studies have shown that exposure to Ex-527 effectively reduces SIRT1 activity [43–45], and produces maximal p53 acetylation, but does not induce significant toxicity in untreated keratinocytes at a dose of 1 μM [4, 46].

Keratinocytes that were treated with UVB *plus* heat, in the presence of 1 μM of Ex-257, had significantly higher levels of acetylated p53 protein in comparison with UVB *plus* heat treated samples, resembling the levels of acetylated p53 found in cells treated with UVB alone (Fig. 3a-b). Accordingly, protein expression analysis by immunohistochemistry showed that the percentage of cells that were positive for both CPD and acetylated p53 was significantly increased in UVB *plus* heat treated keratinocytes in the presence of Ex-257 (69 ± 4% vs 28 ± 7%, $p = 0.0001$), compared to exposed cells not treated with the SIRT1 inhibitor (Fig. 3c-d). It is important to note, that the percentage of p53-a382/CPD keratinocytes after UVB *plus* heat together with Ex-527 was comparable to those in samples irradiated with UVB alone (69 ± 4% and 75 ± 4% respectively). Moreover, the presence of SIRT1 appears to correspond to downregulation of *BAX* and the upregulation of *Survivin* observed in UVB *plus* heat treated keratinocytes (Fig. 2b). These results clearly indicate that SIRT1 is important in driving heat-mediated survival of UVB-damaged keratinocytes. However, SIRT1 inhibition did not restore the upregulation of *BAX*, *XPC* and *ERCC1* to levels observed in samples treated with UVB alone. This result suggests that these genes may have returned to baseline levels or might be influenced by factors additional to SIRT1 and/or p53.

SIRT1 inhibition diminished UVB *plus* heat effects on apoptosis and proliferation of keratinocytes

Since UVB *plus* heat causes a significant decrease in apoptosis in keratinocytes, we then determined if SIRT1 inhibition reverses this effect. Less than 5% of untreated NHEKs with or without Ex-527 were apoptotic (Additional file 4: Figure S3). However, the presence of Ex-527 significantly increased cell apoptosis from 7 ± 4% to 23 ± 1% ($p = 0.004$) in UVB *plus* heat, which is similar to levels found in UVB irradiated samples (25 ± 3%) (Fig. 3b). In addition, at 2 days post exposure, in the presence of SIRT1-inhibitor there was a significant decrease in the proportion of keratinocytes that were ki67 positive in UVB *plus* heat treated samples (Fig. 2d and Additional file 3: Figure S2b). Thus, survival and proliferation of DNA damaged cells appears to be ameliorated by the presence of the SIRT1 inhibitor.

Discussion

In this study, we clearly confirm that the exposure of keratinocytes to UVB *plus* heat impairs the p53-mediated cellular stress response. We also show that this phenomenon is a consequence of heat-induced SIRT1

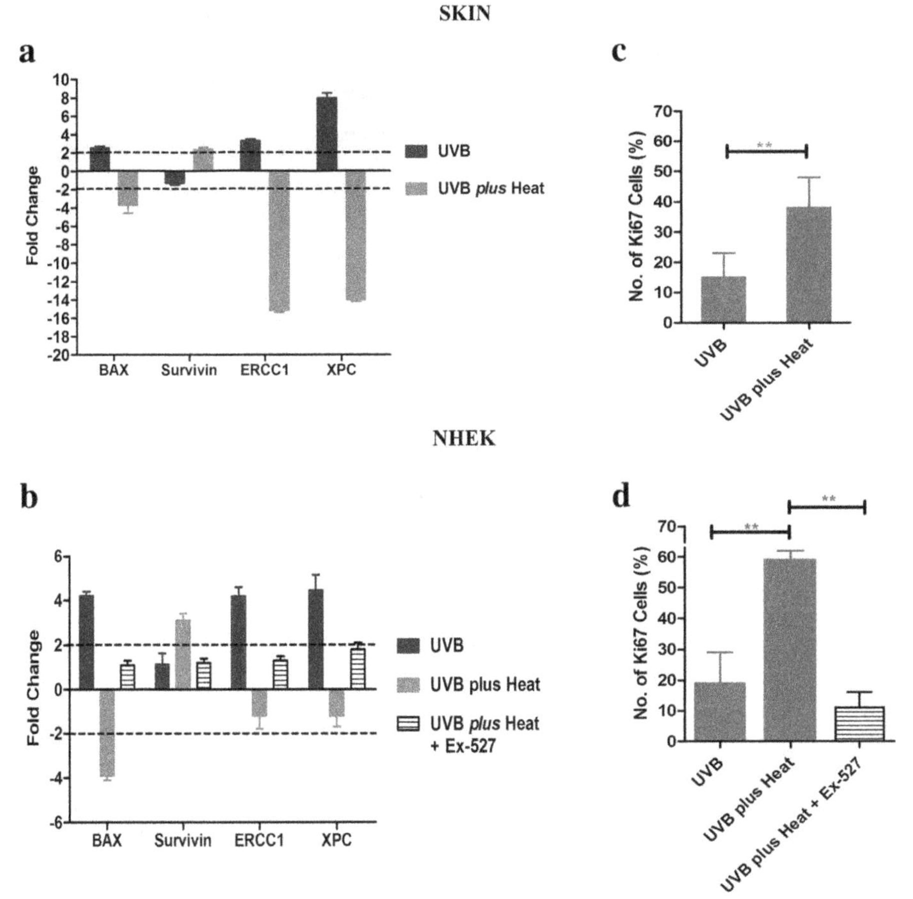

Fig. 2 Effect of UV and/or heat exposure on p53 downstream gene targets and cell proliferation. **a-b** Fold change on mRNA expression of BAX, Survivin, ERCC1 or XPC in keratinocytes of the (**a**) skin and (**b**) in vitro, relative to untreated controls. **c-d** Bar graphs of the percentage mean (+/− SD) of keratinocytes positive for ki67 per field of view either (**c**) in ex vivo skin or (**d**) in vitro. Statistically significant differences are indicated with ** $p < 0.001$ and/or *** for *p*-values $p < 0.0001$

activation in these cells. SIRT1 activation appears to induce post-translational modifications of the p53 protein, affecting the ability of this protein to regulate the expression of downstream gene targets important for regulating DNA damage repair and apoptosis. As a result, keratinocytes containing UVB-induced DNA damage are able to survive and proliferate.

SIRT1 is essential for maintaining chromatin stability but can affect the function of other transcription factors, including HSF-1 and p53, by deacetylation of these protein [26, 47, 48]. In the case of HSF-1, SIRT1-mediated deacetylation of this protein increases its DNA-binding ability, leading to increased expression of heat shock proteins [18, 19, 49]. Conversely, SIRT1-mediated deacetylation of p53 diminishes the ability of this protein to bind to the promoters of its target genes, particularly those required for apoptosis and cell cycle arrest [25, 36, 50].

This study confirmed that SIRT1 is indeed a key molecular event in the UVB *plus* heat-mediated effects on keratinocyte biology. In line with previous observations that SIRT1 activation is inhibited by UV radiation but increased in response to heat stress [19, 24, 26], we observed increased SIRT1 phosphorylation in heat treated but not in UV irradiated samples. The combination of UV *plus* heat also resulted in SIRT1 activation. However, the exact mechanism behind heat-induced activation of SIRT1 is not yet known, and this needs to be assessed in order to fully understand the role of SIRT1 in UVB *plus* heat-mediated survival of DNA damaged keratinocytes.

Interestingly, the presence of the SIRT1 inhibitor (Ex-527) prevented the UVB *plus* heat-mediated survival of DNA damaged keratinocytes. Furthermore, inhibition of SIRT1 in UVB *plus* heat treated keratinocytes induced a significant increase in p53 acetylation and activation of p53 signalling, leading to increased cell apoptosis and a decrease in proliferative keratinocytes. Thus, SIRT1 appears to be indispensable for evasion of apoptosis and survival of UVB *plus* heat treated keratinocytes harbouring DNA damage. By means of post-translational modifications to the p53 protein and consequently, inactivation

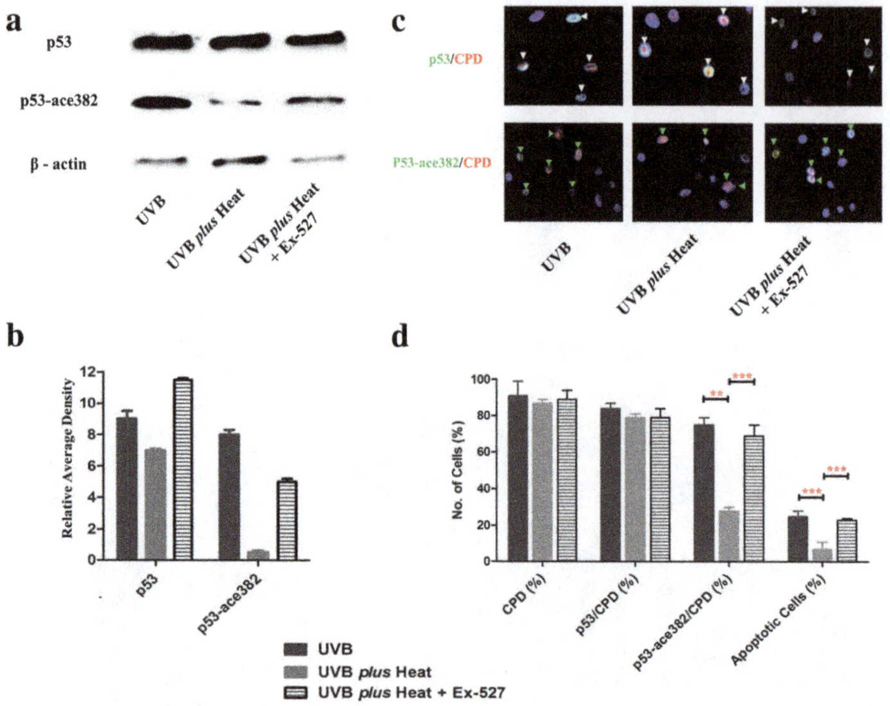

Fig. 3 Inhibition of SIRT1 in UVB plus heat significantly increased acetylated p53 protein expression and apoptosis of keratinocytes in vitro. **a** Immunoblot showing levels of total p53, and acetylated p53 protein in UVB, UVB plus heat and UVB plus heat with the SIRT1 inhibitor (Ex-527). **b** Quantification of protein levels by relative average density standardised by β-actin. **c** Representative immunohistochemical staining of cells positive for CPD and p53 (*white arrows*), CPD and p53-a382 (*green arrows*) in primary keratinocytes exposed to UVB or UVB plus heat with or without SIRT1 inhibitor Ex-527. All images are at 400X magnification. **d** Bar graphs of percentage mean (+/− SD) of DNA damaged (CPD), apoptotic, p53 or p53-a382 positive primary keratinocytes exposed to UVB or UVB plus heat with or without Ex-527. Statistically significant differences are indicated with ** for $p < 0.001$ and/or *** for *p*-values $p < 0.0001$ respectively

of p53 signalling, heat-mediated SIRT1 activation appears to negate the ability of UVB *plus* heat keratinocytes to mount an appropriate response to UVB-induced DNA damage.

Despite the significant impact of SIRT1 activation on p53 signalling, increased levels of phosphorylated SIRT1 were found to have no effect on the levels of the p53 protein, i.e. there were no significant differences in the level of p53 protein in UVB or UVB *plus* heat treated samples. Thus, the diminished efficiency of p53-mediated cellular stress response in UVB *plus* heat treated samples does not appear to arise from changes in p53 protein transcription nor its translocation to the nucleus. Therefore, lack of an appropriate p53-mediated DNA damage response in keratinocytes after UVB *plus* heat exposure appears to be a consequence of SIRT1-imposed post-translational modifications to the p53 protein.

The interference of the p53-mediated surveillance of DNA damage via deacetylation appears to be one of the primary effects of UVB plus heat exposure in keratinocytes. One of the most notable consequences of SIRT1-induced deacetylation and therefore, inactivation of p53 in UVB plus heat treated keratinocytes, was the significant downregulation of ERCC1 and XPC, which are responsible for the recognition and repair of CPDs [51–53], as the products of these genes are responsible for the recognition of distortions in the DNA helix and activation of global genome nucleotide excision repair pathways (GG-NER) [54, 55]. In particular, the *XPC* promoter contains a putative p53 response element and elevated XPC expression after UV irradiation occurs in a p53-dependent manner [56–58]. Thus, the persistence of CPD could be a result of the lack of effective recognition of the existing damage, preventing the removal of CPDs and resulting in impaired clearance of DNA lesions. This finding is of particular importance considering a recent study showed that a significant percentage of 'normal' epidermal keratinocytes harbour UV-signature mutations in genes that are key drivers of squamous cell carcinoma [59]. By affecting the ability of keratinocytes to recognise and repair DNA damage, consecutive exposure to UVB plus heat stress may induce further accumulation of mutations in these 'normal' cells, fuelling their transformation into a malignant phenotype. However, a more comprehensive study on the effects of UVB plus heat-mediated SIRT1 activation on the mediators of the nucleotide excision repair system, including XPA, is necessary to provide an improved understanding of the effects of SIRT1 deacetylation on the nucleotide excision repair mechanisms overall. More importantly, further studies are required to determine whether heat stress can indeed exacerbate UVB-induced skin carcinogenesis.

It is important to note that the survival mechanism we observed in our UVB *plus* heat treated keratinocytes are in direct contradiction to previous reports. A few studies have shown that prior heat treatment protects human and murine keratinocytes against UVB-induced DNA damage, as a consequence of pre-activated heat shock proteins [9, 11–13]. However, the mechanisms involved in our experiments, where heat is added after UVB, appear to be primarily driven by heat-mediated post-translational modifications to the p53 protein. Nevertheless, heat shock response mediators, particularly HSP90, were found upregulated in UVB *plus* heat treated keratinocytes at 4 h post exposure (data not shown), suggesting that the heat shock response is functional despite repeated exposure to multiple stressors. Given the importance of HSPs in resisting UVB-induced apoptosis, UVB *plus* heat treatment therefore, provides keratinocytes with additional capacity to survive and proliferate.

Interestingly, in the presence of SIRT1 inhibitor (Ex-527), UVB *plus* heat treated cells did not show similar upregulated levels of HSP90 expression in vitro and in ex vivo skin (data not shown). Thus, SIRT1 activation appears to be required for the full induction of the heat shock response. A similar observation indicating that SIRT1 can affect the regulation of the heat shock response has also been reported previously [19]. In their study, Westerheide and colleagues observed diminished HSP90 expression when HeLa cells were exposed to nicotinamide, another Sirt1-inhibitor drug. In addition, they found that SIRT1 deacetylates HSF-1, increasing its DNA binding affinity to the promoters of HSPs. This result indicates that SIRT1 may act as an upstream regulator of the HSF-1-mediated heat shock response, and thus elucidates the importance of this particular Sirtuin protein in thermal stress response. However, the exact mechanism as to how heat induces SIRT1 activation needs to be fully determined.

It is also important to note that while we found evidence to show that UVB *plus* heat induces survival of DNA damaged keratinocytes, these observations are that of a UVB followed by heat exposure model. Heat stress and UVB radiation occur simultaneously in the environment. Thus, activation of SIRT1, and its subsequent effects on the p53-mediated cellular stress response and the heat shock response, must be confirmed in a UV and heat concurrent exposure model. Nonetheless, we propose that heat in the environment would similarly affect UVB irradiated cells, i.e. it will aid in the survival of DNA damaged keratinocytes.

Conclusions

In conclusion, our study uncovered a survival pathway intrinsically induced by UVB *plus* heat exposure and mediated by SIRT1 activation. In addition, we provide additional evidence that exposure to high temperatures, subsequent to UV irradiation, impairs effective cell arrest, DNA repair and/or apoptosis of DNA damaged keratinocytes, indicating that subsequent UV and heat may potentially act synergistically to create pre-cancerous lesions. However, translational studies using mouse models may be required to determine whether heat treatment will enhance UVB-induced tumourigenesis.

Additional files

Additional file 1: Figure S1. Exposure to UVB plus heat significantly decreased acetylated p53 levels in keratinocytes. Immunohistochemical staining of nuclear DNA (DAPI, blue), CPD (red) and active caspase (casp-3), phosphorylated SIRT1 (SIRT1-p), total p53 or acetylated p53 (p53-a382) (green) in primary keratinocytes (NHEK) in vitro either untreated, or exposed to heat, UV or UVB plus heat.

Additional file 2: Table S1. Keratinocytes expressing SIRT1 only after UVB and/or heat exposure.

Additional file 3: Figure S2. Exposure to UVB plus heat induced an increase in the number of keratinocytes expressing Ki67. (a) Immunohistochemical staining of nuclear DNA (DAPI, blue), Ki67 (red) and cytokeratin (CytoK) (green) in UV or UVB plus heat treated skin. (b) Fluorescent immunocytochemistry staining of nuclear DNA (DAPI, blue) and Ki67 (green) in primary keratinocytes (NHEK) in vitro.

Additional file 4: Figure S3. SIRT1 inhibitor (Ex-527) does not induce toxicity to NHEK. Levels of cell apoptosis in untreated keratinocytes with or without Ex-527.

Abbreviations

CPD: Cyclobutane pyrimidine dimers; NHEK: Primary normal human epidermal keratinocytes; UVB: Ultraviolet radiation B

Acknowledgments

We extend our thanks to Mr. Michael Morici, Ms. Tenielle Porter and the ECU Melanoma Research Team for their assistance and support in the laboratory.

Funding

This study was funded by Edith Cowan University. The funding body was not involved in the design of the study and collection, analysis, interpretation of data and in writing the manuscript.

Author contributions

LC, EG and MZ participated in the study design, analysis of the results and wrote the manuscript. SK, AD and PD provided the skin models and made revisions to the manuscript. All authors read and approved the final manuscript.

Competing interest

We certify that there is no conflict of interest with any organization, financial or otherwise, regarding the material discussed in this manuscript.

Ethics approval and consent to participate

The collection and commercialisation of skin models (NativeSkin) for research purposes were authorised by the French Ministry of Research and French Ethical Committee (Comité de Protection des Personnes (CPP)). The use of NativeSkin and NHEK cell lines for all experiments presented in the manuscript was approved by the ECU Research Ethics Committee.

Author details

[1]School of Medical Science, Edith Cowan University, 270 Joondalup Drive, Joondalup, Perth, WA 6027, Australia. [2]GENOSKIN Centre Pierre Potier, Oncopole, Toulouse, France. [3]School of Pathology and Laboratory Medicine, University of Western Australia, Crawley, WA, Australia.

References

1. Madan V, Lear JT, Szeimies RM. Non-melanoma skin cancer. Lancet. 2010; 375(9715):673–85.
2. Welsh MM, Karagas MR, Kuriger JK, Houseman A, Spencer SK, Perry AE, et al. Genetic determinants of UV-susceptibility in non-melanoma skin cancer. PLoS One. 2011;6(7):e20019.
3. Liu L, Rezvani HR, Back JH, Hosseini M, Tang X, Zhu Y, et al. Inhibition of p38 MAPK signaling augments skin tumorigenesis via NOX2 driven ROS generation. PLoS One. 2014;9(5):e97245.
4. Herbert KJ, Cook AL, Snow ET. SIRT1 inhibition restores apoptotic sensitivity in p53-mutated human keratinocytes. Toxicol Appl Pharmacol. 2014;277(3):288–97.
5. van der Leun JC, Piacentini RD, de Gruijl FR. Climate change and human skin cancer. Photochem Photobiol Sci. 2008;7(6):730–3.
6. Freedman DM, Kitahara C, Linet M, Alexander B, Neta G, Little M, et al. Ambient temperature and risk of first primary basal cell carcinoma: a nationwide United States cohort study. J Photochem Photobiol B Biol. 2015; 148:284–9.
7. Calapre L, Gray ES, Ziman M. Heat stress: a risk factor for skin carcinogenesis. Cancer Lett. 2013;337(1):35–40.
8. Maytin EV, Wimberly JM, Kane KS. Heat shock modulates UVB-induced cell death in human epidermal keratinocytes: evidence for a hyperthermia-inducible protective response. J Invest Dermatol. 1994;103(4):547–53.
9. Trautinger F, Kindas-Mugge I, Barlan B, Neuner P, Knobler RM. 72-kD heat shock protein is a mediator of resistance to ultraviolet B light. J Invest Dermatol. 1995;105(2):160–2.
10. Kane KS, Maytin EV. Ultraviolet B-induced apoptosis of keratinocytes in murine skin is reduced by mild local hyperthermia. J Invest Dermatol. 1995; 104(1):62–7.
11. Maytin EV. Heat shock proteins and molecular chaperones: implications for adaptive responses in the skin. J Invest Dermatol. 1995;104(4):448–55.
12. Jantschitsch C, Kindas-Mugge I, Metze D, Amann G, Micksche M, Trautinger F. Expression of the small heat shock protein HSP 27 in developing human skin. Br J Dermatol. 1998;139(2):247–53.
13. Jantschitsch C, Trautinger F. Heat shock and UV-B-induced DNA damage and mutagenesis in skin. Photochem Photobiol Sci. 2003;2(9):899–903.
14. Calapre L, Gray ES, Kurdykowski S, David A, Hart P, Descargues P, et al. Heat-mediated reduction of apoptosis in UVB-damaged keratinocytes in vitro and in human skin ex vivo. BMC Dermatol. 2016;16(1):6.
15. Jang SY, Kim SY, Bae YS. p53 deacetylation by SIRT1 decreases during protein kinase CKII downregulation-mediated cellular senescence. FEBS Lett. 2011;585(21):3360–6.
16. Kim DH, Jung YJ, Lee JE, Lee AS, Kang KP, Lee S, et al. SIRT1 activation by resveratrol ameliorates cisplatin-induced renal injury through deacetylation of p53. Am J Physiol Renal Physiol. 2011;301(2):F427–35.
17. Kume S, Haneda M, Kanasaki K, Sugimoto T, Araki S, Isono M, et al. Silent information regulator 2 (SIRT1) attenuates oxidative stress-induced mesangial cell apoptosis via p53 deacetylation. Free Radic Biol Med. 2006; 40(12):2175–82.
18. Donmez G, Arun A, Chung CY, McLean PJ, Lindquist S, Guarente L. SIRT1 protects against alpha-synuclein aggregation by activating molecular chaperones. J Neurosci. 2012;32(1):124–32.
19. Westerheide SD, Anckar J, Stevens SM Jr, Sistonen L, Morimoto RI. Stress-inducible regulation of heat shock factor 1 by the deacetylase SIRT1. Science. 2009;323(5917):1063–6.
20. Chou WW, Chen KC, Wang YS, Wang JY, Liang CL, Juo SH. The role of SIRT1/AKT/ERK pathway in ultraviolet B induced damage on human retinal pigment epithelial cells. Toxicol in Vitro. 2013;27(6):1728–36.
21. Gonfloni S, Iannizzotto V, Maiani E, Bellusci G, Ciccone S, Diederich M. P53 and Sirt1: routes of metabolism and genome stability. Biochem Pharmacol. 2014;92(1):149–56.
22. Wilking MJ, Singh C, Nihal M, Zhong W, Ahmad N. SIRT1 deacetylase is overexpressed in human melanoma and its small molecule inhibition imparts anti-proliferative response via p53 activation. Arch Biochem Biophys. 2014;563:94–100.
23. Lou G, Liu Y, Wu S, Xue J, Yang F, Fu H, et al. The p53/miR-34a/SIRT1 positive feedback loop in Quercetin-induced apoptosis. Cell Physiol Biochem. 2015;35(6):2192–202.
24. Raynes R, Brunquell J, Westerheide SD. Stress Inducibility of SIRT1 and its role in Cytoprotection and cancer. Genes Cancer. 2013;4(3–4):172–82.
25. Glozak MA, Seto E. Histone deacetylases and cancer. Oncogene. 2007;26(37):5420–32.
26. Cao C, Lu S, Kivlin R, Wallin B, Card E, Bagdasarian A, et al. SIRT1 confers protection against UVB- and H2O2-induced cell death via modulation of p53 and JNK in cultured skin keratinocytes. J Cell Mol Med. 2009;13(9B):3632–43.
27. van Leeuwen IM, Higgins M, Campbell J, McCarthy AR, Sachweh MC, Navarro AM, et al. Modulation of p53 C-terminal acetylation by mdm2, p14ARF, and cytoplasmic SirT2. Mol Cancer Ther. 2013;12(4):471–80.
28. Xu Y, Li N, Xiang R, Sun P. Emerging roles of the p38 MAPK and PI3K/AKT/mTOR pathways in oncogene-induced senescence. Trends Biochem Sci. 2014;39(6):268–76.
29. Chakraborty A, Uechi T, Kenmochi N. Guarding the 'translation apparatus': defective ribosome biogenesis and the p53 signaling pathway. Wiley Interdiscip Rev RNA. 2011;2(4):507–22.
30. Chipuk JE, Green DR. Cytoplasmic p53: bax and forward. Cell Cycle. 2004; 3(4):429–31.
31. Chung, KW, Choi YJ, Park MH, Jang EJ, Kim DH, Park, BH, et al. Molecular insights into SIRT1 protection against UVB-Induced skin fibroblast senescence by suppression of oxidative stress and p53 acetylation. J Gerontol A Biol Sci Med Sci. 2015;70(8):959-68.
32. Winter M, Moser MA, Meunier D, Fischer C, Machat G, Mattes K, et al. Divergent roles of HDAC1 and HDAC2 in the regulation of epidermal development and tumorigenesis. EMBO J. 2013;32(24):3176–91.
33. Murphy M, Mabruk MJ, Lenane P, Liew A, McCann P, Buckley A, et al. Comparison of the expression of p53, p21, Bax and the induction of apoptosis between patients with basal cell carcinoma and normal controls in response to ultraviolet irradiation. J Clin Pathol. 2002;55(11):829–33.
34. D'Costa AM, Denning MF. A caspase-resistant mutant of PKC-delta protects keratinocytes from UV-induced apoptosis. Cell Death Differ. 2005;12(3):224–32.
35. Piao MJ, Hyun YJ, Cho SJ, Kang HK, Yoo ES, Koh YS, et al. An ethanol extract derived from *Bonnemaisonia hamifera* scavenges ultraviolet B (UVB) radiation-induced reactive oxygen species and attenuates UVB-induced cell damage in human keratinocytes. Mar Drugs. 2012;10(12):2826–45.
36. Lee JT, Gu W. SIRT1: regulator of p53 Deacetylation. Genes Cancer. 2013; 4(3–4):112–7.
37. Chen WY, Wang DH, Yen RC, Luo J, Gu W, Baylin SB. Tumor suppressor HIC1 directly regulates SIRT1 to modulate p53-dependent DNA-damage responses. Cell. 2005;123(3):437–48.
38. Rezvani HR, Rossignol R, Ali N, Benard G, Tang X, Yang HS, et al. XPC silencing in normal human keratinocytes triggers metabolic alterations through NOX-1 activation-mediated reactive oxygen species. Biochim Biophys Acta. 2011;1807(6):609–19.
39. Bria E, Furlanetto J, Carbognin L, Brunelli M, Caliolo C, Nortilli R, et al. Human epidermal growth factor receptor 2-positive breast cancer: heat shock protein 90 Overexpression, Ki67 proliferative index, and Topoisomerase II-alpha co-amplification as predictors of pathologic complete response to Neoadjuvant chemotherapy with Trastuzumab and Docetaxel. Clin Breast Cancer. 2015;15(1):16–23.
40. Katzenberger T, Petzoldt C, Holler S, Mader U, Kalla J, Adam P, et al. The Ki67 proliferation index is a quantitative indicator of clinical risk in mantle cell lymphoma. Blood. 2006;107(8):3407.
41. Kanitakis J, Narvaez D, Euvrard S, Faure M, Claudy A. Proliferation markers Ki67 and PCNA in cutaneous squamous cell carcinomas: lack of prognostic value. Br J Dermatol. 1997;136(4):643–4.

42. Putri RI, Siregar NC, Siregar B. Overexpression and amplification of Murine double minute 2 as a diagnostic tool in large lipomatous tumor and its correlation with Ki67 proliferation index: an institutional experience. Indian J Pathol Microbiol. 2014;57(4):558–63.
43. Gertz M, Fischer F, Nguyen GT, Lakshminarasimhan M, Schutkowski M, Weyand M, et al. Ex-527 inhibits Sirtuins by exploiting their unique NAD+ –dependent deacetylation mechanism. Proc Natl Acad Sci U S A. 2013; 110(30):E2772–81.
44. Peck B, Chen CY, Ho KK, Di Fruscia P, Myatt SS, Coombes RC, et al. SIRT inhibitors induce cell death and p53 acetylation through targeting both SIRT1 and SIRT2. Mol Cancer Ther. 2010;9(4):844–55.
45. Ido Y, Duranton A, Lan F, Weikel KA, Breton L, Ruderman NB. Resveratrol prevents oxidative stress-induced senescence and proliferative dysfunction by activating the AMPK-FOXO3 cascade in cultured primary human keratinocytes. PLoS One. 2015;10(2):e0115341.
46. Solomon JM, Pasupuleti R, Xu L, McDonagh T, Curtis R, DiStefano PS, et al. Inhibition of SIRT1 catalytic activity increases p53 acetylation but does not alter cell survival following DNA damage. Mol Cell Biol. 2006;26(1):28–38.
47. Cheng HL, Mostoslavsky R, Saito S, Manis JP, Gu Y, Patel P, et al. Developmental defects and p53 hyperacetylation in Sir2 homolog (SIRT1)-deficient mice. Proc Natl Acad Sci U S A. 2003;100(19):10794–9.
48. Botta G, De Santis LP, Saladino R. Current advances in the synthesis and antitumoral activity of SIRT1-2 inhibitors by modulation of p53 and pro-apoptotic proteins. Curr Med Chem. 2012;19(34):5871–84.
49. Liu DJ, Hammer D, Komlos D, Chen KY, Firestein BL, Liu AY. SIRT1 knockdown promotes neural differentiation and attenuates the heat shock response. J Cell Physiol. 2014;229(9):1224–35.
50. Yi J, Luo J. SIRT1 and p53, effect on cancer, senescence and beyond. Biochim Biophys Acta. 2010;1804(8):1684–9.
51. Amundson SA, Patterson A, Do KT, Fornace AJ Jr. A nucleotide excision repair master-switch: p53 regulated coordinate induction of global genomic repair genes. Cancer Biol Ther. 2002;1(2):145–9.
52. Ford JM. Regulation of DNA damage recognition and nucleotide excision repair: another role for p53. Mutat Res. 2005;577(1–2):195–202.
53. Fitch ME, Cross IV, Ford JM. p53 responsive nucleotide excision repair gene products p48 and XPC, but not p53, localize to sites of UV-irradiation-induced DNA damage, in vivo. Carcinogenesis. 2003;24(5):843–50.
54. Min JH, Pavletich NP. Recognition of DNA damage by the Rad4 nucleotide excision repair protein. Nature. 2007;449(7162):570–5.
55. Sugasawa K, Okamoto T, Shimizu Y, Masutani C, Iwai S, Hanaoka F. A multistep damage recognition mechanism for global genomic nucleotide excision repair. Genes Dev. 2001;15(5):507–21.
56. Adimoolam S, Ford JM. p53 and DNA damage-inducible expression of the xeroderma pigmentosum group C gene. Proc Natl Acad Sci U S A. 2002; 99(20):12985–90.
57. Tan T, Chu G. p53 binds and activates the xeroderma pigmentosum DDB2 gene in humans but not mice. Mol Cell Biol. 2002;22(10):3247–54.
58. Barckhausen C, Roos WP, Naumann SC, Kaina B. Malignant melanoma cells acquire resistance to DNA interstrand cross-linking chemotherapeutics by p53-triggered upregulation of DDB2/XPC-mediated DNA repair. Oncogene. 2014;33(15):1964–74.
59. Martincorena I, Roshan A, Gerstung M, Ellis P, Van Loo P, McLaren S, et al. Tumor evolution. High burden and pervasive positive selection of somatic mutations in normal human skin. Science. 2015;348(6237):880–6.

24

Knowledge, attitudes and practices of the medical personnel regarding atopic dermatitis in Yaoundé, Cameroon

Emmanuel Armand Kouotou[1,2,3*], Jobert Richie N. Nansseu[4], Alexandra Dominique Ngangue Engome[1,2], Sandra Ayuk Tatah[2,5] and Anne Cécile Zoung-Kanyi Bissek[1]

Abstract

Background: Atopic dermatitis (AD) is a chronic, relapsing and pruritic inflammatory skin disease whose management remains unclear to most non-dermatologists. This study aimed to assess the knowledge, attitudes and practices (KAP) of the medical staff regarding AD in Yaoundé, Cameroon.

Methods: This was a cross-sectional study conducted from January to April 2014 in 20 health facilities located in Yaoundé, the capital city of Cameroon. All medical staff who provided their consent were included in the study. A score was established for each of the KAP categories, and subsequently grouped into 4 classes considering a score <50, 50-<65, 65-<85 or ≥85%, respectively.

Results: We enrolled 100 medical personnel, 62% of whom were females. Overall, the level of knowledge on AD was moderate (65%). Allergy was the main cause of AD, stated by 64% of participants. Only 43% personnel cited the genetic cause. Asthma was mentioned by 78% as an associated pathology. Regarding attitudes, the majority (84%) thought that AD is equally common among Black and Caucasian populations; 42% of participants believed that evolution is favorable when appropriate medical treatment is prescribed. These attitudes were considered wrong (64%). Similarly, the general level of practice was inadequate: 50%.

Conclusion: Levels of knowledge, attitudes and practices of the medical staff regarding AD were poor, implying that management of this condition is non optimal in our setting.

Keywords: Atopic dermatitis, KAP study, Medical staff, Cameroon

Background

Atopic Dermatitis (AD) is a chronic, relapsing and pruritic inflammatory skin disease [1]. It is a condition that predominantly affects children especially of a certain age, in developed countries and increasingly in the developing world. An epidemiological study conducted at the Yaoundé General Hospital (Cameroon) by Zoung-Kanyi et al. found that allergic skin diseases were more common in children aged 0–5 years with AD as the leading one [2].

* Correspondence: kouotoea@yahoo.fr; kearm_tosss@yahoo.fr
[1]Department of Internal Medicine and Specialties, Faculty of Medicine and Biomedical Sciences, University of Yaoundé I, P.O. Box: 8314, Yaoundé, Cameroon
[2]Yaoundé University Teaching Hospital, Yaoundé, Cameroon
Full list of author information is available at the end of the article

Onset of this condition occurs mostly in the first months of life. Indeed, 60–70% of cases start before the age of 6 months. Mesrati et al. in a pediatric dermatology unit in Tunisia noticed that 7.5% of consultations concerned AD [3], which contrasts with a prevalence of 10–25% reported in Western countries [4]. The young and immature immunity of the child underlies this increased susceptibility to outbreaks of AD, and consequently the high prevalence of AD in this age group. Indeed, AD is caused by defects in epidermal and cutaneous barriers which allow penetration of environmental molecules in contact with the skin. This results in a cutaneous inflammaxtion of which T-cells are responsible, directed against environmental allergens (extrinsic AD) and/or cutaneous auto-antigens (intrinsic AD). Moreover, AD can occur either in a context of atopy (predisposition to atopic states, known as extrinsic AD) or not (intrinsic AD) [5].

Evolution of the disease remains difficult to appreciate over years, although an improvement of signs is observed in regularly monitored patients. In fact, AD is usually characterized by surges and remissions at unpredictable frequencies, varying from one person to another with or without the influence of any driving factor, making it difficult to infer on the final issue. Following the exponential increase in AD in both developed and developing countries, restructuring of various aspects of its management has become essential to prevent complications.

But prior to this restructuring, an assessment of the knowledge and practices of the medical staff is mandatory, which will identify their weaknesses and subsequently enable improvement of their capacities. To the best of our knowledge, no study has already assessed the knowledge, attitudes and practices (KAP) of the medical personnel towards AD in Cameroon, a developing country. With the ultimate goal of improving the management of AD in Cameroonian hospitals, we undertook the present study which purposed to assess the KAP of medical professionals practicing in Yaoundé (Cameroon) with respect to AD.

Methods

From January to April 2014, we conducted a cross-sectional study including the medical staff practicing in the city of Yaoundé. Five out of the seven existing health districts of Yaoundé were selected for this study and a total of 20 health facilities were visited. The choice of health districts and health facilities was arbitrary, taking into account the convenience for the investigators and accessibility of health facilities. The study population was comprised medical staff responsible for consultations in the selected health facilities: doctors (general practitioners and specialists/pediatricians) and nurses. At each visit to the study sites, all consulting staff irrespective of sex, seniority/experience, who consented to participate, were included. Our sampling was consecutive throughout the study period.

Before the study began, an ethical clearance was obtained from the Ethical Review Board of the Faculty of Medicine and Biomedical Sciences of the University of Yaoundé I, Cameroon. Authorizations were equally issued by health authorities of the selected health districts as well as directors of selected health facilities. The procedures were in compliance with the current revision of Helsinki Declaration. All aspects and procedures of the study were fully presented to each potential participant, and we included only those who voluntarily signed the consent form. Anonymity of participants and confidentiality of collected data were respected.

This study used as reference model the international consensus on management of AD [6]. An anonymous pre-tested and standardized questionnaire was used for data collection. All participants received the questionnaire to be filled; then the investigator returned on an appointed day to retrieve the questionnaire, after ensuring that this has been properly and extensively completed. The questionnaire, in addition to questions about age, gender, specialty and seniority in job/work experience, consisted of a set of 45 questions divided into three parts:

- Knowledge: theoretical clinical knowledge (primary lesions, localization, associated pathologies, causes); clinical knowledge based on recognition of iconography (Additional file 1); knowledge on prevention (information or advice to give to patients/parents in order to prevent an AD surge/relapse);
- Attitudes: perceptions of medical staff regarding the frequency of AD (specifically depending on race), evolution of AD with treatment, contribution of relatives in AD management and capacity of medical personnel to efficiently manage AD in our setting;
- Practice: number of cases of AD seen during consultations, prescription given for surges/relapses, route of administration of prescribed drugs, frequency of drug administration and monitoring of treatment.

The paper from Essi et al. on KAP studies [7] was used to establish scores for each part of the questionnaire. According to the sections (Knowledge, Attitudes, and Practice), the categories are distributed as follows:

- Knowledge: very poor (score <50%); poor (score: ≥50 and <65%); moderate (score: ≥65 and <85%); good (score ≥85%);
- Attitudes: harmful (score <50%); wrong (score: ≥50 and <65%); approximate (score: ≥65 and <85%); right (score ≥85%);
- Practices: harmful (score <50%); inadequate (score: ≥50 and <65%); average (score: ≥65 and <85%); adequate (score ≥85%).

Data were recorded and coded using Microsoft Excel 2007, then analyzed with SPSS v. 20 (IBM SPSS Inc., Chicago, Illinois, USA). Results are presented as frequency (percentage) for categorical variables and mean ± standard deviation (SD) for quantitative variables. To compare qualitative variables, we used the chi-square test. The level of statistical significance was set at $p < 0.05$.

Results

Characteristics of the study population

We included 100 participants, predominantly females (62/100; 62.0%), giving a M/F sex ratio of 0.6/1. Our sample consisted of specialists (40/100; 40%), namely pediatric residents (20/100; 20%) and pediatricians (20/100; 20%), general practitioners (38/100, 38%) and State Registered Nurses (22/100; 22%).

Knowledge

General knowledge

Definition of AD

The majority of participants (75/100; 75%) were able to accurately define AD (Table 1).

Associated pathologies

In our series, 78% (78/100) and 58% (58/100) respectively thought that asthma and conjunctivitis can occur in a patient with AD (Table 1).

Causes

Allergy was cited as the main cause of AD by 64% (64/100) of our participants, and genetics by 43% (43/100) (Table 1).

Evolution

Most participants 77% (77/100) described AD as a chronic disease; 54% (54/100) thought the condition is rather acute and 46% (46/100) thought it is both acute and chronic (Table 1).

Theoretical clinical knowledge

Primary lesions in AD

Concerning primary lesions of AD, the majority of health care providers cited xerosis cutis (86%; 86/100), erythema (81%; 81/100) and desquamation (58%; 58/100) as the main signs observed in AD (Table 2).

Sites in infants and young adults

In infants (0–5 years old), participants declared that the face (44/100; 44%) and torso (48/100; 48%) were the most likely localizations for AD (Table 2). On the other hand, the face (76/100; 76%) and trunk (58/100; 58%) were declared not to be privileged sites of AD in young adults (25–34 years old). Also, a little over half of participants (59/100; 59%) believed the lower limbs were a preferred site of AD lesions in adults (35 years old and above) (Table 2).

Table 1 General knowledge of medical staff

Question	Right response Number (%)		Wrong response Number (%)	
General knowledge (*N* = 100)				
Definition				
AD is chronic and inflammatory	75	(75)	25	(25)
AD is chronic or inflammatory	7	(7)	93	(93)
AD is inflammatory and acute	13	(13)	87	(87)
AD is inflammatory or acute	2	(2)	98	(98)
I do not know	3	(3)	97	(97)
Associated pathologies				
Asthma is an associated pathology	78	(78)	22	(22)
Conjunctivitis is an associated pathology	58	(58)	42	(42)
Chronic cough is an associated pathology	16	(16)	84	(84)
There is no associated pathology	12	(12)	88	(88)
Causes				
The cause is psychological	2	(2)	98	(98)
The cause is allergic	64	(64)	36	(36)
The cause is genetic	43	(43)	57	(57)
The cause is infectious	18	(18)	82	(82)
I do not know	5	(5)	95	(95)
Evolution (*n* = 100)				
Evolution could be acute	54	(54)	46	(46)
Evolution could be chronic	77	(77)	23	(23)
Evolution is acute and chronic	46	(46)	54	(54)
Evolution is exclusively acute	1	(1)	99	(99)
Evolution is exclusively chronic	14	(14)	86	(86)

Table 2 Clinical theoretical knowledge as medical personnel

Question	Right response Number (%)		Wrong response Number (%)	
Theoritical clinical knowledge (*n* = 100)				
Primary lesions				
Xerosis cutis is a sign of AD	86	(86)	14	(14)
Erythema is a sign of AD	81	(81)	19	(19)
Desquamation is a sign of AD	58	(58)	42	(42)
Diffuse ulcerations is are signs of AD	17	(17)	83	(83)
Moist skin is a sign of AD	13	(13)	87	(87)
Cyanosis is a sign of AD	2	(2)	98	(98)
Sites in children (0–5 years old)				
The face is a site of AD	44	(44)	56	(56)
The torso is a site of AD	48	(48)	52	(52)
The lower limb is a site of AD	32	(32)	68	(68)
Sites in adults (25 years old and above)				
The face is a site of AD	24	(24)	76	(76)
The torso is a site of AD	42	(42)	58	(58)
The upper limb is a site of AD	79	(79)	21	(21)
The lower limb is a site of AD	41	(41)	59	(59)

Clinical knowledge based on iconography

Pictures 1 (80/100; 80%), 4 (75/100; 75%) and 5 (67/100; 67%) were selected for the diagnosis of AD while pictures 9 (15/100; 15%), 11 (15/100; 15%) and 13 (20/100; 20%) were not (Additional file 1).

Prevention

The majority of participants (95/100; 95%) said they provide patients with advice and information about prevention. Furthermore, 91 (91) and 88 (88%) participants thought that cotton clothing are recommended and a relapse requires a new consultation, respectively.

Attitudes

Occurrence of AD based on race

AD is a disease that affects both Blacks and Caucasians alike according to 84% (84/100) of the medical staff.

Opinion on evolution of AD

For 59% (59/100) of our sample, AD is a disease which evolves towards complete remission when patients receive the right treatment (Table 3).

Patient care by the relatives

A total of 42 participants (42%) thought that patients could be taken care of by their relatives (Table 3).

Management in our setting

In our series, 85% (85/100) thought that management of AD could be adequately provided in our setting (Table 3).

Practice

Of the 100 participants, 91% (91/100) reported having encountered cases of AD during consultations. Table 4 shows their usual practice for every patient with this pathology.

Half of our sample (51/100; 51%) said they had received between 1 and 10 cases of AD per month at their consultations while 25% (25/100) reported having consulted more than 20 cases of AD.

Over half (79/100) of our sample chose to prescribe a medication for a patient with AD.

When a patient came to consult for AD, 88% (88/100) of the staff prescribed corticosteroids, most often topical (80/83; 96.4%) and to be applied 2 times a day (46/88; 52.3%).

Management of xerosis cutis and pruritus

Xerosis cutis was supposed to be treated as declared by 81% (81/100) of the staff interviewed. For complaints of pruritus, 90% (90/100) of participants prescribed antihistamines and frequently associated antihistamines and corticosteroids, 63% (63/100) (Table 4).

Association of knowledge, attitudes and practices of medical staff

Score of knowledge among medical staff

The level of knowledge was conditioned by experience of the specialists. Indeed, more than half of pediatricians had a moderate level of knowledge (14/20; 70%), while 50% of residents had a poor level of knowledge (10/20; 50%). General practitioners had poor to moderate levels of knowledge about AD (Table 5).

Table 3 Attitudes of medical personnel

Question	Right response Number (%)		Wrong response Number (%)	
Opinion on occurrence of ad depending on race ($N = 100$)				
AD mostly affects Blacks	3	(3)	97	(97)
AD equally affects Caucasians and Blacks	84	(84)	16	(16)
No idea	13	(13)	87	(87)
Opinion on the evolution of ad with treatment ($N = 100$)				
Discouraging evolution	21	(21)	79	(79)
Favorable evolution	59	(59)	41	(41)
No idea	20	(20)	80	(80)
Opinion on contribution of relatives in management of ad ($n = 100$)				
Discouraging contribution	28	(28)	72	(72)
Favorable contribution	42	(42)	58	(58)
No idea	30	(30)	70	(70)
Opinion on ability to adequately manage ad in our setting ($N = 100$)				
AD can be managed	85	(85)	15	(15)
AD cannot be managed	7	(7)	93	(93)
No idea	8	(8)	92	(92)

Table 4 Practice of medical staff in case of AD relapses

Question	Right Response Number (%)
Number ad cases seen during consultations ($N = 100$)	
1-10 cases	51 (51)
11-20 cases	13 (13)
> 20 cases	25 (25)
No cases	11 (11)
*Drug prescription for ad relapse ($N = 100$)	
Corticosteroids	88 (88)
Antihistamines (AH)	64 (64)
Antifungal	14 (14)
Antibiotics	12 (12)
Corticosteroids + AH	56 (56)
Management of xerosis cutis: yes	81 (81)
Drug prescription in case of pruritus	
Antihistamines (AH)	90 (90)
Corticosteroids + AH	63 (63)
*Administration route of corticosteroids ($N = 100$)	
Oral	17 (20.2)
Topical	80 (96.4)
Oral + Topical	12 (70.6)
Administration modalities of topical corticosteroids ($n = 88$)	
1 application/day	38 (43.2)
2 applications/day	46 (52.3)
3 applications/day	4 (4.5)
Duration of the topical corticosteroid treatment ($N = 100$)	
< 2 weeks	43 (43)
2 weeks	30 (30)
1 month	12 (12)
> 1 month	0 (0)

*More than one answer was possible

Score for attitudes among medical staff

Less than half (40/100) of pediatricians had a right attitude towards AD, Fifty percent of pediatric residents had an approximate score, General practitioners had approximate to harmful attitudes and nurses had approximate attitudes in relation to AD (Table 5).

Score for practices among medical staff

Practices by all the professional categories were inadequate (Table 5).

After making an overall score for each parameter (knowledge, attitudes and practices), we observed that the medical staff of Yaoundé had a moderate level of knowledge (65%) with wrong attitudes (64%) and inadequate practices (50%) concerning AD.

Discussion

This study on AD enabled us to assess the knowledge of medical professionals, their attitudes and clarify their different practices. A total of 100 subjects agreed to answer the questionnaire. Levels of knowledge, attitudes and practices were respectively 65%, 64% and 50%. It clearly appears thus that urgent measures need to be taken to strengthen our medical staff capacities in order to improve management of AD in Cameroonian hospital settings.

Knowledge of the medical staff

Overall, most of the medical personnel had already heard about AD and was able to define it correctly. They were also able to recognize the characteristic lesions of the condition, probably as a result of their experience. The most frequently mentioned cause of AD was allergy (64%) in contrast to the genetic cause (43%). These results are significantly different from those found in the

Table 5 Scores of health care personnel according to the professional category

Consultant*	Scores**											
	very poor/harmful/harmful			poor/wrong/inadequate			moderate/approximate/average			good/right/adequate		
	K	A	P	K	A	P	K	A	P	K	A	P
Pediatricians	0 (0)	0 (0)	4 (20)	4 (20)	6 (30)	16 (80)	14 (70)	6 (30)	0 (0)	2 (10)	8 (40)	0 (0)
Residents	0 (0)	4 (20)	5 (25)	10 (50)	5 (25)	15 (75)	9 (45)	10 (50)	0 (0)	2 (5)	1 (5)	0 (0)
General practitioners	1 (2.6)	10 (26.3)	15 (39.5)	18 (47.4)	12 (31.6)	23 (60.5)	18 (47.4)	10 (26.3)	0 (0)	0 (0)	6 (15.8)	0 (0)
Nurses	2 (9.1)	2 (9.1)	9 (41.0)	11 (50)	2 (9.1)	12 (54.5)	9 (45)	7 (31.8)	1 (4.5)	1 (0)	11 (50)	0 (0)
Total	3 (3)	16 (16)	33 (33)	43 (43)	25 (25)	66 (66)	50 (50)	33 (33)	1 (1)	4 n	26 (26)	0 (0)

*Figures represent the number (percentage); **The scores were classified into: very poor/harmful/harmful = less than 50%; poor/wrong/inadequate = less than 65%; moderate/approximate/average = less than 85%; good/right/adequate = more than 85% correct answers; K = Knowledge; A = Attitude; P = Practice

French national survey of professional practices on the treatment of AD [8]. In this survey, the genetic cause was indeed cited by almost all; regarding the allergic cause, two sources were cited by the different categories of professionals (allergists, dermatologists, general practitioners and pediatricians), namely food and inhaled allergens [8]. The psychological cause meanwhile was rarely mentioned by those participating in our survey, which mirrors findings from the French national survey indicating that 80% of physicians rarely or never suggested a psychological cause [8].

The medical staff demonstrated some confusion when asked about chronicity of AD because 77% of the staff declared that evolution could be chronic while 14% said it was exclusively chronic. Furthermore, half of our sample thought that this evolution could be acute. This significant confusion could be explained by the fact that in AD, the pruritic erythema is usually attributed to an acute pathology.

The medical staff had average knowledge on prevention. Pure cotton clothing was proposed by 90% of the staff as a preventive method. This choice of clothing is one of the recommendations of the 2005 consensus on the management of AD in children [6]. Most often, the staff believed a patient must return for consultation at every relapse of AD (87%) while 15% thought that the prescribed treatment would be sufficient to handle every relapse. Also, 63% of participants declared that moisturizing body lotions were prescribed for prevention. Certainly the 2005 consensus conference on the management of AD is in favor of keeping the skin moisturized permanently; however the medical professional must ensure that the chosen lotion or cream is conducive for treatment of xerosis cutis [6]. Furthermore 54% of our participants encouraged the use of antiseptic solutions for baths which is in contradiction with the 2013 consensus on AD, bolstering that the use of antiseptics for baths is indicated only for superinfected AD [9]. The moderate level of knowledge on AD in our sample (65%) already predicted an inappropriate management of the condition. This can be justified by the dearth of information on AD in our setting where it is considered a foreign pathology.

Attitudes and practices of the medical staff

Half of our prescribers reported meeting between 1 and 10 cases of AD per month at consultations while only 25% had already received more than 20 cases/month. This result is contrary to those from the French survey where among various professional categories, 2 (pediatricians and allergists) saw more than 30 cases per month while only half of GPs (55%) saw less than 10 cases of AD per month [8]. AD is a disease that equally affects Blacks and Caucasians according to 84% of our sample, a somewhat contradictory result given that only 54% said they had not encountered many cases.

For 59% of our participants, AD usually has a favorable evolution when properly treated whereas 21% felt the outcome is actually unfavorable. Yet, AD classically involves intermittent periods of relapse and recovery even when properly treated. Overall, the staff had wrong attitude in relation to AD.

In case of AD relapses, our medical staff most frequently said they prescribe corticosteroids; 80% of these participants chose a topical corticosteroid, which is higher than those of the French study where dermatologists and general practitioners generally prescribed topical corticosteroid as first-line treatment in 60% and 28% of cases, respectively [8]. Moreover, in our study 56% reported prescribing a corticosteroid and an antihistamine in case of AD relapse but from the 2005 consensus conference on the treatment of AD, antihistamines have no place in the treatment of AD [6]. The 2013 consensus from the experts recommends the use of sedating antihistamines in case of intense pruritus [9].

Regarding the application of topical corticosteroid, half of medical staff recommended 2 applications per day while only 42% thought that the application of a topical corticosteroid once daily would be sufficient. According to Aubert et al., the use of corticosteroids differs depending on symptomatic variations in the patient and should be reasonable in order to avoid the risk of dependence or addiction [10]. Xerosis cutis is the sign in AD which prompted prescription of a treatment in 81% of our sample. Almost all prescribers said pruritus requires prescription of an antihistamine. Also, a combination of antihistamines and corticosteroids is systematic according to 63% of participants, although the 2005 consensus on AD states that administration of a topical corticosteroid alone would be effective because of its antipruritic and anti-inflammatory properties [6]. Clearly, the medical personnel adopted a poor practice in cases of AD most probably influenced by the moderate knowledge and inadequate attitude towards the condition.

The non-random selection of health facilities and the relatively small number of enrolled participants may constitute limits to the generalization of our results. Furthermore, many medical staff had not agreed to take part in this study and some were absent during our multiple visits to the facilities. Nevertheless, the use of the gradation developed by Essi et al. [7] allowed us to have a clear idea of the level of knowledge, attitudes and practices of our participants.

Conclusion

This study allowed us to point out the moderate level of knowledge, wrong attitudes and inadequate practices of medical staff consulting in Yaoundé as far as AD is concerned, which suggests a poor quality of care delivered to patients with AD in our milieu, and a move towards emergence of complications. Management guidelines on this condition must be created and made available to our healthcare providers along with organization of regular continuous medical education sessions for them. Larger scale studies are needed throughout the country, to have a more precise mapping of the level of knowledge, attitudes and practices regarding AD in order to improve its management locally.

Acknowledgments
The authors gratefully acknowledge all the medical personnel who have volunteered to participate in the present study.

Funding
This research did not receive any specific grant from funding agencies in the public, commercial, or not-for-profit sectors.

Authors' contributions
EAK and ACZB conceived and designed the study. EAK and ADNE collected the data. EAK, ADNE and JRNN analyzed and interpreted the data. EAK, JRNN and SAT drafted the manuscript. EAK, JRNN, ADNE, SAT and ACZB reviewed and revised the manuscript. All authors read and approved the final version of the manuscript.

Competing interests
The authors declare that they have no competing interests.

Author details
[1]Department of Internal Medicine and Specialties, Faculty of Medicine and Biomedical Sciences, University of Yaoundé I, P.O. Box: 8314, Yaoundé, Cameroon. [2]Yaoundé University Teaching Hospital, Yaoundé, Cameroon. [3]Biyem-Assi District Hospital, Yaoundé, Cameroon. [4]Department of Public Health, Faculty of Medicine and Biomedical Sciences, University of Yaoundé I, Yaoundé, Cameroon. [5]Department of Paediatrics and Specialties, Faculty of Medicine and Biomedical Sciences, University of Yaoundé I, Yaoundé, Cameroon.

References

1. Atherton D. Essential aspects of atopic dermatitis, Journal of the academy of dermatology, vol. 24(6). Berlin: Springer-Verlay; 1991. p. 104.
2. Zoung-Kanyi AC, Kouotou E, Njamnshi AK. Epidemiologie des dermatoses à l'hopital Général de Yaoundé. Health Sci Dis. 2009;10(4):145–9.
3. Mesrati H, Chaabane M, Amouri M, Hariz W, Mseddi M. Motifs de consultation des enfants en age préscolaire dans un service de dermatopédiatrie. J annder. 2011;092:186–8.
4. Dammak A, Guillet G. Dermatite atopique de l'enfant. J Pediatr Pueric. 2011;24:84–102.
5. Nicolas JF, Nosbaum A, Berard F. Comprendre la dermatite atopique. In: Réalités thérapeutiques en dermato-vénérologie # 213. 2012.
6. Société Française de Dermatologie. Prise en charge de la dermatite atopique de l'enfant. Conférence de consensus. Ann Dermatol Venereol. 2005;132:1S19–33.
7. Essi Marie José, Njoya Oudou. L'Enquête CAP (Connaissances, Attitudes, Pratiques) en Recherche Médicale. Health Sci Dis. 2013;14(2):135–6.
8. Barbarot S, Beauchet A, Zaid S, Lacour JP. Prise en charge de la dermatite atopique de l'enfant par les dermatologues, pédiatres, médecins généralistes et allergologues: enquête nationale de pratique. Ann Dermatol Venereol. 2005;132:1S283–95.
9. Lebwohl MG, Del Rosso JQ, Abramovits W, Berman B. Pathways to managing Atopic Dermatitis:Consensus From the Experts. J Clin Aesthet Dermatol. 2013(7 Suppl):S2–S18.
10. Aubert H, Barbarot S. Non adhésion et corticothérapie. Ann Dermatol Venereol. 2012;139(S7-S12):2–6.

25

Elucidating mechanistic insights into drug action for atopic dermatitis: a systems biology approach

Indhupriya Subramanian, Vivek K. Singh* and Abhay Jere

Abstract

Background: Topical Betamethasone (BM) and Pimecrolimus (PC) are widely used drugs in the treatment of atopic dermatitis (AD). Though the biomolecules and biological pathways affected by the drugs are known, the causal inter-relationships among these pathways in the context of skin is not available. We aim to derive this insight by using transcriptomic data of AD skin samples treated with BM and PC using systems biology approach.

Methods: Transcriptomic datasets of 10 AD patients treated with Betamethasone and Pimecrolimus were obtained from GEO datasets. We used a novel computational platform, eSkIN (www.persistent.com/eskin), to perform pathway enrichment analysis for the given datasets. eSkIN consists of 35 skin specific pathways, thus allowing skin-centric analysis of transcriptomic data. Fisher's exact test was used to compute the significance of the pathway enrichment. The enriched pathways were further analyzed to gain mechanistic insights into the action of these drugs.

Results: Our analysis highlighted the molecular details of the mechanism of action of the drugs and corroborated the known facts about these drugs i.e. BM is more effective in triggering anti-inflammatory response but also causes more adverse effect on skin barrier than PC. In particular, eSkIN helped enunciate the biological pathways activated by these drugs to trigger anti-inflammatory response and its effect on skin barrier. BM suppresses pathways like TNF and TLRs, thus inhibiting NF-κB while PC targets inflammatory genes like IL13 and IL6 via known calcineurin-NFAT pathway. Furthermore, we show that the reduced skin barrier function by BM is due to the suppression of activators like AP1 transcription factors, CEBPs.

Conclusion: We thus demonstrate the detailed mechanistic insight into drug action of AD using a novel computational approach.

Keywords: Atopic dermatitis, Computational approach, Transcriptomic data analysis

Background

Atopic dermatitis (AD) is one of the most common disorders of skin that affects approximately 20% of children and 3% adults worldwide [1]. The pathophysiology of AD includes breakdown of the skin barrier, which in turn, initiates immunological response and inflammation [1]. The current treatment for AD involves topical application of corticosteroids or calcineurin inhibitors [2]. Betamethasone valerate (BM) and Pimecrolimus (PC) are two of the most commonly used drugs for the treatment of atopic dermatitis.

BM, a corticosteroid, is known to suppress the inflammation, but fails to adequately restore the damaged skin barrier which subsequently leads to secondary skin infections. BM binds to its corticosteroid receptor in skin and perturbs various biomolecules in keratinocytes involved in processes like inflammation, keratinocyte differentiation, proliferation and cellular adhesion [3]. On the other hand, PC, a topical calcineurin inhibitor (TCI), causes mild suppression of inflammation, but is more efficient in restoring the skin barrier. PC is known to mediate its action through NFAT signaling pathways [2].

US FDA issues TCI drugs with a boxed warning owing to a potential risk of malignancy, in spite of various studies disproving any such association [4]. This favors the use

* Correspondence: vivek_ksingh@persistent.com
LABS, Persistent Systems Limited, 9A/12, Erandwane, Pune, Maharashtra 411004, India

of topical corticosteroids as an alternate treatment for AD, even though it suffers from impaired skin barrier and risk of secondary skin infections as side effects. This raises the need to have a complete mechanistic insight into the action of these drugs, which can then be used to understand the factors responsible for side effects and develop better treatment for AD.

A central piece for gaining mechanistic insight into drug action is to understand the biomolecular interactions and pathways that are impacted by the drug, which in turn, determine the therapeutic efficiency and adverse effects. In this study, we have used eSkIN, a novel systems biology based computational platform specially designed to aid skin omics research. eSkIN contains a comprehensive model of skin with 35 manually-curated skin-specific pathways and 2600+ genes. This allows skin-centric analysis and interpretation of omics data, which to the best of our knowledge, is not available in other commonly used software applications (e.g. *DAVID* [5, 6] and GSEA [7]).

We present the detailed mechanistic analysis of BM and PC highlighting the biomolecular interactions and pathways involved in their mechanism of action and adverse effects. Publicly available transcriptomic data from patients treated with BM and PC [2] were used for this study and the data were analyzed using eSkIN platform. We report that distinct pathways are affected by these drugs to bring about their therapeutic effect, and we also further elucidate the importance of these pathways in the context of skin physiology.

Methods

Transcriptomic data

Transcriptomic data from lesional AD skin samples of 10 patients, before and after topical treatment of BM and PC twice daily for three weeks, were used in this study [2]. The data was downloaded from NCBI GEO (Gene Expression Omnibus) database using following accession number: GSE32473.

Normalization and quality check

The datasets of BM and PC were analyzed separately. All the samples were normalized as per Jensen et al., [2]. Briefly, each sample was normalized with 50th percentile (median) of that sample. To ensure quality of the input data, only probe sets with present or marginal calls in at least 70% of samples per analysis group were considered. Median expression values of probes were assigned to gene.

Data analysis

eSkIN (www.persistent.com/eskin) was used to perform skin-centric analysis of the transcriptomic data owing to the availability of 35 manually-curated skin-specific pathways (Additional file 1: Table S1) and 2600+ genes in this platform. The 35 pathways represent following functional categories of skin physiology: Basic skin physiology, Epidermal formation, Pigmentation and Stress response. The eSkIN pathways include molecular interactions that detail the roles played by various biomolecules (e.g. genes, proteins and small molecules) in a particular pathway.

We computed the Log_2 fold change of the genes with respect to baseline (before topical treatment) samples of respective drug. Two fold change was used as a threshold to identify differentially expressed genes i.e. up-regulated genes $\geq +1$ Log_2 fold change and down-regulated genes ≤ -1 Log_2 fold change. Sensitivity analysis of fold change cutoff was performed by increasing and decreasing one fold change of the default value to understand its effect on our analysis (see Additional files 2, 3 and 4). As observed, the key pathways contributing towards the drug action are captured by all the three fold change cutoffs. Hence, for further analysis we used the default cutoff (Log_2 fold change = 1).

Pathway enrichment analysis using eSkIN

Pathway enrichment analysis is based on the assumption that behavior of the genes involved in the same biological pathways is correlated. Using statistical methods, it helps to identify the most perturbed pathways based on an input set of genes [8]. Such analysis is widely used to gain insight into functional roles of differentially expressed genes [9, 10]. Statistical methods like Fisher's test, hypergeometric, binomial, bayesian and chi-squared are widely used in pathway enrichment analysis [6].

We used the skin-centric knowledge-base of eSkIN as the backend database for performing pathway enrichment analysis. This facilitates the identification of skin-specific pathways that are perturbed due to the treatment and thus, helps in understanding the skin-centric effects of the treatment. eSkIN uses Fisher's exact test for computing the significance of the enrichment of pathways. Fisher's exact test with following parameters is used for computing *p*-value.

$$p = \frac{\binom{a+b}{a}\binom{c+d}{c}}{\binom{n}{a+c}} = \frac{(a+b)!(c+d)!(a+c)!(b+d)!}{a!b!c!d!n!} \quad (1)$$

In Eq. (1), a = number of unique differentially expressed genes (DEGs) in a pathway in eSkIN knowledge-base, b = number of unique DEGs in eSkIN knowledge-base excluding DEGs in that pathway, c = number of unique non-DEGs in that pathway, d = number of unique genes in eSkIN knowledge-base that are non-DEG and not part of that pathway, n = a + b + c + d, and $\binom{n}{k}$ represents binomial coefficient. The *p*-value from Fisher's exact test is a measure of the chance of random association between differentially expressed genes and a pathway. Smaller the p-value, lower is the random chance, and thus, higher is the likelihood that a pathway is significantly enriched.

Furthermore, eSkIN eliminates the need to average out sample level information as it allows analysis of multiple samples simultaneously. The enriched pathways (i.e. eSkIN p-value < 0.05) in BM and PC treated samples were further analyzed by overlaying the transcriptomic data on these pathways using Gene Expression Overlay feature of eSkIN. This feature of eSkIN allows pathway enrichment analysis and visualization of transcriptomic data in the context of skin related pathways. The genes are colored based on their expression levels, and thus, helps in exploration of the enriched pathways in the context of their molecular interactions. This provides insight into the various signaling events triggered by the drugs that are discussed in the Results and Discussion sections.

Comparative pathway enrichment analysis using DAVID

For comparing our results with DAVID (https://david.ncifcrf.gov/) [5], we assigned median expression values of the biological replicates (samples) to the genes. Our default cutoff i.e. fold change of 2 (Log2 fold change = 1) was used to identify the differentially expressed genes.

We performed DAVID enrichment analysis using GO biological processes (GO_BP_FAT) and KEGG pathways as the annotation datasets. Significantly enriched processes based on similar criterion to that of eSkIN (i.e. p-value < 0.05), were considered for comparison.

Results

To gain mechanistic insight into the action of BM and PC, skin-centric transcriptomic data analysis was performed using eSkIN (Refer Methods). It is well-known that BM is more effective in curbing inflammatory effects of AD but also known to cause more adverse effects especially on skin barrier formation as compared to PC [2]. Our analysis provides new insights in the form of detailed account of the pathways that explains the molecular perturbations after drug treatments. Tables 1 and 2 provide a brief account of our key findings that adds value to the previously reported findings by Jensen et al., 2012 [2]. The findings are further discussed elaborately in this section.

BM causes large-scale perturbations in inflammatory response as compared to PC

As evident from Fig. 1a, the total number of differentially expressed genes (DEG) is higher in BM samples (approximately 1000–2000 genes) than that in PC samples (approximately 500–1000 genes), thus, indicating that BM has more profound effect on skin processes than PC. Similar trend is evident for Inflammation and Keratinocyte Differentiation pathways (see Fig. 1b-c).

Our pathway enrichment analysis shows that the pathways associated with inflammation (e.g. Inflammation, Immune Response and Chemokine Signaling) and skin barrier (e.g. Keratinocyte Differentiation, Wound Healing and Barrier Formation) are enriched (see Fig. 2), thus, corroborating the already reported findings. It is interesting to note that same set of pathways are enriched by both

Table 1 Key findings from our analysis: Genes and pathways perturbed by BM

Gene/Pathway	Role in skin pathways	Impact derived from eSkIN
TNF pathway	TNF pathway via NF-κB regulates the transcription of inflammatory cytokines, adhesion molecules, MMP9 and SELE.	TNF and its receptors are downregulated after treatment with BM, thus effecting anti-inflammatory effect.
TLRs	TLRs play important role in inflammation by activating NF-κB, which in turn, activates inflammatory cytokines.	Downregulated after treatment with BM, thus bringing about anti-inflammatory effect.
IL4 pathway	Involved in T-cell and eosinophil chemotaxis	Downregulated after treatment with BM, thus contributes towards anti-inflammatory effect.
LOR, FLG, TGM5 and CDSN	Important skin barrier proteins	Upregulated after treatment with BM; contributes towards restoration of skin barrier functions.
IVL, Keratins, LCEs, desmocollins and desmogleins	Important skin barrier proteins	Downregulated after treatment with BM representing the damage to skin barrier; CD44, AKT1, PKC-δ, HRAS and MAP2K3 involved in pathway leading to transcriptional activation of barrier proteins are also downregulated in BM samples.
S100 family proteins	Important anti-microbial peptides that help in protecting the skin from infections.	Downregulated after treatment with BM, thus leading to impaired barrier function.
VEGF	Wound healing and cell migration, vascular permeability, angiogenesis, cell invasion and coagulation	Downregulated after treatment with BM, thus affecting wound healing and other cellular processes through PLC-γ and MAPK cascade.
H2AFX, RAD51, BRCA2, MCM3, DHFR, HMOX1, GINS1 and PCNA	Genes involved in DNA repair	Downregulated after treatment with BM, thus affecting DNA repair processes.

Table 2 Key findings from our analysis: Genes and pathways perturbed by PC

Gene/Pathway	Role in skin pathways	Impact derived from eSkIN
TGF-β	Plays important role in inflammation via SMADs, and regulates IFNG, IL2, CCL4, CXCL2 and MMP2 that are involved in T-cell chemotaxis and B-cell maturation	Downregulated after treatment with PC, thus contributes towards anti-inflammatory effect.
IL13 receptor (IL13RA2)	Important regulator of chemokines through JAK-STAT pathway	Downregulated after treatment with PC, thus contributes towards anti-inflammatory effect.
LOR, FLG, TGM5 and CDSN	Important skin barrier proteins	Upregulated after treatment with PC, thus contributes towards restoration of barrier functions.

BM and PC, however, the detailed analysis clearly differentiates the mechanisms with which these drugs act on skin.

Additionally, pathways such as Basal Layer Formation and cellular pathways like Cell Migration, Cell Adhesion, Proteasomal Degradation, Autophagy, DNA Damage and Repair, Lipid Synthesis and ROS (Reactive Oxygen Species) Generation were also enriched in certain BM and PC samples.

BM mediates its anti-inflammatory effect via TNF, TLRs and IL4 pathways

BM, a corticosteroid, is known to activate glucocorticoid receptors (NR3C1) on skin, which in turn, inhibit the activity or transcription of various triggers of inflammation like IL1-β, IL4, IL11, TNF-α, TGF-β, MMPs (MMP1, 2 and 9), IFN-γ and VEGF [3]. Below, we present the inflammation-specific biomolecular interactions of these triggers in the context of transcriptomic data of BM treated samples, and relate them to key components of inflammatory response including the activation of T-cell, B-cell, eosinophils and monocytes.

Our analysis of Inflammation pathway shows that NR3C1 can inhibit TNF pathway, albeit with an unclear mechanism [11]. Its involvement in anti-inflammatory response of BM is evident from the fact that TNF, its receptor TNFRSF1A and TRADD are downregulated (Additional file 5: Figure S2). TNF pathway is known to play a major role in activating NF-κB (NFKB1) [11], and

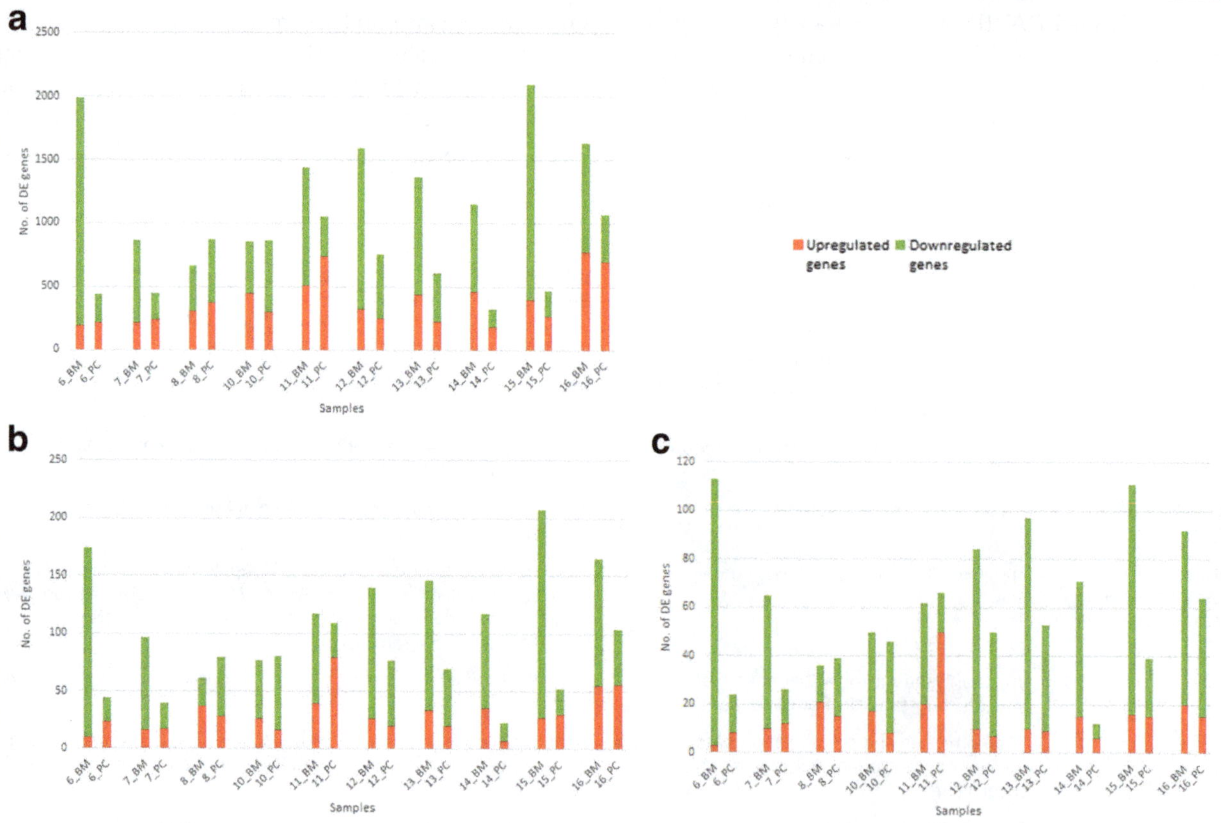

Fig. 1 Differential gene expression in BM and PC samples. Differential gene expression with respect to (**a**) complete BM and PC datasets; (**b**) effect on Inflammation pathway; and (**c**) effect on Keratinocyte Differentiation pathway

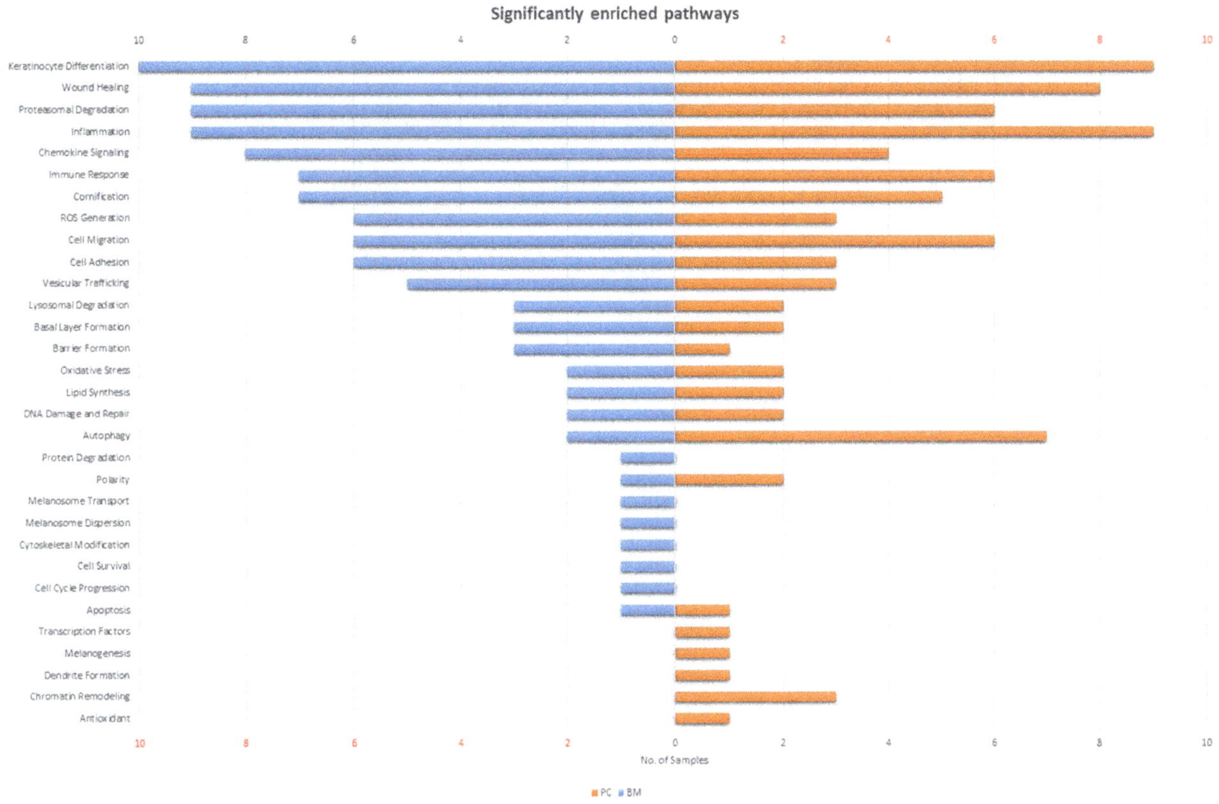

Fig. 2 Significantly enriched eSkIN pathways in BM and PC samples. The length of the bars denote the number of samples in which the pathways are enriched. Pathways with eSkIN p-value < 0.05 are considered to be significantly enriched

thus, its inhibition results in deactivation of NF-κB (Fig. 3a).

NF-κB is one of the important factors in the transcription of inflammatory cytokines, and its deactivation affects inflammation by downregulating the expression of following genes: (i) inflammatory markers: CXCL1, CXCL9, CXCL10, IL18, CCL2, CCL5, CCL13 and CD86; (ii) adhesion molecules: ICAM1 and VCAM1; (iii) matrix metalloproteinases responsible for degradation of collagen: MMP9; and (iv) factors causing accumulation of leukocytes at the site of inflammation: SELE [12, 13]. Although NF-κB is significantly down regulated only in 2 out of 10 samples, it is indeed down regulated in all the other samples albeit in lower magnitude (see Fig. 3b and Additional file 6: Figure S3). However, as reported by Chen et al., a small change in expression level of NF-κB can result in significant change in the expression of its target genes [14], which is also observed in our study. Thus, this implicates NF-κB dependent anti-inflammatory effect as an important mechanism by which BM brings about its anti-inflammatory effect. Moreover, it is interesting to note that NF-κB also regulates the expression of TNF with the help of SMAD4 [12], thereby adding further to its anti-inflammatory effect.

eSkIN also shows that TLRs (TLR1 and TLR2), which are known to promote atopic dermatitis [15], are downregulated by BM. TLRs activate NF-κB through IRAK4, and thus downregulation of TLRs lead to suppression of inflammation by diminishing NF-κB dependent inflammation, as discussed above (Additional file 7: Figure S4) [16]. Moreover, eSkIN depicts that NR3C1 can also directly inhibit the activity of NF-κB through activation of IκB (IKBKB) [3]. However, IκB did not show significant change in its expression level in BM samples (Additional file 8: Figure S5), thus indicating that this is not a likely route taken by BM to bring about its anti-inflammatory effect.

eSkIN also depicts a route for NR3C1 mediated inhibition of IL4 pathway and IFN-γ (IFNG) pathway. Although, the transcriptomic data indicated downregulation of IL4 and its receptors in BM samples, IFN-γ pathway seems to be unaffected (Additional file 9: Figure S6a). Thus, implicating IL4 pathway as an effector of BM drug action. Our analysis indicate that IL4 pathway through JAK-STAT mechanism can regulate the transcription of CXCL6, CXCL16, CCL8, CCL24, CCL25 and CCL26 which play a major role in T-cell and eosinophil chemotaxis (Additional file 9: Figure S6b) [17]. The chemokines and cytokines downstream of this pathway are down

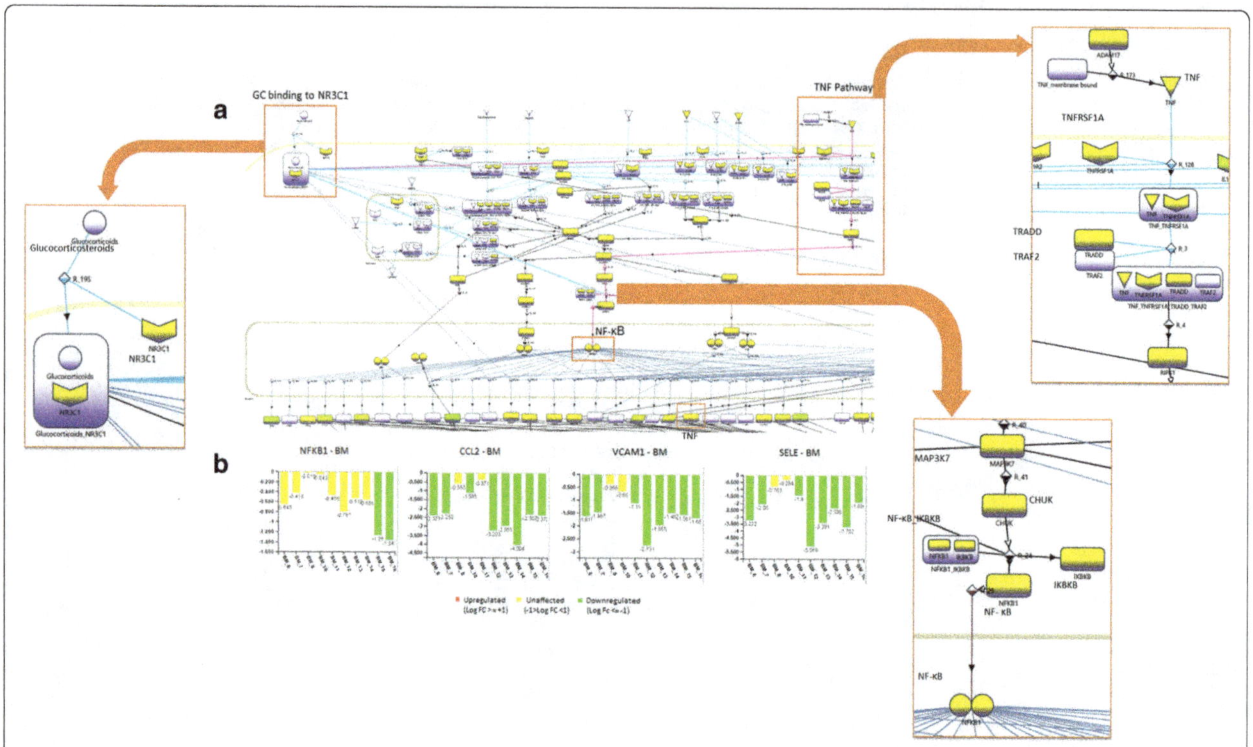

Fig. 3 TNF mediated anti-inflammatory effect of BM. (**a**) Section of eSkIN Inflammation pathway showing NR3C1 mediated inhibition of TNF and the downstream repression of inflammatory markers via NF-κB; (**b**) Expression profiles showing various genes regulated by NF-κB. Important genes/proteins in the pathway are labelled for clarity

regulated in most of the BM treated samples (Additional file 10: Figure S7). This indicates that IL4 mediated suppression of inflammation may also be contributing to anti-inflammatory effect of BM.

PC suppresses inflammation via IL13, IL6 and VEGF pathways

PC is a calcineurin inhibitor and inhibits the activity of NFAT (NFATC1) [4]. NFAT along with AP1 family of transcription factors is known to regulate the transcription of IL2, IL4, IL5, IL8, IL13, GM-CSF, TNF-α and IFN-γ, which are important inflammatory triggers [18, 19]. The transcriptomic data of PC samples show downregulation of IL13 receptor (IL13RA2), but, it also show downregulation of receptors of additional inflammatory triggers, namely IL6 and TGF-β. At the downstream, IL13 regulate the transcription of CCL8 and CCL26 via STAT6, and TGF-β regulate the transcription of CXCL2 via SMAD4. We observed all these downstream chemokines to be downregulated in PC samples (see Additional file 11: Figure S8). Moreover, the transcription of following chemokines and adhesion molecules: CXCL1, CXCL9, CXCL10, CCL2, SELE, ICAM1 and VCAM1, are also downregulated, but, their causal route could not be deciphered from this data.

Additional pathways responsible for anti-inflammatory effect of BM and PC

a) It is known that JAK-STAT cascade helps in the transcription of genes responsible for leukocyte, eosinophil and T-cell migration [20, 21]. Our analysis shows that BM and PC affects this activity through certain common triggers (i.e. IL6, IL4, and IL27) as is evident from downregulation of their respective receptors (in particular, IL6R, IL4R and IL27RA). PC also shows few specific triggers like IL13 and IL12 (downregulation of IL13RA2 and IL12RB) (Additional file 12: Figure S9).
b) Chemokine Signaling is known to affect processes like adhesion, migration, phagocytosis, immune response and anaphylaxis. Our analysis shows that most of the signaling cascades like RAS-RAF pathway, MAPK cascade and JAK-STAT pathway, triggered by various chemokines and growth factors like HBEGF and AREG [22, 23], show profound under expression in BM samples but mild under expression in PC samples (data not shown).

Restoration of skin barrier by BM and PC

Keratinocyte differentiation is central to the formation of healthy skin barrier. BM is known to efficiently inhibit the primary cause of AD i.e. inflammation, but it also affects the skin barrier leading to secondary complications like skin atrophy and infection.

Our analysis corroborates the fact that BM and PC upregulate several key skin barrier formation genes such as Loricrin (LOR), Filaggrin (FLG), TGM5 and CDSN (Additional file 13: Figure S10a) as a measure to restore barrier functions [2]. However, it is also observed that most of the other barrier formation proteins like involucrin (IVL), LCEs (LCE3D), TGM1, TGM3 and DSG3 are under expressed in BM samples while they are mostly unaffected by PC (Additional file 13: Figure S10b).

BM adversely affects the synthesis of barrier proteins through AP1 family and CEBPs

We explored the possible causative pathway that could lead to the impairment of skin barrier by BM. It is known that calcium acts as a key trigger for epidermal differentiation through PLC-γ (PLCG1), which regulates the transcription of barrier proteins. Our analysis depicts another, calcium independent route, to activate PLC-γ through AKT1-PKN2 complex which is activated by CD44 [24] (Fig. 4a). This pathway further activates several transcriptional regulators including AP1 family of transcription factors like JUN and FOS, CEBP-β (CEBPB), SP1 and HSPB1. These regulators play a major role in the transcription of barrier proteins like keratins, transglutaminases, loricrin, involucrin, filaggrin, LCEs, desmogleins, desmocollins, family of S100 proteins [25]. The molecular details feature of eSkIN shows that the genes involved in this pathway like CD44, AKT1, PKC-δ, HRAS and MAP2K3 are mostly downregulated in BM samples, thus, implying the role of this pathway in BM triggered skin barrier impairment (see Fig. 4b).

Other transcriptional regulators involved in the activation of skin barrier proteins like JUND and FOSL1, are also found to be downregulated. Furthermore, CEBP-α (CEBPA), an important transcription factor involved in the transcription of IVL and desmocollins [26], is also under expressed in BM samples (Additional file 14: Figure S11). TGFA pathway mediates this transcriptional regulation of CEBP-α [27]. The proliferation markers like MYC and ERK (MAPK1) present in this pathway are also under expressed in BM samples (data not shown).

Keratinocyte Differentiation pathway also indicates that the anti-microbial peptides S100A7, S100A8 and S100A9 are under expressed in BM samples (Additional file 15: Figure S12). While S100A7 transcription is mediated by JUN [28], S100A8 and S100A9 transcription is mediated by STAT3 via IL4 pathway (Additional file 15: Figure S12) [29]. This further explains the compromised skin barrier functions upon treatment with BM, leading to skin infection [2].

On the contrary, PC has mild effect on barrier proteins and their regulation, and thus, helps in restoring skin barrier in AD patients.

In addition to the profile of skin barrier proteins observed in Keratinocyte Differentiation pathway, Barrier Formation genes like CTTN, CDC42, GRHL3 and AHR which are involved in the formation of tight junctions [30] are under expressed in BM samples. PC samples does not show significant enrichment of this pathway in most of the samples (Additional file 16: Figure S13).

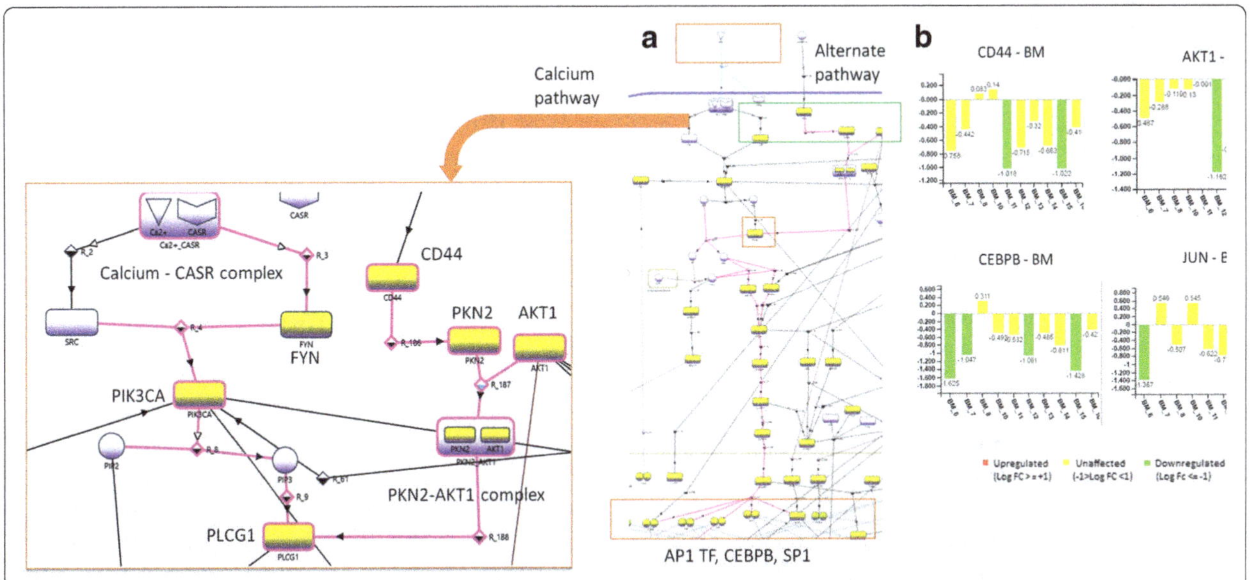

Fig. 4 AP1 and CEBP mediated skin barrier impairment by BM. (**a**) eSkIN Keratinocyte Differentiation pathway depicting the effect of BM on synthesis of skin barrier proteins; (**b**) Expression profiles of key genes in this pathway. Important genes/proteins in the pathway are labelled for clarity

Additional pathways responsible for effect on skin barrier by BM and PC

a) Wound Healing pathway of eSkIN shows that VEGF (VEGFA), an important trigger for cellular processes like cell migration, vascular permeability, angiogenesis, cell invasion and coagulation, is significantly more under expressed in BM than in PC (Additional file 17: Figure S14). VEGFA activates various pathways like PI3K (PIK3CA), PLC-γ and MAPK cascade, thus, impacting the normal physiological processes that are responsible for wound healing [31]. Fibronectin (FN1), another protein involved in wound healing, is downregulated as well in BM samples [32].
b) Similarly, Basal Layer Formation pathway shows that proteins like integrins, LAMA5 and collagens like COL4A1 [33] are under expressed in BM samples. On the contrary, most of these proteins show an upregulated trend in PC dataset (Additional file 18: Figure S15).

This further illustrates that BM affects the skin barrier formation by influencing the synthesis of barrier proteins, antimicrobial proteins and basal layer proteins. Such behavior is not observed in PC samples.

Cellular functions affected by BM and PC

Lipid Synthesis pathway is of interest as lipids are an integral part of skin barrier. Application of BM is known to impair the fatty acids and lipid content of skin [34]. Lipid Synthesis pathway shows that lipid transporters like LDLR and ABCA12 [35, 36] show downregulated trend (Additional file 19: Figure S16a), which might hinder the transportation of cholesterol and other lipids to skin. Enzymes like SPTLC2, SGMS2 and SMPD2 involved in the conversion of fatty acids to glucosylceramides [36] are also downregulated (Additional file 19: Figure S16b). Moreover, genes involved in the synthesis of fatty acids or lipids like LXR (NR1H2), SCD, FASN and HMGCR [37, 38] are downregulated (Additional file 20: Figure S17a), while genes involved in the metabolism of lipids like LPL and APOC1 [39] are showing an upregulated trend (Additional file 20: Figure S17b).

DNA Damage and Repair is differentially affected in BM and PC dataset. While most of the genes are unaffected by PC, genes involved in DNA repair like H2AFX, RAD51, BRCA2, MCM3, DHFR, HMOX1, GINS1 and PCNA [40–42] are under expressed in BM (Additional file 21: Figure S18). Similarly, CDK1, CDKN1A, CCNB1 and E2F family of proteins, involved in cell cycle progression [43] show a downregulated trend in BM samples.

Though Autophagy and Proteasomal Degradation pathways are enriched in most of the BM and PC samples, we could not establish any relevance of this to the action of these drugs.

Comparison of eSkIN results with DAVID

To evaluate the performance of eSkIN pathway enrichment analysis, we compared the results with the most widely used functional enrichment tool, DAVID (https://david.ncifcrf.gov/) [5]. BM and PC samples were analyzed separately in DAVID. We obtained 409 differentially expressed genes in BM and 49 genes in PC datasets that were used as input for DAVID analysis (refer Methods for details).

Comparison of pathway enrichment for BM dataset

The enriched processes for BM dataset yielded 781 GO Biological Processes (GO BP) terms and 24 KEGG pathways (see Additional file 22). We observe that Immune response, Defense response, Inflammatory response, Keratinocyte differentiation, Skin development and Keratinization are enriched amongst the GO terms. Amongst KEGG pathways, Drug metabolism, Steroid hormone biosynthesis, Chemokine signaling pathway and NF-kappa B signaling pathways are enriched.

eSkIN uses a comprehensive manually curated skin centric knowledge-base for its analysis, and thus we observe a limited set of only relevant pathways (26 pathways) to be enriched. The pathways related to skin physiology, which are enriched in DAVID analysis are also obtained using eSkIN analysis (see Table 3), thus, corroborating the capability of eSkIN to perform skin-centric pathway enrichment analysis.

However, GO BP terms cannot be further explored in terms of the molecular interactions between these genes (or their protein products) to derive mechanistic insights into the action of the drugs. On the other hand, eSkIN allows further exploration of the enriched pathways in terms of the molecular interactions in them, and thus, helps in deriving mechanistic insights into drug action (see Table 1). Though KEGG Pathways can be explored in similar context, the enriched KEGG pathways (Drug metabolism, Steroid hormone biosynthesis Chemokine signaling pathway and NF-kappa B signaling pathways) are not directly relevant to our analysis.

Comparison of pathway enrichment for PC

The enriched processes for PC dataset yielded 62 GO BP terms and 0 KEGG pathways (see Additional file 22). We observe that skin related processes like Epidermis development, Skin development, Keratinocyte differentiation, Immune response and Defense response are enriched amongst the GO terms. As is evident from Table 3, the corresponding pathways are also enriched in eSkIN. Moreover, owing to the capability of eSkIN to highlight

Table 3 Comparison of pathways enriched in eSkIN and DAVID analysis

S.No.	Important pathways enriched in eSkIN	Related processes/pathways enriched in BM samples		Related processes/pathways enriched in PC samples	
		GO_BP_FAT	KEGG	GO_BP_FAT	KEGG
1.	Keratinocyte differentiation, Cornification, Basal layer formation	keratinocyte differentiation, skin development, keratinization, skin epidermis development	–	epidermis development, skin development, keratinocyte differentiation, epidermal cell differentiation, keratinization	–
2.	Inflammation	inflammatory response, regulation of inflammatory response, T-cell activation	TNF signaling pathway, NF-κB signaling pathway, Inflammatory bowel disease	–	–
3.	Immune response	Immune response, defense response, Innate immune response	–	Immune response, defense response, Innate immune response	–
4.	Chemokine signaling	Chemokine mediated signaling pathway and chemokine production	Chemokine signaling pathway, Cytokine-cytokine receptor interaction	–	–
5.	DNA Damage and Repair	DNA integrity checkpoint	–	–	–
6.	Cell Adhesion, Cell Migration	Cell adhesion, leukocyte cell-cell adhesion, cell migration, regulation of cell migration, leukocyte migration	Cell adhesion molecules (CAMs)	Cell migration, leukocyte migration	–

molecular interactions of the enriched pathways, insights into mechanistic action of PC were obtained (see Table 2).

Discussion

In this study, we analyzed transcriptomic datasets of AD patients treated with Betamethasone and Pimecrolimus. We used a novel systems biology based approach to understand the detailed molecular level differences in the mechanism of action of the drugs. Though the pathway enrichment analysis broadly showed similar set of pathways being enriched by both BM and PC, a detailed molecular level study showed that these drugs opt different mechanisms to control the disorder. Fig. 5 provides an overview of the routes taken by these drugs.

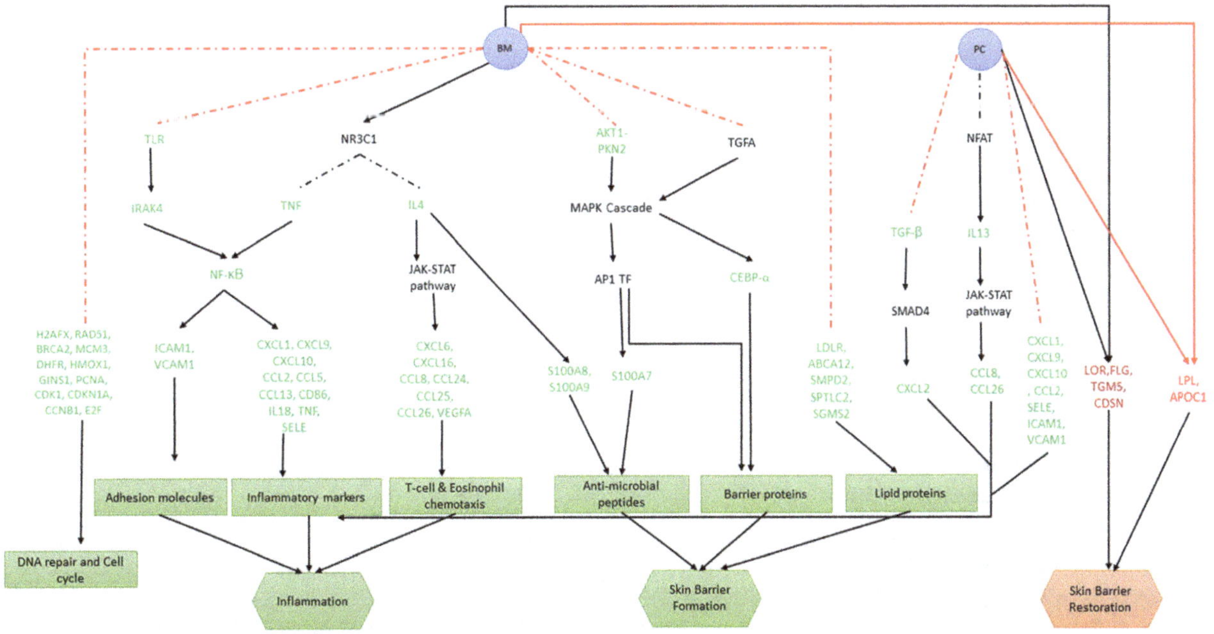

Fig. 5 Pathways perturbed by BM and PC and their role in the action of these drugs. Solid lines depict activation or stimulation while the dotted lines represent inhibition. Colors of the lines denote known mechanism (black) and unknown mechanism (red). Colors of the gene names denote downregulation (green) and upregulation (red). This clearly shows that BM has a larger impact on inflammation than PC. But it is also evident that, unlike PC, BM negatively affects the skin barrier functions

We highlighted the role of TLRs, TNF and IL4 to trigger the anti-inflammatory response and AKT1-PKN2 and TGFA via MAPK cascade to affect the skin barrier proteins in AD patients, when treated with BM. Stojadinovic et al. have shown the role of glucocorticoids in various cellular processes like inflammation, innate immunity, cell migration, tissue remodeling, cell differentiation and cell death in keratinocytes [3]. Our analysis further adds value to the above mentioned finding by elaborating on the pathways that trigger various cellular responses, particularly in AD patients. We also depict the impact of BM on lipids and DNA damage and repair proteins thus leading to an impaired barrier function.

Under PC treatment, we show that TGF- and IL13 could be the plausible pathways involved in anti-inflammatory response. Through our comparative study of the two drugs, we show that the molecular signatures of barrier proteins under PC clearly contributes towards restoration of barrier.

Novel insight into disease manifestation during drug treatment

The mechanistic analysis of transcriptomic data of BM and PC treated samples also allowed us to understand the manifestation of disease during the treatment by these drugs. This provides new avenue towards future direction of drug discovery efforts in this area.

In particular, EDN1 (Endothelin 1), which is positively correlated with AD clinical severity [44, 45], is observed to be mostly upregulated in BM while PC shows mild upregulation. This implies a risk of disease manifestation even after treatment by BM or PC. By leveraging the molecular interaction maps of eSkIN, we elucidate that in the downstream, EDN1 activates PLCB2 [46], which in turn, triggers the MAPK cascade involved in cell migration and inflammation (see Fig. 6a). We believe that treatment by BM or PC, if supplemented with a drug targeting EDN1 or downstream proteins, can bring synergistic therapeutic effect in AD care.

Furthermore, it is interesting to note that the suppressors of cytokine family (SOCS), SOCS1 and SOCS3 are downregulated even after the treatment with BM and PC. SOCS proteins are known to contribute towards disease manifestation in psoriatic skin [47]. Our analysis shows that SOCS3 inhibits STAT3 activation via JAK1 [48] (Fig. 6b). However, their role in AD manifestation is not very well studied. Based on our analysis using eSkIN, it appears that downregulation of SOCS could be contributing towards the manifestation of AD, and thus, it may be worthwhile to explore it as a drug target for future drug discovery efforts.

Conclusion

Our study suggested the causal biomolecular interrelationships involved in the action of BM and PC on human skin, apart from highlighting the existing evidence on these drugs in the context of skin-associated functional networks. It is evident that BM downregulates

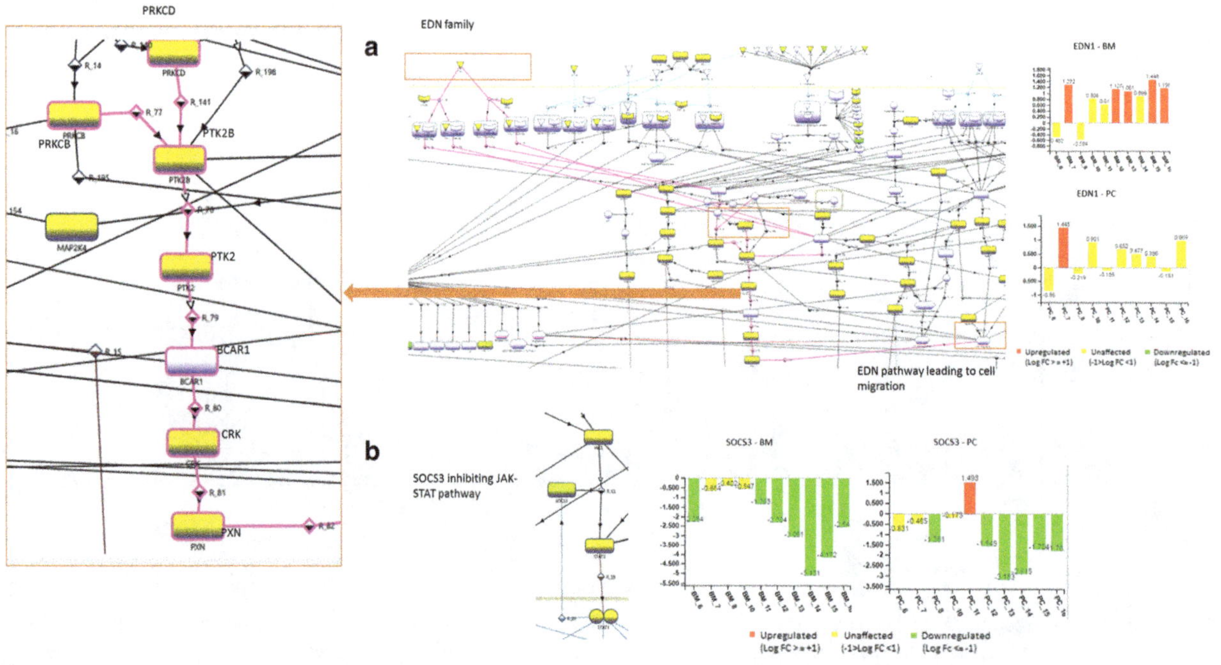

Fig. 6 Factors implicated in manifestation of disease during drug treatment. (**a**) EDN1 mediated; (**b**) SOCS3 mediated. Important genes/proteins in the pathway are labelled for clarity

molecules involved in inflammation, T-cell & eosinophil chemotaxis, adhesion, DNA repair and cell cycle, while PC targets a smaller section of inflammatory genes. Also, both BM and PC upregulate few important barrier proteins to restore the skin barrier functions. However, BM also downregulates many other barrier components which is largely unaffected by PC, thus, accounting for the impaired skin barrier due to the treatment with BM. It should be noted that the results reported in this study are based on 10 AD patients' data that were available in NCBI GEO database, and needs further validation in a larger cohort.

Additional files

Additional file 1: Table S1. List of 35 pathways of eSkIN and their categorization. (DOCX 13 kb)

Additional file 2: Sensitivity analysis to evaluate the effect of fold change cutoff on pathway enrichment analysis. (DOCX 12 kb)

Additional file 3: Pathway enrichment analysis for different fold change cutoffs. Table and charts of pathway enrichment analysis for different fold change cutoffs. (XLSX 30 kb)

Additional file 4: Figure S1. Comparison of enriched pathways at three different fold change cutoffs (Log_2 fold change (FC) = 0.5, 1 and 1.5). (TIFF 3928 kb)

Additional file 5: Figure S2. Expression profile of genes involved in TNF pathway in BM samples. (TIFF 4333 kb)

Additional file 6: Figure S3. Expression profile of genes regulated by NF-κB in BM samples. (TIFF 12640 kb)

Additional file 7: Figure S4. Section of eSkIN Inflammation pathway showing TLR mediated activation of NF-κB and the expression profile of genes involved in this pathway. (TIFF 12017 kb)

Additional file 8: Figure S5. Section of eSkIN Inflammation pathway showing NR3C1 mediated inhibition of NF-κB through IκB (highlighted in pink) and the expression profile of IκB. (TIFF 7299 kb)

Additional file 9: Figure S6. Sections of eSkIN Inflammation pathway showing: (a) activation of JAK-STAT pathway by IL4 and IFN-γ and their expression profiles (b) genes regulated by STAT6. (TIFF 9845 kb)

Additional file 10: Figure S7. Expression profile of genes activated by IL4 via JAK-STAT pathway. (TIFF 5004 kb)

Additional file 11: Figure S8. Expression profile of inflammatory genes that show downregulation in PC samples. (TIFF 10440 kb)

Additional file 12: Figure S9. Section of eSkIN Immune Response pathway showing various activators of JAK-STAT pathway and their expression profile in BM and PC samples. (TIFF 10437 kb)

Additional file 13: Figure S10. Expression profile of skin barrier proteins in BM and PC samples. (a) Expression profile of genes that are upregulated in both BM and PC in order to restore barrier functions; (b) Expression profile of skin barrier genes that show treatment specific difference in their expressions. (TIFF 8378 kb)

Additional file 14: Figure S11. Expression profile of important transcription factors of barrier proteins in BM. (TIFF 5538 kb)

Additional file 15: Figure S12. Expression profile of anti-microbial peptides in BM samples and a section of eSkIN pathway showing their transcriptional regulation by IL4. (TIFF 5747 kb)

Additional file 16: Figure S13. Expression profile of junction proteins that show treatment specific difference in their expressions. (TIFF 6474 kb)

Additional file 17: Figure S14. Section of eSkIN Wound Healing pathway showing VEGF mediated activation of cellular functions like focal adhesion, actin remodeling, cell migration, vascular permeability, angiogenesis, degradation of collagen, cell invasion and blood coagulation, and expression profile of VEGF in BM and PC samples. (TIFF 12210 kb)

Additional file 18: Figure S15. Expression profile of basal layer genes that show treatment specific difference in their expressions. (TIFF 12463 kb)

Additional file 19: Figure S16. Sections of eSkIN Lipid Synthesis pathway showing: (a) lipid transporters and their expression profiles in BM samples (b) enzymes involved in fatty acid conversion and their expression profiles in BM samples. (TIFF 5067 kb)

Additional file 20: Figure S17. Sections of eSkIN Lipid Synthesis pathway showing: (a) the genes involved in the synthesis of lipids and fatty acids and their expression profiles in BM samples (b) genes involved in lipid metabolism and their expression profiles in BM samples. (TIFF 7877 kb)

Additional file 21: Figure S18. Section of eSkIN DNA Damage and Repair pathway showing the genes involved in DNA repair mechanisms and their expression profiles in BM samples. (TIFF 10956 kb)

Additional file 22: Pathway enrichment analysis using DAVID. Tables of enriched pathways (*p*-value < 0.05) using GO biological process (GO_BP_FAT) and KEGG pathways as annotation datasets in DAVID. BM and PC datasets were analyzed separately. (XLSX 168 kb)

Abbreviations

AD: Atopic dermatitis; BM: Betamethasone valerate; DEG: Differentially expressed genes; GEO: Gene Expression Omnibus; PC: Pimecrolimus; ROS: Reactive oxygen species; TCI: Topical calcineurin inhibitor; US FDA: US Food and Drug Administration

Acknowledgements

The authors acknowledge the eSkIN team for making eSkIN available for the present study. We thank Council of Scientific and Industrial Research (CSIR) for funding eSkIN project.

Funding

Not applicable

Authors' contributions

AJ, VS and IS conceived and designed the study. IS and VS performed the experiments. All authors contributed in analyzing the results and writing the manuscript. All authors have given approval to the final version of the manuscript.

Competing interests

All authors are employees of Persistent Systems Limited. However, this does not alter the authors' adherence to the journal policies on sharing data and materials.

References

1. Nutten S. Atopic dermatitis: global epidemiology and risk factors. Ann Nutr Metab. 2015;66(Suppl 1):8–16.
2. Jensen JM, et al. Gene expression is differently affected by pimecrolimus and betamethasone in lesional skin of atopic dermatitis. Allergy. 2012;67(3):413–23.
3. Stojadinovic O, et al. Novel genomic effects of glucocorticoids in epidermal keratinocytes: inhibition of apoptosis, interferon-gamma pathway, and wound healing along with promotion of terminal differentiation. J Biol Chem. 2007;282(6):4021–34.

4. Siegfried EC, Jaworski JC, Hebert AA. Topical calcineurin inhibitors and lymphoma risk: evidence update with implications for daily practice. Am J Clin Dermatol. 2013;14(3):163–78.
5. Huang DW, Sherman BT, Lempicki RA. Systematic and integrative analysis of large gene lists using DAVID bioinformatics resources. Nat Protoc. 2009;4(1): 44–57.
6. Huang DW, Sherman BT, Lempicki RA. Bioinformatics enrichment tools: paths toward the comprehensive functional analysis of large gene lists. Nucleic Acids Res. 2009;37(1):1–13.
7. Subramanian A, et al. Gene set enrichment analysis: a knowledge-based approach for interpreting genome-wide expression profiles. Proc Natl Acad Sci U S A. 2005;102(43):15545–50.
8. J.-H. Hung, "Gene set/pathway enrichment analysis," in Data Mining for Systems Biology, H. Mamitsuka, C. DeLisi, and M. Kanehisa, Eds. Humana Press, 2013, pp. 201–213.
9. P. Zhao *et al.*, "Identification of differentially expressed genes in pituitary adenomas by integrating analysis of microarray data," Int J Endocrinol, 2015. Available: https://www.hindawi.com/journals/ije/2015/164087/. Accessed 17 Oct 2017.
10. Wu X, et al. Network expansion and pathway enrichment analysis towards biologically significant findings from microarrays. J Integr Bioinforma. 2016; 9(2):113–25.
11. Bradley JR. TNF-mediated inflammatory disease. J Pathol. 2008;214(2):149–60.
12. Miller LS. Toll-like receptors in skin. Adv Dermatol. 2008;24:71–87.
13. Murphy JE, Robert C, Kupper TS. Interleukin-1 and cutaneous inflammation: a crucial link between innate and acquired immunity. J. Invest. Dermatol. 2000;114(3):602–8.
14. Chen Y, et al. Microarray analysis reveals the inhibition of nuclear factor-kappa B signaling by aristolochic acid in normal human kidney (HK-2) cells. Acta Pharmacol Sin. 2010;31(2):227–36.
15. Kaesler S, et al. Toll-like receptor 2 ligands promote chronic atopic dermatitis through IL-4-mediated suppression of IL-10. J Allergy Clin Immunol. 2014;134(1):92–9.
16. Hari A, Flach TL, Shi Y, Mydlarski PR. Toll-like receptors: role in dermatological disease. Mediat Inflamm. 2010;2010:437246.
17. Bao L, Zhang H, Chan LS. The involvement of the JAK-STAT signaling pathway in chronic inflammatory skin disease atopic dermatitis. JAK-STAT. 2013;2(3):e24137.
18. Im S-H, Rao A. Activation and deactivation of gene expression by Ca2 +/calcineurin-NFAT-mediated signaling. Mol Cells. 2004;18(1):1–9.
19. Medyouf H, Ghysdael J. The calcineurin/NFAT signaling pathway: a novel therapeutic target in leukemia and solid tumors. Cell Cycle Georget Tex. 2008;7(3):297–303.
20. Murata T, Husain SR, Mohri H, Puri RK. Two different IL-13 receptor chains are expressed in normal human skin fibroblasts, and IL-4 and IL-13 mediate signal transduction through a common pathway. Int Immunol. 1998;10(8):1103–10.
21. Wittmann M, Zeitvogel J, Wang D, Werfel T. IL-27 is expressed in chronic human eczematous skin lesions and stimulates human keratinocytes. J Allergy Clin Immunol. 2009;124(1):81–9.
22. New DC, Wong YH. CC chemokine receptor-coupled signalling pathways. Sheng Wu Hua Xue Yu Sheng Wu Wu Li Xue Bao (Shanghai). 2003;35(9):779–88.
23. Pastore S, Mascia F, Mariotti F, Dattilo C, Mariani V, Girolomoni G. ERK1/2 regulates epidermal chemokine expression and skin inflammation. J Immunol Baltim Md 1950. 2005;174(8):5047–56.
24. Bourguignon LYW, Singleton PA, Diedrich F. Hyaluronan-CD44 interaction with Rac1-dependent protein kinase N-gamma promotes phospholipase Cgamma1 activation, ca(2+) signaling, and cortactin-cytoskeleton function leading to keratinocyte adhesion and differentiation. J Biol Chem. 2004; 279(28):29654–69.
25. Eckert RL, et al. Regulation of involucrin gene expression. J. Invest. Dermatol. 2004;123(1):13–22.
26. Efimova T, Deucher A, Kuroki T, Ohba M, Eckert RL. Novel protein kinase C isoforms regulate human keratinocyte differentiation by activating a p38 delta mitogen-activated protein kinase cascade that targets CCAAT/ enhancer-binding protein alpha. J Biol Chem. 2002;277(35):31753–60.
27. Reynolds NJ, et al. Differential induction of phosphatidylcholine hydrolysis, diacylglycerol formation and protein kinase C activation by epidermal growth factor and transforming growth factor-alpha in normal human skin fibroblasts and keratinocytes. Biochem J. 1993;294(Pt 2):535–44.
28. Emberley ED, et al. The S100A7-c-Jun activation domain binding protein 1 pathway enhances prosurvival pathways in breast cancer. Cancer Res. 2005; 65(13):5696–702.
29. Uto-Konomi A, et al. Dysregulation of suppressor of cytokine signaling 3 in keratinocytes causes skin inflammation mediated by interleukin-20 receptor-related cytokines. PLoS One. 2012;7(7):e40343.
30. Jamora C, Fuchs E. Intercellular adhesion, signalling and the cytoskeleton. Nat Cell Biol. 2002;4(4):E101–8.
31. Olsson A-K, Dimberg A, Kreuger J, Claesson-Welsh L. VEGF receptor signalling - in control of vascular function. Nat Rev Mol Cell Biol. 2006;7(5):359–71.
32. Zambruno G, et al. Transforming growth factor-beta 1 modulates beta 1 and beta 5 integrin receptors and induces the de novo expression of the alpha v beta 6 heterodimer in normal human keratinocytes: implications for wound healing. J Cell Biol. 1995;129(3):853–65.
33. Fleischmajer R, et al. Initiation of skin basement membrane formation at the epidermo-dermal interface involves assembly of laminins through binding to cell membrane receptors. J Cell Sci. 1998;111(Pt 14):1929–40.
34. Jensen J-M, et al. Different effects of pimecrolimus and betamethasone on the skin barrier in patients with atopic dermatitis. J Allergy Clin Immunol. 2009;123(5):1124–33.
35. Zhang L, Reue K, Fong LG, Young SG, Tontonoz P. Feedback regulation of cholesterol uptake by the LXR-IDOL-LDLR axis. Arterioscler Thromb Vasc Biol. 2012;32(11):2541–6.
36. Oda Y, Uchida Y, Moradian S, Crumrine D, Elias PM, Bikle DD. Vitamin D receptor and coactivators SRC2 and 3 regulate epidermis-specific sphingolipid production and permeability barrier formation. J. Invest. Dermatol. 2009;129(6):1367–78.
37. Yokoyama A, et al. Induction of SREBP-1c mRNA by differentiation and LXR ligand in human keratinocytes. J. Invest. Dermatol. 2009;129(6):1395–401.
38. Harris IR, et al. Parallel regulation of sterol regulatory element binding protein-2 and the enzymes of cholesterol and fatty acid synthesis but not ceramide synthesis in cultured human keratinocytes and murine epidermis. J Lipid Res. 1998;39(2):412–22.
39. Jiang ZG, Robson SC, Yao Z. Lipoprotein metabolism in nonalcoholic fatty liver disease. J Biomed Res. 2013;27(1):1–13.
40. Malewicz M, et al. Essential role for DNA-PK-mediated phosphorylation of NR4A nuclear orphan receptors in DNA double-strand break repair. Genes Dev. 2011;25(19):2031–40.
41. Yoshida K, Miki Y. Role of BRCA1 and BRCA2 as regulators of DNA repair, transcription, and cell cycle in response to DNA damage. Cancer Sci. 2004; 95(11):866–71.
42. Meng X, Yuan Y, Maestas A, Shen Z. Recovery from DNA damage-induced G2 arrest requires actin-binding protein filamin-a/actin-binding protein 280. J Biol Chem. 2004;279(7):6098–105.
43. Sulaimon SS, Kitchell BE. The basic biology of malignant melanoma: molecular mechanisms of disease progression and comparative aspects. J Vet Intern Med. 2003;17(6):760–72.
44. Aktar MK, Kido-Nakahara M, Furue M, Nakahara T. Mutual upregulation of endothelin-1 and IL-25 in atopic dermatitis. Allergy. 2015;70(7):846–54.
45. Tsybikov NN, Petrisheva IV, Kuznik BI, Magen E. Plasma endothelin-1 levels during exacerbation of atopic dermatitis. Allergy Asthma Proc. 2015;36(4):320–4.
46. Bouallegue A, Daou GB, Srivastava AK. Endothelin-1-induced signaling pathways in vascular smooth muscle cells. Curr Vasc Pharmacol. 2007; 5(1):45–52.
47. Sonkoly E, et al. MicroRNAs: novel regulators involved in the pathogenesis of psoriasis? PLoS One. 2007;2(7):e610.
48. Yamasaki K, et al. Suppressor of cytokine signaling 1/JAB and suppressor of cytokine signaling 3/cytokine-inducible SH2 containing protein 3 negatively regulate the signal transducers and activators of transcription signaling pathway in normal human epidermal keratinocytes. J Invest Dermatol. 2003; 120(4):571–80.

26

Heat-mediated reduction of apoptosis in UVB-damaged keratinocytes in vitro and in human skin ex vivo

Leslie Calapre[1], Elin S. Gray[1], Sandrine Kurdykowski[2], Anthony David[2], Prue Hart[4], Pascal Descargues[2] and Mel Ziman[1,3*]

Abstract

Background: UV radiation induces significant DNA damage in keratinocytes and is a known risk factor for skin carcinogenesis. However, it has been reported previously that repeated and simultaneous exposure to UV and heat stress increases the rate of cutaneous tumour formation in mice. Since constant exposure to high temperatures and UV are often experienced in the environment, the effects of exposure to UV and heat needs to be clearly addressed in human epidermal cells.

Methods: In this study, we determined the effects of repeated UVB exposure 1 kJ/m^2 followed by heat (39 °C) to human keratinocytes. Normal human ex vivo skin models and primary keratinocytes (NHEK) were exposed once a day to UVB and/or heat stress for four consecutive days. Cells were then assessed for changes in proliferation, apoptosis and gene expression at 2 days post-exposure, to determine the cumulative and persistent effects of UV and/or heat in skin keratinocytes.

Results: Using ex vivo skin models and primary keratinocytes in vitro, we showed that UVB *plus* heat treated keratinocytes exhibit persistent DNA damage, as observed with UVB alone. However, we found that apoptosis was significantly reduced in UVB *plus* heat treated samples. Immunohistochemical and whole genome transcription analysis showed that multiple UVB *plus* heat exposures induced inactivation of the p53-mediated stress response. Furthermore, we demonstrated that repeated exposure to UV *plus* heat induced SIRT1 expression and a decrease in acetylated p53 in keratinocytes, which is consistent with the significant downregulation of p53-regulated pro-apoptotic and DNA damage repair genes in these cells.

Conclusion: Our results suggest that UVB-induced p53-mediated cell cycle arrest and apoptosis are reduced in the presence of heat stress, leading to increased survival of DNA damaged cells. Thus, exposure to UVB and heat stress may act synergistically to allow survival of damaged cells, which could have implications for initiation skin carcinogenesis.

Keywords: Heat stress, UVB, Keratinocytes, Apoptosis, p53, DNA damage

* Correspondence: m.ziman@ecu.edu.au
[1]School of Medical Sciences, Edith Cowan University, 270 Joondalup Drive, Joondalup, Perth, WA 6027, Australia
[3]Department of Pathology and Laboratory Medicine, University of Western Australia, Crawley, WA, Australia
Full list of author information is available at the end of the article

Background

The anatomical location of epidermal keratinocytes makes them vulnerable to the effects of UV radiation and temperature fluctuations [1]. UV radiation, particularly UVB, can induce DNA damage, in the form of cyclobutane pyrimidine dimers (CPD), and is a known risk factor for skin carcinogenesis [2, 3]. Moreover, it is well-known that UV irradiation of normal keratinocytes activates the p53 tumour suppressor protein, which is crucial for regulating cell cycle arrest, apoptosis and nuclear excision repair of UV-induced DNA damage [4–8].

Heat stress also causes DNA damage and has been observed to deaminate cytosine and hydrolise glycosyl bonds, leading to genome instability [9–11]. In addition, exposure to heat stress can induce formation of reactive oxygen species, which can, cause G to T transversion mutations [11–14]. Heat stress can also trigger extensive denaturation, degradation and aggregation of critical intracellular proteins [15, 16], leading to defective DNA replication, transcription and repair, thus affecting cell survival and apoptosis [17–19]. The deleterious effect of heat on cellular processes is normally countered by activation of a conserved heat shock response [20–22], which stabilises cells by interacting with pro-survival signalling pathways such as PI3K/Akt [20, 23, 24].

Continuous exposure to heat stress independently or concurrently with UV radiation is commonly experienced in several geographical locations. Furthermore, a previous report has shown increased risk of non-melanoma skin cancers in geographical areas with high environmental temperature [25]. However, little work has been done to show the consequences of repeated exposure of keratinocytes to both high temperatures and UV [26]. Previous studies have shown that pre-treatment with heat shock at 38–42 °C, prior to UVB irradiation, increases cell survival and decreases UVB-induced DNA damage of normal murine and human keratinocytes [27–30]. However, it is important to note that these previously described experiments involved a singular exposure to heat then UV. Other studies have shown that repeated and simultaneous exposure to UVB and heat stress increased the rate of cutaneous tumour formation in mice [31, 32]. Thus, the effects of multiple simultaneous exposures to heat and UVB need to be clearly addressed in human keratinocytes, and molecular changes in response to UVB *plus* heat remain to be characterised.

In this study, we investigated the effects of heat stress alone, or immediately after UVB radiation, on primary keratinocyte cultures in vitro and in an ex vivo human skin model. Given that exposure to UVB radiation and/or heat stress is often repeatedly experienced in nature, we particularly aimed to determine the effects of multiple exposures to these environmental stressors. Thus, to determine whether heat alleviates or exacerbates the effects of UVB irradiation, we looked at the level of DNA damage, apoptosis and cell proliferation in keratinocytes two days after repeated UVB and/or heat treatment. To detail the molecular events underpinning the observed cellular changes, a whole genome gene expression array was performed in heat and/or UVB treated samples, and pathways activated by UVB *plus* heat were identified. Moreover, we investigated the expression of key proteins involved in the affected molecular pathways activated in DNA-damaged cells.

Methods

Cell lines

Primary adult human epidermal keratinocytes (NHEK-c, Promocell) were cultured in vitro using Keratinocyte Growth Medium 2 (Promocell) supplemented with $CaCl_2$ (0.06 mM) and penicillin/streptomycin (Sigma-Aldrich, AUSTRALIA).

Skin model

NativeSkin® (Genoskin, France) models are ex vivo punch biopsies of normal human skin embedded in a matrix and fixed in a cell culture insert. Twelve skin models were generated from non-sun exposed skin of a donor. The skin biopsies were reported as clear of any lesions. Informed consent from donors and ethics approval was obtained for commercialisation and experimental use of the skin biopsies.

UVB radiation and heat exposure

A UV cabinet fitted with a TL20W/01 RS SLV Narrowband UVB lamp (Philips, GERMANY), with a spectral output between 305–315 nm, was used to administer UVB irradiation at a dose of 1 kJ/m^2. Cells were covered with a thin layer of pre-warmed PBS (37 °C) and ex vivo skins were maintained in their nourishing matrix during the irradiation process. PBS was removed and replaced with culture immediately following UVB exposure. Heat stress involved culture in a normal CO_2 incubator, with temperature maintained at 39 °C for three hours. The temperature used in the experiments was based on previous measurements of skin surface temperature of miners, who are prone to intense heat stress, in the Pilbara region of Western Australia (unpublished data). For UVB *plus* heat exposures, cells and skin models were exposed to 1 kJ/m^2 of UVB followed by 3 h of heat stress (39 °C) once per day, for four consecutive days. Cell proliferation, apoptosis and whole genome expression profiles were analysed two days after the last exposure.

To analyse proliferation and apoptosis, primary keratinocytes at passage 4–6 were seeded in a 6-well plate at 200,000 cells/well, and in LabTek Chambered Microscopic slides (Thermofisher, AUSTRALIA) at 100,000 cells/well for immunocytochemistry analysis. Cells were at 50 % confluence at the point of first UVB and/or heat exposures. Each experiment was performed in triplicate and each set of experiments included untreated cells which underwent similar handling.

For the skin model experiments, NativeSkin® was placed in a 6-well plate provided with media and then incubated overnight prior to initial UVB and/or heat exposures. Experiments were performed in duplicate. Untreated skins underwent similar processing and handling to the treated skins but were not exposed to any UVB radiation and were kept at 37 °C throughout the experiments. These samples were considered experimental controls.

Cell count and apoptosis assay – NHEK

Treated primary NHEK cells were trypsinised two days post UVB and/or heat exposure, centrifuged at 300 g for 5 min, resuspended in 500 μL media, and counted in a Vi-Cell™ Viability Analyser (Beckman-Coulter). The level of apoptosis for exposed primary cells was determined using Annexin V-FITC Apoptosis Detection Kit I (BD Pharmingen, USA) and cells were stained as per the manufacturer's instructions. Samples were analysed using the Gallios™ flow cytometer (Beckman-Coulter). For each sample, 10,000 events were acquired. Annexin $V^{+}PI^{-}$cells represented early apoptotic populations and Annexin $V^{+}PI^{+}$ cells represented either late apoptotic or secondary necrotic populations.

Immunohistochemistry – skin proliferation and apoptosis

For immunohistochemistry, the formalin-fixed paraffin-embedded (FFPE) skin tissues were de-waxed at 58 °C for 20 min, and deparaffinised with xylene and hydrated with a graded series of ethanol. Sections were microwaved for 15 min in sodium citrate buffer for antigen retrieval, permeabilised with 0.025 % Triton-X, blocked with 1 % BSA in TBS and incubated with antibodies either thymine dimer/cyclobutane pyrimidine dimer (CPD) (mouse monoclonal, 1:500 dilution; Kamiya Biomedical, USA), active-caspase-3 (rabbit monoclonal, 1:50 dilution; Abcam, USA), p53 antibody (rabbit monoclonal, 1:50 dilution; Abcam, USA), acetylated p53-382 (rabbit polyclonal, 1:250 dilution, Abcam, USA), SIRT1 (mouse monoclonal, 1:250 dilution, Abcam, USA) or SIRT1-p (rabbit monoclonal, 1:250). Anti-pan-cytokeratin (mouse monoclonal 1:50; Abcam, USA) was used to label keratinocytes. Anti-mouse Alexa Fluor 550 and anti-rabbit Alexa Fluor 488 secondary antibodies were used for detection. The stained tissues were mounted using Prolong Gold Mounting media with DAPI.

To determine percentages of keratinocytes positive for certain markers, three sections, which are considered as experimental triplicates, were analysed per biological duplicate (n=2 × 3-sections) and five random fields-of-view were quantified to generate a value of positive cells per section. The number of cells in each of the 6 sections were analysed for standard errors.

Ex vivo gene expression analysis

RNA was isolated from skin tissues using an AllPrep RNA/DNA Mini Kit (SABioscience, AUSTRALIA). RNA extracted from samples was sent to the Australian Genome Research Facility (Melbourne, Australia) where it was reversed transcribed to cDNA and hybridised to the Human HT-12 Expression v4 BeadChip (Illumina, USA) for whole genome expression profiling. This microarray targets 47,231 probes derived from genes in the NCBI RefSeq database. The relative expression of each gene was calculated as fold-change and p-value relative to untreated tissue using R version 3.1.1. Ingenuity Pathway Analysis (IPA) (Qiagen, USA) annotated the effects of altered gene expression on cell function and upstream signalling pathways. Significant transcription regulators and cellular functions were identified as enriched and significant using fold changes and p-values.

Statistical analyses

Two-way ANOVA was used to analyse differences across treatment groups, while parametric unpaired t-tests were used to detect differences between specific treatment groups in all experimental categories, i.e. proliferation, apoptosis and gene expression, with p-values <0.05 considered significant.

Results

UVB *plus* heat exposed keratinocytes exhibit persistent DNA damage but significantly less apoptosis in vitro

We first examined the presence of DNA damage in UVB and/or heat exposed keratinocytes by labelling the DNA with anti-thymine dimer antibody (CPD). The number of DNA damaged cells (CPD-positive keratinocytes) was calculated as a percentage of the total number of keratinocytes per field of view (representative pictures of the IHC staining for each sample are shown in Figure S1). None of the untreated cells had detectable CPD, while 26 ± 7 % (mean ± SD) of heat treated keratinocytes had DNA damage (Fig. 1a). By contrast, 83 ± 9 % and 72 ± 5 % of keratinocytes showed DNA damage in UVB and UVB *plus* heat treated samples respectively, which was significantly greater than the number of CPD-positive cells in heat exposed keratinocytes ($p \leq 0.001$for both).

We next quantified the number of cells surviving after multiple exposures to UVB and/or heat, and also determined what proportion of these were apoptotic and/or necrotic cells (Fig. 1b and Table S1). Heat treated keratinocytes had a slightly higher cell count (5.4×10^{6}) and higher percentage of apoptotic cells (9 ± 4 %) than untreated cells (4×10^{6} and 7 ± 3 % respectively). By

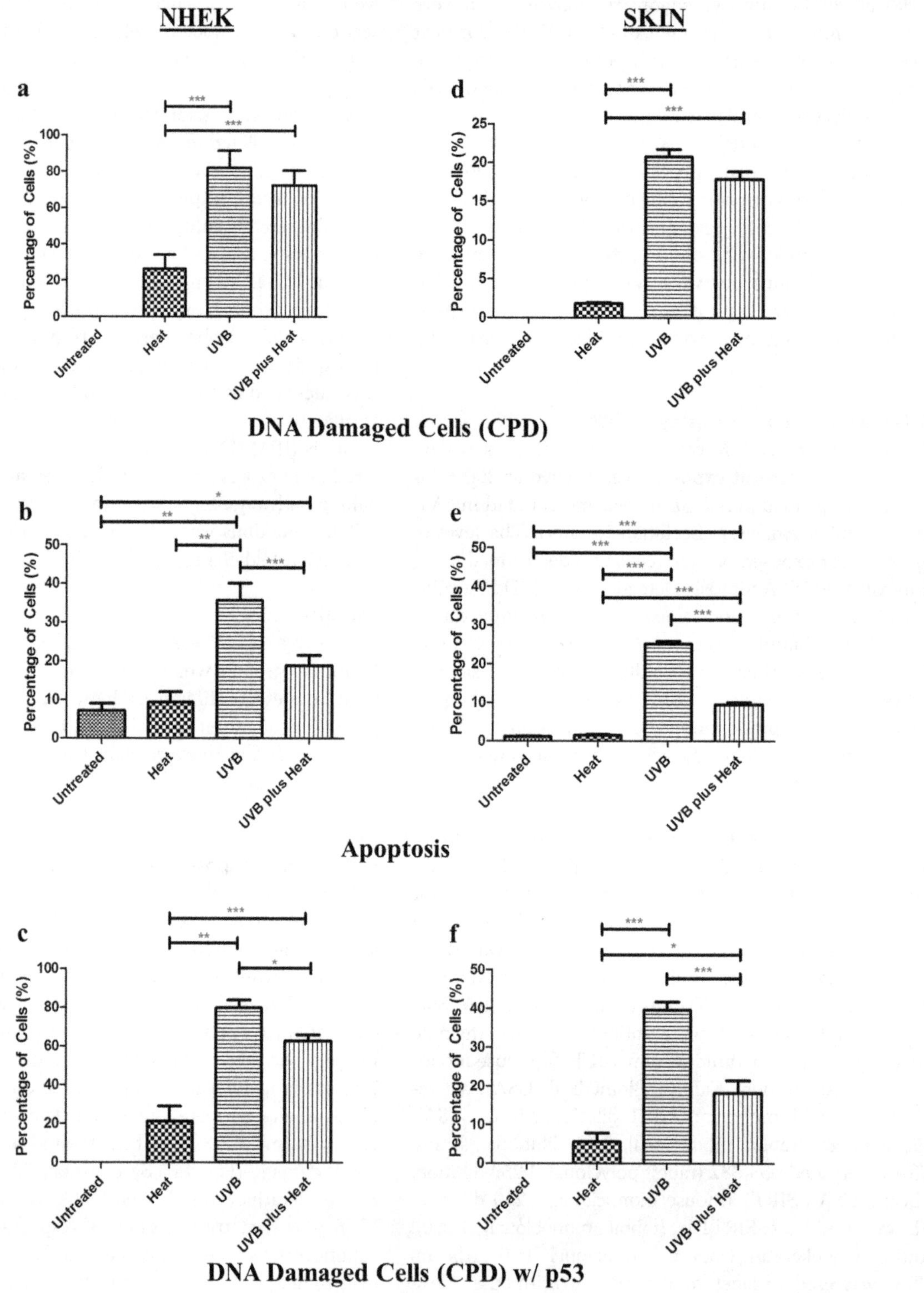

Fig. 1 Effects of UVB and/or heat stress on DNA damage and apoptosis in keratinocytes in vitro and in an ex vivo skin model. Bar graphs of mean ± SD percent keratinocytes that (a and d) harboured DNA damage (CPD), (b and e) were apoptotic, or (c and f) harboured DNA damage and expressed p53 in (**a**–**c**) NHEK or (**d**–**f**) skin per field of view. Statistically significant differences are indicated with *, ** or *** for *p*-values <0.05, <0.01 or ≤0.001 respectively

contrast, UVB treated cells had the lowest cell count (1.15×10^6), with significantly higher number of necrotic (50 ± 4 %) and apoptotic (35 ± 8 %) cells relative to untreated (p=0.004) or heat treated (p=0.02) samples. Remarkably, UVB *plus* heat treated keratinocytes exhibited a higher cell count (2.25×10^6) and significantly reduced numbers of necrotic (23 ± 5 %, p=0.04) and apoptotic cells (19 ± 4 %, $p \leq 0.001$) relative to those treated with UVB alone. Thus, heat appears to diminish the level of cell death induced by UV irradiation. Overall, these results show that multiple consecutive exposures to UVB followed immediately by heat stress reduce apoptosis and necrosis, and increases survival of keratinocytes.

Primary keratinocytes treated with UVB *plus* heat showed diminished p53 response in vitro

We then assessed the presence of p53 in keratinocytes showing persistent DNA damage, to determine the efficiency of the cellular stress response in these cells (Fig. 1c). The number of p53/CPD-positive keratinocytes was calculated as a percentage of the total number of CPD-positive keratinocytes per field of view. In the heat treated samples, approximately 21 ± 8 % of CPD positive cells were also p53 positive. By contrast, 83 ± 6 % of CPD-positive keratinocytes in UVB irradiated samples expressed p53, confirming that repeated UVB treatment activates this cellular stress response [6]. Interestingly, despite having similar numbers of CPD positive cells as UVB exposed cells, only 63 ± 4 % of UVB *plus* heat treated cells were p53-positive, which was significantly lower than that of UVB irradiated samples (p=0.01).

UVB *plus* heat exposure induced DNA damage but lower numbers of apoptotic keratinocytes in an ex vivo skin model

Given the observed changes in apoptosis and cell survival after UVB *plus* heat stress in primary NHEK cells in vitro, we next examined if similar effects were induced in these cells in an ex vivo human skin model. As in the in vitro experiments, we first looked at the level of DNA damage and apoptosis in exposed skin samples by labelling with antibodies to CPD (Fig. 1d). Untreated skins were found to be negative for CPD, while 2 ± 1 % of heat treated epidermal keratinocytes had DNA damage. After multiple exposures, UVB and UVB *plus* heat treated epidermal keratinocytes had significantly higher numbers of cells with DNA damage, at 23 ± 1 % and 18 ± 2 % respectively (p=0.001 for both).

To determine the level of apoptosis after several exposures to UVB and/or heat, we labelled epidermal keratinocytes with cleaved (active) caspase-3 protein, a marker of apoptosis (Fig. 1e). Approximately 1 ± 1 % of keratinocytes were apoptotic in both the untreated and heat treated skins. As expected, UVB irradiated skins showed a significant increase ($p \leq 0.001$) in the number of apoptotic keratinocytes (24 ± 1 %) relative to untreated and heat treated samples. UVB *plus* heat treated skins had significantly less apoptotic keratinocytes (9 ± 1 %) than UVB irradiated samples ($p \leq 0.001$), suggesting possible impairment of apoptosis response mechanisms in UVB *plus* heat treated skin samples, as observed in NHEK cells in vitro.

UVB *plus* heat exposure diminished cellular stress responses in DNA damaged epidermal keratinocytes

We next assessed the presence of p53 in epidermal cells with DNA damage to determine the efficiency of the cellular stress response in these cells (Fig. 1f). In the heat treated skins, among the 2 ± 1 % CPD-positive cells, approximately 5 ± 6 % were p53 positive. By contrast, 39 ± 2 % of CPD-positive keratinocytes in UVB irradiated samples expressed p53, suggesting that significantly higher proportions of damaged cells have an active cellular stress response, even at 2 days after multiple exposures. Interestingly, and as observed in vitro, the percentage of p53-positive keratinocytes with DNA damage (18 ± 3 %) was significantly lower in UV *plus* heat treated skins than in UV irradiated samples (p=0.006). These results suggest that the efficiency of the p53-mediated apoptosis response to DNA damage is diminished when UVB treatment is followed by heat exposure.

UVB and UVB *plus* heat differentially affect expression of the genes involved in proliferation/survival and apoptosis in epidermal keratinocytes

To further understand the observed effects of multiple exposures to UVB *plus* heat and to characterise molecular events that govern such changes, we analysed the whole genome expression profiles of the exposed skin samples. Gene expression fold changes and p-values were calculated for each sample relative to untreated controls and considered significant when fold changes were ≥2 or <0.5 relative to untreated control samples and p-values were <0.05. Heat treated skin samples had only 7 significantly differentially expressed genes relative to controls. By contrast, UVB irradiated skins had 629 differentially expressed genes, while UVB *plus* heat treated samples had 4966.

In order to determine the biological significance of the observed changes in gene expression, we reviewed the data through the use of Ingenuity Pathway Analysis (IPA) software (Table S2). Due to the low number of affected genes, the functional annotations observed in heat treated samples were not significant. UVB irradiated skin samples showed significant upregulation of apoptosis related genes ($p \leq 0.001$) and a significant downregulation of genes involved in cell viability ($p \leq 0.001$) relative to untreated samples. Notably, UVB *plus* heat treated samples showed a significant downregulation in the expression of genes associated with apoptosis ($p \leq 0.001$), as well as an increase in expression of cell viability (p=0.001) and mismatch repair of DNA (p=0.004) related genes.

We next focused on 28 genes found to be the most differentially expressed and associated with the functional pathways highlighted above. Hierarchical clustering of these genes revealed a clear segregation between UVB and UVB *plus* heat treated samples, and two distinct groups of genes became apparent (Fig. 2). Group 1 consisted of

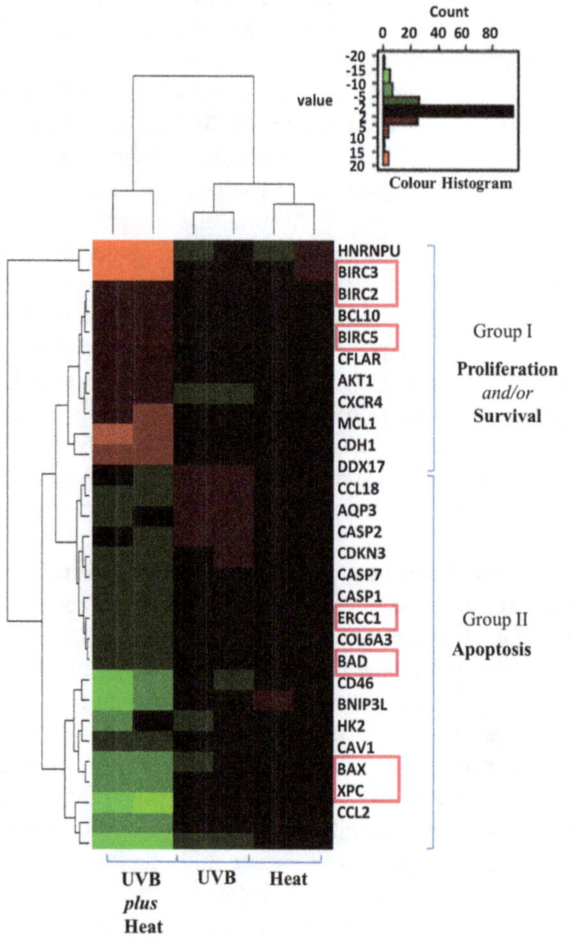

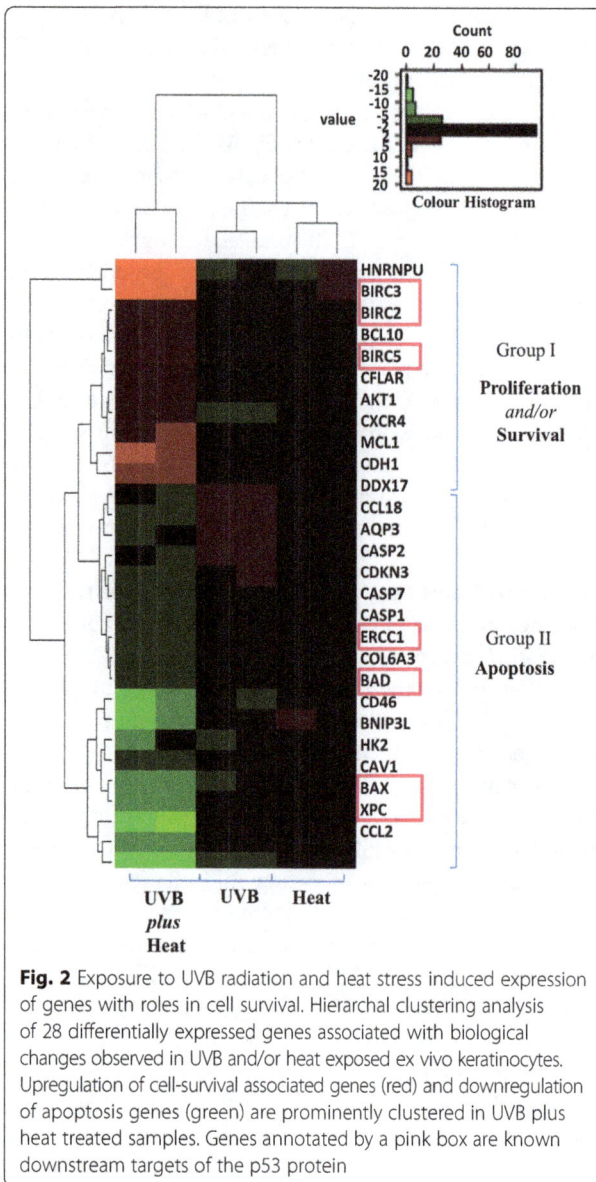

Fig. 2 Exposure to UVB radiation and heat stress induced expression of genes with roles in cell survival. Hierarchal clustering analysis of 28 differentially expressed genes associated with biological changes observed in UVB and/or heat exposed ex vivo keratinocytes. Upregulation of cell-survival associated genes (red) and downregulation of apoptosis genes (green) are prominently clustered in UVB plus heat treated samples. Genes annotated by a pink box are known downstream targets of the p53 protein

cluster of genes associated with the regulation of cell apoptosis, such as BAX and BAD, as well as DNA repair, such as XPC and ERCC1. These genes were downregulated in UVB *plus* heat but were either less affected or upregulated in UVB alone. By contrast, Group 2 was formed by genes associated with proliferation and survival pathways, particularly BIRC2, BIRC3 and survivin (BIRC5). These genes were upregulated in UVB *plus* heat but not affected or downregulated in UVB treated samples.

Upstream regulatory factors important for cell survival are activated by UVB *plus* heat

Using IPA upstream analysis, we then examined the activity of key transcription factors and signalling pathways that govern cell apoptosis, survival and proliferation to determine if these were significantly affected. In particular, we looked for factors that would affect the observed gene expression changes in the activity of TP53, given its role in cell cycle regulation, apoptosis and DNA repair as well as the fact that damaged keratinocytes in UVB *plus* heat treated skins showed persistent significantly lower levels of p53 protein.

As expected, UVB exposed samples showed significant activation of cell cycle arrest and pro-apoptotic transcription regulators, particularly TP53 and CDKN1A (Table 1). By comparison, in UVB *plus* heat treated samples, TP53 activity was significantly reduced ($p \leq 0.001$) and no upregulation of CDKN1A activity was apparent. In addition, classical upstream regulators of survival such as NFkB, ERK, PI3K and Akt were significantly inhibited in UVB exposed skin samples, but were not similarly affected in UVB *plus* heat. Likewise, HSF-1 was found highly activated only in UVB *plus* heat treated samples. We did not, however, observe HSF-1 activity after heat treatment alone; previous literature suggests that this gene is only upregulated at time points early after heat treatment [33]. Thus, consecutive exposure to UVB *plus* heat may have an enhanced effect on the activity of HSF-1 such that its activation was still apparent when measured 2 days after multiple consecutive treatments as performed in these experiments. Overall, our functional and upstream analysis confirms that cell cycle arrest and pro-apoptotic signalling were reduced after consecutive UVB and heat exposure, while proliferation and survival signalling were upregulated.

UVB *plus* heat induced upregulation of SIRT1 protein and a significant decrease in acetylated p53 in NHEK cells in vitro and in the skin models

SIRT1 is known to deacetylate p53 at lysine residue K382 of its c-terminal domain, which can diminish the ability of p53 to act as transcriptional modulator of its downstream gene targets [34–37]. We also observed persistent significant activation of histone deacetylases, particularly SIRT1, in our IPA analysis results (Table 1). Thus, we hypothesised that heat-induced interference in p53 signalling may be due to SIRT1-mediated deacetylation of p53.

Of note, phosphorylation of SIRT1 is important for the activation, stability and deacetylase function of the protein. Therefore, first we quantified the number of CPD containing keratinocytes that were positive for total (SIRT1) and phosphorylated SIRT1 (SIRT1-p) in vitro and in the skin model. We show that in fact all SIRT1 positive cells had the phosphorylated form of the protein in heat and UVB *plus* heat treated samples (Figure S2).

We, therefore, next assessed the number of CPD positive cells with p53 acetylated at lysine 382 (p53-a382). The number of p53-a382/CPD or SIRT1-p/CPD positive keratinocytes was calculated as a percentage of the total number of CPD-positive keratinocytes per field of view (Fig. 3).

Table 1 Upstream regulators significantly activated in UVB *plus* heat

Upstream regulators	z score *(p value)*		Function	Reference
	UVB	UVB *plus* Heat		
Pro-apoptotic signalling				
TP53	3.25 *(4×10^{-6})*	-2.04 *(3.8×10^{-14})*	Cell arrest and/or apoptosis	[8, 52]
CDKN1A	2.60 *(5×10^{-9})*		Inhibit cell proliferation and cell cycle progression	[53]
Proliferation and Survival				
NFkB (complex)	-2.87 *(2×10^{-4})*	-1.34 *(1×10^{-2})*	Cell survival	[54]
ERK	-2.42 *(7×10^{-3})*	-1.77 *(1×10^{-3})*	Cell survival and proliferation	[55, 56]
PI3K (complex)	-2.19 *(3×10^{-3})*	-0.69 *(1×10^{-2})*	Cell survival and proliferation	[57, 58]
Akt	-1.99 *(7×10^{-2})*		Cell survival and proliferation	[59, 60]
Others				
HSF-1		1.98 *(2×10^{-8})*	Heat shock response regulator	[37, 61]
SIRT1		2.16 *(8×10^{-4})*	Cell proliferation and protection	[40]
Hdac (Histone deacetylases)		3.36 (2×10^{-2})	p53 deacetylation and inhibition of nuclear translocation	[39, 62, 63]

There was no CPD or acetylated p53 protein staining observed in the untreated primary NHEK cells in vitro (Figure S3). In the heat treated samples, only a small percentage (4 ± 1 %) of CPD-positive keratinocytes were positive for p53 acetylation in vitro (Fig. 3b), and none of the damaged cells were positive for acetylated p53 in skin keratinocytes (Fig. 3c). By contrast, 33 ± 2 % of damaged keratinocytes in UVB *plus* heat treated NHEK in vitro showed significantly lower p53 acetylation than in NHEK irradiated with UVB alone (79 ± 10 %, p=0.01). Similarly, in the skin models, DNA-damaged keratinocytes of the UVB *plus* heat treated samples showed significantly lower levels of acetylated p53 (10 ± 3 %) relative to UVB irradiated samples (68 ± 2 %, p=0.02).

Interestingly, in the heat treated samples, 93 ± 10 % of CPD-positive cells were positive for SIRT1-p in vitro (Fig. 3d), and all damaged cells showed SIRT1-p in the skin models (Fig. 3e). By contrast, 54 ± 5 % and 57 ± 5 % of damaged cells in UVB *plus* heat treated cells showed SIRT1-p protein, in vitro and in skin samples respectively. There was no SIRT1-p staining noted in UVB exposed cells. Noticeably, there was an overall negative relationship between the number of SIRT1-p/CPD positive cells and the number of acetylated p53/CPD positive cells in UVB *plus* heat treated samples. These results suggest that exposure to heat stress, in addition to UV, significantly inactivates p53 via SIRT1-mediated deacetylation of this protein.

Discussion

In this study, we showed that the response to UVB-mediated cellular damage is diminished in the presence of heat and, for the first time, provide a molecular mechanism that explains these effects. NHEK cells in vitro and ex vivo epidermal keratinocytes that were repeatedly irradiated with UVB showed higher level of cellular damage and significant activation of cellular stress responses and pro-apoptotic signalling, evident by p53 activation and the high level of caspase-3, a protease involved in apoptosis of damaged cells [38–41], even at two days post-exposure. By contrast, keratinocytes with multiple heat and UVB exposures exhibited significant inactivation of the p53-mediated stress response and showed reduced numbers of apoptotic and necrotic cells at similar time point. Moreover, we show that SIRT1-mediated deacetylation of p53 is a possible mediator of these effects.

Previous studies have shown that singular pre-treatment with heat stress (38-41 °C), prior to UVB (290–320 nm) exposure, increases viability and decreases thymine dimer formation in murine and human keratinocytes, suggesting heat-mediated protection of UVB-damaged keratinocytes [27–30]. By contrast, we found that with repeated exposure to UVB and high temperature, heat did not reduce DNA damage (presence of CPDs) but rather promoted the survival of keratinocytes containing these UVB-induced DNA lesions. Moreover, our results show that persistent heat-mediated survival and reduction of cell arrest, apoptosis and necrosis of damaged keratinocytes in UVB *plus* heat treated samples appears to be mediated by inactivation of p53 signalling.

The p53 protein is an important transcription factor involved in maintaining genome integrity upon exposure to UV, either by enforcing a G1 cell cycle arrest, inducing apoptosis or enhancing nuclear excision repair of damaged cells [6, 42]. While gene expression of TP53 was not significantly affected or the mRNA level reduced after multiple UVB and heat exposures,

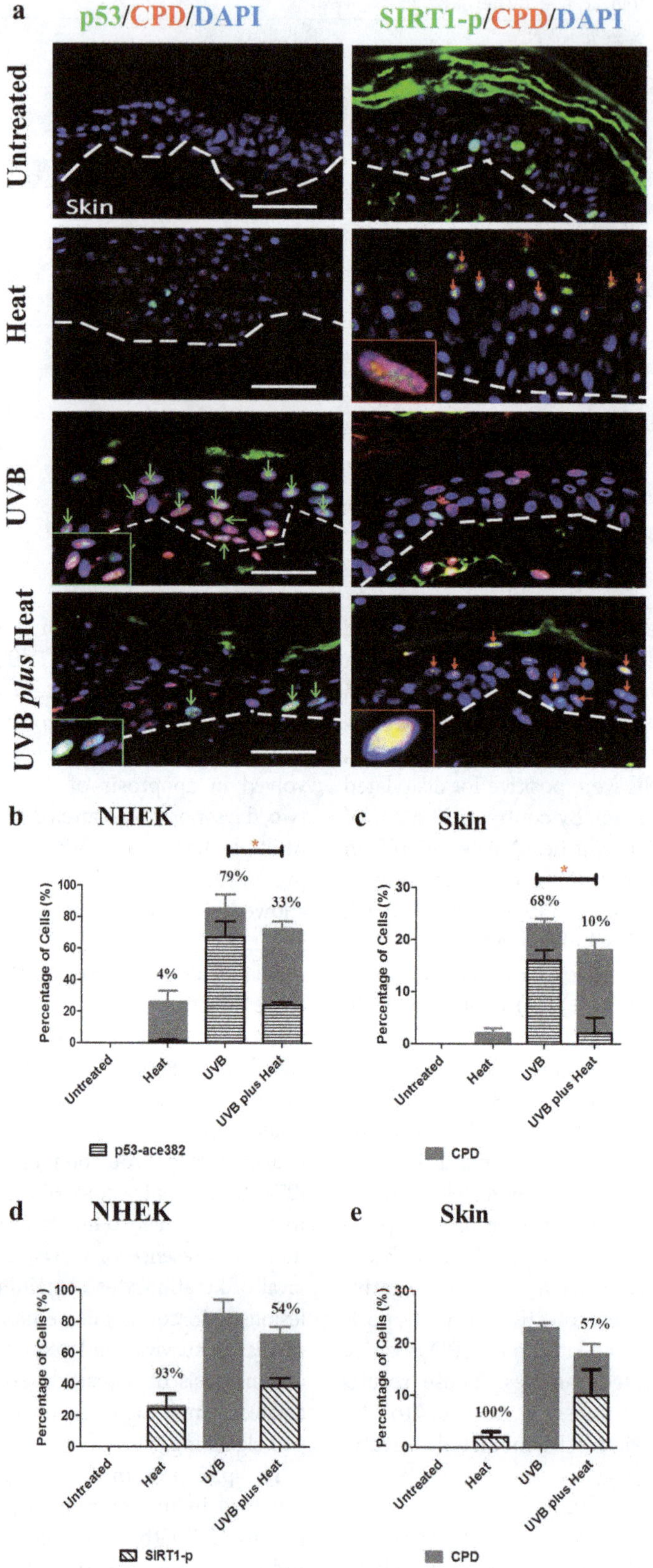

Fig. 3 (See legend on next page.)

(See figure on previous page.)
Fig. 3 Exposure to UVB plus heat induced a significant decrease in acetylated p53 and an increase in SIRT1 protein levels in NHEK and in skin models. **a** Immunohistochemical staining of CPD (red), p53-a382 or SIRT1-p (green) and DAPI (blue) in untreated or UVB and/or heat treated ex vivo skin keratinocytes. Inset images are an enlarged view of SIRT1/DNA damaged (CPD positive) keratinocytes, which are also indicated by red arrows. Broken lines denote the epidermal/dermal border. Scale bar (white line) =100 μm. **b–e** Bar graphs of mean ± SD percent keratinocytes with CPD and positive for (**b** and **c**) p53-a382 or (**d** and **e**) SIRT1-p per field of view in (**b** and **d**) primary NHEK or (**c** and **e**) in skin models. Statistically significant differences are indicated with * for *p*-values <0.05

the expression levels of the majority of its downstream gene targets, particularly BAX and survivin, were consistent with inactivation of the p53 protein. As transcription of BAX and survivin is regulated via binding of p53 to their promoters [43, 44], this set of results suggests possible impairment of the DNA-binding capability of p53.

We also noted a significant activation of SIRT1 in UVB *plus* heat treated samples. The number of damaged cells with phosphorylated SIRT1 protein corresponded to the number of damaged cells that were negative for p53 acetylation at K382 in UVB *plus* heat treated samples. Thus, inactivation of p53 signalling, observed after multiple exposures to UVB and heat, may be attributed to the SIRT1-mediated post-translational modification of the p53 protein. SIRT1 is a histone deacetylase that can deacetylate p53 and significantly reduce its DNA binding capability, which can lead to deregulation of p53 dependent genes [8, 36, 45, 46]. It is important to note that SIRT1 activity is downregulated by UV [47, 48], but is consistently increased after heat shock [34–36]. Thus, heat stress may activate SIRT1 in damaged cells, which leads to deacetylation and inactivation of p53, and diminishing the capacity of the p53 protein to bind and regulate transcription of its downstream target genes.

The discrepancy between our findings and previous studies is likely a result of the differences in the exposure models. It is important to note that previous studies adhered to a single heat-then-UVB exposure experimental protocol, with a four-hour interval between heat and UVB exposures [28, 49, 50]. Pre-treatment to heat stress prior to UVB irradiation was shown to activate the heat shock response and increase expression of HSP70 protein in keratinocytes [17, 51], and thus these cells were thought to have been provided with a pre-established protective mechanism against UVB-induced DNA damage. By contrast, our study was based on repeated UVB and heat exposures, with heat exposure following immediately after UVB. In the environment, UVB and heat stress often occur concurrently and can, therefore, synchronously affect epidermal cells. Thus, the exposure model used here may have affected the ability of keratinocytes to mount an appropriate response to UVB-mediated DNA damage, presumably via impairment of p53-mediated cell apoptosis. In addition, the use of narrowband UVB instead of broadband UVB lamps may have contributed to the different factors activated in keratinocytes as a result of UVB *plus* heat exposure. This study was originally conceptualised to determine if extreme heat, in addition to UV, can have major effects on epidermal cell biology. Narrowband UVB was used in this study as it has previously been shown to induce higher frequency of skin cancer in mice [52], and thus was more fitting in creating an exposure model where the consequent UV- and/or temperature-induced damage are high.

Nevertheless, further studies are required to establish direct association between p53 and SIRT1 activity in UVB *plus* heat treated cells. In this study, we were particularly interested in the overall and persistent effects of repeated UVB *plus* heat, in order to assess potential outcomes of these exposures. To better define the pathways directly involved in UVB *plus* heat-mediated cell survival, molecular mechanisms need to be assessed at earlier stages of the cellular stress response. In addition, while the use of ex vivo skin preserved the close interaction of keratinocytes and melanocytes as an epidermal-melanin unit, which ensures protection against UVB and other stressors [53], and provided for accurate measures of clinically relevant changes in keratinocytes after UVB and/or heat exposures, this study was largely disadvantaged by small sample size. This limitation will also need to be addressed in future studies in order to concretely define the effects of UV and heat exposure on keratinocyte biology, particularly in defining heat-induced alterations in the genetic or molecular profiles of these cells.

Conclusions

In conclusion, this study showed for the first time that multiple exposures to heat stress, in addition to UVB, prevents DNA-damaged human keratinocytes from undergoing apoptosis, as a result of inactivation of the p53 function. The results suggest that exposure to UVB and heat stress may act synergistically to allow survival of damaged cells, which could have implications for initiation of skin carcinogenesis. Knowledge of the effects of UVB *plus* heat stress on skin carcinogenesis can be utilised to decrease risk exposures particularly for people exposed to combinations of these environmental hazards in workplaces such as the mining, construction and petroleum industries.

Additional files

Additional file 1: Figure S1. Immunohistochemical staining of cytokeratin (CytoK) or CPD (red), p53 or active caspase-3 (green) and DAPI (blue) in untreated or UVB and/or heat treated NHEK or ex vivo skin. Inset images are an enlarged view of CPD/p53 positive and CytoK/Casp-3 cells. Arrows indicate cells expressing CPD/p53 (orange) and CytoK/Casp-3 (white). H and E staining of untreated or UVB and/or heat treated ex vivo skin. Broken lines denote the epidermal/dermal border. Scale bar (white line) =100 μm. (JPG 713 kb)

Additional file 2: Figure S2. (a) Immunohistochemical staining of SIRT1-p (green), total SIRT1 (red) and DAPI (nucleus, blue) in skin samples or primary keratinocytes that were either untreated, or exposed to heat, UVB or UVB plus heat. Broken lines denote the epidermal/dermal border. Scale bar (white line) =100 μm. Inset images are enlarged view of SIRT1/SIRT1-p positive cells, which are also indicated by red arrows. (b) Bar graphs of mean ± SD percent keratinocytes carrying phosphorylated and normal SIRT1 protein in ex vivo skin. (JPG 367 kb)

Additional file 3: Figure S3. Exposure to UVB plus heat induced a significant decrease in acetylated p53 levels in NHEK and in skin models. Immunohistochemical staining of CPD (red), p53-a382 or SIRT1-p (green) and DAPI (blue) in untreated or UVB and/or heat treated NHEK. Cells co-expressing p53-a382/CPD are also indicated by green arrows. Scale bar (white line) =100 μm. (JPG 304 kb)

Abbreviations
CPD, cyclobutane pyrimidine dimers; IPA, ingenuity pathway analysis; NHEK, primary normal human epidermal keratinocytes.

Acknowledgments
We extend our thanks to Dr David Raven of Saint John of God Hospital Pathology Department and Miss Christie Chee of Clinipath for advice and assistance with tissue sections. We also thank A/Prof Jacques Oosthuizen and Dr Joe Mates from Edith Cowan University for the data on surface skin temperature of miners in WA, the ECU Melanoma Research team for assistance, and special thanks to Ms Sophie Zeigler for assistance with statistical analysis of gene expression data.

Funding
This study was funded by Edith Cowan University.

Authors' contributions
LC, EG and MZ participated in the study design, analysis of the results and wrote the manuscript. SK, AD and PD provided the skin models and made helpful suggestions to the manuscript. PH contributed to the study design. All authors read and approved the final manuscript.

Competing interests
We certify that there is no conflict of interest with any organisation, financial or otherwise, regarding the material discussed in this manuscript.

Author details
[1]School of Medical Sciences, Edith Cowan University, 270 Joondalup Drive, Joondalup, Perth, WA 6027, Australia. [2]GENOSKIN Centre Pierre Potier, Oncopole, Toulouse, France. [3]Department of Pathology and Laboratory Medicine, University of Western Australia, Crawley, WA, Australia. [4]Telethon Kids Institute, University of Western Australia, 100 Roberts Road, Subiaco, Perth 6008, Australia.

References
1. D'Costa AM, Denning MF. A caspase-resistant mutant of PKC-delta protects keratinocytes from UV-induced apoptosis. Cell Death Differ. 2005;12(3):224–32.
2. Matsunaga T, Hieda K, Nikaido O. Wavelength dependent formation of thymine dimers and (6–4) photoproducts in DNA by monochromatic ultraviolet light ranging from 150 to 365 nm. Photochem Photobiol. 1991;54(3):403–10.
3. Besarutinia A, Bates SE, Synold TW, Pfeifer GP. Similar mutagenecity of photoactivated porphyrins and ultraviolet a radiation in mouse embryonic fibroblasts: involvement of oxidative lesions in mutagenesis. Biochemistry. 2004;43:15557–66.
4. Brash DE. Roles of the transcription factor p53 in keratinocyte carcinomas. Br J Dermatol. 2006;154 Suppl 1:8–10.
5. Terzian T, Torchia E, Dai D, Robinson S, Murao K, Steigman R, Gonzalez V, Boyle G, Powell M, Pollock P et al. p53 prevents progression of nevi to melanoma predominantly through cell cycle regulation. Pigment Cell Melanoma Res. 2010;23:781–94.
6. Ozaki T, Nakagawara A. Role of p53 in cell death and human cancers. Cancers. 2011;3:994–1013.
7. Benjamin CL, Ullrich SE, Kripke ML, Ananthaswamy HN. p53 tumor suppressor gene: a critical molecular target for UV induction and prevention of skin cancer. Photochem Photobiol. 2008;84(1):55–62.
8. Beckerman R, Prives C. Transcriptional regulation by p53. Cold Spring Harb Perspect Biol. 2010;2(8):a000935.
9. Lindahl T, Nyberg B. Heat-induced deamination of cytosine residues in deoxyribonucleic acid. Biochemistry. 1974;13(16):3405–10.
10. Poltev VI, Shulyupina NV, Bruskov VI. The formation of mispairs by 8-oxyguanine as a pathway of mutations induced by irradiation and oxygen radicals. J Mol Recognit. 1990;3(1):45–7.
11. Bruskov VI, Malakhova LV, Masalimov ZK, Chernikov AV. Heat-induced formation of reactive oxygen species and 8-oxoguanine, a biomarker of damage to DNA. Nucleic Acids Res. 2002;30(6):1354–63.
12. Smirnova VS, Gudkov SV, Chernikov AV, Bruskov VI. [The formation of 8-oxoguanine and its oxidative products in DNA in vitro at 37 degrees C]. Biofizika. 2005;50(2):243–52.
13. Takahashi A, Matsumoto H, Nagayama K, Kitano M, Hirose S, Tanaka H, Mori E, Yamakawa N, Yasumoto J, Yuki K et al. Evidence for the involvement of double-strand breaks in heat-induced cell killing. Cancer Res. 2004; 64(24):8839–45.
14. Ehrlich M, Norris KF, Wang RY, Kuo KC, Gehrke CW. DNA cytosine methylation and heat-induced deamination. Biosci Rep. 1986;6(4):387–93.
15. Chinnathambi S, Tomanek-Chalkley A, Bickenbach JR. HSP70 and EndoG modulate cell death by heat in human skin keratinocytes in vitro. Cells Tissues Organs. 2008;187(2):131–40.
16. Bivik C, Rosdahl I, Ollinger K. Hsp70 protects against UVB induced apoptosis by preventing release of cathepsins and cytochrome c in human melanocytes. Carcinogenesis. 2007;28(3):537–44.
17. Roti Roti JL. Heat-induced alterations of nuclear protein associations and their effects on DNA repair and replication. Int J Hyperthermia. 2007;23(1):3–15.
18. Wong RS, Kapp LN, Krishnaswamy G, Dewey WC. Critical steps for induction of chromosomal aberrations in CHO cells heated in S phase. Radiat Res. 1993;133(1):52–9.
19. Hunt CR, Pandita RK, Laszlo A, Higashikubo R, Agarwal M, Kitamura T, Gupta A, Rief N, Horikoshi N, Baskaran R et al. Hyperthermia activates a subset of ataxia-telangiectasia mutated effectors independent of DNA strand breaks and heat shock protein 70 status. Cancer Res. 2007;67(7):3010–7.
20. De Maio A. Heat shock proteins: facts, thoughts, and dreams. Shock. 1999;11(1):1–12.
21. De Maio A. Extracellular heat shock proteins, cellular export vesicles, and the stress observation system: a form of communication during injury, infection, and cell damage. It is never known how far a controversial finding will go! dedicated to Ferruccio Ritossa. Cell Stress Chaperones. 2011;16(3):235–49.
22. Dai C, Dai S, Cao J. Proteotoxic stress of cancer: implication of the heat-shock response in oncogenesis. J Cell Physiol. 2012;227(8):2982–7.
23. Akerfelt M, Trouillet D, Mezger V, Sistonen L. Heat shock factors at a crossroad between stress and development. Ann N Y Acad Sci. 2007;1113:15–27.

24. Echchgadda I, Roth CC, Cerna CZ, Wilmink GJ. Temporal gene expression kinetics for human keratinocytes exposed to hyperthermic stress. Cells. 2013;2(2):224–43.
25. van der Leun JC, Piacentini RD, de Gruijl FR. Climate change and human skin cancer. Photochem Photobiol Sci. 2008;7(6):730–3.
26. Calapre L, Gray ES, Ziman M. Heat stress: a risk factor for skin carcinogenesis. Cancer Lett. 2013;337(1):35–40.
27. Maytin EV. Heat shock proteins and molecular chaperones: implications for adaptive responses in the skin. J Invest Dermatol. 1995;104(4):448–55.
28. Kane KS, Maytin EV. Ultraviolet B-induced apoptosis of keratinocytes in murine skin is reduced by mild local hyperthermia. J Invest Dermatol. 1995;104(1):62–7.
29. Trautinger F, Knobler RM, Honigsmann H, Mayr W, Kindas-Mugge I. Increased expression of the 72-kDa heat shock protein and reduced sunburn cell formation in human skin after local hyperthermia. J Invest Dermatol. 1996;107(3):442–3.
30. Maytin EV, Murphy LA, Merrill MA. Hyperthermia induces resistance to ultraviolet light B in primary and immortalized epidermal keratinocytes. Cancer Res. 1993;53(20):4952–9.
31. Bain JA, Rusch HP, Kline BE. The effect of temperature upon ultraviolet carcinogenesis with wavelengths 2,800-3,400 A. Cancer Res. 1943;3:610–2.
32. Freeman RG, Knox JM. Influence of temperature on ultraviolet injury. Arch Dermatol. 1964;89:858–64.
33. Dai C, Whitesell L, Rogers AB, Lindquist S. Heat shock factor 1 is a powerful multifaceted modifier of carcinogenesis. Cell. 2007;130(6):1005–18.
34. Westerheide SD, Anckar J, Stevens Jr SM, Sistonen L, Morimoto RI. Stress-inducible regulation of heat shock factor 1 by the deacetylase SIRT1. Science. 2009;323(5917):1063–6.
35. Fritah S, Col E, Boyault C, Govin J, Sadoul K, Chiocca S, Christians E, Khochbin S, Jolly C, Vourc'h C. Heat-shock factor 1 controls genome-wide acetylation in heat-shocked cells. Mol Biol Cell. 2009;20(23):4976–84.
36. Raynes R, Pombier KM, Nguyen K, Brunquell J, Mendez JE, Westerheide SD. The SIRT1 modulators AROS and DBC1 regulate HSF1 activity and the heat shock response. PLoS One. 2013;8(1):e54364.
37. Li Y, Matsumori H, Nakayama Y, Osaki M, Kojima H, Kurimasa A, Ito H, Mori S, Katoh M, Oshimura M et al. SIRT2 down-regulation in HeLa can induce p53 accumulation via p38 MAPK activation-dependent p300 decrease, eventually leading to apoptosis. Genes Cells. 2011;16(1):34–45.
38. Bratton SB, Salvesen GS. Regulation of the Apaf-1-caspase-9 apoptosome. J Cell Sci. 2010;123(Pt 19):3209–14.
39. Cagnol S, Mansour A, Van Obberghen-Schilling E, Chambard JC. Raf-1 activation prevents caspase 9 processing downstream of apoptosome formation. J Signal Transduct. 2011;2011:834948.
40. Porter AG, Janicke RU. Emerging roles of caspase-3 in apoptosis. Cell Death Differ. 1999;6(2):99–104.
41. Bushell M, McKendrick L, Janicke RU, Clemens MJ, Morley SJ. Caspase-3 is necessary and sufficient for cleavage of protein synthesis eukaryotic initiation factor 4G during apoptosis. FEBS Lett. 1999;451(3):332–6.
42. Harris SL, Levine AJ. The p53 pathway: positive and negative feedback loops. Oncogene. 2005;24(17):2899–908.
43. Wang Z, Fukuda S, Pelus LM. Survivin regulates the p53 tumor suppressor gene family. Oncogene. 2004;23(49):8146–53.
44. Yi J, Luo J. SIRT1 and p53, effect on cancer, senescence and beyond. Biochim Biophys Acta. 2010;1804(8):1684–9.
45. Yuan J, Luo K, Liu T, Lou Z. Regulation of SIRT1 activity by genotoxic stress. Genes Dev. 2012;26(8):791–6.
46. Lou G, Liu Y, Wu S, Xue J, Yang F, Fu H, Zheng M, Chen Z. The p53/miR-34a/SIRT1 positive feedback loop in quercetin-induced apoptosis. Cell Physiol Biochem. 2015;35(6):2192–202.
47. Cao C, Lu S, Kivlin R, Wallin B, Card E, Bagdasarian A, Tamakloe T, Wang WJ, Song X, Chu WM et al. SIRT1 confers protection against UVB- and H2O2-induced cell death via modulation of p53 and JNK in cultured skin keratinocytes. J Cell Mol Med. 2009;13(9B):3632–43.
48. Chou WW, Chen KC, Wang YS, Wang JY, Liang CL, Juo SH. The role of SIRT1/AKT/ERK pathway in ultraviolet B induced damage on human retinal pigment epithelial cells. Toxicology in vitro. 2013;27(6):1728–36.
49. Jantschitsch C, Kindas-Mugge I, Metze D, Amann G, Micksche M, Trautinger F. Expression of the small heat shock protein HSP 27 in developing human skin. Br J Dermatol. 1998;139(2):247–53.
50. Maytin EV, Wimberly JM, Kane KS. Heat shock modulates UVB-induced cell death in human epidermal keratinocytes: evidence for a hyperthermia-inducible protective response. J Invest Dermatol. 1994;103(4):547–53.
51. Jantschitsch C, Trautinger F. Heat shock and UV-B-induced DNA damage and mutagenesis in skin. Photochem Photobiol Sci. 2003;2(9):899–903.
52. Yogianti F, Kunisada M, Ono R, Sakumi K, Nakabeppu Y, Nishigori C. Skin tumours induced by narrowband UVB have higher frequency of p53 mutations than tumours induced by broadband UVB independent of Ogg1 genotype. Mutagenesis. 2012;27(6):637–43.
53. Costin GE, Hearing VJ. Human skin pigmentation: melanocytes modulate skin color in response to stress. FASEB J. 2007;21(4):976–94.
54. Piva R, Belardo G, Santoro MG. NF-kappaB: a stress-regulated switch for cell survival. Antioxid Redox Signal. 2006;8(3-4):478–86.
55. Pognonec P. ERK and cell death: overview. FEBS J. 2010;277(1):1.
56. von Kriegsheim A, Pitt A, Grindlay GJ, Kolch W, Dhillon AS. Regulation of the Raf-MEK-ERK pathway by protein phosphatase 5. Nat Cell Biol. 2006;8(9):1011–16.
57. Chalhoub N, Baker SJ. PTEN and the PI3-kinase pathway in cancer. Annu Rev Pathol. 2009;4:127–50.
58. Hafner C, Landthaler M, Vogt T. Activation of the PI3K/AKT signalling pathway in non-melanoma skin cancer is not mediated by oncogenic PIK3CA and AKT1 hotspot mutations. Exp Dermatol. 2010;19(8):e222–27.
59. Lee ER, Kim JH, Choi HY, Jeon K, Cho SG. Cytoprotective effect of eriodictyol in UV-irradiated keratinocytes via phosphatase-dependent modulation of both the p38 MAPK and Akt signaling pathways. Cell Physiol Biochem. 2011;27(5):513–24.
60. Dent P. Crosstalk between ERK, AKT, and cell survival. Cancer Biol Ther. 2014;15(3):245–46.
61. Dai C, Santagata S, Tang Z, Shi J, Cao J, Kwon H, Bronson RT, Whitesell L, Lindquist S. Loss of tumor suppressor NF1 activates HSF1 to promote carcinogenesis. J Clin Invest. 2012;122(10):3742–754.
62. Aarenstrup L, Flindt EN, Otkjaer K, Kirkegaard M, Andersen JS, Kristiansen K. HDAC activity is required for p65/RelA-dependent repression of PPARdelta-mediated transactivation in human keratinocytes. J Invest Dermatol. 2008;128(5):1095–106.
63. Place RF, Noonan EJ, Giardina C. HDAC inhibition prevents NF-kappa B activation by suppressing proteasome activity: down-regulation of proteasome subunit expression stabilizes I kappa B alpha. Biochem Pharmacol. 2005;70(3):394–406.

Perinatal probiotic supplementation in the prevention of allergy related disease: 6 year follow up of a randomised controlled trial

Melanie Rae Simpson[1*], Christian Kvikne Dotterud[1,2], Ola Storrø[1], Roar Johnsen[1] and Torbjørn Øien[1]

Abstract

Background: Perinatal probiotics supplementation has been shown to be effective in the primary prevention of atopic dermatitis (AD) in early childhood, although the long term effects of probiotics on AD and other allergic diseases is less certain. We have previously reported a significant reduction in the cumulative incidence of AD at 2 years after maternal probiotic supplementation. In this study we present the effects of perinatal probiotics given to women from a general population on allergy related diseases in their offspring at 6 years.

Methods: Four hundred and fifteen pregnant women were randomised to receive probiotic or placebo milk in a double-blinded trial from 36 week gestation until 3 months postpartum. Probiotic milk contained *Lactobacillus rhamnosos GG, L. acidophilus La-5* and *Bifidobacterium animalis* subsp. *lactis* Bb-12. At 6 years, children were re-assessed for AD, atopic sensitisation, asthma and allergic rhinoconjunctivitis (ARC).

Results: At 6 years, 81 and 82 children were assessed for AD in the probiotic and placebo groups, respectively. In a multiple imputation analysis, there was as trend towards a lower cumulative incidence of AD in the probiotic group compared to the placebo group (OR 0.64, 95 % CI 0.39-1.07, $p = 0.086$; NNT = 10). This finding was statistically significantly in the complete case analysis (OR 0.48, 95 % CI 0.25-0.92, $p = 0.027$, NNT = 6). The prevalence of asthma and atopic sensitisation, and the cumulative incidence of ARC were not significantly affected by the probiotic regime at 6 years of age.

Conclusions: Maternal probiotic ingestion alone may be sufficient for long term reduction in the cumulative incidence of AD, but not other allergy related diseases.

Keywords: Allergy, Asthma, Atopic dermatitis, Paediatrics, Prevention, Probiotics, Rhinitis

Background

Atopic dermatitis (AD), asthma and allergic rhinoconjunctivitis (ARC) are a major cause of chronic disease in childhood. A revised version of the "hygiene hypothesis" suggests that the pattern of colonisation and the diversity of the intestinal microbiota may be an important factor in the increased prevalence of these diseases observed over the past several decades [1–3]. Subsequently, probiotics have been investigated in the prevention and treatment of allergy related diseases [3–8], with the strongest evidence emerging for the primary prevention of atopic dermatitis [3–5]. Throughout this paper we refer AD, asthma and ARC as "allergy related diseases", recognising that not all presentations of these conditions are related to a classic IgE-mediated inflammatory process.

Randomised controlled trials (RCTs) testing probiotics in the prevention of childhood allergy related disease are heterogeneous and have used a variety of bacterial strains, administration regimes and varying ages of follow-up.

* Correspondence: melanie.simpson@ntnu.no
[1]Department of Public Health and General Practice, Faculty of Medicine, Norwegian University of Science and Technology (NTNU), Postboks 8905, MTFS, 7491, Trondheim, Norway
Full list of author information is available at the end of the article

Using information from the first published follow up for each trial, a recent meta-analysis concluded that probiotic administration is protective against the development of AD in infancy [3]. Among the studies with follow-up at or beyond 5 years of age, the greatest protective benefit of probiotics against AD appears to be in early childhood and it is less certain if this effect persists until school age [9–25]. Only one of these studies did not specify a maternal or family history of atopy as an inclusion criteria [9, 10], and there is therefore a particular need for further longer term follow-up studies to determine the ongoing effect of perinatal probiotics in general populations.

The Probiotics in the Prevention of Allergy among Children in Trondheim (ProPACT) study is a double-blinded RCT investigating the effect of maternal probiotic supplementation on childhood allergy related diseases in a general population. The initial results of the ProPACT study demonstrated a clinically significant reduction in the cumulative incidence of AD at 2 years (OR 0.51, 95 % CI 0.30 – 0.87, $p = 0.013$), with the greatest reduction seen in children not considered at "high risk" for allergy related disease based on a negative family history [26]. Probiotic supplementation did not significantly affect the incidence of asthma, ARC or atopic sensitisation at 2 year of age, although the diagnosis of the former two diseases is uncommon and controversial at such a young age.

The participating children were re-contacted and reassessed at 6 years of age for the presence of allergy related diseases and allergic sensitisation. The aim of the current paper was to investigate the effect of maternal perinatal probiotic supplementation on the cumulative incidence of AD and ARC and prevalence of asthma and atopic sensitisation at 6 years of age.

Methods

Participants and design

The ProPACT study has been described in detail previously [26]. Briefly, 415 women living in Trondheim, Norway, were randomised to receive daily probiotic supplementation or placebo from 36 weeks gestation until 3 months postpartum. Probiotic supplementation consisted of 250 mL of low fat fermented milk containing 5×10^{10} colony-forming units (CFUs) of *Lactobacillus rhamnosus GG* (LGG) and *Bifidobacterium animalis* subsp. *lactis* Bb-12 (Bb-12) and 5×10^{9} CFU of *L. acidophilus* La-5 (La-5). The equivalently tasting placebo milk was sterile and contained no probiotic bacteria. The study milk was consumed by the women both pre- and postnatally, and the children did not receive any probiotic supplementation as a part of this study.

Participants were requested to complete questionnaires regarding lifestyle factors during pregnancy and at 6 weeks, 1 year and 2 years postpartum. These questionnaires detailed family history of allergy related diseases, dietary and parental smoking habits, housing conditions, family structure and the general health of the children. A child health questionnaire focusing on the presence of allergic symptoms and antibiotic use was completed at 1, 2 and 6 years. Information regarding mode of delivery was unavailable, although assumed to be unaffected by the intervention regime. Those who had not initially responded to the 6 year child health questionnaire were re-sent this questionnaire in October 2013, when the children were between 8 and 10 years of age and responders to this re-sent questionnaire were considered "late responders".

Families were encouraged to attend a clinical examination for AD prior to 1 year if the child developed an itchy rash which lasted for more than 4 weeks. At 2 and 6 years, all children were invited to attend a clinical examination, including a structured interview, and allergy testing consisting of skin-prick testing (SPT) and specific IgE (sIgE). This examination was conducted by specially trained nurses at the 6 year follow-up who were unaware of treatment allocation. Participants were unblinded after the publication of the 2 year follow-up results [26]. Prior to this, the participants and investigators were blinded to treatment allocation which was conducted by the Department of Applied Clinical Research at the Norwegian University of Science and Technology through a computer-generated randomisation list without restrictions.

The trial was approved by the Regional Committee for Medical Research Ethics for Central Norway (Ref. 097–03) and the Norwegian Data Inspectorate (Ref. 2003/953-3 KBE) and the trial protocol is registered in ClinicalTrials.gov (identifier NCT00159523). Parents gave their written consent.

Outcomes

The primary outcomes of interest were: cumulative incidence of atopic dermatitis (AD) and allergic rhinoconjunctivitis (ARC), and the 12 month prevalence of asthma. Children who attended the clinical examination(s) were assessed for AD using the UK Working Party (UKWP) diagnostic criteria [27]. Children who were assessed under these criteria as having AD at any point up to 6 years were considered to ever have had AD in the cumulative incidence estimate.

The cumulative incidence of ARC was defined by a positive answer to the question "Has your child *ever* had hay fever or allergic rhinoconjunctivitis?" in the 1, 2 or 6 year questionnaire. Current asthma was defined as a positive answer to both questions "Has your child *ever* been diagnosed with asthma by a doctor?" and "In the past 12 months, has your child been treated with tablets, inhalers or other medications for wheezing, chest tightness or asthma?". These questionnaire based definitions were used in order to minimise the proportion of participants with missing data and vary from the clinical examination based definitions presented in the 2 year follow-up article (Additional file 1: Table S1). Prompted by the findings of other probiotic trials, we include here the cumulative incidence of wheeze defined by a positive answer to both questions "Has your child *ever* had whistling in the chest?" and "Has your child *ever* had episodes of wheezing or tightness in the chest?" and a history of a lower respiratory tract infection, subcategorised into bronchitis and pneumonia, in the 1, 2 or 6 year questionnaire.

Atopic sensitisation was assessed as a secondary endpoint and was defined as any SPT wheal ≥ 3 mm or any sIgE level ≥ $0.35kUL^{-1}$. Both SPT and sIgE testing was performed as described previously [26] according to the ISAAC II procedure [28] for the following allergens: mite, mould, cat and dog dander, birch, timothy (grass) and mugwort pollen, egg white, codfish, hazelnut, peanut and cow's milk.

Statistical analysis

All statistical analyses were conducted using Stata/IC 13.1. The sample size calculation and randomisation procedure has been previously reported [26]. Due to the presence of missing data, the intention to treat (ITT) analysis strategy [29] included a main analysis using multiple imputations by chained equations (MICE) under the assumption that the data is missing at random (MAR) and a pattern mixture model (PMM) analysis to assess the sensitivity of the conclusions to this assumption. One hundred (m = 100) imputed data sets were created for the MICE analysis using the following predictor variables: treatment allocation, family history of atopy, siblings, sex, paternal smoking, antibiotic use within the first year of life, parentally reported eczema, protocol compliance and disease outcomes at 2 and 6 years of age. Further details regarding the MI model are provided in Additional file 1. A complete case analysis is also presented which includes participants who submitted the 6 year health questionnaire and or attended the 6 year clinical interview.

Univariate logistic regression was used to assess the impact of maternal probiotic supplementation on each of the outcomes for both multiple imputed datasets and complete case analyses. Although potential confounders should be balanced in an RCT, an alternate logistic regression model including family history, sex and siblings was assessed because of their previously reported associations with allergic disease and slight imbalance in the latter two.

A missing not at random (MNAR) sensitivity analysis was conducted using the pattern-mixture model version of the user written Stata command *rctmiss*. A detailed explanation of this analysis is provided in the Additional file 1.

Results

Participants

Participating families were recruited between September 2003 and September 2005, and the initial 6 year follow up occurred from December 2009 to December 2011. The 6 year child health questionnaire was completed by 281 (67.7 %) families and 163 (39.3 %) attended the clinical interview (Fig. 1), with no significant difference in attendance rates between the probiotic and placebo groups. Mean age of follow-up at the clinical examination was 6.3 years (SD 0.2 years) in both probiotic and placebo arms. The mean age of completion of the questionnaire was also comparable between treatment arms among both initial and late responders (data not shown).

The baseline data and characteristics of participants randomised to receive probiotic supplementation or placebo showed minimal differences between the treatment groups (Table 1). Differences considered to be of potential influence due to reported association with childhood allergic diseases included the higher proportion of males (49.7 vs 41.8 %) and children with older siblings (44.0 vs 39.0 %) in the probiotic group compared to the placebo group.

Characteristics of participants followed-up at 6 years

Compared to those lost to clinical follow up, the children who attended the 6 year clinical examination had older mothers, were less likely to have a father who smoked during their first year of life and to have received fish before 6 months of age, and were more likely to have a family history of atopy, an older sibling and study protocol compliance (Table 1). Additionally, the children sensitised and or diagnosed with AD at 2 years were more likely to have attended the 6 year examination (Table 1). Similar differences were observed between children with and without a completed 6 year questionnaire (details provided in Additional file 1: Table S2).

Atopic dermatitis

A trend towards a lower cumulative incidence of UKWP diagnosed AD in the probiotic group with an odds ratio (OR) of 0.64 (95 % CI 0.39-1.07, $p = 0.086$; NNT = 10) was observed in the MICE analysis (Table 2). This finding was statistically significantly in the complete case analysis (OR 0.48, 95 % CI 0.25-0.92, $p = 0.027$; NNT = 6). The adjustment for the covariates family history, sex and presence of older siblings resulted in inconsequential changes in the calculated OR estimates and did not substantially improve the precision of the estimate (data not shown).

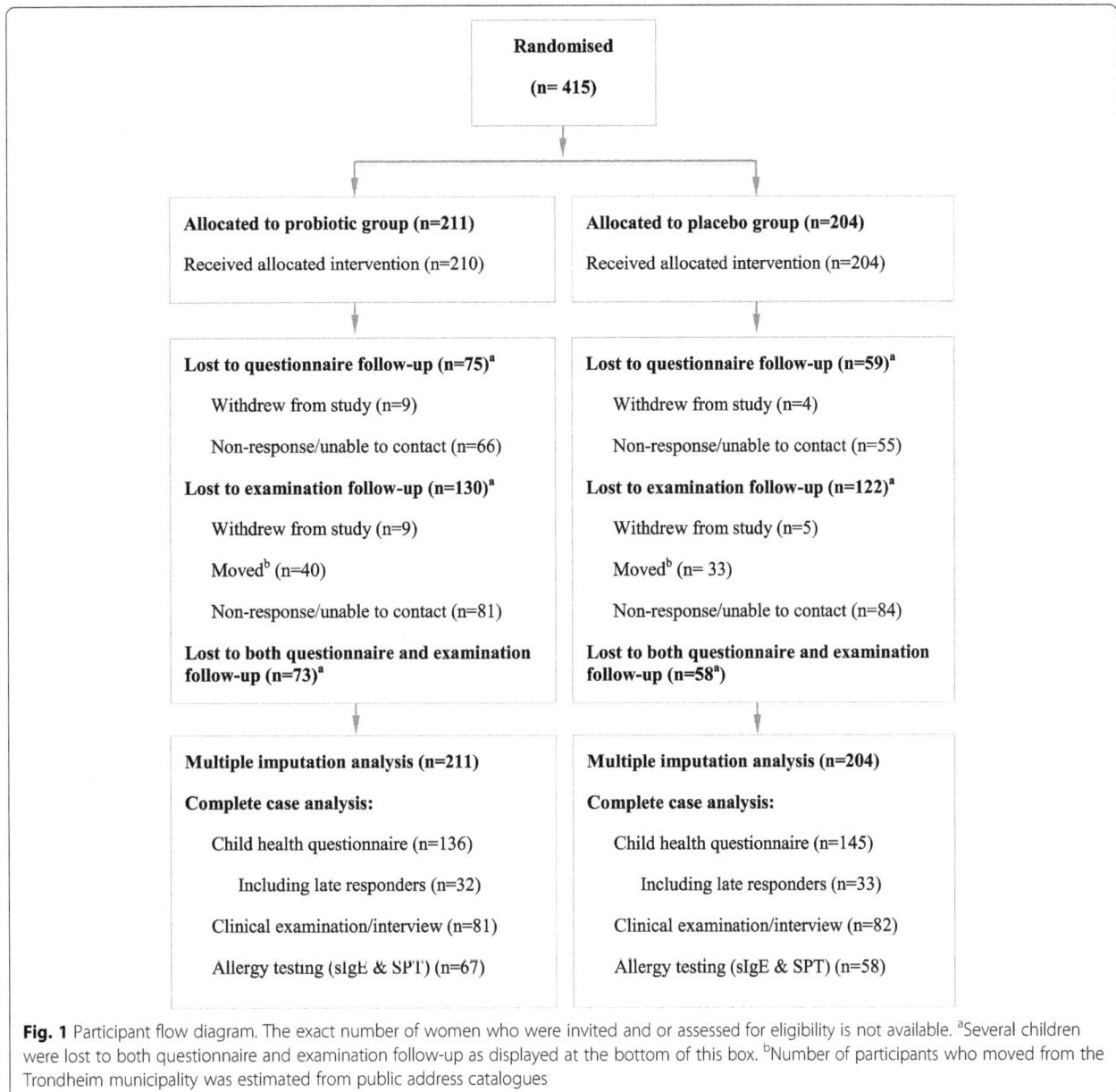

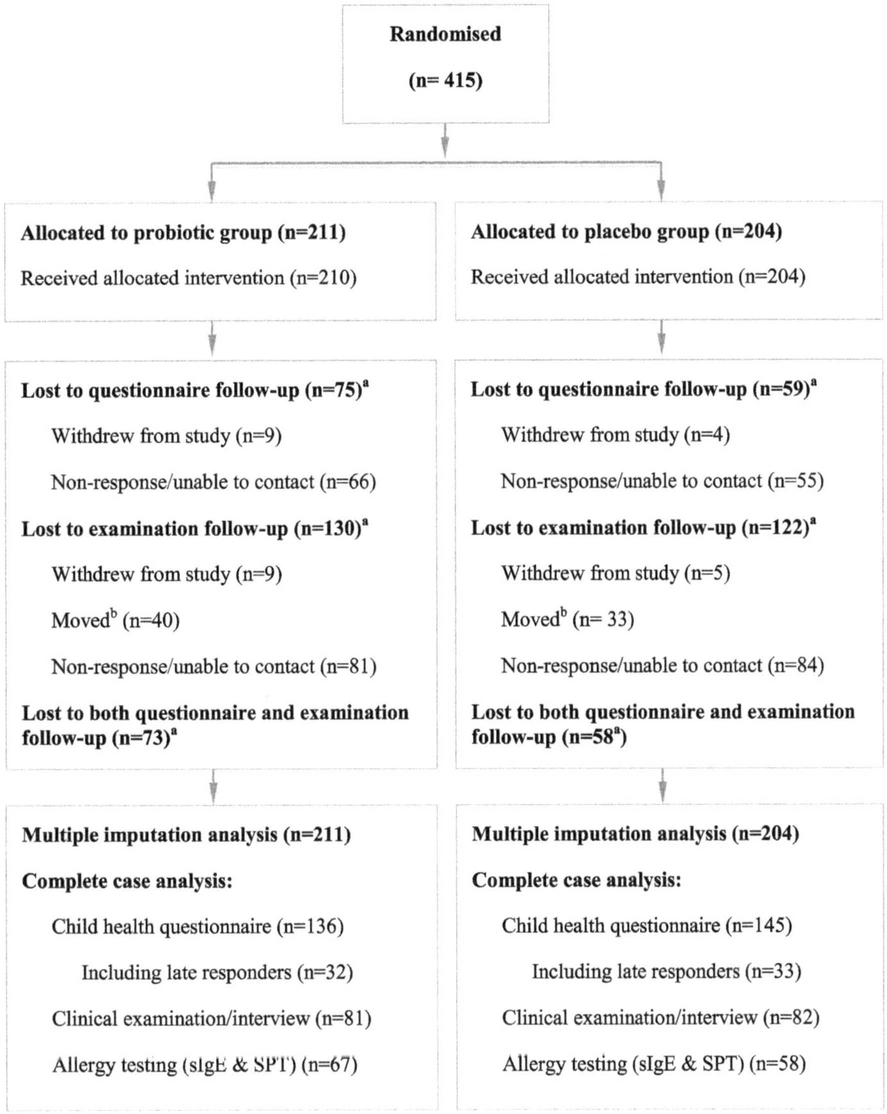

Fig. 1 Participant flow diagram. The exact number of women who were invited and or assessed for eligibility is not available. [a]Several children were lost to both questionnaire and examination follow-up as displayed at the bottom of this box. [b]Number of participants who moved from the Trondheim municipality was estimated from public address catalogues

Allergic rhinoconjunctivitis, asthma, sensitisation and lower respiratory tract infections

There was no statistically significant difference observed between the cumulative incidence of ARC, 12 month prevalence of asthma or current atopic sensitisation in the MICE or complete case analyses (Table 2). Parental reported cumulative incidence of wheeze and lower respiratory tract infections were not influenced by the probiotic regime in observed cases or imputed estimates. There was a trend towards a lower cumulative incidence of pneumonia in the probiotic group (OR 0.41, 95 % CI 0.17-1.04, $p = 0.062$, Table 2) which was not statistically significant in the MICE analysis.

Sensitivity analysis

The results of the sensitivity analysis are provided in the Additional file 1. Briefly, if children with AD were more likely to be lost to follow-up in the probiotic group than the placebo group, then the preventative effect of probiotics would have been weakened.

Discussion

Maternal probiotic supplementation given to a general population of women appears to have an ongoing preventative effect on the cumulative incidence of AD until school age, however this did not reach statistical significance in the MICE analysis. There was no observed

Table 1 Baseline data, characteristics and allergy related disease at 2 years

	Comparison of treatment groups				Comparison of drop out cases				
	Probiotic ($n = 211$)		Placebo ($n = 204$)		Attended 6 yr examination		Drop-outs		
	n[a]		n[a]		n[a]		n[a]		*p*-value[b]
Baseline data and characteristics									
Age, mother (years), mean ± SD	191	30.1 (3.9)	189	30.3 (4.4)	162	30.7 (3.9)	218	29.8 (4.2)	0.024
Education, mother (yrs), mean ± SD	183	15.3 (2.2)	181	15.2 (2.3)	156	15.2 (2.1)	208	15.2 (2.4)	0.968
Education, father (yrs), mean ± SD	184	14.8 (2.7)	179	14.7 (2.4)	156	14.7 (2.5)	207	14.8 (2.6)	0.561
Birth weight (g), mean ± SD	187	3662 (478)	176	3596 (474)	161	3626 (466)	202	3635 (486)	0.814
Sex (male), n (%)	193	96 (49.7)	191	80 (41.8)	163	76 (46.6)	221	100 (45.3)	0.151
Premature, n (%)	189	5 (2.7)	185	7 (3.8)	162	5 (3.1)	212	7 (3.3)	1.000[c]
Siblings, n (%)	207	91 (44.0)	200	78 (39.0)	163	82 (50.3)	244	87 (35.7)	0.003
Atopy in family, n (%)	207	152 (73.4)	200	148 (74.0)	163	127 (77.9)	244	173 (70.9)	0.115
Smoking mother[d], n (%)	204	16 (7.8)	200	19 (9.5)	163	13 (8.0)	241	12 (9.1)	0.686
Smoking father[d], n (%)	203	35 (17.2)	198	38 (19.2)	163	21 (12.8)	238	52 (21.8)	0.022
Breastfed ≥ 3 months, n (%)	168	164 (97.6)	166	162 (97.6)	155	153 (98.7)	179	173 (96.7)	0.293[c]
At least one pet at home[d], n (%)	207	52 (25.1)	200	53 (26.5)	163	47 (28.8)	244	58 (23.7)	0.253
Used antibiotics[d], n (%)	161	35 (21.7)	159	34 (21.4)	152	34 (22.4)	168	35 (20.8)	0.739
Fish ≤ 6 mo., n (%)	163	35 (21.5)	165	27 (16.4)	155	22 (14.2)	173	40 (23.1)	0.039
Vegetables ≤ 6 mo., n (%)	166	84 (50.6)	166	105 (63.3)	156	90 (57.7)	176	99 (56.3)	0.791
Protocol compliance[e], n (%)	150	130 (86.7)	148	128 (86.5)	147	134 (91.2)	151	124 (82.1)	0.022
Allergy related disease at 2 years									
Atopic dermatitis, n(%)	138	29 (21.0)	140	48 (34.3)	145	52 (35.9)	133	25 (18.8)	0.001
Allergic sensitisation[f], n(%)	131	20 (15.3)	133	15 (11.3)	140	26 (18.6)	124	9 (7.3)	0.007

[a]N: number of observed cases for each variable differs based on the source of information; [b]p-values for attendees versus dropouts calculated using t-test for continuous variables and χ^2 for binary variables; [c]Fisher's exact test used to calculate *p*-values for binary variables with frequency <=5 in one or more cell of the contingency table; [d]Exposure to smoking, household pets or antibiotics reported anytime during the first year of life or during pregnancy; [e]Compliance defined as consumption of 250 mL of study on ≥50 % of days, no consumption of other probiotic products and breast feeding for ≥ 3 months; [f]Positive skin prick test and or specific IgE level, if only one negative test result was available, the child was considered not sensitised

Table 2 Prevalence and cumulative incidence at 6 years of allergy related diseases, wheeze and lower respiratory tract infections in the probiotic and placebo groups

	Imputed estimates			Observed cases				
Allergy related disease	Probiotic, n=211	Placebo, n=204	Odds ratio (95 % CI)[a]	Probiotic		Placebo		Odds ratio
	% (95 % CI)	% (95 % CI)		n/n	% (95 % CI)	n/n	% (95 % CI)	(95 % CI)[a]
Current disease								
Asthma	2.3 (0.0-4.7)	0.9 (0.0-2.5)	1.68 (0.21-13.20)	3/136	2.2 (0.7-6-7)	1/145	0.7 (0.0-4.8)	3.25 (0.33-31.6)
Allergic sensitisation	30.0 (21.2-38.8)	28.0 (18.8-37.1)	1.11 (0.62-1.96)	23/80	28.8 (19.7-39.8)	19/78	24.4 (16.0-35.3)	1.25 (0.62-2.54)
Cumulative incidence								
Atopic dermatitis	29.3 (21.2-37.4)	39.1 (30.2-48.0)	0.64 (0.39-1.07)[b]	22/81	27.2 (17.3-37.1)	36/82	43.9 (32.9-54.9)	0.48 (0.25-0.92)[c]
ARC	21.6 (14.6-28.6)	18.8 (12.0-25.7)	1.19 (0.66-2.16)	22/134	16.4 (10.1-22.8)	20/145	13.8 (8.1-19.5)	1.22 (0.64-2.37)
Wheeze	39.0 (30.9-47.1)	45.8 (37.4-54.1)	0.75 (0.47-1.22)	46/132	34.9 (26.7-43.0)	55/142	38.7 (30.7-46.8)	0.85 (0.52-1.38)
LRTI (any)	30.6 (22.2-39.1)	36.8 (29.1-44.5)	0.76 (0.47-1.23)	33/128	25.8 (18.1-33.4)	40/138	29.0 (21.4-36.6)	0.85 (0.50-1.46)
Bronchitis	23.6 (16.3-30.9)	27.6 (20.2-35.0)	0.81 (0.48-1.36)	29/130	22.3 (15.1-29.5)	32/139	23.0 (16.0-30.1)	0.96 (0.54-1.70)
Pneumonia	10.2 (4.5-15.9)	15.4 (9.4-21.4)	0.61 (0.29-1.32)	7/129	5.4 (1.5-9.4)	17/141	12.1 (6.6-17.5)	0.42 (0.17-1.04)[d]

ARC: allergic rhinoconjunctivitis; LRTI: Lower respiratory tract infection; [a]Unadjusted logistic regression odds ratio; Significant or near significant *p*-values: [b]p=0.086, [c]p=0.027 and [d]p=0.062

effect of probiotics on the cumulative incidence of ARC, the 12 month prevalence of asthma or current atopic sensitisation.

A significant proportion of cases of allergy related diseases occur in children who are otherwise considered not to be at "high risk" and therefore primary prevention strategies must also be assessed in general populations [30]. This long term follow-up of the ProPACT trial is an important addition to the literature concerning probiotics in the prevention of allergic disease as one of few studies to recruit participants from a general population [7, 8, 29]. The only other RCT to have reported long term follow-up in a general population observed no benefit of their probiotic regime on the prevalence of any allergic disease or the cumulative incidence of questionnaire defined AD at 8–9 years of age [9, 10]. Their regime included *Lactobacillus paracasei* spp *paracasei* F19 supplementation given to children during weaning. In comparison, our study involved pre- and postnatal supplementation of a mixture of probiotics which included the *L. rhamnosus GG* (LGG) strain. Both LGG and pre- and postnatal regimes were found to be associated with reduced RR of AD on sub-group analysis in a meta-analysis [3]. Additionally, we report UK Working Party diagnostic criteria defined AD which is a more extensively validated method of diagnosis [31, 32].

Looking to other trials, five RCTs have assessed the cumulative incidence of AD at 5 years of age or beyond in "high risk" populations [11–23]. The trial presented by Kalliomaki et al. [11–13] and the *Lactobacillus rhamnosus* (HN001) arm of the study by Wickens et al. [14–16] report a significant reduction in the cumulative incidence of AD, which is sustained, although reduced, at follow-up at 6 years. Together with the current study, these trials indicate that the beneficial effect of probiotics on AD is most pronounced in infancy and may continue into early childhood. Furthermore, they suggest that we are observing a true primary preventative effect, rather than an intervention which delays the onset of AD. Contrastingly, the preventative effect of probiotics seen at 2 years in the large RCT published by Kukkonen/Kuitunen et al. [17, 18] showed no trend towards ongoing benefit on follow-up at 5 years. The *Bifidobacterium animalis* subsp. *lactis* (HN019) arm of Wickens et al. [14–16] and 2 other trials [19–23] demonstrated no significant effect of probiotics on the cumulative incidence of AD at any follow-up time point from 1 to 7 years of age. It is interesting to note that all of the studies with an observed ongoing effect administered a *L. rhamnosus* strain pre- and postnatally, and that if the child was breastfed, the postnatal supplementation was given solely to the mother during the first months with the exception of Kalliomaki et al. [11–13] where approximate 57 % of participants opted to give the probiotic or placebo capsules directly to the newborn children. In contrast, studies without an ongoing effect have either administered probiotic species other than *L. rhamnosus* and or specified that the probiotic supplements were to be given directly to the children regardless of breastfeeding. Further research is required to investigate if these observations are coincidental or represent strain and or regime specific effects.

The lack of effect on asthma, ARC and atopic sensitisation may reflect a true lack of effect or that the current study is under-powered to observed smaller differences in less frequent diseases. This is a universal problem for probiotic trials reporting asthma as an outcome [8]. Two recent meta-analyses concluded that there is not enough evidence to support perinatal probiotic supplementation in the prevention of childhood asthma or wheeze [7, 8]. Reassuringly, neither our study nor these meta-analyses found that probiotics increased the risk of asthma or wheeze, a concern which arose after long term follow-up by Kalliomaki et al. [8, 11] Whilst one of these meta-analyses suggested that probiotics may increase lower respiratory tract infections [8], our study does not support this conclusion. On the contrary, we observe a trend towards lower cumulative incidence of pneumonia in the probiotic group. Atopic sensitisation was found to be significantly reduced in a sub-group meta-analysis of regimes which combined pre- and postnatal administration [7]. Consistent with the ProPACT study, none of the individual longer term follow-up studies have observed a significant effect of probiotics on sensitisation at school age. Interestingly, *Lactobacillus acidophilus* was found to be associated with an increased rate of atopic sensitisation in a multivariate meta-regression analysis [7]. This observation requires further investigation and may, in part, explain the lack of effect of the probiotic regime on sensitisation in the ProPACT trial.

The major limiting factor of this RCT is the high proportion of missing data which naturally raises concerns regarding the generalisability of the results and introduction of bias. Following the four point ITT analysis strategy recommended by White et al. [29] we have attempted to follow-up all participants, performed a primary analysis using MICE and a sensitivity analysis using PMM. Both of the latter two models account for all randomised participants under a range of assumptions about the cause of missingness and in doing so attempt to minimise bias from covariate-related and outcome-related drop-out, respectively. The reasons for loss to follow-up are primarily unknown, however very few participants actively withdrew from the study. An estimated 73 participants had moved from the study region, which would have precluded their attendance at the clinical examination in a presumably random manner. A number of these participants were followed-up through the questionnaire. In terms of generalisability, the original ProPACT population was similar to the total PACT population, which in turn was representative of the general population in Trondheim, Norway [26]. At the 6 year follow-up, the remaining participants were more likely to have a family history of atopy, older siblings and a pet and less likely to have a father who smoked. As these differences were not large we believe that the results are still generalisable to westernised populations where there is a reasonably high rate of allergy related disease. The PMM sensitivity analysis is particularly pertinent in this case because atopic sensitisation and or a diagnosis of AD at 2 years are associated with both attendance at the 6 year clinical examination and a diagnosis of AD at 6 years. This raises suspicions that the data is partially MNAR which would lead to biased estimates under both the complete case and multiple imputations analysis models. The PMM analysis suggests that results of this study for ARC, asthma and atopic sensitisation would have only been affected if there was an unrealistically strong association between disease and missingness in a single treatment arm. On the other hand, the magnitude of the preventative effect attributed to probiotics for AD at 6 years must be considered with caution, as the observed benefit is sensitive to the assumption that the relationship between AD and loss to follow-up is essentially identical in both the probiotic and placebo groups. Regardless of whether the outcome variables are partially MNAR, the MICE estimates are expected to be less biased than the complete case analysis. Another limitation is that the participants were informed of their treatment allocation and the observed reduction in AD after publication of the results from the 2 year follow-up in 2010 [26], although we do not believe that this to have significantly affected the current results. Firstly, the knowledge of treatment allocation has not affected participant behaviour with equal numbers from the probiotic and placebo groups attending the clinical follow-up at 6 years. Secondly, the UKWP diagnosis was based on assessment by research nurses who were unaware of treatment allocation.

Conclusions

In conclusion, we have previously shown that perinatal maternal probiotic supplementation is effective in reducing the cumulative incidence of AD in children up to 2 years of age. The current study does not conclusively demonstrate an ongoing benefit, however there is a strong trend towards a reduced cumulative incidence at 6 years. This would suggest that perinatal probiotics prevent and do not mere delay the onset of AD in childhood. The cumulative incidence of ARC and prevalence of asthma and atopic sensitisation were unaffected by the probiotic regime at 6 years of age.

Abbreviations

AD: Atopic dermatitis; ARC: Allergic rhinoconjunctivitis; ProPACT: Probiotics in the Prevention of Allergies among Children in Trondheim; sIgE: Specific immunoglobulin E; SPT: Skin prick test; UKWP: UK Working Party diagnostic criteria for atopic dermatitis; ISAAC: International Study of Asthma and Allergies in Childhood; ITT: Intention to treat; MICE: Multiple imputation by chained equations; MAR: Missing at random; MNAR: Missing not at random; PMM: Pattern mixture model.

Competing interests

T.Ø., O.S., C.K.D and M.R.S. participated in seminars sponsored by Tine BA. All other authors declare that they have no conflict of interest.

Authors' contributions

OS, RJ and TØ designed the study and directed its implementation. MRS conducted the statistical analysis and drafted the manuscript. CKD contributed to the interpretation of results and writing of the manuscript. All authors were involved in the interpretation of the results, revision of draft manuscript and have approved the final manuscript.

Acknowledgements

We thank all the children and their parents for their participation in this study along with the project assistants, Guri Helmersen and Else Bartnes, Dr Anne Rø, and the midwives of the Trondheim region.

Funding sources

This study was funded by the Norwegian University of Science and Technology, the Norwegian Research Council, Nidarosfondet and Siemens Medical Solutions Diagnostics AS. Tine BA sponsored the study through supply of study milk and logistics of its distribution. Employees from funding sources played no role in the study design, data collection, data analysis, interpretation of the study results, or writing of the manuscript.

Author details

[1]Department of Public Health and General Practice, Faculty of Medicine, Norwegian University of Science and Technology (NTNU), Postboks 8905, MTFS, 7491, Trondheim, Norway. [2]Department of Dermatology, St Olavs Hospital, Trondheim University Hospital, Trondheim, Norway.

References

1. Rautava S, Ruuskanen O, Ouwehand A, Salminen S, Isolauri E. The hygiene hypothesis of atopic disease–an extended version. J Pediatr Gastroenterol Nutr. 2004;38(4):378–88.
2. Wold AE. The hygiene hypothesis revised: is the rising frequency of allergy due to changes in the intestinal flora? Allergy. 1998;53(46 Suppl):20–5.
3. Pelucchi C, Chatenoud L, Turati F, Galeone C, Moja L, Bach JF, et al. Probiotics supplementation during pregnancy or infancy for the prevention of atopic dermatitis: a meta-analysis. Epidemiology. 2012;23(3):402–14.
4. Panduru M, Panduru NM, Salavastru CM, Tiplica GS. Probiotics and primary prevention of atopic dermatitis: a meta-analysis of randomized controlled studies. J Eur Acad Dermatol Venereol. 2015;29(2):232–42.
5. Fiocchi A, Pawankar R, Cuello-Garcia C, Ahn K, Al-Hammadi S, Agarwal A, et al. World allergy organization-McMaster university guidelines for allergic disease prevention (GLAD-P): probiotics. World Allergy Organ J. 2015;8(1):4.
6. Szajewska H. Early nutritional strategies for preventing allergic disease. Isr Med Assoc J. 2012;14(1):58–62.
7. Elazab N, Mendy A, Gasana J, Vieira ER, Quizon A, Forno E. Probiotic administration in early life, atopy, and asthma: a meta-analysis of clinical trials. Pediatrics. 2013;132(3):e666–676.
8. Azad MB, Coneys JG, Kozyrskyj AL, Field CJ, Ramsey CD, Becker AB, et al. Probiotic supplementation during pregnancy or infancy for the prevention of asthma and wheeze: systematic review and meta-analysis. BMJ. 2013;347:f6471.
9. West CE, Hammarstrom ML, Hernell O. Probiotics during weaning reduce the incidence of eczema. Pediatr Allergy Immunol. 2009;20(5):430–7.
10. West CE, Hammarstrom ML, Hernell O. Probiotics in primary prevention of allergic disease–follow-up at 8–9 years of age. Allergy. 2013;68(8):1015–20.

11. Kalliomaki M, Salminen S, Poussa T, Isolauri E. Probiotics during the first 7 years of life: a cumulative risk reduction of eczema in a randomized, placebo-controlled trial. J Allergy Clin Immunol. 2007;119(4):1019–21.
12. Kalliomaki M, Salminen S, Poussa T, Arvilommi H, Isolauri E. Probiotics and prevention of atopic disease: 4-year follow-up of a randomised placebo-controlled trial. Lancet. 2003;361(9372):1869–71.
13. Kalliomaki M, Salminen S, Arvilommi H, Kero P, Koskinen P, Isolauri E. Probiotics in primary prevention of atopic disease: a randomised placebo-controlled trial. Lancet. 2001;357(9262):1076–9.
14. Wickens K, Stanley TV, Mitchell EA, Barthow C, Fitzharris P, Purdie G, et al. Early supplementation with Lactobacillus rhamnosus HN001 reduces eczema prevalence to 6 years: does it also reduce atopic sensitization? Clin Exp Allergy. 2013;43(9):1048–57.
15. Wickens K, Black PN, Stanley TV, Mitchell E, Fitzharris P, Tannock GW, et al. A differential effect of 2 probiotics in the prevention of eczema and atopy: a double-blind, randomized, placebo-controlled trial. J Allergy Clin Immunol. 2008;122(4):788–94.
16. Wickens K, Black P, Stanley TV, Mitchell E, Barthow C, Fitzharris P, et al. A protective effect of Lactobacillus rhamnosus HN001 against eczema in the first 2 years of life persists to age 4 years. Clin Exp Allergy. 2012;42(7):1071–9.
17. Kukkonen K, Savilahti E, Haahtela T, Juntunen-Backman K, Korpela R, Poussa T, et al. Probiotics and prebiotic galacto-oligosaccharides in the prevention of allergic diseases: a randomized, double-blind, placebo-controlled trial. J Allergy Clin Immunol. 2007;119(1):192–8.
18. Kuitunen M, Kukkonen K, Juntunen-Backman K, Korpela R, Poussa T, Tuure T, et al. Probiotics prevent IgE-associated allergy until age 5 years in cesarean-delivered children but not in the total cohort. J Allergy Clin Immunol. 2009;123(2):335–41.
19. Taylor AL, Dunstan JA, Prescott SL. Probiotic supplementation for the first 6 months of life fails to reduce the risk of atopic dermatitis and increases the risk of allergen sensitization in high-risk children: a randomized controlled trial. J Allergy Clin Immunol. 2007;119(1):184–91.
20. Prescott SL, Wiltschut J, Taylor A, Westcott L, Jung W, Currie H, et al. Early markers of allergic disease in a primary prevention study using probiotics: 2.5-year follow-up phase. Allergy. 2008;63(11):1481–90.
21. Jensen MP, Meldrum S, Taylor AL, Dunstan JA, Prescott SL. Early probiotic supplementation for allergy prevention: long-term outcomes. J Allergy Clin Immunol. 2012;130(5):1209–11. e1205.
22. Abrahamsson TR, Jakobsson T, Bottcher MF, Fredrikson M, Jenmalm MC, Bjorksten B, et al. Probiotics in prevention of IgE-associated eczema: a double-blind, randomized, placebo-controlled trial. J Allergy Clin Immunol. 2007;119(5):1174–80.
23. Abrahamsson TR, Jakobsson T, Bjorksten B, Oldaeus G, Jenmalm MC. No effect of probiotics on respiratory allergies: a seven-year follow-up of a randomized controlled trial in infancy. Pediatr Allergy Immunol. 2013;24(6):556–61.
24. Gorissen D, Rutten N, Oostermeijer C, Niers L, Hoekstra M, Rijkers G, et al. Preventative effects of selected probiotc strains on the development of asthma and allergic rhinitis in childhood. The Panda study. Clin Exp Allergy. 2014;44:1431–3.
25. Niers L, Martin R, Rijkers G, Sengers F, Timmerman H, van Uden N, et al. The effects of selected probiotic strains on the development of eczema (the PandA study). Allergy. 2009;64(9):1349–58.
26. Dotterud CK, Storro O, Johnsen R, Oien T. Probiotics in pregnant women to prevent allergic disease: a randomized, double-blind trial. Br J Dermatol. 2010;163(3):616–23.
27. Williams HC, Burney PG, Hay RJ, Archer CB, Shipley MJ, Hunter JJ, et al. The U.K. Working Party's diagnostic criteria for atopic dermatitis. I. Derivation of a minimum set of discriminators for atopic dermatitis. Br J Dermatol. 1994;131(3):383–96.
28. Weiland SK, Bjorksten B, Brunekreef B, Cookson W, Von Mutius E, Strachan D. Phase II of the international study of asthma and allergies in childhood (ISAAC II): rationale and methods. Eur Respir J. 2004;24(3):406–12.
29. White IR, Horton NJ, Carpenter J, Pocock SJ. Strategy for intention to treat analysis in randomised trials with missing outcome data. BMJ. 2011;342:d40.
30. Williams HC. Prevention of Atopic Eczema: a dream not so far away? Arch Dermatology. 2002;138:391–2.
31. Williams HC, Burney PG, Pembroke AC, Hay RJ. Validation of the U.K. diagnostic criteria for atopic dermatitis in a population setting. Brit J Dermatol. 1996;135:12–7.
32. Brenninkmeijer EEA, Schram ME, Leeflang MM, Bos JD, Spuls P. Diagnostic criteria for atopic dermatitis: a systematic review. Epidemiology and Health Services Research. 2007;158:754–65.

Real-world health outcomes in adults with moderate-to-severe psoriasis in the United States: a population study using electronic health records to examine patient-perceived treatment effectiveness, medication use, and healthcare resource utilization

April W. Armstrong[1*], Shonda A. Foster[2], Brian S. Comer[2], Chen-Yen Lin[2], William Malatestinic[2], Russel Burge[2,3] and Orin Goldblum[2]

Abstract

Background: Little is known regarding real-world health outcomes data among US psoriasis patients, but electronic health records (EHR) that collect structured data at point-of-care may provide opportunities to investigate real-world health outcomes among psoriasis patients. Our objective was to investigate patient-perceived treatment effectiveness, patterns of medication use (duration, switching, and/or discontinuation), healthcare resource utilization, and medication costs using real-world data from psoriasis patients.

Methods: Data for adults (≥18-years) with a dermatology provider-given diagnosis of psoriasis from 9/2014–9/2015 were obtained from dermatology practices using a widely used US dermatology-specific EHR containing over 500,000 psoriasis patients. Disease severity was captured by static physician's global assessment and body surface area. Patient-perceived treatment effectiveness was assessed by a pre-defined question. Treatment switching and duration were documented. Reasons for discontinuations were assessed using pre-defined selections. Healthcare resource utilization was defined by visit frequency and complexity.

Results: From 82,621 patients with psoriasis during the study period, patient-perceived treatment effectiveness was investigated in 2200 patients. The proportion of patients reporting "strongly agree" when asked if their treatment was effective was highest for biologics (73%) and those reporting treatment adherence (55%). In 16,000 patients who received oral systemics and 21,087 patients who received biologics, median treatment duration was longer for those who received biologics (160 vs. 113 days, respectively). Treatment switching was less frequent among patients on systemic monotherapies compared to those on combination therapies. The most common reason for discontinuing biologics was loss of efficacy; the most common reason for discontinuing orals was side effects. In 28,754 patients, higher disease severity was associated with increased healthcare resource utilization (increased visit frequency and complexity). When compared between treatment groups ($n = 10{,}454$), healthcare resource utilization was highest for phototherapy. Annual medication costs were higher for biologics ($21,977) than oral systemics ($3413).

(Continued on next page)

* Correspondence: armstrongpublication@gmail.com
[1]Department of Dermatology, Keck School of Medicine, University of Southern California, Los Angeles, CA 90033, USA
Full list of author information is available at the end of the article

(Continued from previous page)

Conclusions: Real-world research using a widely implemented dermatology EHR provided valuable insights on patient perceived treatment effectiveness, patterns of medication usage, healthcare resource utilization, and medication costs for psoriasis patients in the US. This study and others utilizing EHRs for real-world research may assist clinical and payer decisions regarding the management of psoriasis.

Keywords: Electronic health records, EHR, Psoriasis, Dermatology, Treatment effectiveness, Outcomes, Switching, Discontinuation, Healthcare resource utilization, Costs

Background

Psoriasis is an immune-mediated disease that affects 3.2% of adults in the United States (US) [1, 2]. The estimated percentages of patients in the US with mild, moderate, or severe psoriasis are 83.3, 11.4, and 5.3%, respectively [3]. Psoriasis is associated with significant morbidity and clinically significant comorbidities including diabetes, cardiovascular disease, metabolic syndrome, autoimmune diseases, and psychiatric impairment [4–10]. The disease impacts overall quality of life and productivity due to its physical and psychological components [11]. Currently, retrospective research in psoriasis is limited by knowledge gaps that exist in commonly used data sources, but electronic health records (EHR) may help address this problem [12].

Population studies in psoriasis have typically relied on claims databases or publicly available national databases [12]. However, these databases often lack point-of-care data collected at actual clinic visits. Furthermore, these databases are often not specialty-specific and therefore do not ask clinically relevant questions to a particular specialty [12]. Disease registries or post-marketing drug registries collect useful and structured information [13–16], but these registries may have circumscribed focus, assess a characteristically or geographically limited population, and/or require substantial human resources and financial support [12]. Specialty-specific EHRs provide an opportunity to conduct research from a large, diverse population using clinically relevant data that are collected at point-of-care as part of a typical provider consultation. Because specialty-specific EHRs are completed by specialist providers, the specialty-specific data are much less likely to be subject to misclassification errors compared to data collected by non-specialist providers. EHR systems that collect large amounts of structured data from diverse dermatology practices can fill substantial knowledge gaps not filled with claims databases, publicly available national databases, or data from single institutions [12].

In this study, we used point-of-care, real-world clinical data from a widely used dermatology-specific EHR in the US to examine patient-perceived treatment effectiveness, patterns of medication use (duration, switching, and/or discontinuation), healthcare-resource utilization, and medication costs among psoriasis patients.

Methods

Data source

Data were collected from Electronic Medical Assistant (EMA) Dermatology, a HIPAA-compliant dermatology-specific cloud-based EHR (Modernizing Medicine, Inc., Boca Raton, Florida, US). EMA is a widely implemented dermatology-specific EHR platform, used by over 4500 dermatology providers (30% of the market share) across the US. EMA houses data for over 500,000 psoriasis patients from 49 US states and 2 territories. Dermatology providers input data directly into this EHR during clinical visits at point-of-care. Data were de-identified to ensure patient privacy. Research using de-identified records was approved by the New England Independent Review Board.

Study design

This multicentre, longitudinal, observational cohort study retrospectively examined adults (≥ 18 years) with psoriasis who visited participating dermatology practices in the US during the study period (September 1, 2014-September 1, 2015).

Study population

The study population included adults who were diagnosed with psoriasis by a dermatologist, were classified as having moderate-to-severe psoriasis, and visited a dermatology provider during the study period. Patients were considered to have "moderate-to-severe" disease if they were scored ≥3 on the static physician's global assessment (sPGA [0 = very clear, 5 = very severe]), ≥ 3% body surface area (BSA), received phototherapy, oral systemics (methotrexate, acitretin, cyclosporine, or apremilast), or biologic therapies (etanercept, adalimumab, infliximab, ustekinumab, or secukinumab) during the study period or 6 months prior to study initiation. Patients were categorized into the following treatment groups for analyses: topical treatments, phototherapy, oral systemic treatments (methotrexate, acitretin, cyclosporine, and apremilast), biologic treatments (i.e., etanercept, adalimumab, infliximab, ustekinumab, and secukinumab), combination treatments, and other interventions. Other interventions included patients who were not on topical, phototherapy, oral systemic, biologic, combination therapies commonly used for psoriasis, or patients not receiving psoriasis treatment during the study period. At the time of the study, limited data were available for secukinumab, and data were not available for ixekizumab or brodalumab.

Patient-perceived treatment effectiveness

Patient-perceived treatment effectiveness was assessed by patient response to the following question at follow-up: "I believe this treatment is effective in clearing my skin of psoriasis." Responses were graded on a 5-point Likert scale (1 = "strongly agree," 5 = "strongly disagree"). Adherence was determined by a "yes" or "no" patient response in EMA to the following question: "The treatment was followed as directed."

Patterns of medication usage: duration, switching, and discontinuation

Medication duration Median duration was defined as the amount of time that a patient is on a study drug of interest. Medication duration was calculated for biologics (etanercept, adalimumab, and ustekinumab) and oral systemic medications (methotrexate, apremilast, acitretin, and cyclosporine) during the study period. Patients who received biologic (etanercept, adalimumab, and ustekinumab) or oral systemic medications (methotrexate, apremilast, acitretin, and cyclosporine) at any time during the study period were included in the analysis.

Changing systemic medications Starting treatment was defined as the earliest treatment that a patient was on during the study period. A single treatment switch was defined as any change in treatment group. Patients that switched more than once were classified as undergoing multiple switches. Time on treatment was defined as the overall time documented in EMA on a given treatment prior to the first switch during the study period.

Reasons for discontinuing treatment Providers documented the reasons for treatment discontinuation after conversations with the patient. The providers selected from "loss of efficacy," "side effects," "inability to comply with treatment regimen," "inability to afford treatment," "patient fear or risk," or "unknown." Providers could select more than one reason.

Healthcare resource utilization

Visit frequency Visit frequency was defined as the number of patient visits during the study period.

Visit complexity Visit complexity was defined as a function of annual combined visit and procedure costs using evaluation and management (E/M) (Additional file 1: Table S1) and Current Procedural Terminology (CPT) codes. Separately, annual visit costs were also calculated using only E/M codes.

Medication costs Medication costs were calculated as average medication costs per patient per year (using standard National Average Drug Acquisition Cost pricing). Patients who received biologic (etanercept, adalimumab, and ustekinumab) or oral systemic medications (methotrexate, apremilast, acitretin, and cyclosporine) during the study period were included in the analysis, and those receiving combination treatment were counted more than once. Treatments were excluded if pricing data were unavailable (i.e. secukinumab, infliximab).

Data analyses Data are presented as numbers and percentages, mean ± standard deviation (SD), or median (interquartile range [IQR]), where appropriate. All analyses were performed using R (version 3.2.2) [17]. To be included in the patient-perceived treatment effectiveness analyses, patients had to be on a given oral or biologic treatment for at least 6 months, except for cyclosporine for which patients were included regardless of treatment duration because cyclosporine is often used intermittently. Patient-perceived overall treatment effectiveness was evaluated with stratification by treatment group first and then further stratification by adherence. Only the most recent treatment satisfaction responses were used for patient-perceived treatment effectiveness analyses. Visit frequency and complexity were assessed in relation to maximum sPGA, maximum BSA, or treatment documented during the study period. Treatment group comparisons for visit frequency and costs only included patients that did not switch treatments during the study period.

Results

Patient-perceived treatment effectiveness

From 82,621 adult patients with psoriasis during the study period, patient-perceived treatment effectiveness was investigated in 2200 patients with psoriasis. Patient perceived treatment effectiveness response choices for the question "I believe this treatment is effective in clearing my skin of psoriasis" included "strongly agree," "somewhat agree," "neither agree or disagree," "somewhat disagree," and "strongly disagree." Demographics and clinical characteristics for this patient population are listed in Additional file 1: Table S2. Mean age, comorbidities, and race were similar across the categories of patient-perceived treatment effectiveness. Overall 50% of patients strongly agreed that their treatment was effective compared to 32% reporting "somewhat agree" and 7% reporting "neither agree nor disagree" (Table 1). Biologics users reported highest agreement with the statement their treatment was effective (73%), followed by phototherapy (61%), and then oral systemics (57%).

Results for patient-perceived treatment effectiveness were also examined following stratification by treatment adherence (Table 2). Among patients who provided information on treatment effectiveness, 53% reported treatment adherence, 3% reported non-adherence, and 44% had no adherence data. Patients who were reported to be adherent to their treatments were more likely to perceive their treatments to be effective (84% in the adherent group compared to 62% in the non-adherent group). Similarly, those who were reported to be non-adherent to their treatment were more likely to perceive their treatment to be ineffective (23%) compared to the adherent patients (10%).

Patterns of medication usage: duration, switching, and discontinuation

We evaluated medication duration in 21,087 patients on biologics and 16,000 patients on oral systemics. Overall, patients on biologics had longer median duration on treatment compared to patients on oral systemic medications (160 days [IQR, 57–279] vs. 113 days [IQR, 50–217]; biologics vs orals, respectively).

We also examined medication use patterns for patients who started on monotherapies or combination therapies (Table 3). Overall, patients who started on monotherapies were least likely to switch with 58% of patients treated with topicals, 37% of patients treated with biologics, and 33% of patients treated with oral systemics reporting no treatment switch. Median treatment duration for patients that did not switch therapies was 327 days for topicals, 238 days for biologics, and 159 days for oral systemics. Switching multiple times during the study period was most common among patients who were on combination therapies. For example, patients treated with oral systemic + biologic + phototherapy, biologic + phototherapy, and oral systemic + phototherapy combinations experienced multiple treatment switches (100, 75, and 68%, respectively).Among 427 patients who reported discontinuing treatment, no major differences were observed for age, gender, or comorbidity with respect to treatment groups (Additional file 1: Table S3). Discontinuations were highest from biologic treatment (52%), followed by oral systemic treatment (34%), and phototherapy (6%), with 9% of patients reporting multiple discontinuations. Overall, the most common reasons reported for discontinuing treatment were loss of efficacy (60%) and side effects (27%) (Table 4). When discontinuation reasons were stratified by treatment, the most common reasons for discontinuing treatment were loss of efficacy for biologics (74%) and phototherapy (55%), and side effects for oral systemics (48%).

Healthcare resource utilization

Visit frequency Visit frequency is a measure of healthcare resource utilization. We evaluated visit frequency in patients with data available for maximum disease severity and/or treatment. Among 28,754 patients who had sPGA data, those with severe psoriasis (sPGA of 4 or 5) had a greater frequency of visits compared to those with mild-to-moderate psoriasis (sPGA of 0–3) (Fig. 1a and Additional file 1: Table S4). Among 27,150 patients who had BSA data, the distribution of the visit frequency data reflected a trend consistent with the sPGA data (Results not shown).

Visit frequency during the study period was also stratified for 10,454 patients based on treatment groups (Fig. 1c/d and Additional file 1: Table S5). Patients receiving phototherapy had the highest median number of visits during the one- year study period (49). Biologics and oral systemic treatments both had a median of 3 visits over the 12-months study period. Patients receiving topical treatments alone or other interventions had the lowest median visit frequencies, 2 and 1, respectively.

Visit complexity Visit complexity was defined by patient annual healthcare costs using both visit and procedure costs. This definition was based upon the assumption that patients with greater healthcare costs have greater visit complexity. As with visit frequency, we evaluated visit complexity in patients with data available for maximum disease severity and/or treatment. Patients with a severe psoriasis (sPGA of 4 or 5) had the highest annual combined costs of visits and procedures with $161.70 and

Table 1 Patient-perceived treatment effectiveness stratified according to treatment groups

	Total (n)	Strongly Agree n (%)	Somewhat Agree n (%)	Neither Agree nor Disagree n (%)	Somewhat Disagree n (%)	Strongly Disagree n (%)
Total	2200	1099 (50.0)	706 (32.1)	161 (7.3)	150 (6.8)	84 (3.8)
Topical	1336	524 (39.2)	492 (36.8)	128 (9.6)	126 (9.4)	66 (4.9)
Phototherapy	175	106 (60.6)	63 (36.0)	†	†	†
Oral systemics	199	113 (56.8)	50 (25.1)	18 (9.1)	†	†
Biologics	478	350 (73.2)	96 (20.1)	†	12 (2.5)	†

n, number of patients; †Patient counts < 5 hidden to comply with HIPAA privacy rule. Additional cells hidden as needed to prevent recalculation of hidden values

Table 2 Patient-perceived treatment effectiveness overall and stratified according to treatment group and treatment adherence

	Adherence		Strongly Agree	Somewhat Agree	Neither Agree nor Disagree	Somewhat Disagree	Strongly Disagree
Treatment		n (%)	n (%)	n (%)	n (%)	n (%)	n (%)
Total	Yes	1176 (53.5)	608 (51.7)	375 (31.9)	76 (6.5)	74 (6.3)	43 (3.7)
	No	66 (3.0)	12 (18.2)	29 (43.9)	10 (15.2)	7 (10.6)	8 (12.1)
	Unknown	958 (43.5)	479 (50.0)	302 (31.5)	75 (7.8)	69 (7.2)	33 (3.4)
Topical	Yes	738 (55.2)	306 (41.5)	267 (36.2)	67 (9.1)	63 (8.5)	35 (4.7)
	No	58 (4.3)	9 (15.5)	27 (46.6)	8 (13.8)	6 (10.3)	8 (13.8)
	Unknown	540 (40.4)	209 (38.7)	198 (36.7)	53 (9.8)	57 (10.6)	23 (4.3)
Phototherapy	Yes	88 (50.3)	54 (61.4)	†	†	†	†
	No	†	†	†	†	†	†
	Unknown	87 (49.7)	52 (59.8)	†	†	†	†
Oral Systemics	Yes	90 (45.2)	54 (60.0)	†	†	†	†
	No	†	†	†	†	†	†
	Unknown	106 (53.3)	58 (54.7)	†	13 (12.3)	†	†
Biologics	Yes	254 (53.1)	191 (75.2)	52 (20.5)	†	5 (2.0)	†
	No	5 (1.0)	†	†	†	†	†
	Unknown	219 (45.8)	157 (71.7)	43 (19.6)	8 (3.7)	6 (2.7)	5 (2.3)

n number of patients
†Patient counts < 5 hidden to comply with HIPAA privacy rule. Additional cells hidden as needed to prevent recalculation of hidden values

$150.92, respectively (Table 5). The distribution of the data in patients with BSA data available reflected a trend consistent with the sPGA data (Results not shown). Similar results were observed for patients with data available for sPGA (Additional file 1: Table S6) and BSA (Results not shown) when comparing disease severity to only annual visit costs.

Annual combined costs of visits and procedures were also compared between the different treatment groups (Table 6). Patients who received phototherapy had the highest median annual combined visit and procedure costs ($3217.98). Patients who received other interventions had the lowest median annual combined visit and procedure costs ($108.88). A comparison of treatment groups by only annual visit costs indicated that patients who received oral systemics had the highest median annual visit costs ($217.76) while patients receiving topicals or other interventions had the lowest median annual visit costs ($108.88 for both) (Additional file 1: Table S7).

Medication cost Medication costs were investigated for patients on oral systemic medications ($n = 16{,}000$) and those on biologic medications ($n = 21{,}087$). Patients on biologics had numerically higher average drug costs per patient relative to patients on oral systemics ($21,976.6 vs. $3412.71, respectively).

Discussion

Health outcomes of psoriasis patients in the real world are critical to inform clinical practice. However, these data are scarce in the US. This is due at least in part to difficulties in synthesizing data across disparate EHR systems. Studies using structured, point-of-care clinical data that are supplied directly by dermatology providers can provide in-depth understanding of clinical interactions occurring at the visit-level in the real world.

This study uses real-world, point-of-care data obtained from dermatology providers on a widely used dermatology specific EHR-platform in the US in order to address clinically relevant questions in patients with moderate-to-severe psoriasis. Many data elements are unique to the present study, such as patient-perceived treatment effectiveness and collection of validated psoriasis outcome measures.

Patient-perceived treatment effectiveness affects clinical decision-making in substantial ways because patient input during clinical encounters often influence management plans. In this study, the majority of patients under the care of dermatology providers agreed that their treatments were effective. Specifically, those receiving biologic medications reported the highest rate of strong agreement that the treatment "is effective in clearing my skin of psoriasis." The results derived from EMA for patient-perceived treatment effectiveness on biologics are in agreement with published studies [18]. Of note, greater patient-perceived treatment effectiveness was associated with treatment adherence. Because perceived treatment effectiveness and treatment adherence are interdependent, addressing treatment adherence directly with patients during visits is paramount.

The finding from this study that the majority of psoriasis patients thought their treatment was effective differs somewhat from a previous study [19]. The previous

Table 3 Changes in treatment group from starting treatment for patients treated with monotherapy or combination therapy

Starting treatment group[a]	New treatment group	Percentage switched n (%)	Median (days)[b]	IQR
Topical, *n* = 44,603	Phototherapy	1613 (3.6)	48.0	0.0–296.0
	Oral Systemic	2232 (5.0)	139.0	14.0–327.3
	Biologic	2841 (6.4)	135.0	15.0–283.0
	Oral Systemic + Biologic	9 (0.0)	30.0	0.0–48.0
	Multiple Switch	11,927 (26.7)	79.0	7.0–243.0
	No Switch	25,981 (58.2)	327.0	174.8–365.0
Phototherapy, *n* = 5248	Topical	2438 (46.5)	84.0	33.0–185.0
	Oral Systemic	19 (0.4)	113.0	53.0–149.0
	Biologic	18 (0.3)	79.0	44.3–142.5
	Oral Systemic + Phototherapy	45 (0.9)	56.0	5.0–239.0
	Biologic + Phototherapy	17 (0.3)	76.0	21.0–189.0
	Other Interventions	665 (12.7)	35.0	3.0–97.0
	Multiple Switch	726 (13.8)	98.0	45.0–182.0
	No Switch	1320 (25.2)	160.0	55.0–350.7
Oral Systemic, *n* = 7116	Topical	1751 (24.6)	105.0	21.0–219.0
	Oral Systemic	7 (0.1)	0.0	0.0–111.0
	Biologic	6 (0.1)	34.5	7.0–134.8
	Oral Systemic + Phototherapy	19 (0.3)	2.0	0.0–166.5
	Oral Systemic + Biologic	73 (1.0)	35.0	0.0–100.0
	Other Interventions	445 (6.3)	33.0	0.0–136.0
	Multiple Switch	2459 (34.6)	117.0	45.0–215.5
	No Switch	2356 (33.1)	159.0	61.0–299.1
Biologic, *n* = 11,767	Topical	1857 (15.8)	191.0	83.0–290.2
	Oral Systemic	5 (0.0)	317.0	0.0–342.2
	Biologic	5 (0.0)	42.0	39.0–87.0
	Biologic + Phototherapy	15 (0.1)	7.0	0.0–204.9
	Oral Systemic + Biologic	80 (0.7)	204.8	39.5–302.5
	Other Interventions	800 (6.8)	0.0	0.0–186.6
	Multiple Switch	4669 (39.7)	112.0	15.0–227.0
	No Switch	4336 (36.9)	238.0	139.0–319.8
Oral Systemic + Phototherapy, *n* = 146	Topical	10 (6.9)	52.5	36.5–141.5
	Phototherapy	10 (6.9)	165.0	146.8–240.6
	Oral Systemic	14 (9.6)	88.5	31.0–132.8
	Multiple Switch	99 (67.8)	90.0	40.5–156.0
	No Switch	13 (8.9)	54.0	20.0–144.0
Biologic + Phototherapy, *n* = 65	Biologic	9 (12.0)	91.0	28.0–227.0
	Multiple Switch	56 (74.7)	70.0	38.8–148.0
Oral Systemic + Biologic, *n* = 350	Oral Systemic	18 (5.1)	81.5	3.8–210.5
	Biologic	54 (15.2)	144.5	49.8–227.0
	Multiple Switch	237 (66.8)	94.0	35.0–189.0
	No Switch	41 (11.6)	140.1	48.0–298.5
Oral Systemic + Biologic + Phototherapy, *n* = 5	Multiple Switch	5 (100.0)	137.0	109.0–196.0
Other Interventions, *n* = 13,200	Topical	1782 (13.5)	25.5	0.0–140.0

Table 3 Changes in treatment group from starting treatment for patients treated with monotherapy or combination therapy *(Continued)*

Starting treatment group[a]	New treatment group	Percentage switched n (%)	Median (days)[b]	IQR
	Phototherapy	408 (3.1)	0.0	0.0–0.0
	Oral Systemic	491 (3.7)	0.0	0.0–86.0
	Biologic	1488 (11.3)	12.0	0.0–158.3
	Multiple Switch	4835 (36.6)	13.0	0.0–102.5
	No Switch	4196 (31.8)	265.0	115.9–365.0

IQR interquartile range

[a]Patient numbers provided for starting treatment as documented in EMA for the study period

[b]For patients tracked in EMA prior to the study initiation date, their first visit date was captured and time on treatment was normalized to account for overall time documented in EMA

study consisted of randomly selected psoriasis patients regardless of provider type; more than half of these patients reported dissatisfaction with their treatment [19]. Two factors may contribute to the differences in findings. First, it is likely that patients under the care of dermatology providers are more likely to be satisfied with their treatments than patients cared for by generalists. Second, temporal differences in the study periods can affect the findings because the availability of advanced therapies for psoriasis has improved over time.

We investigated changes in treatments including switching and discontinuation. The data showed that both treatment switching and discontinuation were common in the study population. Switching was lowest in patients treated with topical therapies even though the highest proportion of those on topical therapies reported that they did not perceive their topical treatment to be effective. One potential explanation is that, even though topical therapies may only be modestly effective, patients continue on them due to perception of these therapies being safer. This explanation is supported by results from Armstrong and colleagues [19] indicating that a high proportion of psoriasis patients participating in National Psoriasis Foundation (NPF) Surveys with all spectrum of disease severity chose to receive topical treatment alone due to "fewer adverse events than other treatments". Another potential explanation is that certain providers may have a higher threshold for what may trigger a therapeutic escalation from topical medications alone to initiating systemic therapies.

Across treatment categories, the most frequent reasons reported for discontinuation of treatment were loss of efficacy and side effects. Those on biologics or oral systemics reported the highest frequencies for treatment discontinuation. Among patients who discontinued biologics and oral systemics, the most common reason for discontinuing biologics was loss of efficacy, and the most common reason for discontinuing oral medications was side effects. Similarly, Levin and colleagues [20] also observed that discontinuations were most frequently due to lack of efficacy for biologics and adverse events for traditional systemic therapies. These results may help providers better understand why patients continue, discontinue, or switch treatments. In addition, these results highlight the need for newer treatments (biologics and oral) that are more capable of providing long-term disease control.

With regards to healthcare resource utilization, patients with more severe disease had greater visit frequency and visit complexity compared to those with milder psoriasis. Therefore, concerted efforts at controlling psoriasis severity are important not only to reduce physical and psychosocial burden, but also to reduce overall healthcare resource utilization. The association between severity and visit complexity (measured as cost) is consistent with findings by Evans [21]. Evans reported that patients with moderate-to-severe psoriasis have 5-fold higher total healthcare costs versus patients with mild psoriasis [21].

In addition, healthcare resource utilization also varied across treatment groups. Notably, being on oral therapies

Table 4 Reasons for discontinuing treatments ($n = 528$)

Treatment	Patient/Fear Risk n (%)	Inability to afford treatment n (%)	Inability to comply n (%)	Loss of efficacy n (%)	Side effects n (%)
Total	30 (5.7)	28 (5.3)	13 (2.5)	314 (59.5)	143 (27.1)
Phototherapy	†	†	†	18 (54.5)	8 (24.2)
Oral systemics	†	†	†	81 (39.9)	98 (48.3)
Biologics	17 (5.8)	16 (5.5)	7 (2.4)	215 (73.6)	37 (12.7)

n number of patients

†Patient counts hidden to comply with the HIPAA privacy rule. Additional cells hidden as needed to prevent recalculation of hidden values

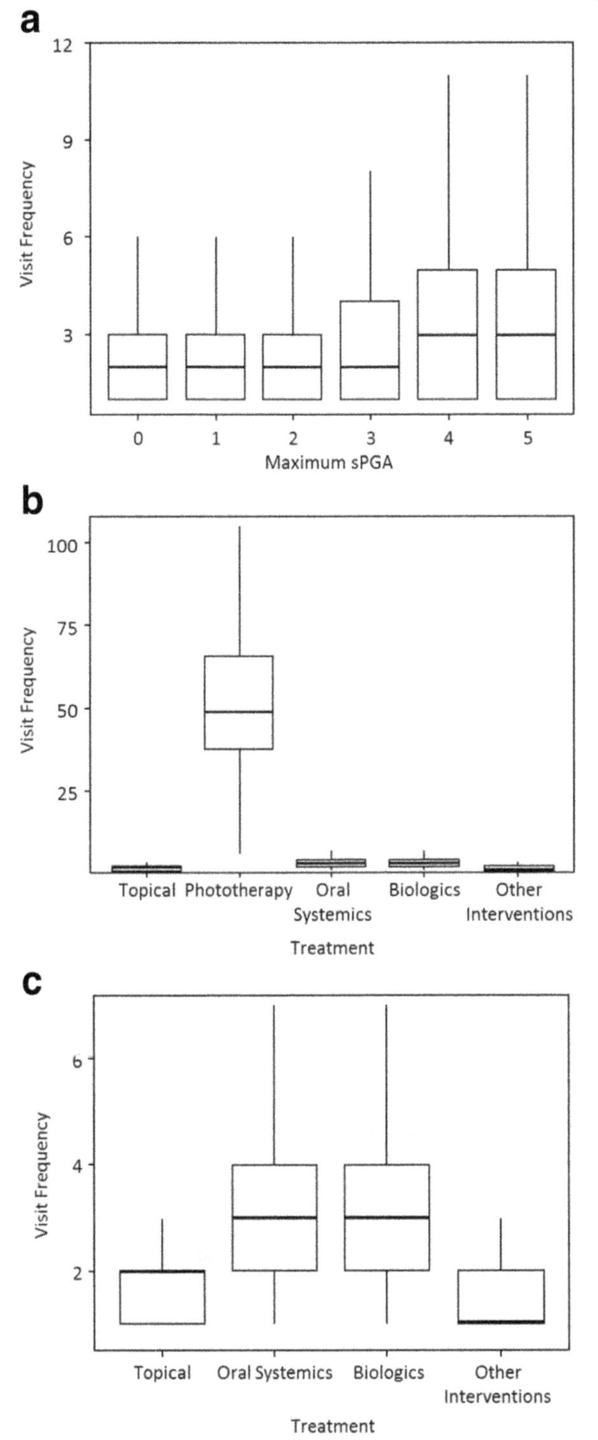

Fig. 1 Visit frequency stratified according to maximum sPGA (**a**), treatment (**b**), and treatment with phototherapy excluded (**c**)

Table 5 Annual combined visit and procedure costs stratified according to maximum sPGA

	Minimum ($)	Maximum ($)	Median ($)	IQR ($)
Maximum sPGA				
0	20.12	892.56	88.40	73.30–109.60
1	20.12	5633.94	104.93	73.30–146.60
2	20.12	10,317.27	108.88	73.30–182.18
3	20.12	15,619.27	109.60	75.46–219.20
4	20.12	17,735.86	161.70	108.88–293.20
5	7.91	9353.18	150.92	108.88–300.94

sPGA static physicians global assessment, *IQR* interquartile range

required highest visit complexity, possibly due to the need for more intense monitoring and management, greater frequency of laboratory evaluation, and greater incidence of adverse events [22]. While treatment with biologics was associated with higher costs, biologic medication duration was longer than oral systemics. Phototherapy was associated with the highest visit frequency, which was expected due to the regularity of visits necessary for in-office light treatments. These results highlight the differences in healthcare resource utilization and costs associated with differing levels of disease severity and treatments.

This pilot study highlights the potential for using an EHR such as EMA to conduct real-world health outcomes research. A unique advantage of a dermatology-specific EHR is the minimization of the risk of misclassification because the data are entered directly by dermatology providers. This is supported by a prior study which reported psoriasis diagnoses (as ≥3 ICD-9 codes) provided by dermatologists had a 97.7% positive prediction value [23]. Both combination therapy data and patient adherence data were limited. In addition, documented medications reflect prescription behaviours and may not accurately represent ultimate utilization by patients. Our grouping of apremilast with other oral systemics may affect cost and healthcare utilization data.

Conclusions

This study used point-of-care, real-world data from a widely implemented US EHR platform to examine several clinically relevant and important questions including patient-perceived treatment effectiveness, medication duration, reasons for switching/discontinuation of treatments, healthcare resource utilization, and costs. With continued

Table 6 Annual combined visit and procedure costs stratified according to treatment groups

Treatment	Minimum ($)	Maximum ($)	Median ($)	IQR ($)
Topical	7.91	1999.68	117.50	73.30–214.16
Phototherapy	144.46	15,119.08	3217.98	1456.65–5678.06
Oral Systemics	25.51	1821.80	217.76	146.60–293.20
Biologics	25.51	1128.32	168.52	108.88–246.22
Other Interventions	20.12	936.07	108.88	73.30–182.18

IQR interquartile range

development and improvement, EHRs with structured and validated data can serve as a powerful tool for real-world research. Real-world research using EHRs provides valuable insights and help clinicians and payers address questions on treatment patterns, costs of care, real-world effectiveness of treatments, and patient satisfaction in clinical practice.

Abbreviations

BSA: Body surface area; CPT: Current procedural terminology; E/M: Evaluation and management; EHR: Electronic health records; EMA: Electronic Medical Assistant; FDA: Food and Drug Administration; HIPAA: Health Insurance Portability and Accountability Act; IQR: Interquartile range; n: Number of patients; SD: Standard deviation; sPGA: Static physician global assessment

Acknowledgements

Modernizing Medicine, Inc. provided assistance with conceptualization and acquisition of data for this study.

Funding

The study was funded by Eli Lilly and Company.

Authors' contributions

AWA, SAF, WM, and OG were involved with conception and/or design of the study. All authors were involved in analyses and/or interpretation of results provided by Modernizing Medicine per initial study design. All authors were involved in drafting and critical revision of the manuscript. All authors read and approved the final manuscript.

Competing interests

A.W. Armstrong: Investigator and/or consultant to Amgen, AbbVie, Janssen, Eli Lilly, Novartis, Valeant, Regeneron, Sanofi, and Modernizing Medicine. S. A. Foster, B. S. Comer, C-Y. Len, W. Malatestinic, R. Burge, and O. Goldblum: All employees and stockholders of Eli Lilly and Company.

Author details

[1]Department of Dermatology, Keck School of Medicine, University of Southern California, Los Angeles, CA 90033, USA. [2]Eli Lilly and Company, Indianapolis, IN, USA. [3]College of Pharmacy, University of Cincinnati, Cincinnati, OH, USA.

References

1. Boehncke WH, Schon MP. Psoriasis. Lancet. 2015;386(9997):983–94.
2. Rachakonda TD, Schupp CW, Armstrong AW. Psoriasis prevalence among adults in the United States. J Am Acad Dermatol. 2014;70(3):512–6.
3. Vanderpuye-Orgle J, Zhao Y, Lu J, Shrestha A, Sexton A, Seabury S, Lebwohl M. Evaluating the economic burden of psoriasis in the United States. J Am Acad Dermatol. 2015;72:961–7. e965
4. Edson-Heredia E, Zhu B, Lefevre C, Wang M, Barrett A, Bushe CJ, Cox A, Wu JJ, Maeda-Chubachi T. Prevalence and incidence rates of cardiovascular, autoimmune, and other diseases in patients with psoriatic or psoriatic arthritis: a retrospective study using clinical practice research datalink. J Eur Acad Dermatol Venereol. 2015;29:955–63.
5. Famenini S, Sako EY, Wu JJ. Effect of treating psoriasis on cardiovascular co-morbidities: focus on TNF inhibitors. Am J Clin Dermatol. 2014;15:45–50.
6. Fried RG, Friedman S, Paradis C, Hatch M, Lynfield Y, Duncanson C, Shalita A. Trivial or terrible? The psychosocial impact of psoriasis. Int J Dermatol. 1995;34:101–5.
7. Nguyen T, Wu JJ. Relationship between tumor necrosis factor-α inhibitors and cardiovascular disease in psoriasis: a review. Permanente J. 2014;18:49–54.
8. Sommer DM, Jenisch S, Suchan M, Christophers E, Weichenthal M. Increased prevalence of the metabolic syndrome in patients with moderate to severe psoriasis. Arch Dermatol Res. 2006;298:321–8.
9. Wu JJ, Choi YM, Bebchuk JD. Risk of myocardial infarction in psoriasis patients: a retrospective cohort study. J Dermatolog Treat. 2015;26:230–4.
10. Wu JJ, Nguyen TU, Poon K-YT, Herrinton LJ. The association of psoriasis with autoimmune diseases. J Am Acad Dermatol. 2012;67:924–30.
11. Rapp SR, Feldman SR, Exum ML, Fleischer AB Jr, Reboussin DM. Psoriasis causes as much disability as other major medical diseases. J Am Acad Dermatol. 1999;41(3 Pt 1):401–7.
12. Armstrong AW, Reddy SB, Garg A. Novel approach to utilizing electronic health records for dermatologic research: developing a multi-institutional federated data network for clinical and translational research in psoriasis and psoriatic arthritis. Dermatol Online J. 2012;18(5):2.
13. Davison NJ, Warren RB, Mason KJ, McElhone K, Kirby B, Burden AD, Smith CH, Payne K, Griffiths CEM. Identification of factors that may influence the selection of first-line biological therapy for people with psoriasis: a prospective, multicentre cohort study. Br J Dermatol. 2017; 177(3):828–36.
14. Iskandar IY, Ashcroft DM, Warren RB, Yiu ZZ, McElhone K, Lunt M, Barker JN, Burden AD, Ormerod AD, Reynolds NJ, et al. Demographics and disease characteristics of patients with psoriasis enrolled in the British Association of Dermatologists biologic interventions register. Br J Dermatol. 2015;173(2):510–8.
15. Iskandar IYK, Ashcroft DM, Warren RB, Evans I, McElhone K, Owen CM, Burden AD, Smith CH, Reynolds NJ, Griffiths CEM. Patterns of biologic therapy use in the management of psoriasis: cohort study from the British Association of Dermatologists biologic interventions register (BADBIR). Br J Dermatol. 2017;176(5):1297–307.
16. Burden AD, Warren RB, Kleyn CE, McElhone K, Smith CH, Reynolds NJ, Ormerod AD, Griffiths CE. The British Association of Dermatologists' biologic interventions register (BADBIR): design, methodology and objectives. Br J Dermatol. 2012;166(3):545–54.
17. Ihaka R, Gentleman R. R: a language for data analysis and graphics. J Comput Graph Stat. 1996;5(3):299–314.
18. Lebwohl MG, Kavanaugh A, Armstrong AW, Van Voorhees AS. US perspectives in the Management of Psoriasis and Psoriatic Arthritis: patient and physician results from the population-based multinational assessment of psoriasis and psoriatic arthritis (MAPP) survey. Am J Clin Dermatol. 2016; 17(1):87–97.
19. Armstrong AW, Robertson AD, Wu J, Schupp C, Lebwohl MG. Undertreatment, treatment trends, and treatment dissatisfaction among patients with psoriasis and psoriatic arthritis in the United States: findings from the National Psoriasis Foundation surveys, 2003-2011. JAMA Dermatol. 2013;149(10):1180–5.
20. Levin AA, Gottlieb AB, Au SC. A comparison of psoriasis drug failure rates and reasons for discontinuation in biologics vs conventional systemic therapies. J Drugs Dermatol. 2014;13(7):848–53.
21. Evans C. Managed care aspects of psoriasis and psoriatic arthritis. Am J Manag Care. 2016;22(8 Suppl):s238–43.
22. Papoutsaki M, Costanzo A. Treatment of psoriasis and psoriatic arthritis. BioDrugs. 2013;27(Suppl 1):3–12.
23. Besen J, McDermott L, Lam C, Legler A, Burris K, Garg A. Validation and comparison of psoriasis case-finding algorithms using international classification of diseases nosology. J Psoriasis Psoriatic Arthritis. 2016;1(3): 123–7.

Effect of 12-*O*-tetradecanoylphorbol-13-acetate-induced psoriasis-like skin lesions on systemic inflammation and atherosclerosis in hypercholesterolaemic apolipoprotein E deficient mice

Marie Madsen[1], Peter Riis Hansen[2], Lars Bo Nielsen[1,3], Karsten Hartvigsen[1,5], Anders Elm Pedersen[4], Jan Pravsgaard Christensen[4], Annemarie Aarup[1] and Tanja Xenia Pedersen[1*]

Abstract

Background: Risk of cardiovascular disease is increased in patients with psoriasis, but molecular mechanisms linking the two conditions have not been clearly established. Lack of appropriate animal models has hampered generation of new knowledge in this area of research and we therefore sought to develop an animal model with combined atherosclerosis and psoriasis-like skin inflammation.

Methods: Topical 12-*O*-tetradecanoylphorbol-13-acetate (TPA) was applied to the ears twice per week for 8 weeks in atherosclerosis-prone apolipoprotein E deficient ($ApoE^{-/-}$) mice.

Results: TPA led to localized skin inflammation with increased epidermal thickness, infiltration of inflammatory-like cells and augmented tissue interleukin-17F levels. Systemic effects of the topical application of TPA were demonstrated by increased plasma concentration of serum amyloid A and splenic immune modulation, respectively. However, atherosclerotic plaque area and composition, and mRNA levels of several inflammatory genes in the aortic wall were not significantly affected by TPA-induced skin inflammation.

Conclusions: TPA-induced psoriasis-like skin inflammation in atherosclerosis-prone $ApoE^{-/-}$ mice evoked systemic immune-inflammatory effects, but did not affect atherogenesis. The results may question the role of psoriasis-induced inflammation in the pathogenesis of atherosclerosis in psoriasis patients.

Keywords: Psoriasis, Atherosclerosis, Inflammation, $ApoE^{-/-}$ mouse, Interleukin-17, Immune cells

Background

Psoriasis is a chronic inflammatory disease of the skin estimated to affect 2–4 % of adults in the western population, but with a varying prevalence due to factors including geography and age [1]. Epidemiological studies have demonstrated that psoriasis is associated with increased risk of cardiovascular disease, e.g., myocardial infarction, stroke, and cardiovascular death [2–6]. This association has led to recommendations for screening and aggressive management of traditional cardiovascular risk factors in psoriasis patients [7]. Indeed, cardiovascular risk factors including hyperlipidaemia, obesity, smoking, hypertension, and diabetes are also more frequently observed in psoriasis patients and the comorbidities are often underdiagnosed and undertreated [8–10].

The leading cause of cardiovascular death is atherosclerosis [11]. Like psoriasis, atherosclerosis is a chronic inflammatory disease and common immunological pathways may causally link the two diseases [10–13]. Thus, psoriasis per se may be an independent risk factor for cardiovascular disease, but it remains to be proven whether psoriasis-driven systemic

* Correspondence: tanjax@sund.ku.dk
[1]Department of Biomedical Sciences, University of Copenhagen, Copenhagen, Denmark
Full list of author information is available at the end of the article

inflammation accelerates atherosclerosis. The lack of appropriate models to study potential causal links between psoriasis and cardiovascular disease has hampered such investigations. Therefore, development of an animal model with psoriasis-like skin lesions and atherosclerosis would provide a valuable tool for investigations of putative shared disease mechanisms and potential new therapeutic targets aimed at both diseases. Shared immunological pathways in psoriasis and atherosclerosis include T helper cell 1 (Th1)-mediated inflammation, alterations in angiogenesis, and dysfunction of the endothelium [11]. Moreover, interleukin (IL)-17-producing cells have been found to have a key role in the pathogenesis of both psoriasis and atherosclerosis, even though the exact role of Th17 cells in atherogenesis remains debated [14].

Presently, only few studies have examined vascular changes in mice with experimentally induced psoriasis-like skin lesions and these have exclusively been performed in atherosclerosis-resistant (normocholesterolaemic) mice. Hence, the former studies have assessed vascular parameters other than established atherosclerosis, e.g., inflammatory cell infiltration, reactive oxygen species formation, endothelial dysfunction, and thrombogenicity [15, 16]. To enable investigations of potential causal links between psoriasis and atherosclerosis, we aimed to develop a mouse model combining the two diseases. The hypercholesterolaemic apolipoprotein E deficient ($ApoE^{-/-}$) mouse is a well-established model for atherosclerosis [17, 18]. Thus, $ApoE^{-/-}$ mice develop extensive atherosclerotic lesions detectable from approximately 10 weeks of age when on a chow diet [17]. The phorbol ester 12-*O*-tetradecanoylphorbol-13-acetate (TPA) is a protein kinase C activator, which after application to the skin induces inflammation and epidermal hyperplasia that recapitulate some of the hallmarks of psoriasis [19, 20]. To investigate whether TPA-induced skin inflammation would induce sufficient deregulation of the systemic immune-inflammatory homeostasis to affect the extent and composition of atherosclerotic plaques we therefore examined the latter after repeated applications of TPA to the ears of $ApoE^{-/-}$ mice. Since atherosclerosis is a disease that progresses slowly, we applied TPA for 8 weeks, as has been done by others [21]. Topical TPA applications induced psoriasis-like skin lesions and unequivocal signs of increased systemic inflammation but had no effect on the development of atherosclerosis in this model.

Methods

Mice and topical application

Female $ApoE^{-/-}$ mice were purchased from Taconic (Ry, Denmark), model n° APO-F (B6.129P2-$ApoE^{tm1Unc}$ N11). Two separate, but similar, studies were conducted, i.e., a pilot study with $n = 5–7$ mice/group (study 1) followed by a full-scale study with $n = 15$ mice/group (study 2). Mice had access to water and standard diet ad libitum (Altromin 1314, Brogaarden, Gentofte, Denmark) and were housed with 12 h light/dark cycles in a temperature- and humidity-controlled room at 21–23 °C at the University of Copenhagen.

At the age of 11 weeks, mice received 2 topical applications/week (20 µl/ear) of either vehicle (acetone) or TPA (Sigma-Aldrich, Brøndby, Denmark; dissolved in acetone at a 0.1 µg/µl concentration). Applications were given on both ears and the mice received 16–17 applications during a total of 8 weeks. Mice were terminated either 3–4 (study 1) or 2 (study 2) days after the last TPA application. Ear thickness was measured prior to each TPA application using a digimatic thickness gauge (Mitutoyo, Illinois, US). All measurements were performed by the same investigator. At study termination, mice were anaesthetized subcutaneously with a 0.1 ml/10 g mouse dose of either a mixture of fentanyl (0.079 mg/mL), fluanisone (2.5 mg/mL), and midazolam (1.25 mg/mL) (study 1), or a mixture of tiletamine (1.63 mg/mL), zolazepam (1.63 mg/mL), xylazin (2.61 mg/mL), and butorphanol tartrate (0.065 mg/mL) (study 2). Subsequently, blood was collected and mice were perfused with ice-cold saline.

Skin histology

Half of an 8 mm biopsy of the right ear was prepared for histology by fixation for one week at room temperature in 10 % neutral buffered formalin ("Lillie" formaldehyde solution 4 %, Hounisen, Skanderborg, Denmark) and embedded in paraffin. Cross-sections of 4 µm were deparaffinized and rehydrated prior to staining with Mayer's hematoxylin and eosin (Rigshospitalet, Copenhagen, Denmark), rinsing and dehydration. Digital images were obtained with a light microscope (Leica Microsystems, Ballerup, Denmark).

Protein analysis from serum and skin samples

Blood was collected in heparinized microtubes (capiject; Terumo Medical Coorporation, Elkton, US) prior to the first TPA/acetone application (baseline sample, submandibular vein) and again at study termination (retro-orbital vein). Plasma was collected after centrifugation for 10 min at 1000 × *g* at 4 °C, aliquoted, and stored at −80 °C until use. Plasma cholesterol was measured in duplicates using the CHOD-PAP reagent from Roche (Roche Diagnostics, Denmark). For protein analyses of ear lysates, an 8 mm biopsy of the left ear was snap-frozen in liquid nitrogen. Using a tissue homogenizer (Precellys 24, Bertin Technologies, Montigny le Bretonneux, France), the biopsies were crushed in cell lysis buffer (Cell Signaling Technology,

The Netherlands) containing freshly added protease inhibitors (complete protease inhibitor with Halt, Thermo Scientific, Rockford, US). Tissue lysates were collected after 15 min of centrifugation at 15,000 × *g* and total protein concentration was measured with the Pierce BCA protein assay kit (Thermo Scientific), according to the manufacturer's instructions. Murine IL-22 and IL-17F (R&D Systems, Minneapolis, US) and serum amyloid A (SAA) (Tridelta, Kildare, Ireland) were measured by commercial ELISA according to the manufacturer's instructions. Mouse interferon-γ (IFNγ), tumor necrosis factor- α (TNFα), keratinocyte-derived cytokine (KC), IL-1β, IL-2, IL-4, IL-5, IL-6, IL-10, IL-12p70, and total IL-12 were measured with the ProInflammatory 7-Plex and Th1/Th2 9-Plex MSD MULTI-spot Assay Systems (Meso Scale Discovery, Rockville, US) according to the manufacturer's instructions. For each assay, a volume of 1.7–5 μl heparinized plasma or a total protein amount of 12–200 μg of ear lysate was used.

Aortic arch atherosclerosis (*en face*) and aortic arch mRNA

The relative amount of atherosclerosis was measured *en face* in the aortic arch (from the heart to the 7th rib), and the same tissue was used for RNA extraction and quantitative real-time PCR. The aortic arch (from the heart to the 7th rib) was snap-frozen in liquid nitrogen. For *en face* analysis, the aortic arch was opened longitudinally, and images of the luminal surface were acquired with a digital camera connected to a dissecting microscope and analysed using the Leica IM50 software (Leica Microsystems). For mRNA analysis, total RNA was extracted from the aortic arch using TRIzol (Life Technologies, Naerum, Denmark) and examined on an Agilent 2100 Bioanalyzer (Agilent Technologies, Santa Clara, US). RNA concentration was measured using a NanoDrop 1000 Spectrophotometer (Thermo Scientific) before cDNA synthesis of 250 ng RNA/aorta using the High Capacity cDNA Reverse Transcription Kit (Life Technologies). Real-time quantitative PCR was performed on a TaqMan (Life Technologies). Primer and probe information can be found in Additional file 1.

Aortic root histology

The apex of the heart was cut off and the remaining part fixed in Lillie's formalin at 4 °C overnight prior to being snap-frozen in Tissue-Tek O.C.T. (Sakura Finetek, Leiden, Netherlands) in ice-cold isopentane. The aortic root was sectioned on a cryostat (Leica) at −18 to −25 °C. Ten μm sections were collected on SuperFrost Plus slides (Menzel-Gläser; Thermo Scientific) for a total of 900 μm starting from where an aortic valve cusp was first visible. The atherosclerotic plaque area was measured, where all three aortic valve cusps were visible to ensure that quantifications were performed at the same anatomical site in each mouse. Masson's Trichrome staining was performed according to the manufacturer's instructions (Sigma-Aldrich), and was used to detect collagen/fibrosis. Immunohistochemical staining was performed with monoclonal rat anti-mouse macrophages/monocytes (MOMA-2 MCA519, 1:500; AbD Serotec, Kidlington, UK). Corresponding antibody isotype control was run with monoclonal rat IgG2b (MAB0061, 1:500, R&D systems). For detection, we used a biotinylated secondary antibody rabbit anti-rat (E0468, 1:2000; Dako, Glostrup, Denmark). The staining procedure included blocking of endogenous peroxidase with 0.5 % H_2O_2, blocking of unspecific antibody binding with 2 % BSA, brown positive staining using a horse-raddish peroxidase approach (Vectastain Elite ABC kit; VectorLab) followed by diaminobenzidine (DAB+, Dako), and counterstaining with Mayer's hematoxylin (Sigma-Aldrich). Digital photos of histological sections were acquired using a slide scanner (Pannoramic, 3DHISTECH, Budapest, Hungary or Axio Scan.Z1, Zeiss, Birkerød, Denmark), and quantified using the Visiomorph software (Visiopharm, Hørsholm, Denmark).

Flow cytometry

Single-cell splenocyte preparations were made by gently forcing splenic tissue through a 70 μm mesh using a 3-ml syringe plunger and ice-cold Hanks Buffered Salt Solution (HBSS, Panum, Denmark). Splenocytes were pelleted at 300×*g* for 8 min, washed once in HBSS, and counted using methylene violet and the 'Countess' (Invitrogen). Half of the mice were euthanized in one day and the other half the following day, and each day we made a pool of splenocytes from control mice and from TPA mice. These pools were used for setup and for making 'fluorescence minus one' (FMO)-controls. Four different flow cytometry analyses were carried out (see Additional files 2 and 3 for more information on antibodies applied together with the corresponding representative figures for gating strategies). Cell surface staining was accomplished using standard techniques in 100 μl in V-bottom 96-well microplates (TPP Techno Plastic Products, Trasadingen, Switzerland). Briefly, $1–2 \times 10^6$ splenocytes were pelleted and blocked with 50 μl FACS buffer (0.1 % sodium azide and 2 % bovine serum albumin in phosphate-buffered saline, PBS) containing FcBlock (1:100; Cat. n° 101302, BioLegend) for 5 min to block Fcγ receptors on the splenocytes. Without washing, staining antibodies were added in 50 μl FACS buffer and incubated for an additional 20 min at 4 °C in the dark. Next, splenocytes were washed, fixed with paraformaldehyde in PBS, and analysed within 24 h using LSRII flow cytometer (BD Biosciences, Albertslund, Denmark). For intracellular staining of Foxp3 (regulatory T-cells), we followed eBioscience's protocol for staining of intracellular/nuclear proteins after cell surface markers (CD4 and CD25) had been stained using the above protocol. To assess changes in $CD4^+$ helper T-cell bias due to the TPA application, we followed the manufacturer's protocol for the Mouse Th1/Th2/Th17 Phenotyping Kit (Cat. n° 560758, BD Biosciences). In order to investigate parallel changes in $CD8^+$ cytotoxic T-cell bias, an anti-CD8 antibody was added to splenocytes as described in the manufacturer's protocol. Briefly, for individual mice, two cultures with 10×10^6 splenocytes were seeded in RP-10 media (RPMI-1640 media containing 2 mM L-glutamine, 10 % heat-inactivated fetal bovine serum, 10 mM HEPES buffer, 0.1 mM non-essential amino acids, 100 U/ml penicillin, and 100 μg/ml streptomycin) containing the BD GolgiStop reagent. Splenocytes in one culture were stimulated with 50 ng/ml TPA and 1 μg/ml Ionomycin for 4 h at 37 °C, whereas the second culture was left unstimulated. Splenocytes were harvested, washed, counted, and 1.2×10^6 splenocytes were fixed using BD Cytofix buffer, washed, permeabilized using BD Perm/Wash buffer, and stained using the kit's antibody cocktail, followed by staining with the anti-CD8 antibody. Stimulated and unstimulated cells were then washed in FACS buffer prior to flow cytometric analysis.

Statistics

Results are shown as mean ± SEM or mean ± SD for normally distributed data or median [interquartile range (IQR)] for non-normally distributed data. Differences between groups were analysed with parametric or non-parametric t-tests, and multiple t-tests with correction for multiple comparisons were used when appropriate. A p-value <0.05 was considered significant. Data were analysed using the Graphpad Prism version 6.05 (GraphPad Software, California, US).

Results

Long-term application of TPA induces ear swelling and local inflammation in $ApoE^{-/-}$ mice

To induce psoriasis-like skin inflammation, hypercholesterolaemic $ApoE^{-/-}$ mice received twice weekly topical applications on both ears of either TPA or vehicle (control), for 8 weeks. TPA led to a skin reaction characterized by scaly skin and redness (Fig. 1a), and by a marked increase in ear thickness throughout the application period ($p < 0.001$ at all time points after baseline, TPA vs. control, Fig. 1b). The ear thickness in control mice was not affected by vehicle application. Histological examination of hematoxylin and eosin-stained ear cross-sections revealed that TPA induced epidermal thickening and local inflammation as assessed by the presence of inflammatory cells in the dermis (Fig. 1a). To investigate whether the TPA-induced histological features were accompanied by changes in local levels of inflammatory mediators, we measured protein levels of selected cytokines in ear lysates. Levels of IL-17F were significantly higher in ear lysates from TPA-treated mice as compared to those from control mice (16.2 [12.1–24.1] pg/mg total protein vs. 0 [0.0–0.5] pg/mg total protein, $p = 0.003$, Fig. 1c), indicating that topical TPA application induced a local immune response with infiltration of IL-17F producing cells. We found no difference in protein levels of IL-12 and KC. Protein levels of the cytokines IL-1β, −2, −4, −5, −6, −10, −12p70, −22, and IFNγ, and TNFα were below the ELISA detection limits in all ear lysates.

Topical TPA application elicits systemic inflammatory modulations

To investigate whether topical application of TPA would induce not only a local immune response, but also systemic effects, we measured plasma levels of SAA and inflammatory cytokines (IL-1β, −2, −4, −5, −6, −10, and -12p70, and IFNγ, and TNFα), and performed flow cytometry of spleens from TPA and control mice. Plasma SAA levels were higher in TPA-treated vs. control mice (4.1 [3.1–6.7] μg/ml vs. 2.8 [2.7–3.0] μg/ml, $p < 0.0001$, Fig. 2a), whereas the other measured cytokines either were below ELISA detection limits, or showed no difference between the two groups (data not shown). TPA application caused larger spleens compared to vehicle application (5.4 ± 0.2 vs. 4.6 ± 0.2 mg wet weight/body weight, $p = 0.0039$); however, this difference was not reflected in absolute splenocyte numbers ($105 \pm 8 \times 10^6$ vs. $98 \pm 7 \times 10^6$ cells, $p > 0.05$). Flow cytometry analyses revealed a significantly higher amount of $CD11b^+$ cells in spleens from TPA-treated mice compared to control mice (12.0 ± 1.2 vs. $7.9 \pm 0.7 \times 10^6$ cells, $p = 0.009$, Fig. 2b). In mouse spleen, CD11b is expressed primarily by inflammatory monocytes, macrophages, neutrophils, and some subpopulations of dendritic cells [22]. Additional flow cytometry analyses of the spleens did not reveal differences in cytotoxic ($CD8^+$) or helper ($CD4^+$) T-cell populations (data not shown). However, detailed analyses of activated $CD4^+$ and $CD8^+$ T-cell populations, based on expression pattern of CD62L and CD44, revealed significantly expanded effector ($CD44^+CD62L^-$) and memory ($CD44^+CD62L^+$) $CD4^+$ T-cell populations in the TPA mice compared to control mice (Fig. 2c). In addition, the memory ($CD44^+CD62L^+$) $CD8^+$ T-cell population was also expanded in the TPA mice (Fig. 2d). There were corresponding reductions of naïve $CD4^+$ and $CD8^+$ T-cell populations (data not shown). Using TPA/ionomycin-stimulation of splenocytes, we detected similar expression of intracellular IFN-γ, IL-4, and IL-17 (Th1, Th2, and Th17 signature cytokines, respectively) in $CD4^+$ cells from TPA and control mice (data not shown). However, in the

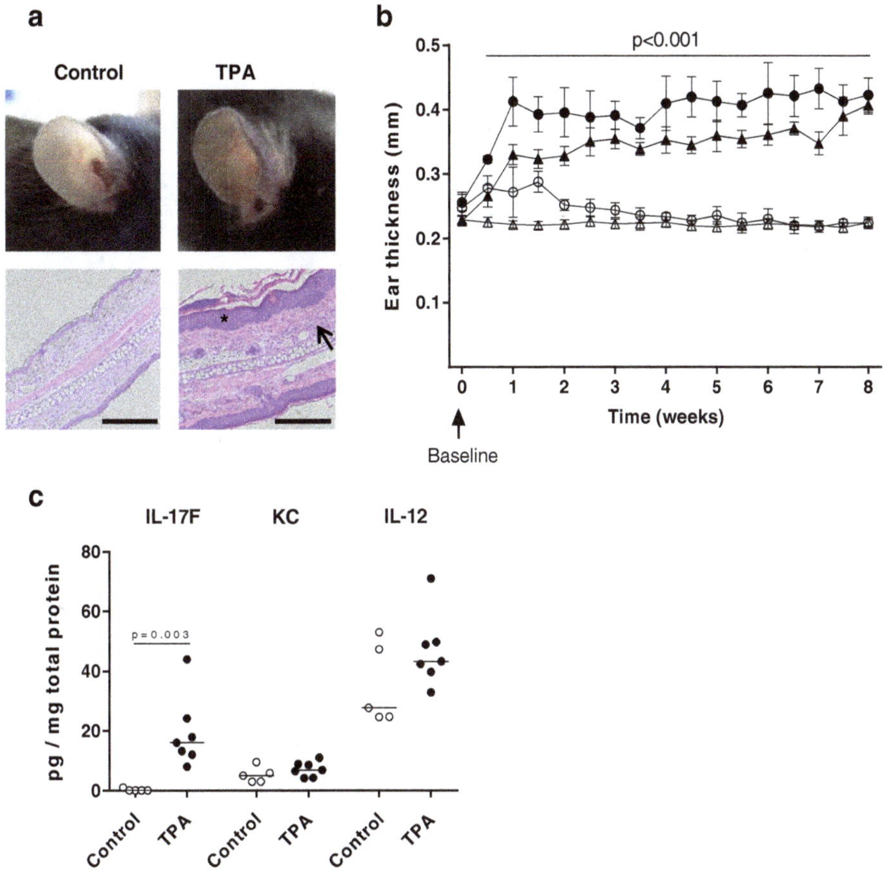

Fig. 1 Topical 12-*O*-tetradecanoylphorbol-13-acetate (TPA) induces local skin inflammation with increased skin thickness and interleukin (IL)-17F levels. **a** Representative photos illustrating the red and scaly appearance of ears after TPA application as compared to control ears, and representative hematoxylin and eosin-stained ear cross-sections at 10× magnification. Scale bar = 200 μm. TPA led to epidermal hyperproliferation (*star*) and dermal inflammation (*arrow*). **b** Ear thickness (mm) was measured twice weekly in ApoE$^{-/-}$ mice after TPA or vehicle application. Data from two separate, but similar studies with vehicle or TPA application on both ears were included; study 1: $n = 5$–7/group (*unfilled circle: control, filled circle*: TPA), study 2: $n = 15$/group (*unfilled triangle: control, filled triangle*: TPA). The depicted values in **b** are mean ± SD, i.e., mean value of right and left ear for each mouse. $p < 0.001$, control vs. TPA at all time points except at baseline; multiple *t*-test corrected for multiple comparisons was applied. **c** Measurement of interleukin IL-17F, IL-12, and keratinocyte-derived cytokine (KC) in ear tissue homogenates after 8 weeks of TPA or vehicle application in study 1. Data is depicted as pg cytokine per mg total protein (median values, unpaired non-parametric *t*-test)

CD8$^+$ cells, we found a significantly higher percentage of IFN-γ expression (Tc1-cells) in TPA mice (Fig. 2e). There was a corresponding reduction of uncommitted CD8$^+$ cells, but no differences in IL-4 and IL-17 expression in the CD8$^+$ cells (data not shown). In a separate analysis, we found significantly elevated percentages of splenic CD4$^+$Foxp3$^+$CD25$^-$ regulatory T-cells (Tregs) in TPA mice compared to control mice (Fig. 2f). There were no differences in natural CD4$^+$Foxp3$^+$CD25$^+$ Tregs or activated CD4$^+$CD25$^+$Foxp3$^-$ T-cells (data not shown).

Topical application of TPA does not accelerate atherosclerosis in ApoE$^{-/-}$ mice

Atherosclerotic plaque area in the aortic root as well as in the aorta *en face* was similar in TPA-treated and control mice (Figs. 3a and b). Also, we found no differences in plasma cholesterol levels (Additional file 4) or in the composition of the plaques in the aortic root, as assessed by histological staining for macrophages and collagen (Fig. 3c). To investigate whether more subtle inflammatory changes had occurred in the arterial wall, we measured aortic arch mRNA expression of several genes involved in atherogenesis, i.e., macrophage markers (F4/80, murine monocyte chemoattractant protein-1 [MCP-1]), adhesion molecules (intercellular adhesion molecule 1 [ICAM-1], vascular cell adhesion molecule 1 [VCAM-1]), and inducible nitric oxide synthase [iNOS]). None of these genes were differentially expressed between TPA and control mice (Fig. 3d).

Discussion

In the present study, we demonstrated that long-term topical TPA application in hypercholesterolaemic ApoE$^{-/-}$ mice induced skin inflammation with psoriasis-like

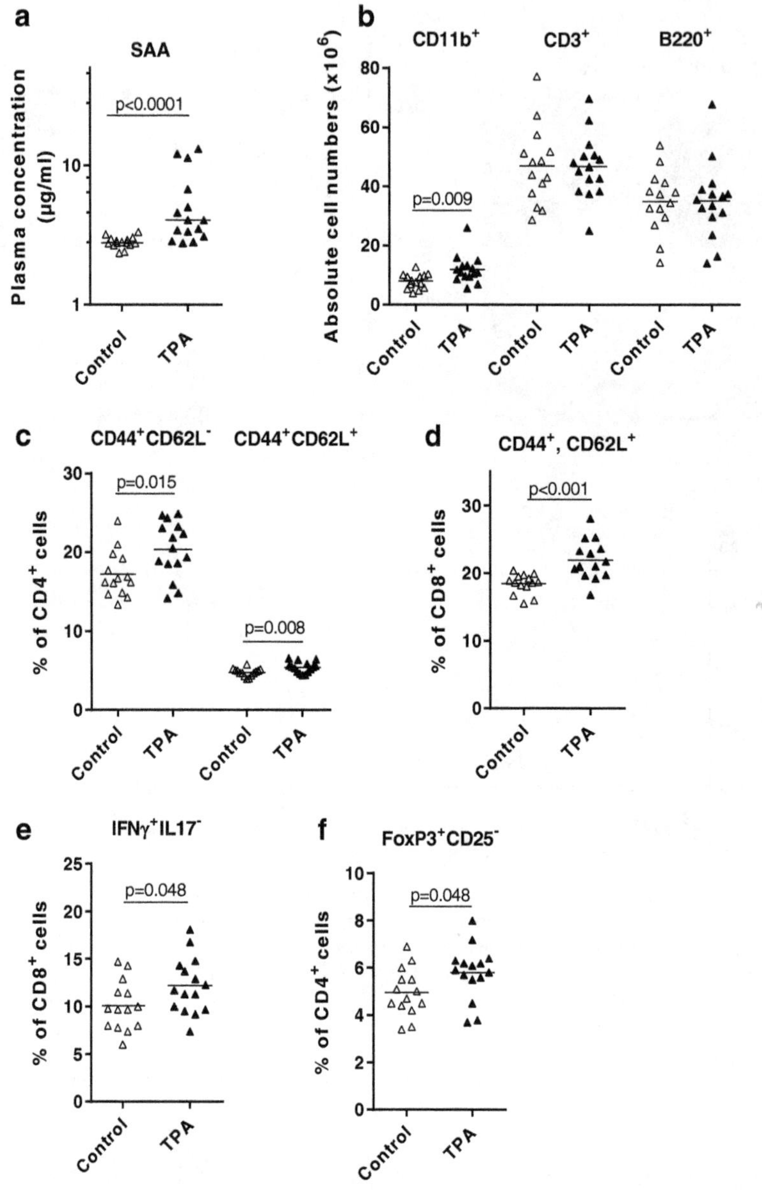

Fig. 2 Topical 12-*O*-tetradecanoylphorbol-13-acetate (TPA) application induces systemic inflammation. **a** Serum amyloid A (SAA) levels (µg/ml) measured in plasma after 8 weeks of topical application on both ears with either TPA or vehicle (control). Note: the y-axis is displayed as a log10 scale. Values are depicted as median and statistical differences analysed by non-parametric *t*-test. **b-f** Spleen flow cytometry data. Symbols and horizontal bars indicate individual mice and group averages, respectively, and parametric t-tests were used to detect statistical differences. **b** Levels of $CD11b^+$ cells, T-cells ($CD3^+$), and B-cells ($B220^+$). **c** Effector and memory $CD4^+$ T-cells ($CD44^+CD62L^-$ and $CD44^+CD62L^+$ cells, respectively), and **d** memory $CD8^+$ T-cells ($CD44^+CD62L^+$ cells). **e** Tc1 cells ($IFN\gamma^+IL17^-$). **f** Regulatory T-cells ($Foxp3^+CD25^-$). *Unfilled and filled triangles* represent control and TPA mice, respectively, from study 2. $N = 14–15$ mice/group; one control mouse was omitted from flow cytometry data due to abnormal values (i.e., above 3xSD)

features, i.e., epidermal thickening and increased local IL-17F levels in the skin, presumably reflecting skin infiltration of IL-17F-producing immune cells. TPA application also led to systemic effects, as identified by higher plasma levels of SAA and splenic weight, and altered splenic cellular populations. These systemic immunomodulatory effects of TPA-induced dermatitis, however, did not affect the area and composition of atherosclerotic plaques, and had no effect on aortic expression of a range of inflammatory genes.

Despite strong epidemiological associations, it is unclear which mechanisms mediate the increased risk of cardiovascular disease in patients with psoriasis. In patients with psoriasis, clinical data from treatment studies with antibodies against TNFα and IL-17, suggest that Th1 and Th17 cells play a significant role in

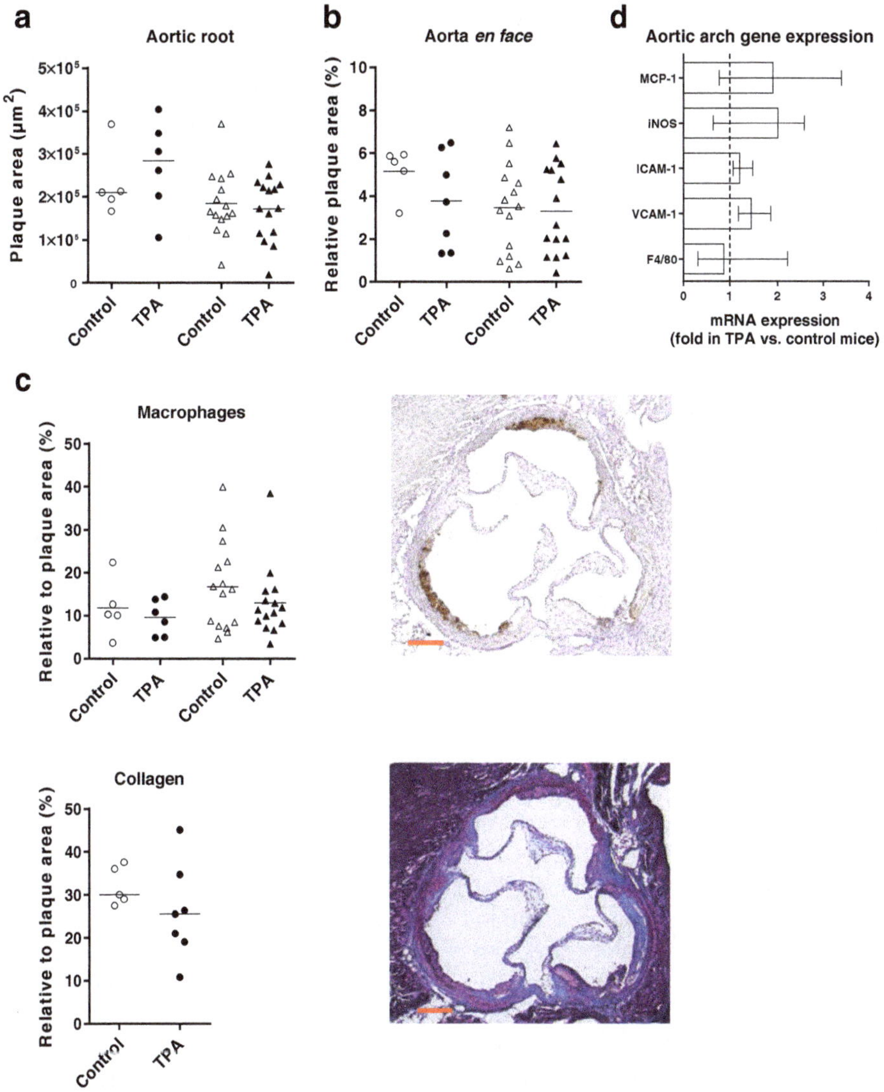

Fig. 3 Topical 12-*O*-tetradecanoylphorbol-13-acetate (TPA) application does not affect atherogenesis in apolipoprotein E deficient (ApoE$^{-/-}$) mice. Plaque areas measured in control and TPA mice in: **a** cross sections of the aortic root (µm^2), and **b** the aortic arch *en face* (% of the aortic arch area); data represent mean values, parametric *t*-test. In **a**, the number of sections quantified were *n* = 4–7/mouse in study 1, and *n* = 1–4/mouse in study 2. **c** Quantification of the level of macrophages and monocytes (MOMA-2, *brown*) and collagen content (Trichrome, *blue*) in aortic root plaque (depicted as % of the total plaque area in the aortic root, mean values, parametric t-tests). Data from study 1 (*n* = 5–7/group) are shown as follows: control: *unfilled circle*; TPA: *filled circle*, and from study 2 (*n* = 10–15/group) as control: unfilled triangle; TPA: filled triangle. Also shown representative photos of the two aortic root stainings, with scale bar = 200 µm. **d** mRNA levels of the macrophage marker F4/80, vascular adhesion molecule 1 (VCAM-1), intercellular adhesion molecule 1 (ICAM-1), inducible nitric oxide synthase (iNOS), and monocyte chemoattractant protein 1 (MCP-1) in the aortic arch as measured by real-time quantitative PCR. The expression levels were normalized to the housekeeping gene glycealdehyde-3-phosphate-dehydrogenase (GAPDH). Subsequently, fold expression in TPA mice relative to control mice was calculated and depicted (control mice set to 1 and depicted as a dotted line). Ten mice/group from study 2 were randomly selected for this analysis. Results are shown as median (IQR), and statistical differences were analysed with non-parametric *t*-test

development and progression of psoriasis [23]. Moreover, IL-17A, IL-17C, and IL-17F protein levels are increased in psoriatic lesions in humans as well as in some mouse models of psoriasis, e.g., after TPA application in transgenic mice with skin-specific expression of vascular endothelial growth factor, and in the imiquimod (a toll-like receptor 7 and 8 ligand and potent immune stimulator) model [24, 25]. KC, the proposed murine functional analogue of human IL-8, is a pro-inflammatory chemokine that has also been shown to play a role in human psoriasis pathogenesis [26]. In our study, we found higher levels of IL-17F, and similar levels of KC in TPA mice compared to vehicle-treated mice. Thus, our data indicate that in ApoE$^{-/-}$ mice, the

TPA-induced skin lesions involve IL-17F-producing cells, but our negative results for the range of other investigated inflammatory cytokines in the ear lysates suggest that important differences exist between the immuno-inflammatory mechanisms in human psoriasis compared to the TPA model.

To assess whether the TPA-induced cutaneous lesions affected the mice systemically, we measured plasma levels of SAA and selected cytokines. SAA is a circulating acute phase protein in humans and in mice (where expression of C-reactive protein [CRP] is negligible) and hepatic SAA production is stimulated by IL-1, IL-6, and TNFα [27]. Plasma levels of SAA and CRP have been reported to be up-regulated in psoriasis patients [28, 29]. In our study, plasma levels of SAA were significantly higher in $ApoE^{-/-}$ mice with TPA-induced skin inflammation as compared to vehicle-treated mice. None of the other investigated cytokines were increased in plasma, and most were below detection limit of our assays. These findings indicate that topical application of TPA induced a relatively low-grade systemic inflammation which may be comparable to the relatively modest increases of circulating levels of inflammatory markers that have been found in patients with psoriasis [30]. Flow cytometric analyses of the spleen revealed that topical application of TPA increased the number of $CD11b^+$ cells and also caused more subtle changes with expanded populations of effector ($CD44^+CD62L^-$) $CD4^+$ T-cells and memory ($CD44^+CD62L^+$) $CD4^+$ and $CD8^+$ T-cells, together with a relative increase in Tc1-cells and Tregs. Interestingly, hyper-activated effector T-cells and a considerable number of Tregs are present in psoriatic skin lesions, where the ability of Tregs to suppress inflammation may be diminished by mechanisms dependent on IL-6, but the relevance of our findings to these abnormalities in patients with psoriasis are unclear at present [31, 32]. Notwithstanding, the immunomodulatory effects on spleen cell populations after TPA application in the present study did not lead to increased atherosclerosis and it is possible that the strength and specificity of these effects were insufficient to affect atherogenesis in this model.

Only very few studies have been published that examined mechanisms by which psoriatic skin lesions may influence vascular biology. The KCTie2 doxycycline-repressible murine model of psoriasis with transgenic expression in keratinocytes of the angiopoietin receptor Tie2 was reported to develop systemic inflammation and aortic root vasculitis in one third of the mice at 12 months of age and these mice had shortened time to occlusive thrombus formation in a model of photochemical carotid artery thrombosis [16]. Very recently, results from a $K14\text{-}IL\text{-}17A^{ind/+}$ mouse model with keratinocyte overexpression of IL-17A were published and these animals developed very severe psoriasis-like skin lesions and displayed increased vascular oxidative stress, endothelial dysfunction, hypertension, left ventricle hypertrophy, and markedly reduced survival as compared to controls [15]. In both studies, the psoriatic skin inflammation therefore significantly affected the vascular system, but it was not possible to assess the effect of skin inflammation on atherogenesis since these mouse models were normocholesterolaemic and thus resistant to development of atherosclerosis. In our study, we used the hypercholesterolaemic atherosclerosis-prone $ApoE^{-/-}$ mouse, and atherosclerosis was measured both in the aorta *en face* and in aortic root cross sections. We found no evidence that the TPA-induced skin inflammation and systemic inflammatory changes significantly influenced atherosclerotic plaque size, plaque composition or aortic arch mRNA levels of inflammatory mediators. Of note, similar results have previously been obtained in $ApoE^{-/-}$ mice with chronic dermatitis induced by croton-oil, the compound from which TPA was originally isolated. However, in that study, mice were challenged only once per 4 weeks, with 8 applications in total, there was no evidence of sustained systemic inflammation, and atherosclerosis was assessed exclusively by aortic *en face* lesion area [33]. Our results add considerably to these earlier data by showing that although experimental induction of psoriasis-like skin lesions led to systemic inflammation, atherosclerosis in the $ApoE^{-/-}$ model was not significantly affected. This finding should be interpreted in light of the limitations of our study, e.g., the inflammatory status of the $ApoE^{-/-}$ model may represent an overwhelming stimulus that abrogates the influence of skin lesions, the immunostimulatory effects of TPA are unlikely to reproduce all abnormalities found in psoriasis, and the relatively small area of psoriasis-like skin lesions in the model, where the ears measure approximately 1 cm^2 on each side thus representing about 6 % of total mouse body surface area [34]. Indeed, a maximum severity psoriasis lesion with 6 % of total body area involvement corresponds to a Psoriasis Area Severity Index (PASI, the most widely used tool to clinically assess psoriasis severity) of 5, compatible with mild-to-moderate disease [35]. On the other hand, we found that these skin lesions elicited unequivocal signs of increased systemic inflammation and it is notable that even mild psoriasis has been associated with increased risk of myocardial infarction and stroke [2, 3]. If TPA had also been applied to the back skin, the systemic inflammatory response might have been stronger. However, we decided against this procedure, since the $ApoE^{-/-}$ mouse is on a C57Bl6/j background and has patches on the back skin, where the cycle of hair follicles is not synchronized after the age of approximately 10 weeks. When analysing effects of TPA application over 8 weeks hereafter, this 'patching' makes is impossible to compare skin lesions on the same anatomical site in different mice. Also, topical application of imiquimod has been suggested to be a more representative model of psoriasis [25]. However, all animal models of psoriasis carry inherent limitations and although keratinocyte signal transduction after stimulation with TPA or imiquimod shows similarities, e.g., with involvement of nuclear factor kappa B (NF-kB) and signal transducer and activator of transcription 3 (STAT3) pathways, important differences between imiquimod-induced skin inflammation and psoriatic plaques were recently demonstrated [36, 37].

Conclusions

In summary, we have investigated a new mouse model that potentially allows for long-term studies of effects of psoriasis-like skin lesions in hypercholesterolaemic mice. Our data suggest that in ApoE$^{-/-}$ mice, TPA-induced psoriasis-like skin lesions lead to both local and systemic inflammation, but despite these effects, we found no alteration in atherosclerotic plaque development. Thus, additional animal models are needed to examine the hypothesis that psoriasis can promote cardiovascular disease.

Additional files

Additional file 1: Primers used for quantitative real-time PCR. (DOCX 14 kb)

Additional file 2: Antibodies used for flow cytometry. (DOCX 16 kb)

Additional file 3: Flow cytometry gating strategy. A. Gating strategy in Fig. 2b: Detection of CD3$^+$, B220$^+$, and CD11b$^+$ cells. B. Gating strategy in Fig. 2c and d: Detection of effector and memory CD4$^+$ and CD8$^+$ T-cells. C. Gating strategy in Fig. 2e: Mouse Th1/Th2/Th17 Phenotyping Kit plus CD8 staining. D. Gating strategy Fig. 2f: Detection of regulatory T-cells (Tregs).

Additional file 4: Mouse body weight and plasma cholesterol. Mean ± SEM, unpaired parametric test control vs. 12-*O*-tetradecanoylphorbol-13-acetate (TPA) mice at baseline and termination in both studies (no statistical significant differences were found between the two groups of mice).

Abbreviations

ApoE$^{-/-}$, apolipoprotein E deficient; CRP, C-reactive protein; DAB+, diaminobenzidine; FMO, fluorescence minus one; GAPDH, glycealdehyde-3-phosphate-dehydrogenase; HBSS, Hanks Buffered Salt Solution; ICAM-1, intercellular adhesion molecule 1; IFNγ, interferon-γ; IL, interleukin; iNOS, inducible nitric oxide synthase; IQR, interquartile range; KC, keratinocyte-derived cytokine; MCP-1, murine monocyte chemoattractant protein-1; NF-kB, nuclear factor kappa B; PASI, Psoriasis Area Severity Index; SAA, serum amyloid A; STAT3, signal transducer and activator of transcription 3; Th1, T helper cell 1; TNFα, tumor necrosis factor- α; TPA, 12-*O*-tetradecanoylphorbol-13-acetate; Tregs, regulatory T-cells; VCAM-1, vascular cell adhesion molecule 1

Acknowledgements

We wish to thank Bente Emma Møller, Birgitte Sander Nielsen, and Anna Borup for providing excellent technical skills regarding mouse handling, flow cytometry, SAA ELISA, and real-time PCR, and Heidi Marie Paulsen for ear histological processing. Lars Svensson MS PhD from LEO Pharma A/S is acknowledged for scientific contribution to this work. We acknowledge the Core Facility for Integrated Microscopy and the Core Facility for Flow Cytometry, Faculty of Health and Medical Sciences, University of Copenhagen. This study was funded by the LEO Foundation (http://leo-foundation.org/). The funding was received by PRH. The funders had no role in study design, data collection and analysis, decision to publish, or preparation of the manuscript.

Authors' contributions

PRH, LBN, and TXP conceived and designed the study, supervised the experiments, and drafted the manuscript. MM conceived and designed the study, carried out the experiments, analysed all data, and drafted the manuscript. KH, AEP, and JPC carried out the flow cytometry studies and performed the accompanying data analyses. AA participated in the study termination. All authors provided critical revision of the manuscript and have read and approved the final manuscript.

Competing interests

The authors declare that they have no competing interests.

Author details

[1]Department of Biomedical Sciences, University of Copenhagen, Copenhagen, Denmark. [2]Department of Cardiology, Gentofte University Hospital, Gentofte, Denmark. [3]Department of Clinical Biochemistry, Rigshospitalet, Copenhagen University Hospital, Copenhagen, Denmark. [4]Department of International Health, Immunology, and Microbiology, University of Copenhagen, Copenhagen, Denmark. [5]Current Address: Novo Nordisk, Gentofte, Denmark.

References

1. Parisi R, Symmons DPM, Griffiths CEM, Ashcroft DM. Global epidemiology of psoriasis: a systematic review of incidence and prevalence. J Invest Dermatol. 2013;133(2):377–85.
2. Ahlehoff O, Gislason GH, Charlot M, Jørgensen CH, Lindhardsen J, Olesen JB, et al. Psoriasis is associated with clinically significant cardiovascular risk: a Danish nationwide cohort study. J Intern Med. 2011;270(2):147–57.
3. Ahlehoff O, Gislason GH, Jørgensen CH, Lindhardsen J, Charlot M, Olesen JB, et al. Psoriasis and risk of atrial fibrillation and ischaemic stroke: a Danish nationwide cohort study. Eur Heart J. 2012;33(16):2054–64.
4. Armstrong EJ, Harskamp CT, Armstrong AW. Psoriasis and major adverse cardiovascular events: a systematic review and meta-analysis of observational studies. J Am Heart Assoc. 2013;2(2):e000062.
5. Boehncke WH, Boehncke S, Tobin AM, Kirby B. The "psoriatic march": a concept of how severe psoriasis may drive cardiovascular comorbidity. Exp Dermatol. 2011;20:303–7.
6. Gelfand JM, Neimann AL, Shin DB, Wang X, Margolis DJ, Troxel AB. Risk of myocardial infarction in patients with psoriasis. JAMA. 2006;296(14):1735–41.
7. Friedewald VE, Cather JC, Gelfand JM, Gordon KB, Gibbons GH, Grundy SM, et al. AJC editor's consensus: psoriasis and coronary artery disease. Am J Cardiol. 2008;102(12):1631–43.
8. Kimball AB, Szapary P, Mrowietz U, Reich K, Langley RG, You Y, et al. Underdiagnosis and undertreatment of cardiovascular risk factors in patients with moderate to severe psoriasis. J Am Acad Dermatol. 2012;67(1):76–85.
9. Parsi KK, Brezinski EA, Lin T-C, Li C-S, Armstrong AW. Are patients with psoriasis being screened for cardiovascular risk factors? A study of screening practices and awareness among primary care physicians and cardiologists. J Am Acad Dermatol. 2012;67(3):357–62.
10. Pietrzak A, Bartosińska J, Chodorowska G, Szepietowski JC, Paluszkiewicz P, Schwartz RA. Cardiovascular aspects of psoriasis: an updated review. Int J Dermatol. 2013;52(2):153–62.

11. Libby P. Inflammation in atherosclerosis. Nature. 2002;420:868–74.
12. Alexandroff AB, Pauriah M, Camp RDR, Lang CC, Struthers a D, Armstrong DJ. More than skin deep: atherosclerosis as a systemic manifestation of psoriasis. Br J Dermatol. 2009;161(1):1–7.
13. Lowes MA, Bowcock AM, Krueger JG. Pathogenesis and therapy of psoriasis. Nature. 2007;445:866–73.
14. Taleb S, Tedgui A, Mallat Z. IL-17 and Th17 cells in atherosclerosis: subtle and contextual roles. Arterioscler Thromb Vasc Biol. 2015;35(2):258–64.
15. Karbach S, Croxford AL, Oelze M, Schüler R, Minwegen D, Wegner J, et al. Interleukin 17 drives vascular inflammation, endothelial dysfunction, and arterial hypertension in psoriasis-like skin disease. Arterioscler Thromb Vasc Biol. 2014;34(12):2658–68.
16. Wang Y, Gao H, Loyd CM, Fu W, Diaconu D, Liu S, et al. Chronic skin-specific inflammation promotes vascular inflammation and thrombosis. J Invest Dermatol. 2012;132(8):2067–75.
17. Nakashima Y, Plump a S, Raines EW, Breslow JL, Ross R. ApoE-deficient mice develop lesions of all phases of atherosclerosis throughout the arterial tree. Arterioscler Thromb Vasc Biol. 1994;14(1):133–40.
18. Zhang SH, Reddick RL, Piedrahita J a, Maeda N. Spontaneous hypercholesterolemia and arterial lesions in mice lacking apolipoprotein E. Science. 1992;258(5081):468–71.
19. Kulkarni NM, Muley MM, Jaji MS, Vijaykanth G, Raghul J, Reddy NKD, et al. Topical atorvastatin ameliorates 12-O-tetradecanoylphorbol-13-acetate induced skin inflammation by reducing cutaneous cytokine levels and NF-kB activation. Arch Pharm Res. 2015;38(6):1238–47.
20. Stanley PL, Steiner S, Havens M, Tramposch KM. Mouse skin inflammation induced by multiple topical applications of 12-O-tetradecanoylphorbol-13-acetate. Skin Pharmacol. 1991;4:262–71.
21. Nakajima K, Kanda T, Takaishi M, Shiga T, Miyoshi K, Nakajima H, et al. Distinct roles of IL-23 and IL-17 in the development of psoriasis-like lesions in a mouse model. J Immunol. 2011;186:4481–9.
22. Hey YY, O'Neill HC. Murine spleen contains a diversity of myeloid and dendritic cells distinct in antigen presenting function. J Cell Mol Med. 2012;16:2611–9.
23. Martin D a, Towne JE, Kricorian G, Klekotka P, Gudjonsson JE, Krueger JG, et al. The emerging role of IL-17 in the pathogenesis of psoriasis: preclinical and clinical findings. J Invest Dermatol. 2013;133(1):17–26.
24. Hvid H, Teige I, Kvist PH, Svensson L, Kemp K. TPA induction leads to a Th17-like response in transgenic K14/VEGF mice: a novel in vivo screening model of psoriasis. Int Immunol. 2008;20(8):1097–106.
25. Van der Fits L, Mourits S, Voerman JS a, Kant M, Boon L, Laman JD, et al. Imiquimod-induced psoriasis-like skin inflammation in mice is mediated via the IL-23/IL-17 axis. J Immunol. 2009;182(9):5836–45.
26. Pietrzak AT, Zalewska A, Chodorowska G, Krasowska D, Michalak-Stoma A, Nockowski P, et al. Cytokines and anticytokines in psoriasis. Clin Chim Acta. 2008;394(1–2):7–21.
27. Marhaug G, Dowton SB. Serum amyloid A: An acute phase apolipoprotein and precursor of AA amyloid. Baillieres Clin Rheumatol. 1994;8(3):553–73.
28. Beygi S, Lajevardi V, Abedini R. C-reactive protein in psoriasis: a review of the literature. J Eur Acad Dermatol Venereol. 2014;28(6):700–11.
29. Rooney P, Connolly M, Gao W, Mccormick J, Biniecka M, Sullivan O, et al. Notch-1 mediates endothelial cell activation and invasion in psoriasis. Exp Dermatol. 2014;23:113–8.
30. Dowlatshahi EA, Van Der Voort EAM, Arends LR, Nijsten T. Markers of systemic inflammation in psoriasis: a systematic review and meta-analysis. Br J Dermatol. 2013;169:266–82.
31. Goodman W a, Levine AD, Massari JV, Sugiyama H, McCormick TS, Cooper KD. IL-6 signaling in psoriasis prevents immune suppression by regulatory T cells. J Immunol. 2009;183(5):3170–6.
32. Sugiyama H, Gyulai R, Toichi E, Garaczi E, Shimada S, Stevens SR, et al. Dysfunctional blood and target tissue CD4 + CD25high regulatory T cells in psoriasis: mechanism underlying unrestrained pathogenic effector T cell proliferation. J Immunol. 2005;174(1):164–73.
33. Ko KWS, Corry DB, Brayton CF, Paul A, Chan L. Extravascular inflammation does not increase atherosclerosis in apoE-deficient mice. Biochem Biophys Res Commun. 2009;384(1):93–9.
34. Dawson NJ. The surface-area/body-weight relationship in mice. Aust J Biol Sci. 1967;20:687–90.
35. Fredriksson T, Petterson U. Severe psoriasis—oral therapy with a new retinoid. Dermatologica. 1978;157(4):238–44.
36. Andrés RM, Montesinos MC, Navalón P, Payá M, Terencio MC. NF-kB and STAT3 inhibition as a therapeutic strategy in psoriasis: in vitro and in vivo effects of BTH. J Invest Dermatol. 2013;133(10):2362–71.
37. Vinter H, Iversen L, Steiniche T, Kragballe K, Johansen C. Aldara®-induced skin inflammation: studies of patients with psoriasis. Br J Dermatol. 2015;172(2):345–53.

Risk factors associated with abscess formation among patient with leg erysipelas (cellulitis) in sub-Saharan Africa: a multicenter study

Palokinam Vincent Pitché[1*], Bayaki Saka[1], Ahy Boubacar Diatta[2], Ousmane Faye[3], Boh Fanta Diané[4], Abdoulaye Sangaré[5], Pascal Niamba[6], Christine Mandengue[7], Léon Kobengue[8], Assane Diop[2], Fatimata Ly[2], Mame Thierno Dieng[2], Alassane Dicko[3], Maciré Mohamed Soumah[4], Mohamed Cissé[4], Sarah Hamdan Kourouma[5], Isidore Kouassi[5], Taniratou Boukari[1], Sefako Akakpo[1], Dadja Essoya Landoh[9] and Kissem Tchangaï-Walla[1]

Abstract

Background: Abscess formation is a frequent local complication of leg erysipelas. In this study we aimed at identifying factors associated with abscess formation of leg erysipelas in patients in sub-Saharan African countries.

Method: This is a multicenter prospective study conducted in dermatology units in eight sub-Saharan African countries from October 2013 to September 2014. We performed univariate and multivariate analysis to compare characteristics among the group of patients with leg erysipelas complicated with abscess against those without this complication.

Results: In this study, 562 cases of leg erysipelas were recruited in the eight sub-Saharan African countries. The mean age of patients was 43.67 years (SD =16.8) (Range: 15 to 88 years) with a sex-ratio (M/F) of 5/1. Out of the 562 cases, 63 patients (11.2 %) had abscess formation as a complication. In multivariate analysis showed that the main associated factors with this complication were: nicotine addiction (aOR = 3.7; 95 % CI = [1.3 – 10.7]) and delayed antibiotic treatment initiation (delay of 10 days or more) (aOR = 4.6; 95 % CI = [1.8 – 11.8]).

Conclusion: Delayed antibiotics treatment and nicotine addiction are the main risk factors associated with abscess formation of leg erysipelas in these countries. However, chronic alcohol intake, which is currently found in Europe as a potential risk factor, was less frequent in our study.

Keywords: Erysipelas of leg, Lower limbs cellulitis, Abscess formation, Risk factors, Sub-Saharan Africa

Background

Cellulitis is an infection of the deep layers of the skin (dermis and hypodermis), mainly caused by streptococcus species [1]. Its localization on the face has become rare meanwhile; the lower limbs localization is currently more frequent. There are various risk factors associated with lower extremities cellulitis such as; lymphoedema, site of entry, leg oedema, venous insufficiency, traumatic wound, leg ulcers, toe-web intertrigo, excoriated leg dermatosis [2, 3]. Various complications might occur during the course of cellulitis. The local and general complications frequently reported are abscess, superficial necrosis or deep venous thrombosis, these complications might occur as from the first days, but relapse of cellulitis and its sequelae occur sometimes later [4]. Abscess formation is the most frequent local complication [4, 5], furthermore, a study conducted in Europe showed that risk factors identified to be associated with abscess formation were chronic alcohol intake, as well as, delayed antibiotic treatment initiation [6]. In Africa, very few data on the risk factors for abscess formation in cellulitis's patients have been published. In this multicenter study, we aim at identifying risk factors associated with

* Correspondence: vincent.pitche@gmail.com
[1]Service de dermato-vénéréologie, CHU Sylvanus Olympio, Université de Lomé, 08 BP 81056 Lomé 08, Togo
Full list of author information is available at the end of the article

abscess formation among patients presenting with cellulitis of lower extremities in sub-Saharan African countries.

Method

Type and population of the study

This is a multicenter prospective study conducted in dermatology units of eight sub-Saharan African countries. There were six countries from West Africa (Togo, Senegal, Mali, Côte d'Ivoire, Guinea, and Burkina Faso) and two central African countries (Central African Republic and Cameroon). We recruited patients more than 15 years old who attended dermatology consultation for the onset of leg's cellulitis. The study period was twelve months from October, 2013 to September, 2014.

Data collection

A validated questionnaire from two study centers was used to collect data. The variables collected from each patient were:

i) Sociodemographic and anamnesis' data i.e. age, sex, use of non-steroid anti-inflammatory drugs and use of cataplasm before consultation. ii) Clinical data i.e. the site of cellulitis, the degree of pain, the occurrence of fever and/or shivering, cutaneous signs: phlyctenas, and purpura, satellite adenopathy, and skin complications such as abscess formation and necrosis.

During the consultation, patients were asked for the date of onset of cellulitis (debut of at least one of the four following signs and symptoms: pain, redness, swelling of the leg and warm leg) and the date of antibiotic initiation if antibiotic was started before consultation. In general most of patients have started antibiotics the day of the consultation, but few patients had already started antibiotics before the consultation. A patient was considered to have a delay in antibiotic initiation when the period between the onset of cellulitis and antibiotic initiation exceeded 10 days. Patients were followed up during hospitalization to record outcome information. During patient's hospitalization, the onset of an abscess was diagnosed by a physician. Once diagnosed, the abscess was incised and drained.

Other variables were also collected from patients through history taking, as well as trough clinical and biological examinations, they were: iii) In medical history, we searched for chronic alcohol intake, sedentary life style and nicotine addiction: iv) In clinical examination, we looked for point of entry (traumatic wound, vascular ulcers, excoriations, intertrigo of intertie), pitting edema, varicous veins, arteriopathy, previous surgery of the leg, deep venous thrombosis, obesity (BMI ≥30), hypertension, neurologic disorders and/or use of bleaching products; v) in Lab test we performed: Glucose and HIV tests.

Statistical analysis

Data were recorded using Epi Info software version 3.1 and analyzed in SPSS® 20.0 (IBM Corporation, Armonk NY, USA) software. For continuous variables, means and standard deviations were calculated while for categorical variables we calculated proportions. Our primary outcome of interest was patients who had complication of cellulitis with abscess formation compare to those without abscess formation. Chi square or Fisher exact test were used when appropriate in univariate analysis. Multivariate backwards stepwise logistic regression analysis was performed to identify independent risk factors for the dichotomous outcome complication of cellulitis with abscess formation or absence of abscess. All variables significant during univariate analysis at a p-value less than 0.2 were then included in the multivariate analysis to assess the adjusted effect and derive the adjusted odds ratio (aOR) of each on the primary outcome. We allocated the value "1" to the dependent dichotomous variable if cellulitis becomes complicated with abscess formation, and the value 0 otherwise. A 95 % level of confidence was applied throughout.

Ethical issues

Ethics clearance was obtain from each Ethics Committee board of the Universities of the 8 countries participating in this study. The participant signed an informed consent form, after the verbal explanation was delivered by the investigating officers. The survey was anonymous and confidential.

Results

From October, 2013 to September, 2014, a total of 562 cases of leg's cellulitis were recruited in the eight participating countries. The mean age of patients was 43.7 years (SD = 16.8) ranging from15 to 88 years. The sex-ratio (M/F) was 5/1. Out of 562 cases, 63 (11.2 %) had abscess formation as complication. Chronic alcohol intake was found in 2/63 patients (3.2 %), while nicotine addiction was found in 7/63 patients (11.1 %). Meanwhile, 1/63 (1.6 %) patient was infected with HIV. Concerning the point of entry, 12/63 (19 %) had inter-toes intertrigo and 43/63 (68.3 %) had neglected wounds on the legs (Table 1). Delayed antibiotic treatment was found in 492/562 patients (87.5 %) (Table 1).

In univariate analysis, associated factors of abscess formation in patient with cellulitis of the leg were: nicotine addiction (OR = 2.71; 95 % CI = [1.1 – 6.6]), the use of bleaching agents (OR = 0.4; 95 % CI = [0.2 – 0.9]), delayed antibiotics treatment initiation (delay of 10 days or more): OR = 5.2; 95 % CI = [2.2 – 12.1]); the use of non steroid anti-inflammatory drugs before consultation (OR = 2.4; 95 % CI = [1.4 – 4.1]); the use of cataplasms and decoctions before consultation (OR = 2.5; 95 % CI = [1.4 – 4.5]) (Table 1).

Table 1 Risk factors associated with abscess formation of leg erysipelas, univariate analysis

Characteristics	Total	Abscess formation		OR	95 % CI	*P*
	N = 562 (%)	Yes, *n* (%)	No, *n* (%)			
Age						
<25 years	*76 (13.5)*	*10 (13.2)*	*66 (86.8)*	1	-	0.43
25-35 years	*134 (23.9)*	*11 (8.2)*	*123 (91.8)*	0.59	[0.24 – 1.46]	
>35 years	*352 (62.6)*	*42 (11.9)*	*310 (88.1)*	0.89	[0.43 – 1.86]	
Gender						
Male	*223 (39.7)*	*31 (13.9)*	*192 (86.1)*	1.55	[0.92 – 2.62]	0.10
Female	*339 (60.3)*	*32 (9.4)*	*307 (90.4)*	1		
Obesity						
Yes	*230 (40.9)*	*23(10.0)*	*200 (90.0)*	0.81	[0.47 – 1.40]	0.45
No	*332 (59.1)*	*40(12.0)*	*292 (88.0)*	1		
Chronic alcohol intake						
Yes	*18 (3.2)*	*2 (11.1)*	*16 (88.9)*	0.99	[0.22 – 4.41]	0.67
No	*544 (96.8)*	*61 (11.2)*	*483 (88.8)*	1		
Diabetes						
Yes	*27 (4.8)*	*2 (7.4)*	*25 (92.6)*	0.62	[0.14 – 2.69]	0.76
No	*535 (95.2)*	*61 (11.4)*	*474 (88.6)*	1		
Hypertension						
Yes	*81 (14.4)*	*10 (12.3)*	*71 (87.7)*	1.14	[0.55 – 2.34]	0.73
No	*481 (85.6)*	*53 (11.0)*	*428 (89.0)*	1		
Sedentary						
Yes	*85 (15.1)*	*12 (14.1)*	*73 (85.9)*	1.37	[0.70 – 2.70]	0.36
No	*477 (84.9)*	*51 (10.7)*	*426 (89.3)*	1		
Nicotine addiction						
Yes	*29 (5.2)*	*7 (24.1)*	*22 (75.9)*	2.71	[1.11 – 6.63]	0.03
No	*533 (84.8)*	*56 (10.5)*	*477 (89.5)*	1		
HIV infection						
Yes	*16 (2.8)*	*1 (6.2)*	*15 (93.8)*	0.52	[0.07 – 4.01]	0.44
No	*546 (97.2)*	*62 (11.4)*	*484 (88.6)*	1		
Pitting oedema						
Yes	*130 (23.1)*	*20 (15.4)*	*110 (84.6)*	1.65	[0.93 – 2.91]	0.08
No	*432 (76.9)*	*43 (10.0)*	*389 (90.0)*	1		
Varicous vein						
Yes	*19 (3.4)*	*2 (10.5)*	*17 (89.5)*	0.93	[0.21 – 4.21]	0.64
No	*543 (96.6)*	*61 (11.2)*	*482 (88.8)*	1		
Obstructive arteriopathy						
Yes	*5 (0.9)*	*1 (20.0)*	*4 (80.0)*	1.99	[0.22 – 18.14]	0.45
No	*557 (99.1)*	*62 (11.1)*	*495 (88.9)*	1		
Use of bleaching agents						
Yes	*97 (17.3)*	*5 (5.2)*	*92 (94.8)*	0.38	[0.15 – 0.98]	0.04
No	*465 (82.3)*	*58 (12.5)*	*407 (87.5)*	1		

Table 1 Risk factors associated with abscess formation of leg erysipelas, univariate analysis *(Continued)*

Previous history of phlebitis						
Yes	*2 (0.4)*	*0 (0.0)*	*2 (100.0)*	-	-	0.79
No	*560 (99.6)*	*63 (11.2)*	*497 (88.8)*			
Previous history of surgery of the leg						
Yes	*6 (1.1))*	*2 (33.3)*	*4 (66.7)*	4.06	[0.73 – 22.62]	0.14
No	*556 (98.9)*	*61 (11.0)*	*495 (89.0)*	1		
Neurologic disorders						
Yes	*1 (0.2))*	*0 (0.0)*	*1 (100.0)*	-	-	0.88
No	*561 (99.8)*	*63 (11.2)*	*498 (88.8)*			
Intertrigo of intertoe						
Yes	*161 (28.6)*	*12 (7.5)*	*149 (92.5)*	0.55	[0.29 – 1.07]	0.07
No	*401 (71.4)*	*51 (12.7)*	*350 (87.3)*	1		
Neglected wound on the leg						
Yes	*324 (57.7)*	*43 (13.3)*	*281 (86.7)*	1.67	[0.95 – 2.92]	0.07
No	*238 (42.3)*	*20 (8.4)*	*218 (91.6)*	1		
Delayed of antibiotics treatment at onset of erysipelas						
<3 days	*104 (18.5)*	*8 (7.7)*	*96 (92.3)*	1	-	<0.001
3-10 days	*295 (52.5)*	*23 (7.8)*	*272 (92.2)*	1.01	[0.44 – 2.33]	
>10 days	*93 (16.5)*	*28 (30.1)*	*65 (69.9)*	5.17	[2.22 – 12.05]	
Use of non steroidanti inflammatory drugs						
Yes	*207 (36.5)*	*35 (16.9)*	172 (83.1)	2.38	[1.40 – 4.04]	0.001
No	*355 (63.5)*	*28 (7.9)*	327 (92.1)	1		
Use of cataplasms and decoctions before consultation						
Yes	*104 (18.5)*	*21 (20.2)*	*83 (79.8)*	2.51	[1.41 – 4.45]	0.001
No	*458 (81.5)*	*42 (9.2)*	*416 (90.8)*	1		

Furthermore, on multivariate analysis, associated risk factors with abscess formation that remained statistically significant were nicotine addiction (aOR = 3.7; 95 % CI = [1.3 - 10.7]) and delayed antibiotics treatment initiation (delay of 10 days or more: aOR = 4.6; 95 % CI = [1.8 - 11.8]) (Table 2).

Discussion

This was a multicenter prospective study carried out in dermatology units in eight sub-Saharan African countries, aiming at identifying risk factors associated with abscess formation as complication of lower extremities cellulitis. Nicotine addiction and delayed in antibiotic treatment initiation were identified as the risk factors associated with abscess formation of leg cellulitis in these countries. Meanwhile, biological analysis of this skin infection was not performed.

Abscess formation is the most frequent complication of cellulitis. In our study we found 11.2 % of this complication. A meta-analysis of this skin disease conducted within a period of 20 years showed that abscess formation, necrosis and/or deep venous thrombosis complicated 3 % to 12 % of lower limb cellulitis [4]. Krasagakis et al [5] found (46/145) 31.7 % of cases of leg cellulitis to be complicated with abscess formation, while others authors, Picard et al. [6], Mahe et al. [7], Crickx et al. [8] observed 7.9 %, 9.9 % and 3.6 % of cases, respectively. Meanwhile, a monocenter study conducted in Lomé (Togo) detected only (3/67) 4.5 % cases of this complication [9].

Abscess formation is the most frequent, and the main cause of morbidity in lower extremities cellulitis, which prolonged patient's hospitalization and increased the financial coast for both patient and the community.

Table 2 Risk factors associated with abscess formation of erysipelas of the leg, multivariate analysis

Characteristics	aOR	95 % CI for aOR
Nicotine addiction		
	3.75	[1.32 ; 10.70]
Delayed antibiotics treatment at onset of erysipelas		
More than 10 days	4.65	[1.84 ; 11.80]

In our study we identified two risk factors associated with abscess formation of leg cellulitis: delayed antibiotics treatment initiation and nicotine addiction. Delayed antibiotics treatment initiation increases the risk of abscess formation by 1.4 to 4.6 as reported in many other studies [5, 6, 8, 9], thereby, bacteria would become more pathogenic, and invade the deep layers of the skin. We could not give pathophysiological relation between this complication and nicotine addiction. Nevertheless, nicotine addiction could induced an immune depression as in chronic alcoholism, which was not currently found in our study compared to another publication [6].

Furthermore, obesity, diabetes, HIV infection and the use of bleaching products, which are more frequent in sub-Saharan Africa [5, 10], were not found as risk factors associated with local complications and severe cellulitis in this study.

Limitations

This study did not investigate biological aspects of skin infection, which could explain the pathophysiological aspects of abscess formation among patients with leg cellulitis. Also, socioeconomic condition of patients may have influenced the delay in antibiotic initiation. Finally, some recall bias could have occurred during recording of anamnesis information. However, in the eight participating dermatology units, investigation officers have used a validated structured data collection tool, in order to, reduce information bias across countries.

Conclusion

In this study we found that abscess formation is a very frequent complication of leg cellulitis, which is mainly due to nicotine addiction and delayed antibiotics treatment initiation. Knowing these risk factors may help early detection and treatment of this complication.

Competing interests

DEL works for the World Health Organization, country office of Togo. The other authors declare that they have no competing interests.

Authors' contributions

BS: contributed in the management of patients. He participated in data collection and wrote the manuscript. ABD, OF, BFD, AS, PN, CM, LK, AD, FL, MTD, AD, MMS, MC, SHK, IK, TB, SA, KTW: contributed to the clinical and therapeutic management of patients from a dermatological point-of-view. They were involved in data collection and interpretation. They have revised and finalized the manuscript. DEL: Participated in data analysis and interpretation. He was involved in the manuscript writing and its finalization. PVP was responsible for the overall scientific coordination of the study, for data analysis and interpretation, and the preparation of the final manuscript. All the authors had read and approved the final manuscript to be submitted for publication.

Acknowledgments

We would like to thank Mr Issifou Yaya, MPH Epidemiology/Clinical Research, Aix- Marseille University, for his help in statistical analysis. We would like to thank also Dr Ali NAQI, dermatologist, scientific writer for reviewing and copyediting the manuscript.

Author details

[1]Service de dermato-vénéréologie, CHU Sylvanus Olympio, Université de Lomé, 08 BP 81056 Lomé 08, Togo. [2]Service de dermatologie, CHU Le Dantec, Dakar, Université Cheik Anta Diop, Dakar, Sénégal. [3]Service de dermatologie, CNAM, Bamako, Université de Bamako, Bamako, Mali. [4]Service de dermatologie-MST, CHU Donka, Conakry, Université de Conakry, Conakry, Guinée. [5]Centre de dermatologie, CHU Treichville, Université de Cocody, Cocody, Côte d'Ivoire. [6]Service de dermatologie CHU Yaldago Ouédraogo, Ouagadougou, Université de Ouagadougou, Ouagadougou, Burkina Faso. [7]Service de dermatologie, Clinique universitaire des Montagnes, Bangangté, Cameroun. [8]Service de dermatologie, CHU Bangui, Université de Bangui, Bangui, Centrafrique. [9]Division de l'Epidémiologie, Ministère de la santé du Togo, Lomé, Togo.

References

1. Bernard P, Bedane C, Mounier M, Denis F, Bonnetblanc JM. Bacterial dermo-hypodermatitis in adults. Incidence and role of streptococcal etiology. Ann Dermatol Venereol. 1995;122(8):495–500.
2. Dupuy A, Benchikhi H, Roujeau JC, Bernard P, Vaillant L, Chosidow O. Risk factors for erysipelas of the leg (cellulitis): case-control study. BMJ. 1999;318(7198):1591–4.
3. Mokni M, Dupuy A, Denguezli M, Dhaoui R, Bouassida S, Amri M, et al. Risk factors for erysipelas of the leg in Tunisia: a multicenter case-control study. Dermatology. 2006;212(2):108–12.
4. Crickx B. Erysipelas: evolution under treatment, complications. Ann Dermatol Venereol. 2001;128(3 Pt 2):358–62.
5. Krasagakis K, Samonis G, Valachis A, Maniatakis P, Evangelou G, Tosca A. Local complications of erysipelas: a study of associated risk factors. Clin Exp Dermatol. 2011;36(4):351–4.
6. Picard D, Klein A, Grigioni S, Joly P. Risk factors for abscess formation in patients with superficial cellulitis (erysipelas) of the leg. Br J Dermatol. 2013;168(4):859–63.
7. Mahe E, Toussaint P, Lamarque D, Boutchnei S, Guiguen Y. Erysipelas in the young population of a military hospital. Ann Dermatol Venereol. 1999;126(8-9):593–9.
8. Crickx B, Chevron F, Sigal-Nahum M, Bilet S, Faucher F, Picard C, et al. Erysipelas: epidemiological, clinical and therapeutic data (111 cases). Ann Dermatol Venereol. 1991;118(1):11–6.
9. Pitche P, Tchangai-Walla K. Erysipelas of the leg in hospital environment in Lome (Togo). Bull Soc Pathol Exot. 1997;90(3):189–91.
10. Musette P, Benichou J, Noblesse I, Hellot MF, Carvalho P, Young P, et al. Determinants of severity for superficial cellulitis (erysipelas) of the leg: a retrospective study. Eur J Intern Med. 2004;15(7):446–50.

A prospective analysis of pinch grafting of chronic leg ulcers in a series of elderly patients in rural Cameroon

Benjamin Momo Kadia[1,2*], Christian Akem Dimala[3,4,5], Desmond Aroke[4], Cyril Jabea Ekabe[2], Reine Suzanne Mengue Kadia[6] and Alain Chichom Mefire[7]

Abstract

Background: Chronic leg ulcers (CLUs) pose serious public health concerns worldwide. They mainly affect the elderly population. Pinch grafting (PG) could be used to treat a variety of CLUs. However, in Cameroon, there is scarce data on the outcome of PG of CLUs in elderly patients in rural hospitals where most of these patients seek for medical attention and where clinicians rely on unconventional wound dressing methods to treat CLUs. Our objective was to describe the outcome of PG of CLUs in elderly patients in rural Cameroon.

Methods: This was a prospective study conducted in a rural hospital of North West Cameroon. From February 2015 to January 2016, comprehensive historical and clinical data were collected per elderly patient who presented with a chronic leg ulcer necessitating PG. PG was done using a simple procedure and each patient followed up for 8 months. Outcome was described in terms of ulcer healing and pain and donor site complications.

Results: Our series included 13 patients: 8 males (61.54%; 95% CI: 31.58–86.14) and 5 females (38.46%; 95% CI: 13.86–68.42) aged from 69 to 88 years (mean: 77.54 ± 5.70 years). Three patients (23.08%; 95% CI: 5.04–53.81) had associated co-morbidities. All the ulcers were unilateral with durations ranging from 7 to 41 months (mean: 19.46 ± 11.03 months). The ulcers ranged in size from 9.0 to 38.1 cm^2 (mean: 17.66 ± 8.35 cm^2). We registered one (7.69%; 95% CI: 0.19–36.03) graft rejection. Concerning the other ulcers, ten (83.33%; 95% CI: 51.59–97.91) had healed after 12 postoperative weeks while 2 (16.67%; 95% CI: 2.09%–48.41) had healed after 14 postoperative weeks and the mean healing time was 12.33 ± 0.78 weeks. Patients with healed ulcers had reduced ulcer site pain from the immediate postoperative period but there was no significant difference in the mean pain scores before and after graft (6.77 against 4.23, $p = 0.13$). These ulcers remained healed after 8 postoperative months. Each donor site had healed 2 weeks after PG. Donor site problems were minimal and included hypopigmentation.

Conclusion: The outcome of PG of CLUs in our series of older patients was satisfactory. This finding does not discount the role of conservative therapy, but we encourage clinicians in rural Cameroon to consider PG over long-term unconventional conservative therapy in the elderly.

Keywords: Pinch grafting-chronic leg ulcers-elderly

* Correspondence: benjaminmomokadia@yahoo.com
[1]Presbyterian General Hospital Acha-Tugi, Acha-Tugi, Cameroon
[2]Grace Community Health and Development Association, Kumba, Cameroon
Full list of author information is available at the end of the article

Background

Chronic leg ulcers (CLUs) pose serious public health concerns worldwide [1–4]. The global proportion of elderly people is on the rise [5] and this segment of the general population is most affected by CLUs [6, 7]. Consequent to the frailty and usual co-morbid states of older people, CLUs in these persons tend to be difficult to manage [8–11]. Prolonged conservative therapy in a bid to definitively treat CLUs is not always efficacious [12, 13], particularly in elderly patients in whom wound healing is usually indolent and/or incomplete [9, 13]. In sub-Saharan Africa, the challenge of managing CLUs in elderly patients is aggravated by the lack of schemes aimed at improving the health-related quality of life of older people who are traditionally left without appropriate care [13]. In view of these, it is imperative to explore and encourage simple, yet effective methods of treating CLUs in elderly people in sub-Saharan Africa.

Previous reports suggest that pinch grafting (PG) could be used to treat a variety of CLUs [14–16]. Some authors have proposed PG as a complement to conservative wound therapy [16] and as first line transplantation technique [17]. It is a simple, safe and cheap procedure which requires minimal resources [12, 15]. Developed nations have even extended the utility of PG to domiciliary basis with remarkable ulcer healing rates [12, 14, 18]. With regards to Cameroon, there is scarce data on the outcome of PG of CLUs in elderly patients in rural areas where most of these patients live and where clinicians still hugely rely on long-term unconventional wound dressing methods to treat CLUs, which usually involve the prolong use of aggressive detergents as well as traditional natural or synthetic bandages, cotton wool and gauzes that keep the wound dry and retard ulcer healing. The objective of our study was to describe the outcome of PG of CLUs in elderly patients in rural Cameroon.

Methods

This was a prospective study carried out in a Level 1 hospital which is located in a remote village in the North West region of Cameroon. A level 1 hospital is a rural hospital or health center (or a hospital in an extremely disadvantaged urban location) with a small number of beds; it has a sparsely equipped operating room for 'minor' procedures; it provides emergency measures in management of 90–95% of trauma and obstetrics cases; and it conducts referral of other patients for further management at a higher level. A chronic leg ulcer was considered as a wound of the leg that persisted for ≥ 3 months [19]. CLUs requiring PG were defined as leg ulcers that showed no tendency to heal after 3 months of conservative therapy using appropriate wound dressing methods. An elderly patient was defined as a person aged 65 years or above [20, 21]. From January 2015 to January 2016, elderly patients with CLUs necessitating PG were studied. Each patient was assessed by the same 3 General practitioners working in the hospital. Patients who died before the end of the pre-specified postoperative follow-up period were excluded. CLUs were described in terms of 2 broad aspects:

- the ulcer itself: onset, duration, position, multiplicity, tenderness, temperature, size (length X width X $\pi/4$) [22], edge, base, depth, and discharge (if present);
- surrounding tissues: state of adjacent tissue, local circulation and innervation

Ulcer pain was graded using a validated 10 echelon visual analogue scale (VAS).

Ethics approval for this study was obtained from the Institutional Review Board of the Faculty of Health Sciences, University of Buea, Cameroon. All the participants signed an informed consent form prior to data collection for the study.

Pre-graft procedure

Conservative therapy (mainly by ulcer debridement and dressing) was done until enough granulation tissue was generated on the ulcer surfaces. Antibiotics were not systematically used but in 2 of the 13 patients, antibiotics were administered for cellulitis.

Graft procedure

PG in our series was done by the same (2) general practitioners. The anterior aspect of the ipsilateral thigh was used in all cases as the donor site. The site was prepared with Cetrimide solution and Povidone iodine and an area of skin roughly equivalent to the ulcer was demarcated for obtainment of the grafts. The demarcated zone was locally anaesthetized by superficial infiltration with 2% Lidocaine combined with epinephrine. Using a syringe needle inclined to about 30 degrees, tents of skin were raised and cut using a scalpel to harvest multiple small split-thickness grafts whose depths were limited to the dermal layer. These varied from 15 to 35 pinches in our series. The grafts were then put inside a petri dish containing 0.9% saline. Lidocaine combined with epinephrine was applied on the surface of the donor site to achieve faster haemostasis. Vaseline gauze imbibed in 0.9% saline and compressive dressings were then applied on the donor site. The dermal surfaces of the grafts were placed on the ulcer a few mm apart (Fig. 1) and covered with two taut vaseline gauze sheets imbibed with 0.9% saline. Two layers of mild compressive dressing were then applied.

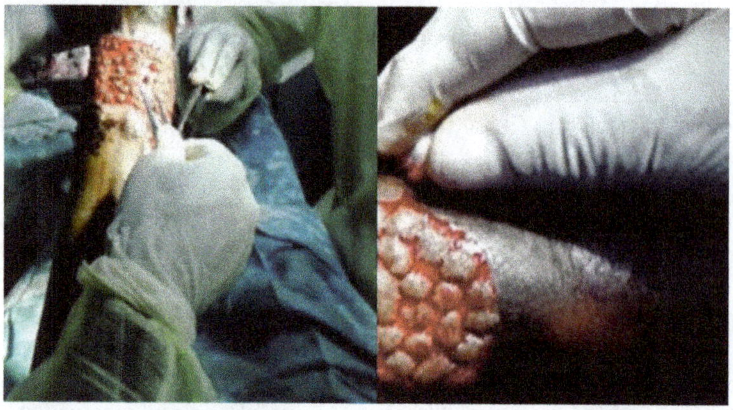

Fig. 1 Grafting of an ulcer

Post-graft procedure

Postoperatively, the patients remained relatively still in bed for one week to avoid shearing forces on the grafts. The donor site was left untouched for a week while the recipient site was uncovered after 5 days and moistened daily with Vaseline gauze imbibed in 0.9% saline. Patients were discharged home after one week of continuous moist dressings of the recipient site, and individually reviewed on outpatient basis: on a weekly basis for the first month, after every two weeks for the second month and then monthly thereafter. Each patient was assessed over 8 postoperative months. Outcome was described in terms of ulcer healing and pain and donor site complications.

Statistical analysis

The data collected was analyzed using Epi Info version 7 statistical software and means, 95% confidence intervals, proportions and standard deviations were recorded. Means and percentages before and after grafting were compared using the student-t-test.

Results

One patient died at the sixth postoperative month and was excluded from the study. Table 1 summarizes the preoperative characteristics of the remaining 13 patients (92.86% inclusion rate). Our series included 8 males (61.54%; 95% CI: 31.58-86.14) and 5 females (38.46%; 95% CI: 13.86-68.42) aged from 69 to 88 years (mean: 77.54 ± 5.70 years). Three patients (23.08%; 95% CI: 5.04-53.81) had associated co-morbidities. The durations of the ulcers (including the period of conservative therapy) ranged from 7 to 41 months (mean: 19.46 ± 11.03 months). The ulcers ranged in size from 9.0 to 38.1 cm^2 (mean: 17.66 ± 8.35 cm^2). Local circulation in tissues surrounding the ulcers was intact in all the patients except in case 8. Local innervation was conserved in all the affected limbs: neurological examination revealed that muscle tone and power as well as sensation to touch, pain, and vibrations were normal in all the affected limbs.

The pregraft ulcer pain scores ranged from 4 to 9 (mean: 6.77) with 92.31% (95% CI: 63.97%-99.81%) having ulcer pain scores ≥ 5. Nine of the 13 ulcers were traumatic while 4 were probably ischaemic (and ischaemic) ulcers. Nine of the ulcers were due to trauma, and 4 probably due to ischaemia.

In the 12th case, there was partial graft rejection by the fifth postoperative day which progressed to complete graft rejection by the second postoperative week. Concerning the other ulcers, ten (83.33%; 95% CI: 51.59-97.91) had healed after 12 postoperative weeks while 2 (16.67%; 95% CI: 2.09%-48.41) had healed after 14 postoperative weeks. The mean healing time was 12.33 weeks ± 0.78 weeks. The healed ulcers remained healed throughout the follow up period. Post graft, the pain scores ranged from 2-9 (mean: 4.23) and although only 7.69% (95% CI: 0.19–36.03%) of the patients had pain scores ≥ 5, this was not significantly different from the 92.31% of patients with pre-graft pain scores ≥ 5 (p = 0.92 from Fischer's exact test). There was no significant difference in the mean pain scores before and after graft (6.77 against 4.23, $p = 0.13$). None of the patients developed new ulcers during the follow-up period. Donor sites were all healed by the end of the second postoperative week. Donor site problems remained minimal and included mild hypopigmentation (Fig. 2).

Discussion

While re-iterating the important role of PG in the treatment of CLUs in the elderly, the current report, to the best of our knowledge, is the first to assess the technical aspects and long term outcome of PG performed on a series of relatively older patients managed using simple resources at a rural hospital facility of Cameroon. Considering the lower age cut-off for

Table 1 Characteristics of patients

Patient S/N			Variable
	Gender/age	Social habits/comorbidity	Ulcer
1	M/77y		18 month-old superficial traumatic ulcer on medial aspect of middle third of leg with purulent discharge. Ulcer was 13 cm2 in size with an infected soft tissue base. It was severely tender. Adjacent tissue was normal.
2	M/78y		13 month-old deep spontaneous ulcer above medial malleolus. Ulcer had smooth regular sloppy edges, a subcutaneous tissue base and covered an area of 14 cm2. It was warm and moderately tender. Surrounding tissue was normal. Probable aetiology: ischaemia
3	F/75y	• Hypertension	14 month-old superficial traumatic ulcer on medial aspect of middle third of leg. Ulcer had smooth irregular flat edges and covered an area of 21 cm2. It was severely tender and its base consisted of subcutaneous tissue. Surrounding tissue was normal.
4	M/86y		12 month-old superficial traumatic ulcer just above medial malleolus with purulent discharge. Ulcer was 9.0 cm2 in size, mildly tender and had infected soft tissue base with maggots. Surrounding tissue was normal.
5	F/76y		9 month-old deep traumatic ulcer on anterior aspect of middle third of leg with purulent discharge. It covered an area of 23 cm2 with an infected subcutaneous tissue base and was severely tender. Surrounding tissue up to knee level was erythematous, oedematous and severely tender (suggestive of cellulitis)
6	F/77y		25 month-old superficial traumatic ulcer on anterior aspect of middle third of leg. It covered an area of 15 cm2 with a subcutaneous tissue base. It was severely tender. Surrounding tissue was normal.
7	F/70y		41 month-old deep spontaneous ulcer just above lateral malleolus. It covered an area of 20 cm2 with a subcutaneous tissue base. It was severely tender. Surrounding tissue was normal.
8	M/73y		30 month-old superficial traumatic ulcer involving posterior third of distal leg. It was 27 cm2 in size and its base consisted of subcutaneous tissue. It was severely tender. Surrounding tissue was normal.
9	M/81y		39 month-old deep spontaneous ulcer involving almost the entire circumference of the distal third of the leg. It was 38.1 cm2 in size with smooth sloppy (regular) edges and a subcutaneous tissue base. It was cold and severely tender. Surrounding tissue was normal but for faint dorsalis pedis and posterior tibial pulses. Probable aetiology: ischaemia
10	M/83y		18 month-old superficial traumatic ulcer above medial malleolus. Ulcer was 10.0 cm2 in size with a subcutaneous tissue base. It was moderately tender. Surrounding tissue was normal.
11	M/88y		15 month-old superficial spontaneous ulcer on dorsum of foot with serous discharge. Ulcer was 9.3 cm2 in size and moderately tender. Its base was comprised of subcutaneous tissue. Surrounding tissue up to mid leg was erythematous, oedematous and severely tender (suggesting cellulitis). Probable aetiology: ischaemia.
12	M/75y	• Chronic smoking • Diabetes	7 month-old superficial traumatic ulcer just above lateral malleolus with purulent discharge. Ulcer was 11.4 cm2 in size and severely tender. Its base consisted of infected subcutaneous tissue and surrounding tissue was normal.
13	F/69y	• Hypertension	12 month-old superficial traumatic ulcer on posterolateral aspect of distal third of leg. Ulcer measured 18.8 cm2 in size. Its base comprised of subcutaneous tissue. Ulcer was moderately tender. Surrounding tissue was normal.

S/N Serial number, *y* yearsm, *M* male, *F* female

defining older people in the African context [21] and the mean age of our patients, our cohort could be regarded as very elderly. The average healing rate of the ulcers was satisfactory and donor site problems were minimal. The low prevalence of comorbidities could explain in part why such a cohort had a satisfactory outcome. It is, however, worth noting that due to lack of more appropriate measures, our assessment of ulcers (for instance, in terms of neurovascular integrity of surrounding tissues) preoperatively was, in part, subjective and comorbidities may have been underdiagnosed in our series.

Initial conservative therapy is indispensable in achieving sufficient wound granulation which is an important pre-requisite for a skin graft to be supported [23]. A limitation common to most small hospitals like ours is the inability to perform cultures [22] from ulcer swabs which is vital in ruling out ulcer base infection, particularly with group A β-haemolytic streptococci. These microbes are notorious for causing graft failure [23]. The

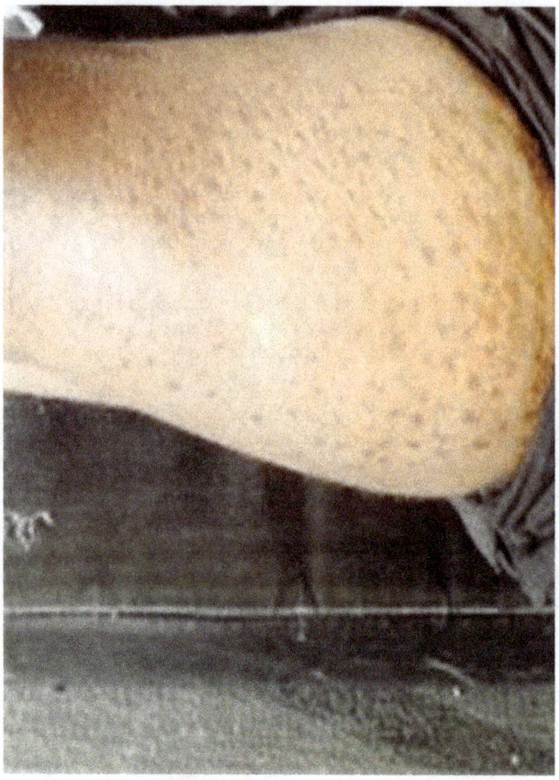

Fig. 2 Hypo-pigmented donor site

complete graft rejection we encountered was possibly due to residual infection at the ulcer base.

Establishing the aetiology of a chronic ulcer is crucial in individualizing and optimizing health care especially in older patients who usually have underlying comorbidities [2, 4]. Importantly, every chronic ulcer unresponsive to conservative therapy should be biopsied in order to rule out malignant changes [23]. However, even in the presence of robust diagnostic facilities, the aetiologies of most CLUs tend to be unknown [8] or multifactorial [9, 24] and from a practical perspective, verifying the exact aetiology of every chronic ulcer does not always seem to take precedence over performing surgery especially in the event of failing conservative treatment and/or intractable pain. CLUs in our series were predominantly traumatic, which is unusual although consistent with preliminary African reports on relatively younger and more active persons [3]. Traumatic ulcers tend to become chronic in poor settings because of initial unskilled management [13]. The limited size of our cohort prevents us from drawing valid interpretations with regards to the location of CLUs on the right leg in all our patients. Nevertheless, contemporary studies with larger cohorts (although relatively younger patients) did not find CLUs to have a predilection for a particular leg [3, 13].

The surgical approach we utilized is in line with what was proposed by J.S. Davis in 1930[18]. Although a simple procedure that has been used over several years [14], PG in recent times necessitates extreme caution with regards to donor sites because donor-site morbidity post-graft is of growing concern worldwide [10, 25]. We recorded minimal donor site problems in our series possibly because of the moistening effects of Vaseline gauze (imbibed in saline). Literature inclines towards the use of moist dressings for donor and recipient sites because of faster healing when compared to dry dressings [26].

Sufficient new vascularization of the ulcer bed is expected to have occurred by the third to fifth postoperative day [23]. Thus, in our series, recipient sites were partially uncovered by the fifth postoperative day given that grafts will only take on ulcer beds on which they can become vascularized. However, at this stage, moist dressings must be applied with caution because the epidermal-dermal interface of epithelializing wounds is weak and even minimal shear forces could lead to graft failure [23].

Assessing ulcer site pain in our cohort was deemed very necessary because it is reported that ulcer pain seems to receive less attention in ulcer management and thus individual needs might not be adequately addressed [8]. In order to have an appraisal of the ulcer site pain intensity before and after PG, we used a validated VAS with 10 echelons which was simple enough for our elderly patients to comprehend. We observed a rapid general drop in ulcer site pain after grafting which is a reported merit of PG [14].

Well known demerits of PG are altered skin pigmentation and graft contraction (Fig. 3). These are sequelae that are inherent to PG and they are consequent to the thin nature of the harvested grafts [27]. Our choice of donor site as the thigh was advantageous in that the discolouration of the donor site due to healing was subsequently covered by hair growth. Females, however, do not benefit from this advantage. The poor cosmesis of the grafted sites following PG remains a subject of concern. That notwithstanding, the recommended attitude is to concurrently consider aesthetic issues and improvement in life quality as well as functionality in order to have a full appraisal of the therapeutic consequences of any skin graft [28, 29].

There is much controversy with regards to where and how to manage CLUs [3]. Our experience, however, suggests that management of CLUs in very elderly people could be adapted context-wise. The population segment most affected by CLUs (elderly people) is generally inactive and home-ridden. A possible prospect therefore is to assess the role of PG on elderly people at a community level in order to make clearer inferences.

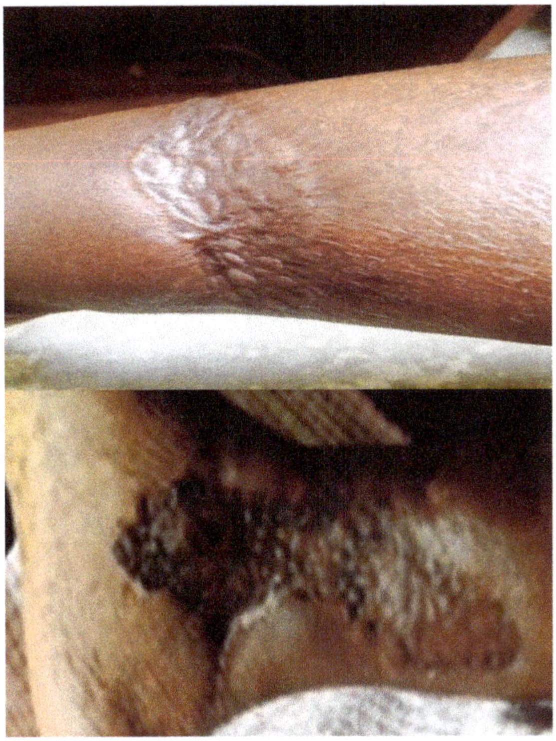

Fig. 3 Healed ulcers post-graft

Conclusions

We describe, to the best of our knowledge, the first report assessing PG of CLUs in older patients in rural Cameroon. PG in our series of relatively older patients (who had a low rate of co-morbidities) in a low-income setting was technically feasible and the outcome was satisfactory. These findings do not discount the role of conservative therapy. However, prolonged unconventional conservative management as definitive treatment for all CLUs in elderly patients may not be worthwhile. More reports on the experience of clinicians on the subject matter could possibly create a platform for progressive refinements in PG procedures and help address the dismal burden of CLUs in elderly patients in rural Cameroon.

Abbreviations

CI: Confidence Interval; CLUs: Chronic leg ulcers; F: Female; M: Male; PG: Pinch Grafting; S/N: Serial number; VAS: Visual Analogue Scale; y: Years

Acknowledgements

We thank all the patients who accepted publication of their data.

Funding

The authors declare that there were no sources of funding for the present investigation.

Authors' contributions

BMK: acquisition of data, data analysis and drafting of manuscript. CAD: reviewed the final manuscript for technical quality. DA: participated in drafting the manuscript. CJE and RSMK edited the initial manuscript. CAM made a critical review of the final manuscript and provided intellectual guidance. All the authors approved the submission of the final manuscript.

Competing interests

The authors declare that they have no competing interests.

Author details

[1]Presbyterian General Hospital Acha-Tugi, Acha-Tugi, Cameroon. [2]Grace Community Health and Development Association, Kumba, Cameroon. [3]Faculty of Epidemiology and Population Health, London School of Hygiene and Tropical medicine, London, UK. [4]Health and Human Development (2HD) Research Group, Douala, Cameroon. [5]Department of Orthopaedics, Southend University Hospital, Essex, UK. [6]Kumba Health District Service, Kumba, Cameroon. [7]Department of Surgery and Obstetrics/Gynaecology, Faculty of Health Sciences, University of Buea, Buea, Cameroon.

References

1. Adeyemi A, Muzerengi S, Gupta I. Leg ulcers in older people: a review of management. Br J Med Pract. 2009;2:21–8.
2. Rayner R, Carville K, Keaton J, Prentice J, Santamaria N. Leg ulcers: atypical presentations and associated comorbidities. Wound Pract Res. 2009;17:168–85.
3. Rahman GA, Adigun IA, Fadeyi A. Epidemiology, etiology, and treatment of chronic leg ulcer: Experience with sixty patients. Ann Afr Med. 2010;9:1–4.
4. Tricco AC, Cogo E, Isaranuwatchai W, Khan PA, Sanmugalingham G, Antony J, Hoch JS, Straus SE. A systematic review of cost-effectiveness analyses of complex wound interventions reveals optimal treatments for specific wound types. BMC Med. 2015;13:90.
5. Retamar P, Lopez-Prieto MD, Rodriguez-Lopez F, de Cueto M, Garcia MV, Gonzalez-Galan V, et al. Predictors of early mortality in very elderly patients with bacteraemia: a prospective multicenter cohort. Int J Infect Dis. 2014;26: 83–7.
6. Briggs M, Jose CS. The prevalence of leg ulceration: a review of the literature. EWMA J. 2003;3:14–20.
7. Adam D, Naik J, Hartshorne T, Bello M, M L. Diagnosis and management of 689 chronic leg ulcers in a single-visit assessment clinic. Eur J Vasc Endovasc Surg. 2003;25:462–8.
8. Hellström A, Nilsson C, Nilsson A, Fagerström C. Leg ulcers in older people: a national study addressing variation in diagnosis, pain and sleep disturbance. BMC Geriatrics. 2016;16:25.
9. Gohel M, Taylor M, Earnshaw J, Heather B, Poskitt K, Whyman M. Risk factors for delayed healing and recurrence of chronic venous Leg ulcers-an analysis of 1324 legs. Eur J Vasc Endovasc Surg Elsevier. 2005;29:74–7.
10. Rogers AD, Atherstone AK, Rode H. Over grafting donor site. East Cent African J Surg. 2009;14:115–6.
11. Ho L, Bailey B, Bajaj P. Pinch grafts in the treatment of chronic venous Leg ulcers. Chir Plast. 1976;3:193–200.
12. Steele K. Pinch grafting for chronic venous leg ulcers in general practice. J R Coll Gen Pract. 1985;35:574–5.

13. Adigun IA, Rahman GA, Fadeyi A. Chronic Leg ulcer in the older Age group: etiology and management. Res J Med Sci Medwell J. 2010;4:107–10.
14. Oien RF, Hansen BU, Hakansson A. Pinch grafting of leg ulcers in primary care. Acta Derm Venereol Scandinavian Univ Press. 1998;78:438–9.
15. Jayaseelan E, Aithal W. Pinch skin grafting in Non-healing leprous ulcers. Int J Lepr. 2004;72:139–42.
16. Christiansen J, Lorens E, Tegner E. Pinch grafting of Leg ulcers: a retrospective study of 412 treated ulcers in 146 patients. Acta Derm Venereol. 1997;77:471–3.
17. Ahnlide I, Bjellerup M. Efficacy of pinch grafting in Leg ulcers of different aetiologies. Acta Derm Ve. 1997;77:144–5.
18. Davis J. The small deep graft. Ann Surg Elsevier. 1930;91:633–5.
19. Agale SV. Chronic Leg Ulcers: Epidemiology, Aetiopathogenesis, and Management. Ulcers. 2013;2013:e413604.
20. Sieber CC. [The elderly patient–who is that?]. Internist (Berl). 2007;48(11): 1190, 1192–4.
21. World Health Organization. Health statistics and information system, Definition of an older or elderly person. Geneva: World Health Organization; 2016.
22. JArroll B, Bourchier R, Gelber P, Jull A, Latta A, Milne R, Oliver F, Tuuta N, Walker N, Waters J. Care of people with chronic leg ulcers: An evidence based guideline. New Zealand: New Zealand Guidelines Group; 1999.
23. Goodacre T. Plastic and reconstructive surgery. In: Norman W, Christopher B, O'connel P (eds.) Bailey and Love's SHORT Practice of Surgery. 25th ed. London. Edward Arnold Ltd; 2008. p394–4091
24. Oien R, Hakansson A, Hansen B. Leg ulcers in patients with rheumatoid arthritis-a prospective study of aetiology, wound healing and pain reduction after pinch grafting. Rheumatology. 2001;40:816–20.
25. Otene C, Olaitan P, Ogbonnaya I, Nnabuko R. Donor site morbidity following harvest of split-thickness grafts in South Eastern Nigeria. J West African Coll Surg. 2011;1:86–96.
26. Wiechula R. The use of moist wound-healing dressings in the management of split-thickness skin graft donor sites: a systematic review. Int J Nurs Pract. 2003;9:S9–17.
27. Shimizu R, Kishi K. Skin Graft. Plastic Surgery International. 2012;2012: e563493.
28. Martin P, S L. Inflammatory cells during wound repair: the good, the bad and the ugly. Trend Cell Biol. 2005;15:599–607.
29. Metcalfe A, Ferguson M. Bioengineering skin using mechanisms of regeneration and repair. Biomaterials. 2007;28:5100–13.

Permissions

All chapters in this book were first published in DERMATOLOGY, by BioMed Central; hereby published with permission under the Creative Commons Attribution License or equivalent. Every chapter published in this book has been scrutinized by our experts. Their significance has been extensively debated. The topics covered herein carry significant findings which will fuel the growth of the discipline. They may even be implemented as practical applications or may be referred to as a beginning point for another development.

The contributors of this book come from diverse backgrounds, making this book a truly international effort. This book will bring forth new frontiers with its revolutionizing research information and detailed analysis of the nascent developments around the world.

We would like to thank all the contributing authors for lending their expertise to make the book truly unique. They have played a crucial role in the development of this book. Without their invaluable contributions this book wouldn't have been possible. They have made vital efforts to compile up to date information on the varied aspects of this subject to make this book a valuable addition to the collection of many professionals and students.

This book was conceptualized with the vision of imparting up-to-date information and advanced data in this field. To ensure the same, a matchless editorial board was set up. Every individual on the board went through rigorous rounds of assessment to prove their worth. After which they invested a large part of their time researching and compiling the most relevant data for our readers.

The editorial board has been involved in producing this book since its inception. They have spent rigorous hours researching and exploring the diverse topics which have resulted in the successful publishing of this book. They have passed on their knowledge of decades through this book. To expedite this challenging task, the publisher supported the team at every step. A small team of assistant editors was also appointed to further simplify the editing procedure and attain best results for the readers.

Apart from the editorial board, the designing team has also invested a significant amount of their time in understanding the subject and creating the most relevant covers. They scrutinized every image to scout for the most suitable representation of the subject and create an appropriate cover for the book.

The publishing team has been an ardent support to the editorial, designing and production team. Their endless efforts to recruit the best for this project, has resulted in the accomplishment of this book. They are a veteran in the field of academics and their pool of knowledge is as vast as their experience in printing. Their expertise and guidance has proved useful at every step. Their uncompromising quality standards have made this book an exceptional effort. Their encouragement from time to time has been an inspiration for everyone.

The publisher and the editorial board hope that this book will prove to be a valuable piece of knowledge for researchers, students, practitioners and scholars across the globe.

Contributors

Laura B von Kobyletzki
Lund University, Institute of Clinical Research in Malmö, Skåne University Hospital, Department of Dermatology, Malmö, Sweden
Karlstad University, Department of Public Health Sciences, Karlstad, Sweden

Åke Svensson
Lund University, Institute of Clinical Research in Malmö, Skåne University Hospital, Department of Dermatology, Malmö, Sweden

Carl-Gustaf Bornehag, Malin Larsson and Cecilia Boman Lindström
Karlstad University, Department of Public Health Sciences, Karlstad, Sweden

Mikael Hasselgren
Örebro University, School of Medicine, Örebro, Sweden
County Council of Värmland, Primary Care Research Unit, Karlstad, Sweden

Bharathi Lingala, Shufeng Li, Ashley Wysong, Allison K Truong, David Kim and Anne Lynn S Chang
Department of Dermatology, Stanford University, Pavilion C, 2nd Floor, 450 Broadway St, Redwood City 94063, CA, USA

James M Mason
School of Medicine, Pharmacy and Health, Durham University, Durham, UK

Julie Carr
Sheffield Children's NHS Foundation Trust, Sheffield, UK

Carolyn Buckley, Steve Hewitt and Phillip Berry
Reckitt Benckiser Healthcare UK, Slough, UK

Josh Taylor
Partizan International, London, UK

Michael J Cork
Academic Unit of Dermatology Research, School of Medicine and Biomedical Sciences, University of Sheffield, Sheffield, UK Department of Dermatology, Sheffield Teaching Hospitals NHS Foundation Trust, Sheffield, UK
Department of Infection and Immunity, The University of Sheffield Medical School, Beech Hill Road, Sheffield S10 2RX, UK

Rhona Auckland
School of Biomedical Sciences, Medical School, Teviot Place, Edinburgh EH8 9AG, UK

Patrick Wassell
Medical School, University of Aberdeen, Polwarth Building, Foresterhill, Aberdeen AB25 2ZD, UK

Susan Hall and Peter Murchie
Centre of Academic Primary Care - Division of Applied Health Sciences, University of Aberdeen, Polwarth Building, Foresterhill, Aberdeen AB25 2ZD, UK

Marianne C Nicolson
ANCHOR Unit, Aberdeen Royal Infirmary, Foresterhill, Aberdeen AB25 2ZN, UK

Ramón Suárez-Medina, Silvia Josefina Venero-Fernández, Esperanza de la Mora-Faife, Gladys García-García, Ileana del Valle-Infante, Liem Gómez-Marrero and Hermes Fundora-Hernández
Instituto Nacional de Higiene, Epidemiología y Microbiología, Infanta No 1158 e/ Llinásy Clavel, Código Postal 10300 La Habana, Cuba

Dania Fabré-Ortiz
Hospital Pediátrico Docente "Juan Manuel Márquez", La Habana, Cuba

Andrea Venn, John Britton and Andrew W Fogarty
Nottingham Biomedical Research Unit, Division of Epidemiology and Public Health, University of Nottingham, Clinical Sciences Building, City Hospital, NG5 1 PB Nottingham, UK

Caroline Biver-Dalle and Eve Puzenat
Department of Dermatology, Besançon University Hospital, Besançon, France

Marc Puyraveau and Frances Sheppard
Clinical Methodology Center, Besançon University Hospital, Besançon, France

Delphine Delroeux
Department of Digestive Surgery, Besançon University Hospital, Besançon, France

Hatem Boulahdour
Department of Nuclear Medicine, Besançon University Hospital, Besançon, France

Fabien Pelletier and Philippe Humbert
Department of Dermatology, Besançon University Hospital, Besançon, France
University of Franche Comté, UMR1098, SFR FED4234, Besançon, France

François Aubin
Department of Dermatology, Besançon University Hospital, Besançon, France
University of Franche Comté, EA3181, SFR FED4234, Besançon, France
Service de Dermatologie, 2 Place Saint-Jacques, 25030, Besançon, cedex, France

Robert L Boggs and Wenzhi Li
Formerly of Pfizer Inc., 3921 Glenlake Garden Drive, Raleigh, NC 27612, USA

Sarolta Kárpáti
Semmelweis University, Budapest, Hungary

Theresa Williams, Ronald Pedersen and Lotus Mallbris
Pfizer Inc, Collegeville, PA, USA

Robert Gniadecki
University of Copenhagen, Copenhagen, Denmark

Valentina S Arsic Arsenijevic and Aleksandra M Barac
Institute of Microbiology and Immunology, University of Belgrade Medical School, Dr Subotica 1, Belgrade, Serbia

Danica Milobratovic
Department of Dermatology, Dermatology Unit, Clinical Center of Serbia; Military Medical Centre, Belgrade, Serbia

Berislav Vekic
Management School, Alfa University, Belgrade, Serbia

Jelena Marinkovic
Institutes for Statistics and Medical Informatics, University of Belgrade School of Medicine, Belgrade, Serbia

Vladimir S Kostic
Institute of Neurology Clinical Centre of Serbia, University of Belgrade, School of Medicine, Belgrade, Serbia

Marianne J Middelveen, Jennie Burke and Peter J Mayne
International Lyme and Associated Diseases Society, Bethesda, MD, USA

Cheryl Bandoski, Eva Sapi and Katherine R Filush
Department of Biology and Environmental Science, University of New Haven, West Haven, CT, USA

Yean Wang and Agustin Franco
Australian Biologics, Sydney, NSW, Australia

Raphael B Stricker
International Lyme and Associated Diseases Society, Bethesda, MD, USA
450 Sutter Street, Suite 1504, San Francisco, CA 94108, USA

Beathe Sitter
Department of Technology, Sør Trøndelag University College, 7004 Trondheim, Norway

Margareta Karin Johnsson
Department of Dermatology, St. Olavs Hospital HF, Trondheim University Hospital, Trondheim, Norway
Department of Cancer Research and Molecular Medicine, Norwegian University of Science and Technology, Trondheim, Norway

Jostein Halgunset
Department of Laboratory Medicine, Children's and Women's Health (LKB), Norwegian University of Science and Technology, Trondheim, Norway
Department of Pathology and Medical Genetics, St. Olavs Hospital HF, Trondheim University Hospital, Trondheim, Norway

Tone Frost Bathen
Department of Circulation and Medical Imaging, Norwegian University of Science and Technology, Trondheim, Norway

Fidelis Mbunda, Phillipo L Chalya and Japhet M Gilyoma
Department of Surgery, Catholic University of Health and Allied Sciences-Bugando, Mwanza, Tanzania

Mabula D Mchembe
Department of Surgery, Muhimbili University of Health and Allied Sciences, Dar Es Salaam, Tanzania

Peter Rambau
Department of Pathology, Catholic University of Health and Allied Sciences- Bugando, Mwanza, Tanzania

Stephen E Mshana
Department of Microbiology, Catholic University of Health and Allied Sciences- Bugando, Mwanza, Tanzania

Benson R Kidenya
Department of Biochemistry and Molecular Biology, Catholic University of Health and Allied Sciences- Bugando, Mwanza, Tanzania

Helen Nankervis, Hywel C Williams, Sherie Smith and Kim S Thomas
Centre of Evidence Based Dermatology, School of Medicine, University of Nottingham, Nottingham, UK

Alison Devine
Glan Clwyd Hospital, Betsi Cadwaladr University Health Board, Bodelwyddan, Rhyl, UK

John R Ingram
Department of Dermatology and Wound Healing, Institute of Infection and Immunity, Cardiff University, Cardiff, Wales

Elizabeth Doney and Finola Delamere
Cochrane Skin Group, Centre of Evidence Based Dermatology, University of Nottingham, Nottingham, UK

Tomasz Jagielski, Aleksandra Ziółkowska, Katarzyna Roeske and Jacek Bielecki
Department of Applied Microbiology, Institute of Microbiology, Faculty of Biology, University of Warsaw, I. Miecznikowa 1, 02-096 Warsaw, Poland

Elżbieta Rup and Anna B Macura
Department of Mycology, Chair of Microbiology, Collegium Medicum, Jagiellonian University, Cracow, Poland

Marion Brusadelli and Géraldine Guasch
Division of Developmental Biology, Cincinnati Children's Hospital Medical Center, 3333 Burnet Avenue, Cincinnati, OH 45229, USA

Adrian J McNairn
Division of Developmental Biology, Cincinnati Children's Hospital Medical Center, 3333 Burnet Avenue, Cincinnati, OH 45229, USA
Department of Biomedical Sciences, College of Veterinary Medicine, Cornell University, Ithaca, NY 14853, USA

Yanne Doucet
Division of Developmental Biology, Cincinnati Children's Hospital Medical Center, 3333 Burnet Avenue, Cincinnati, OH 45229, USA
Department of Dermatology, Columbia University, College of Physicians and Surgeons, New York, NY 10032, USA

Julien Demaude, Charbel Bouez and Lionel Breton
L'OREAL Research and Innovation, 90 rue du General Roguet, 92583, CLICHY, FRANCE

Christopher B Gordon and Armando Uribe-Rivera
Division of Plastic Surgery, Children's Hospital Medical Center, 3333 Burnet Avenue, Cincinnati, OH 45229, USA

Paul F Lambert
University of Wisconsin School of Medicine and Public Health, Madison, WI, USA

Rick Speare
College of Public Health, Medical and Veterinary Sciences, James Cook University, Townsville 4811, Australia
Tropical Health Solutions, 72 Kokoda St, Idalia, Townsville 4811, Australia

Humpress Harrington
Atoifi College of Nursing, Atoifi, Malaita Province, Solomon Islands

Deon Canyon
Office of Public Health Studies, University of Hawaii at Manoa, 1960 East-West Rd, Biomed Building #T103, Honolulu, HI 96822, USA

Peter D Massey
Health Protection, Hunter New England Population Health, Tamworth 2340, Australia

Tarik Benmarhnia, Christophe Léon and François Beck
National Institute for Prevention and Health Education (INPES), 42, Bld de la Libération, St Denis Cedex 93203, France

L. Kemeny
Department of Dermatology and Allergology, University of Szeged, Szeged, Hungary

M. Amaya
Hospital San Lucas, Monterrey, Nuevo Leon, Mexico

P. Cetkovska
Department of Dermatovenereology, Charles University Hospital, Pilsen, Czech Republic

N. Rajatanavin
Division of Dermatology, Ramathibodi Hospital, Mahidol University, Bangkok, Thailand

W-R. Lee
Department of Dermatology, Shuang Ho Hospital, Taipei, Taiwan

A. Szumski, L. Marshall and E. Y. Mahgoub
Global Innovative Pharma, Pfizer, Collegeville, PA, USA

E. Aldinç
Global Innovative Pharma, Pfizer, New York, NY, USA

Anamika Bhattacharyya, Nilu Jain, Sudhanand Prasad, Shilpi Jain, Vishal Yadav and Shamik Ghosh
Vyome Biosciences Pvt. Ltd, Plot# 465, F.I.E., Patparganj Industrial Area, Delhi 110092, India

Shiladitya Sengupta
Medicine and HST, Brigham and Women's Hospital, Harvard Medical School, Room 317, 65 Landsdowne Street, Cambridge, MA 02139, USA

Gefei A. Zhu, Inbar Raber, Shufeng Li, Angela S. Li, Caroline Tan and Anne Lynn S. Chang
Department of Dermatology, Stanford University School of Medicine, 450 Broadway St., Redwood City, CA 94063, USA

Sukolsak Sakshuwong
Department of Computer Science, 353 Serra Mall, Stanford, CA 94305, USA

Hossein Mortazavi and Amirhooshang Ehsani
Autoimmune Bullous Diseases Research Center, Razi Dermatology Hospital, Tehran University of Medical Sciences, Tehran, Iran
Razi Dermtology Hospital, Tehran University of Medical Sciences, Tehran, Iran

Nessa Aghazadeh
Autoimmune Bullous Diseases Research Center, Razi Dermatology Hospital, Tehran University of Medical Sciences, Tehran, Iran
Razi Dermtology Hospital, Tehran University of Medical Sciences, Tehran, Iran
Children's Medical Hospital, Tehran University of Medical Sciences, Tehran, Iran

Ebrahim Arian
Sharif University of Technology, Tehran, Iran

Seyed Sajed Sajjadi
Razi Dermtology Hospital, Tehran University of Medical Sciences, Tehran, Iran

Lara M. Hochfeld, Thomas Anhalt, Marisol Herrera-Rivero, Nadine Fricker, Markus M. Nöthen and Stefanie Heilmann-Heimbach
Institute of Human Genetics, University of Bonn, Sigmund-Freud-Str. 25, 53127 Bonn, Germany
Department of Genomics, Life and Brain Center, University of Bonn, Sigmund-Freud-Str. 25, 53127 Bonn, Germany

Céline S. Reinbold
Human Genomics Research Group, Department of Biomedicine, University of Basel, Hebelstrasse 20, 4031 Basel, Switzerland

Anne M Bruinewoud and Esther WC van der Meer
Department of Public and Occupational Health, EMGO Institute for Health and Care Research, VU University Medical Center, Van der Boechorststraat 7, 1081 BT Amsterdam, The Netherlands

Joost WJ van der Gulden
Department of Primary and Community Care, Centre for Family Medicine, Geriatric Care and Public Health, Radboud University Nijmegen Medical Centre, HB Nijmegen, The Netherlands

Johannes R Anema
Department of Public and Occupational Health, EMGO Institute for Health and Care Research, VU University Medical Center, Van der Boechorststraat 7, 1081 BT Amsterdam, The Netherlands
Body@Work, Research Center Physical Activity, Work and Health, TNO-VU University Medical Center, Amsterdam, The Netherlands
Research Center for Insurance Medicine AMC-UWV-VU University Medical Center, Amsterdam, The Netherlands

Cécile RL Boot
Department of Public and Occupational Health, EMGO Institute for Health and Care Research, VU University Medical Center, Van der Boechorststraat 7, 1081 BT Amsterdam, The Netherlands
Body@Work, Research Center Physical Activity, Work and Health, TNO-VU University Medical Center, Amsterdam, The Netherlands

Leslie Calapre and Elin S. Gray
School of Medical Science, Edith Cowan University, 270 Joondalup Drive, Joondalup, Perth, WA 6027, Australia

Sandrine Kurdykowski, Anthony David and Pascal Descargues
GENOSKIN Centre Pierre Potier, Oncopole, Toulouse, France

Mel Ziman
School of Medical Science, Edith Cowan University, 270 Joondalup Drive, Joondalup, Perth, WA 6027, Australia

School of Pathology and Laboratory Medicine, University of Western Australia, Crawley, WA, Australia

Anne Cécile Zoung-Kanyi Bissek
Department of Internal Medicine and Specialties, Faculty of Medicine and Biomedical Sciences, University of Yaoundé I, Yaoundé, Cameroon

Alexandra Dominique Ngangue Engome
Department of Internal Medicine and Specialties, Faculty of Medicine and Biomedical Sciences, University of Yaoundé I, Yaoundé, Cameroon
Yaoundé University Teaching Hospital, Yaoundé, Cameroon

Emmanuel Armand Kouotou
Department of Internal Medicine and Specialties, Faculty of Medicine and Biomedical Sciences, University of Yaoundé I, Yaoundé, Cameroon
Yaoundé University Teaching Hospital, Yaoundé, Cameroon
Biyem-Assi District Hospital, Yaoundé, Cameroon

Jobert Richie N. Nansseu
Department of Public Health, Faculty of Medicine and Biomedical Sciences, University of Yaoundé I, Yaoundé, Cameroon

Sandra Ayuk Tatah
Yaoundé University Teaching Hospital, Yaoundé, Cameroon
Department of Paediatrics and Specialties, Faculty of Medicine and Biomedical Sciences, University of Yaoundé I, Yaoundé, Cameroon

Indhupriya Subramanian, Vivek K. Singh and Abhay Jere
LABS, Persistent Systems Limited, 9A/12, Erandwane, Pune, Maharashtra 411004, India

Leslie Calapre and Elin S. Gray
School of Medical Sciences, Edith Cowan University, 270 Joondalup Drive, Joondalup, Perth, WA 6027, Australia

Sandrine Kurdykowski, Anthony David and Pascal Descargues
GENOSKIN Centre Pierre Potier, Oncopole, Toulouse, France
Department of Pathology and Laboratory Medicine, University of Western Australia, Crawley, WA, Australia

Prue Hart
Telethon Kids Institute, University of Western Australia, 100 Roberts Road, Subiaco, Perth 6008, Australia

Mel Ziman
School of Medical Sciences, Edith Cowan University, 270 Joondalup Drive, Joondalup, Perth, WA 6027, Australia
Department of Pathology and Laboratory Medicine, University of Western Australia, Crawley, WA, Australia

Melanie Rae Simpson, Ola Storrø, Roar Johnsen and Torbjørn Øien
Department of Public Health and General Practice, Faculty of Medicine, Norwegian University of Science and Technology (NTNU), MTFS, 7491, Trondheim, Norway

Christian Kvikne Dotterud
Department of Public Health and General Practice, Faculty of Medicine, Norwegian University of Science and Technology (NTNU), MTFS, 7491, Trondheim, Norway
Department of Dermatology, St Olavs Hospital, Trondheim University Hospital, Trondheim, Norway

April W. Armstrong
Department of Dermatology, Keck School of Medicine, University of Southern California, Los Angeles, CA 90033, USA

Shonda A. Foster, Brian S. Comer, Chen-Yen Lin, William Malatestinic and Orin Goldblum
Eli Lilly and Company, Indianapolis, IN, USA

Russel Burge
Eli Lilly and Company, Indianapolis, IN, USA
College of Pharmacy, University of Cincinnati, Cincinnati, OH, USA

Marie Madsen, Annemarie Aarup and Tanja Xenia Pedersen
Department of Biomedical Sciences, University of Copenhagen, Copenhagen, Denmark

Peter Riis Hansen
Department of Cardiology, Gentofte University Hospital, Gentofte, Denmark

Lars Bo Nielsen
Department of Biomedical Sciences, University of Copenhagen, Copenhagen, Denmark
Department of Clinical Biochemistry, Rigshospitalet, Copenhagen University Hospital, Copenhagen, Denmark

Anders Elm Pedersen and Jan Pravsgaard Christensen
Department of International Health, Immunology, and Microbiology, University of Copenhagen, Copenhagen, Denmark

Karsten Hartvigsen
Department of Biomedical Sciences, University of Copenhagen, Copenhagen, Denmark
Novo Nordisk, Gentofte, Denmark

Palokinam Vincent Pitché, Bayaki Saka, Taniratou Boukari, Sefako Akakpo and Kissem Tchangaï-Walla
Service de dermato-vénéréologie, CHU Sylvanus Olympio, Université de Lomé, 08 BP 81056 Lomé 08, Togo

Ahy Boubacar Diatta, Assane Diop, Fatimata Ly and Mame Thierno Dieng
Service de dermatologie, CHU Le Dantec, Dakar, Université Cheik Anta Diop, Dakar, Sénégal

Ousmane Faye and Alassane Dicko
Service de dermatologie, CNAM, Bamako, Université de Bamako, Bamako, Mali

Boh Fanta Diané, Maciré Mohamed Soumah and Mohamed Cissé
Service de dermatologie-MST, CHU Donka, Conakry, Université de Conakry, Conakry, Guinée

Abdoulaye Sangaré, Sarah Hamdan Kourouma and Isidore Kouassi
Centre de dermatologie, CHU Treichville, Université de Cocody, Cocody, Côte d'Ivoire

Pascal Niamba
Service de dermatologie CHU Yaldago Ouédraogo, Ouagadougou, Université de Ouagadougou, Ouagadougou, Burkina Faso

Christine Mandengue
Service de dermatologie, Clinique universitaire des Montagnes, Bangangté, Cameroun

Léon Kobengue
Service de dermatologie, CHU Bangui, Université de Bangui, Bangui, Centrafrique

Dadja Essoya Landoh
Division de l'Epidémiologie, Ministère de la santé du Togo, Lomé, Togo

Benjamin Momo Kadia
Presbyterian General Hospital Acha-Tugi, Acha-Tugi, Cameroon
Grace Community Health and Development Association, Kumba, Cameroon

Cyril Jabea Ekabe
Grace Community Health and Development Association, Kumba, Cameroon

Christian Akem Dimala
Faculty of Epidemiology and Population Health, London School of Hygiene and Tropical medicine, London, UK
Health and Human Development (2HD) Research Group, Douala, Cameroon
Department of Orthopaedics, Southend University Hospital, Essex, UK

Desmond Aroke
Health and Human Development (2HD) Research Group, Douala, Cameroon

Reine Suzanne Mengue Kadia
Kumba Health District Service, Kumba, Cameroon

Alain Chichom Mefire
Department of Surgery and Obstetrics/Gynaecology, Faculty of Health Sciences, University of Buea, Buea, Cameroon

Index

www.ingramcontent.com/pod-product-compliance
Lightning Source LLC
Chambersburg PA
CBHW061316190326
41458CB00011B/3820
* 9 7 8 1 6 3 2 4 1 5 7 7 6 *